*Dutta's*

# BEDSIDE CLINICS AND VIVA-VOCE
# IN
# OBSTETRICS AND GYNECOLOGY

**Other books by the same author**
- Textbook of Obstetrics
- Textbook of Gynecology
- Manual in Obstetrics and Gynecology for the Postgraduates

*Dutta's*

# BEDSIDE CLINICS AND VIVA-VOCE IN OBSTETRICS AND GYNECOLOGY

### Seventh Edition 2019

**Hiralal Konar**

(Hons., Gold Medalist)
MBBS (Cal), MD (PGI), DNB (India)
MNAMS, FACS (USA), FRCOG (London)

FOGSI Representative to Asia and Oceania Federation of Obstetrics and Gynecology (AOFOG)
Chairman, Indian College of Obstetricians and Gynaecologists (ICOG–2013)
Professor and Head, Department of Obstetrics and Gynecology
Agartala Government Medical College and GB Pant Hospital, Tripura, India
*Formerly*
Professor Calcutta National Medical College and Hospital, Kolkata, India
Professor and Head, Midnapore Medical College and Hospital, West Bengal University of Health Sciences
Kolkata, India
Rotation Registrar in Obstetrics, Gynecology and Oncology
Northern and Yorkshire Region, Newcastle-upon-Tyne, UK
Examiner of MBBS, DGO, MD and PhD of different Indian Universities
National Board of Examination, New Delhi, India and
Royal College of Physicians, Ireland

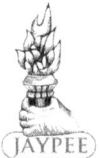

## JAYPEE BROTHERS MEDICAL PUBLISHERS
*The Health Sciences Publisher*
**New Delhi | London**

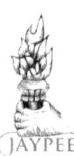

## Jaypee Brothers Medical Publishers (P) Ltd

### Headquarters

Jaypee Brothers Medical Publishers (P) Ltd
4838/24, Ansari Road, Daryaganj
New Delhi 110 002, India
Phone: +91-11-43574357
Fax: +91-11-43574314
Email: jaypee@jaypeebrothers.com

### Overseas Offices

J.P. Medical Ltd
83 Victoria Street, London
SW1H 0HW (UK)
Phone: +44 20 3170 8910
Fax: +44 (0)20 3008 6180
Email: info@jpmedpub.com

Jaypee-Highlights Medical Publishers inc
City of Knowledge, Bld. 235, 2nd Floor, Clayton
Panama City, Panama
Phone: +1 507-301-0496
Fax: +1 507-301-0499
Email: cservice@jphmedical.com

Jaypee Brothers Medical Publishers (P) Ltd
Bhotahity, Kathmandu, Nepal
Phone: +977-9741283608
Email: kathmandu@jaypeebrothers.com

Website: www.jaypeebrothers.com
Website: www.jaypeedigital.com

© Copyright reserved by Mrs Madhusri Konar

The views and opinions expressed in this book are solely those of the original contributor(s)/author(s) and do not necessarily represent those of editor(s) of the book.

All rights reserved. No part of this publication may be reproduced, stored or transmitted in any form or by any means, electronic, mechanical, photocopying, recording or otherwise, without the prior permission in writing of the publishers.

All brand names and product names used in this book are trade names, service marks, trademarks or registered trademarks of their respective owners. the publisher is not associated with any product or vendor mentioned in this book.

Medical knowledge and practice change constantly. This book is designed to provide accurate, authoritative information about the subject matter in question. However, readers are advised to check the most current information available on procedures included and check information from the manufacturer of each product to be administered, to verify the recommended dose, formula, method and duration of administration, adverse effects and contraindications. It is the responsibility of the practitioner to take all appropriate safety precautions. Neither the publisher nor the author(s)/editor(s) assume any liability for any injury and/or damage to persons or property arising from or related to use of material in this book.

This book is sold on the understanding that the publisher is not engaged in providing professional medical services. If such advice or services are required, the services of a competent medical professional should be sought.

Every effort has been made where necessary to contact holders of copyright to obtain permission to reproduce copyright material. If any have been inadvertently overlooked, the publisher will be pleased to make the necessary arrangements at the first opportunity. The **CD/DVD-ROM** (if any) provided in the sealed envelope with this book is complimentary and free of cost. Not meant for sale.

**Inquiries for bulk sales may be solicited at:** jaypee@jaypeebrothers.com

*Bedside Clinics and Viva-Voce in Obstetrics and Gynecology*

*Sixth Edition:* 2016

*Seventh Edition:* **2019**

**ISBN** 978-93-5270-701-0

*Dedicated to*

**The students
of
Obstetrics and Gynecology
past and present**

# Contributors

**Picklu Chowdhury**
Professor and Head
Rampurhat Government
Medical College and Hospital
Birbhum, West Bengal, India

**Aftabuddin Mondal**
Associate Professor
Department of Obstetrics and
Gynecology
Calcutta National Medical College and
Hospital
Kolkata, West Bengal, India

**A Halder**
Assistant Professor
Chittaranjan Seva Sadan
College of Obstetrics, Gynecology
and Child Health
Kolkata, West Bengal, India

**S Basak**
Assistant Professor
Sagar Dutta Medical College and
Hospital
Kolkata, West Bengal, India

**Gita Basu Banerjee**
Professor
Chitta Ranjan Seva Sadan
College of Obstetrics, Gynecology and
Child Health
Kolkata, West Bengal, India

**P Mistri**
Associate Professor
Department of Obstetrics and
Gynecology
Calcutta National Medical College
Kolkata, West Bengal, India

**Rathindranath Roy**
Assistant Professor
Department of Obstetrics and
Gynecology
Institute of Post Graduate Medical
Eduction and Research
Kolkata, West Bengal, India

**S Sengupta**
Assistant Professor
Department of Obstetrics and
Gynecology
North Bengal Medical College and
Hospital
Sushrut Nagar, Darjeeling, West Bengal,
India

# Preface

The examination system all over the world keeps on changing as science and technology continues to evolve and develop. The current examination system is primarily aimed not only to evaluate the factual or theoretical knowledge, but also the conceptual understanding and the analytical power of the candidate. To qualify any examination system, a candidate is expected to demonstrate the skills of clinical examination and data interpretation, the art of communication, decision-making and the management issues. With this sole determination the book *"Bedside Clinics and Viva-Voce in Obstetrics and Gynecology"* has been revised.

A textbook reading has got no alternative for comprehensive knowledge of the subject and understanding the science.

This book is intended for the students at their final phase while preparing for the examination. The book needs to be read and reread to develop a solid grasp of each topic as it contains a huge wealth of the new material.

Exhaustive **case discussions**, commonly presented in the **examination** (both in obstetrics and gynecology) have been made. All the chapters provide innumerable model answers which are framed in a simple, concise and easy-to-reproduce manner. **SBAs** and **MCQs** are still the accepted modes of evaluation throughout the world. 416 MCQs have been discussed in the book.

458 Clinical photographs, sketches, boxes, tables, flowcharts, partographs, cardiotocographs are incorporated to cope up with the need of the changing examination pattern.

Chapters on **Endoscopy** (Laparoscopy and Hysteroscopy) and **Robotic Surgery** in gynecology have been incorporated to keep the readers up-to-date with the progress of science and technology. Similarly, it is enriched with exhaustive number of **imaging studies** [Ultrasonograms: Doppler studies, Magnetic resonance imaging (MRI), Computed tomography (CT) and good-quality skiagrams]. The **index** has been elaborated for ease of quick referencing.

The book is primarily aimed to cover the Indian system of examination (both the University and the National Board). With the growing demand, the current 7th edition has been thoroughly revised and updated to cover the international examinations like the Royal College, London (RCOG), Royal College, Ireland (RCPI), and the American Board of Examinations (USMLE). This revision manual is a high yield concise book that covers all the contemporary examination systems.

*Bedside Clinics and Viva-Voce in Obstetrics and Gynecology* is equally essential for the homeopathic, ayurvedic, and nursing students and also the midwives. The postgraduate students will find it informative and time-saving. Specialists and practitioners will be benefitted as they like to refresh and update their knowledge. Layout of the book is simple. It has been made 'user friendly' making the discussion simple and concise.

The team of experts have been consulted and their experiences have been shared.

Cross references have been made in this book. Most of these are from and within this book in order to avoid the repetition of matters. Second cross references (few) are made to the textbooks (Obstetrics and Gynecology), as felt appropriate for more understanding. This is also meant for those who strive for excellence. List of abbreviations are given in this book which are essential in these days to study the medical science. Pages are left for the candidates to annotate, as they feel, to suit their own needs and style of reading during revision.

Above all, Bedside Clinics is an authoritative, evidence-based synoptic guide mainly for the clinical and viva-voce part of the examination.

I have aimed for brevity and clarity to make reading simple and enjoyable. **Chapter objectives** have been highlighted throughout the book.

Key management points have been highlighted. I would appreciate the readers to write to us: (*h.kondr@gmail.com*) with their suggestions, feedback, and any corrections for the future.

I do hope this book will be of immense value to the students and the clinicians as ever. According to the author's desire, the book is dedicated to the **'Students of Obstetrics and Gynecology – Past and Present'**.

**HIRALAL KONAR**
*P-13, New C.I.T. Road*
*Kolkata – 700 014*
*West Bengal, India*

# Acknowledgments

I am deeply indebted to all the teachers in this country and abroad for their guidance and support in the preparation of this edition (to name a few, I will miss many!). The students from different medical colleges have provided many innovative ideas on how to enhance the book. Their inputs have been invaluable and are sincerely appreciated. While writing such a book, I have consulted a multitude of eminent authors, related publications and many current evidence-based studies, recommendations and guidelines. I do sincerely acknowledge my legacy to all of them including the related authors and publishers.

I express my sincere thanks to Professor KK Kundu, Principal, Agartala Govt. Medical College, Tripura, for all the support for this extensive academic exercise. I am deeply indebted to Dr A Roy, Professor (Retd), for his continued guidance and support while writing this book. Mrs Madhusri Konar, MA, BEd, needs special appreciation for her patient and sincere secretarial job as ever. Her hard work, sacrifice and devotion to this work is a special support to me.

I sincerely acknowledge all the contributors of this edition for sharing their knowledge and experience of teaching.

In organizing this extensive academic compilation, expertise of many of my colleagues have been incorporated. The academic vision and understanding of my colleagues, the faculties of the institution, Agartala Govt Medical College, have been a constant support to me. I am indebted to all of them.

I express sincere thanks to all the students (undergraduates and postgraduates), nursing staff, residents and the teachers of different medical institutions in this country and abroad for their views and suggestions (on e-mail id: h.kondr@gmail.com; and website: www.hiralalkonar.com).

I am indebted to many other departments besides the Obstetrics and Gynecology. Contribution of the Radiology Department is enormous: As I have used numerous images of X-rays, computed tomography (CT) and magnetic resonance Imaging (MRI). Many of the drawings and sketches have been changed by the artistic skill of the experts in the publishing house. I thank all of them. Dr Ms Swapnil Shikha needs special appreciation for her innovative ideas to create the beautiful layouts.

I thank very sincerely all the students, trainee residents in this country and abroad, for their curiosities and queries with the mails that I have received and discussed over the years. This has pushed me for the continued search of knowledge to maintain its excellence.

I thank my colleagues who have generously provided many of the illustrations that appear in this edition. I am grateful to all my patients for their wholehearted support to enrich the book in the true sense of its title.

It goes without saying, such a job would not have been possible without the active support of my family members. Their patience, encouragement and the sacrifice to allow me to carry out the job cannot be expressed in words. I am indebted to them.

Last but not the least, I am grateful to all, who have taught me, most of all, the patients and my beloved students. Md Jakir Hossain deserves special thanks for his hard work of initial composition that was done very carefully.

I thank to the whole team of M/s Jaypee Brothers Medical Publishers (P) Ltd for their watchful care to overcome the potential hurdles. Shri Jitendar P Vij (Group Chairman), Mr Ankit Vij (Managing Director), Mr MS Mani (Group President), Dr Madhu Choudhary (Publishing Head–Education), Ms Pooja Bhandari (Production Head), Ms Sunita Katla (Executive Assistant to Group Chairman and Publishing Manager) deserve special appreciation for their generous support to bring out this edition as per the international standard.

*Hiralal Konar*
*P-13, New C.I.T. Road,*
*Kolkata-700 014*

# Contents

## SECTION I: OBSTETRICS .................................................................................................. 1–370

**Chapter 2:** History Taking and Clinical Examination ................................................. 3–15
- History ........................................................................................................................... 4
- Examination ................................................................................................................. 5
- Obstetric Examination .............................................................................................. 8
- Normal Puerperium ................................................................................................ 11
- Postpartum Exercises ............................................................................................. 13

**Chapter 2:** Obstetric Case Discussions ........................................................................ 16–119
- Case–1 Normal Pregnancy .................................................................................. 18
- Case–2 Primigravida with Floating (Free) Head at Term ....................... 26
- Case–3 Normal Puerperium ............................................................................... 31
- Case–4 Puerperium Normal and Abnormal ............................................... 37
- Case–5 Pregnancy and Labor in a Woman with
  Prior Cesarean Delivery ......................................................................... 41
- Case–6 Anemia in Pregnancy ............................................................................ 48
- Case–7 Diabetes in Pregnancy .......................................................................... 54
- Case–8 Breech Presentation .............................................................................. 59
- Case–9 Prolonged Pregnancy ........................................................................... 65
- Case–10 Fetal Growth Restriction ..................................................................... 68
- Case–11 Pre-Eclampsia and Eclampsia ........................................................... 72
- Case–12 Pregnancy with Maternal Red Cell Alloimmunization .......... 80
- Case–13 Multiple Pregnancy .............................................................................. 86
- Case–14 Intrauterine Fetal Death ...................................................................... 93
- Case–15 Polyhydramnios ..................................................................................... 96
- Case–16 Antepartum Hemorrhage (Placenta Previa) ............................ 100
- Case–17 Abruptio Placentae (Accidental Hemorrhage) ....................... 104
- Case–18 Postpartum Hemorrhage—Prevention
  and Management ................................................................................... 107
- Case–19 Hemorrhage in Early Pregnancy ................................................... 113
- Case–20 Miscarriage (Spontaneous Abortion) .......................................... 117

**Chapter 3:** Single Best Answers and Multiple Choice Questions ................... 120–164

**Chapter 4:** Labor and Delivery ......................................................................................... 165–215
- Maternal Pelvis ....................................................................................................... 166
- Fetal Skull ................................................................................................................. 174
- Mechanism of Labor ............................................................................................ 176
  - Mechanism of Normal Labor ...................................................................... 176
- Labor-Normal, Vaginal Delivery and Management .............................. 180
  - Preterm Labor and Delivery ......................................................................... 191
  - Prelabor Rupture of Membranes (PROM) .............................................. 197
- Labor-Abnormal ..................................................................................................... 198
  - Malposition and Malpresentation .............................................................. 198

- Occiput Posterior Position (OP) .......... 198
- Breech Presentation .......... 202
- Face Presentation .......... 206
- Brow Presentation .......... 209
- Transverse Lie .......... 209
- Cord Prolapse .......... 210
- Compound Presentation .......... 211
- Unstable Lie .......... 212
- Prolonged (Protracted) Labor .......... 212
- Obstructed Labor .......... 214

**Chapter 5: Active Management of Labor .......... 216–234**
- Labor Monitoring—Partography .......... 217
- Intrapartum Electronic Fetal Monitoring—Cardiotocography .......... 229

**Chapter 6: Obsterics Short Questions .......... 235–256**

**Chapter 7: Operative Obstetrics .......... 257–278**
- Dilatation and Evacuation (D and E) .......... 258
- Suction Evacuation .......... 259
- Manual Vacuum Aspiration (MVA) .......... 260
- Episiotomy .......... 261
- Forceps Delivery .......... 263
- Ventouse Delivery .......... 268
- Cesarean Section .......... 269
- Destructive Operations .......... 277

**Chapter 8: Practical Obstetrics .......... 279–337**
- Obstetric Instruments .......... 280
- Specimens .......... 312
- Imaging Studies .......... 316
  - Ultrasonogram .......... 316
  - Magnetic Resonance Imaging (MRI) .......... 323
- Drugs in Obstetrics .......... 324
  - Oxytocics .......... 324
  - Antihypertensives .......... 331
  - Anticoagulants .......... 333
  - Anticonvulsants .......... 333
  - Tocolytic Drugs .......... 336

**Chapter 9: Maternal Health: India and Global Scenario .......... 338–358**
- Maternal Mortality Ratio (MMR), Maternal Mortality Rate and Lifetime Risk .......... 339
- Sustainable Development Goals (SDG 3) .......... 344
- Millennium Development Goals (MDG 4 and 5) and Sustainable Development Goals (SDGs) .......... 345
- National Health Mission (NHM) and Reproductive and Child Health-II (RCH–II) .......... 348

- Janani Shishu Suraksha Karyakram (JSSK) a Government of India (GOI) Scheme ..................350
- Maternal Health Beyond 2030..................357

**Chapter 10:** Drug Therapy, Charts, Illustrations and Medications ..................359–370
- Drug Therapy in Pregnancy and Teratogenicity..................360
- Obstetric Charts and Graphs..................363
- Critical Periods in Embryonic Development ..................365

## SECTION II: GYNECOLOGY ..................371–693

**Chapter 11:** Gynecology Case Discussion ..................373–432
- Case – 1 Fibroid Uterus..................374
- Case – 2 Ovarian Tumor..................381
- Case – 3 Pelvic Organ Prolapse..................392
- Case – 4 Genitourinary Fistula ..................403
- Case – 5 Ureteric Injury in Gynecology..................406
- Case – 6 Rectovaginal Fistula ..................408
- Case – 7 Old Complete Perineal Tear..................410
- Case – 8 Pelvic Infections..................413
- Case – 9 Genital Tuberculosis..................416
- Case – 10 Abnormal Uterine Bleeding (AUB)..................418
- Case – 11 Hydatidiform Mole ..................423
- Case – 12 Uterine Polyp..................428
- Case – 13 Infertility..................430

**Chapter 12:** Special Topics..................433–456
- Physiology of Menstruation ..................434
- Polycystic Ovarian Syndrome ..................440
- Ovulation Induction ..................442
- Endometriosis..................445
- Cervical Intraepithelial Neoplasia (CIN) ..................449
- Amenorrhea ..................453

**Chapter 13:** Gynecology Short Questions..................457–474

**Chapter 14:** Viva-Voce in Gynecology..................475–495
- Gynecology Questions and Answers ..................476

**Chapter 15:** Operative Gynecology ..................496–546
- Dilatation and Curettage..................498
- Dilatation of Cervix..................501
- Dilatation and Insufflation (Rubin's Test) ..................501
- Hysterosalpingography ..................502
- Cervical Biopsy ..................503
- Thermal Cauterization of the Cervix..................504
- Marsupialization of a Bartholin's Cyst ..................504
- Female Sterilization (Tubectomy) ..................505

- Amputation of Cervix .................................................................. 507
- Fothergill's Operation ................................................................. 508
- Operations on the Ovary ........................................................... 509
- Abdominal Hysterectomy ........................................................... 509
- Myomectomy ............................................................................... 516
- Vaginal Hysterectomy ................................................................. 519
- Anterior Colporrhaphy ............................................................... 523
- Colpoperineorrhaphy ................................................................. 523
- Large Loop Excision of Transformation Zone ........................ 525
- Radical Hysterectomy ................................................................ 526
- Endoscopic Surgery in Gynecology ......................................... 528
- Robotics in Gynecology ............................................................. 545

**Chapter 16:** Practical Gynecology .................................................................. 547–649
- Gynecology Instruments ............................................................ 548
- Specimens .................................................................................... 592
- Imaging Studies in Gynecology ................................................ 626
  - Hysterosalpingogram (HSG) ................................................ 626
  - Ultrasonography (USG) ........................................................ 633
  - X-ray ......................................................................................... 640
  - CT scan .................................................................................... 642
  - MRI ........................................................................................... 643
- Drugs in Gynecology
  - Clomiphene Citrate ............................................................... 645
  - Letrozole ................................................................................. 645
  - Danazol ................................................................................... 645
  - Progesterone .......................................................................... 646
  - Combined (Estrogen and Progesterone) Oral Contraceptive Preparations (COC) .................................... 646
  - Tranexamic Acid .................................................................... 648
  - Mifepristone ........................................................................... 648
  - Metformin ............................................................................... 649
  - Methotrexate .......................................................................... 649
  - Cisplatin/Carboplatin ........................................................... 649

**Chapter 17:** Single Best Answer and Multiple Choice Questions ............. 650–688

**Chapter 18:** History in Obstetrics and Gynecology ..................................... 689–693
- Eponyms in Medicine ................................................................ 690

*Index* .................................................................................................................. *695*

# List of Abbreviations Used

| | | | |
|---|---|---|---|
| ABC | Airway, Breathing and Circulation | BPM | Beats Per Minute |
| AC | Abdominal Circumference | BPP | Biophysical Profile |
| ACE | Angiotensin II Converting Enzyme | BRCA | Breast Cancer |
| | | BSO | Bilateral Salpingo-oophorectomy |
| ACTH | Adrenocorticotrophic Hormone | BV | Bacterial Vaginosis |
| AFI | Amniotic Fluid Index | CCT | Controlled Cord Traction |
| AFP | Alpha-fetoprotein | CEA | Carcinoembryonic Antigen |
| AIDS | Acquired Immunodeficiency Syndrome | CEMD | Confidential Enquiry into Maternal Deaths |
| ALT | Alanine Transaminase | CIN | Cervical Intraepithelial Neoplasia |
| AMH | Anti-Müllerian Hormone | COC | Combined Oral Contraceptive |
| AMTSL | Active Management of Third Stage of Labor | CPAP | Continuous Positive Airway Pressure |
| ANA | Antinuclear Antibody | CPD | Cephalopelvic Disproportion |
| ANC | Antenatal Check-up | CPR | Cardiopulmonary Resuscitation |
| ANM | Auxiliary Nurse Midwife | | |
| APH | Antepartum Hemorrhage | CRL | Crown-Rump Length |
| aPL | Antiphospholipid | CRP | C-Reactive Protein |
| APS | Antiphospholipid Syndrome | CRVS | Civil Registration and Vital Statistics |
| APTT | Activated Partial Thromboplastin Time | CS | Cesarean Section |
| ARDS | Acute Respiratory Distress Syndrome | CSF | Cerebrospinal Fluid |
| | | CT | Computed Tomography |
| ARM | Artificial Rupture of Membranes | CTG | Cardiotocography |
| | | CVA | Cerebrovascular Accidents |
| ART | Antiretroviral Therapy | CVP | Central Venous Pressure |
| ART | Assisted Reproductive Technology | CVS | Chorionic Villus Sampling |
| | | CXR | Chest X-ray |
| ASHA | Accredited Social Health Activist | D&C | Dilatation and Curettage |
| | | D&E | Dilatation and Evacuation |
| AST | Aspartate Aminotransferase (Aspartate Transaminase) | DDKs | Disposable Delivery kits |
| | | DHT | Dihydrotestosterone |
| β-hCG | Beta-Human Chorionic Gonadotropin | DIC | Disseminated Intravascular Coagulation |
| BCG | Bacilli Calmette Guerin | DMPA | Depot Medroxyprogesterone Acetate |
| BMI | Body Mass Index | | |
| BP | Blood Pressure | DUB | Dysfunctional Uterine Bleeding |
| BPD | Biparietal Diameter | | |

| | | | |
|---|---|---|---|
| EAS | External Anal Sphincter | HELLP | Hemolysis, Elevated Liver Enzymes and Low Platelets |
| ECG | Electrocardiogram | | |
| ECP | Emergency Contraception Pill | HIE | Hypoxic-ischemic Encephalopathy |
| ECV | External Cephalic Version | | |
| EDD | Estimated Date of Delivery | HIV | Human Immunodeficiency Virus |
| EDF | End-diastolic Flow | | |
| EEG | Electroencephalogram | HLD | High-level Disinfection |
| EFM | Electronic Fetal Monitoring | hMG | Human Menopausal Gonadotropins |
| ERCS | Elective Repeat Cesarean Section | HNPCC | Hereditary Nonpolyposis Colorectal Cancer |
| ERPC | Evacuation of Retained Products of Conception | HPL | Human Placental Lactogen |
| | | HPS | High Performing States |
| ET | Embryo Transfer | HPV | Human Papilloma Virus |
| FBC | Full Blood Count | HRT | Hormone Replacement Therapy |
| FBS | Fetal Blood Sampling | | |
| FDA | Food and Drug Administration | HSV | Herpes Simplex Virus |
| | | IAS | Internal Anal Sphincter |
| FDPs | Fibrin Degradation Products | ICSI | Intracytoplasmic Sperm Injection |
| FGR | Fetal Growth Restriction | | |
| FHR | Fetal Heart Rate | ICTC | Integrated Counseling and Testing Center |
| FHS | Fetal Heart Sound | | |
| FIGO | International Federation of Gynecology and Obstetrics | ICU | Intensive Care Unit |
| | | IFA | Iron Folic Acid |
| FMC | Fetal Movement Counting | IPPV | Intermittent Positive Pressure Ventilation |
| FRU | First Referral Unit | | |
| FS | Female Sterilization | ITP | Idiopathic Thrombocytopenic Purpura |
| FSH | Follicle Stimulating Hormone | | |
| GnRH | Gonadotropin-releasing Hormone | IUCD | Intrauterine Contraceptive Device |
| GOI | Government of India | IUD | Intrauterine Death |
| GTD | Gestational Trophoblastic Disease | IUFD | Intrauterine Fetal Death |
| | | IUGR | Intrauterine Growth Restriction |
| GTN | Gestational Trophoblastic Neoplasia | | |
| | | IUI | Intrauterine Insemination |
| HAART | Highly Active Anti-retroviral Therapy | IUP | Intrauterine Pregnancy |
| | | IUS | Intrauterine System |
| Hb | Hemoglobin | IVF-ET | IVF and Embryo Transfer |
| HBsAg | Hepatitis B Surface Antigen | IVF | Invitro Fertilization |
| HBV | Hepatitis B Virus | IVU | Intravenous Urogram |
| hCG | Human Chorionic Gonadotropin | JSSK | Janani Shishu Suraksha Karyakram |
| HCV | Hepatitis C Virus | LAM | Lactational Amenorrhea Method |
| HDU | High Dependency Unit | | |

| | | | |
|---|---|---|---|
| LAVH | Laparoscopically Assisted Vaginal Hysterectomy | NGO | Nongovernmental Organization |
| LDL | Low-density Lipoprotein | NHM | National Health Mission |
| LH | Luteinizing Hormone | NICE | National Institute for Health and Clinical Excellence |
| LHV | Lady Health Visitor | | |
| LLETZ | Large Loop excision of the Transformation Zone | NICU | Neonatal Intensive Care Unit |
| | | NSAID | Nonsteroidal Anti-inflammatory Drugs |
| LMP | Last Menstrual Period | NST | Nonstress Test |
| LMWH | Low Molecular Weight Heparin | NSV | No-scalpel Vasectomy |
| LNG-IUS | Levonorgestrel-releasing Intrauterine System | NT | Nuchal Translucency |
| | | NTDs | Neural Tube Defects |
| LNG | Levonorgestrel | OAB | Overactive Bladder |
| LOD | Laparoscopic Ovarian Drilling | OCP | Oral Contraceptive Pill |
| | | OGTT | Oral Glucose Tolerance Test |
| LPS | Low-performing States | OHSS | Ovarian Hyperstimulation Syndrome |
| LSCS | Lower Segment Cesarean Section | | |
| | | P/V | Per Vaginum |
| LSIL | Low-grade Squamous Intraepithelial Lesions | PCA | Patient-controlled Analgesia |
| | | PCOS | Polycystic Ovary Syndrome |
| LUNA | Laparoscopic Uterine Nerve Ablation | PCR | Polymerase Chain Reaction |
| | | PDA | Patent Ductus Arteriosus |
| MAP | Mean Arterial Pressure | PEEP | Positive end-expiratory Pressure |
| MAS | Meconium Aspiration Syndrome | | |
| | | PET | Positron Emission Tomography |
| MCA | Middle Cerebral Artery | | |
| MCHC | Mean Corpuscular Hemoglobin Concentration | PFR | Peak Flow Rate |
| | | PFR | Pelvic Floor Repair |
| MCQ | Multiple Choice Question | PHC | Primary Health Center |
| MDG | Millennium Development Goals | PID | Pelvic Inflammatory Disease |
| | | PMB | Postmenopausal Bleeding |
| MDSR | Maternal Death Surveillance and Response | PMR | Perinatal Mortality Rate |
| | | PMS | Premenstrual Syndrome |
| MIS | Minimally Invasive Surgery | PNC | Postnatal Check-up |
| MMR | Maternal Mortality Ratio | PNDT | Prenatal Diagnostic Technique or Test |
| MNM | Maternal Near Miss | | |
| MPA | Medroxyprogesterone Acetate | POC | Products of Conception |
| MRI | Magnetic Resonance Imaging | POF | Premature Ovarian Failure |
| MSAFP | Maternal Serum Alphafetoprotein | POP-Q | Pelvic Organ Prolapse-Quantification |
| MSU | Midstream Urine | POPs | Progestogen Only Pills |
| MTP | Medical Termination of Pregnancy | PPH | Postpartum Hemorrhage |
| | | PPROM | Preterm Premature Rupture of Membranes |
| MVA | Manual Vacuum Aspiration | | |

| | | | |
|---|---|---|---|
| PPTCT | Prevention of Parent-to-child Transmission | STD | Sexually Transmitted Disease |
| PROM | Prelabor Rupture of Membranes | STI | Sexually Transmitted Infection |
| PT | Prothrombin Time | TAH/BSO | Total Abdominal Hysterectomy/Bilateral Salpingo-oopherectomy |
| PTB | Preterm Birth | | |
| PTL | Preterm Labor | TBA | Thermal Balloon Ablation |
| RCH | Reproductive and Child Health | TBA | Traditional Birth Attendant |
| | | TCRE | Transcervical Resection of the Endometrium |
| RCOG | Royal College of Obstetricians and Gynecologists | | |
| | | TDF | Testes-determining Factor |
| RCT | Randomized Controlled Trial | TENS | Transcutaneous Electrical Nerve Stimulation |
| RDS | Respiratory Distress Syndrome | | |
| | | TLH | Total Laparoscopic Hysterectomy |
| RMI | Risk of Malignancy Index | | |
| ROP | Right Occiput Posterior | TOLAC | Trial of Labor After Cesarean |
| RR | Respiratory Rate | TT | Tetanus Toxoid |
| RTI | Reproductive Tract Infection | TTP | Thrombotic Thrombocytopenic Purpura |
| SAMM | Severe Acute Maternal Morbidity | | |
| | | TTTS | Twin-to-twin Transfusion Syndrome |
| SAQ | Short-answer Question | | |
| SBA | Single Best Answer | TVS | Transvaginal Ultrasound |
| SBA | Skilled Birth Attendant | TVT | Tension-free Vaginal Tape |
| SCBU | Special Care Baby Unit | UAE | Uterine Artery Embolization |
| SCC | Squamous Cell Carcinoma | UTI | Urinary Tract Infection |
| SCJ | Squamo Columnar Junction | VBAC | Vaginal Birth After Cesarean |
| SDG | Sustainable Development Goals | VDRL | Venereal Disease Research Laboratory |
| SERM | Selective Estrogen Receptor Modulators | VEGF | Vascular Endothelial Growth Factor |
| SFH | Symphisis Fundal Height | VIN | Vulval Intraepithelial Neoplasia |
| SGOT | Serum Glutamic-oxaloacetic Transaminase | | |
| | | VLP | Virus-like Particles |
| SGPT | Serum Glutamic Pyruvic Transaminase | VTE | Venous Thromboembolism |
| | | VVF | Vesico Vaginal Fistula |
| SHBG | Sex Hormone-binding Globulin | vWF | Von Willebrand Factor |
| | | VZIG | Varicella Zoster IgG |
| SLE | Systemic Lupus Erythematosus | WHO | World Health Organization |
| | | ZDV | Zidovudine |

# OBSTETRICS AND GYNECOLOGY
## MARKS DISTRIBUTION OF 3RD PROFESSIONAL MBBS PART-II EXAMINATION

### 1. WEST BENGAL UNIVERSITY OF HEALTH SCIENCES : KOLKATA — TOTAL MARKS = 200

**(A) THEORY**

| PAPER 1 (40) | PAPER 2 (40) | TOTAL (Paper 1 + 2) (80) | INTERNAL ASSESSMENT (IA) (20) | TOTAL (100) |
|---|---|---|---|---|

**(B) ORAL (30), CLINICAL (50) AND INTERNAL ASSESSMENT (20) = 100**

| OBSTETRICS TABLE VIVA = 20 | | | | | GYNECOLOGY TABLE VIVA = 10 | | | | | TOTAL 20 + 10 = 30 | CLINICAL = 50 | | GRAND TOTAL (80) |
|---|---|---|---|---|---|---|---|---|---|---|---|---|---|
| OBSTETRICS VIVA VOCE = 10 | | | | | GYNECOLOGY VIVA VOCE = 10 | | | | | | LONG CASE (OBST.) (30) | SHORT CASE (GYNE.) (20) | |
| Instrument + Operative (3) | Specimen (2) | X-Ray/ USG (2.5) | Recent Advances/ Problems (2.5) | TOTAL (10) | Instrument + Operative (3) | Specimen (2) | X-Ray/ USG (2.5) | Recent Advances/ Problems + Family Planning (2.5) | | | | | |

| OBSTETRIC MANEUVER (5) | LOG BOOK (5) |
|---|---|

### 2. MAHARASHTRA UNIVERSITY OF HEALTH SCIENCES: NASHIK (MAHARASHTRA) — TOTAL MARKS = 200

**(A) THEORY**

| PAPER 1 (40) | PAPER 2 (40) | TOTAL (Paper 1 + 2) (80) | INTERNAL ASSESSMENT (IA) (20) | TOTAL (100) |
|---|---|---|---|---|

**(B) ORAL (30), CLINICAL (50) AND INTERNAL ASSESSMENT (20) = 100**

| OBSTETRICS TABLE VIVA | GYNECOLOGY TABLE VIVA | FAMILY PLANNING | CLINICAL | | INTERNAL ASSESSMENT | TOTAL |
|---|---|---|---|---|---|---|
| | | | Long case (OBST.) | Short case (GYNE.) | | |
| 10 | 10 | 10 | 40 | 10 | 20 | 100 |

## 3 ALL INDIA INSTITUTE OF MEDICAL SCIENCES : NEW DELHI

A. INTERNAL ASSESSMENT = 150 (continued assessment)
B. EXTERNAL ASSESSMENT = 150 } TOTAL MARKS = 300

(A) THEORY

| EXTERNAL ASSESSMENT 150 | | | |
|---|---|---|---|
| THEORY 75 | ORAL 30 | CLINICAL 45 | TOTAL 150 |
| PAPER 1 = 38 | | PAPER 2 = 37 | TOTAL (Paper 1+ 2) = 75 |

(B) ORAL (30); (C) CLINICAL (45)

| FAMILY PLANNING | CLINICAL | | TOTAL |
|---|---|---|---|
| | OBST. CASE | GYNE. CASE | |
| OBSTETRICS TABLE VIVA | GYNECOLOGY TABLE VIVA | | |
| 10 | 10 | 25 | 20 | 75 |

## 4 RAJIV GANDHI UNIVERSITY OF HEALTH SCIENCES : KARNATAKA

TOTAL MARKS = 500

(A) THEORY

| PAPER 1 100 | PAPER 2 100 | TOTAL (Paper 1 + 2) 200 | INTERNAL ASSESSMENT (IA) 100 | CLINICAL 160 | VIVA 40 | TOTAL 500 |
|---|---|---|---|---|---|---|

(B) INTERNAL ASSESSMENT (IA)

| CONTINUED IA THEORY 60 | IA : CLINICAL AND PRACTICAL 40 | TOTAL 100 |
|---|---|---|

(C) ORAL = (40), CLINICAL = (160) TOTAL = (200)

| OBSTETRICS TABLE VIVA | GYNAECOLOGY TABLE VIVA | FAMILY PLANNING | CLINICAL | | TOTAL |
|---|---|---|---|---|---|
| | | | Obst. case | Gyne. case | |
| 15 | 15 | 10 | 80 | 80 | 200 |

## 5. KERALA UNIVERSITY OF HEALTH SCIENCES : THIRUVANANTHAPURAM (KERALA) — TOTAL MARKS = 200

| (A) THEORY | PAPER 1 | PAPER 2 | TOTAL (Paper 1 + 2) | INTERNAL ASSESSMENT (IA) | TOTAL |
|---|---|---|---|---|---|
| | 40 | 40 | 80 | 20 | 100 |

(B) ORAL = 30, (C) CLINICAL = 50 (D) INTERNAL ASSESSMENT = 20  TOTAL : 100

| | OBSTETRICS VIVA | GYNECOLOGY VIVA | CLINICAL | | INTERNAL ASSESSMENT | TOTAL |
|---|---|---|---|---|---|---|
| | | | Obst. case | Gyne. case | | |
| | Log Book 10 | Viva 10 | 25 | 25 | 20 | 100 |

## 6. RANI DURGABATI UNIVERSITY OF HEALTH SCIENCES : JABALPUR (M.P) — TOTAL MARKS = 200

| (A) THEORY | PAPER 1 (40) | PAPER 2 (40) | TOTAL (Paper 1 + 2) (80) | INTERNAL ASSESSMENT (IA) (20) | TOTAL (100) |
|---|---|---|---|---|---|

(B) ORAL (40), CLINICAL (40) AND INTERNAL ASSESSMENT (20)  TOTAL : 100

| OBSTETRICS VIVA TABLE | GYNECOLOGY VIVA TABLE | FAMILY PLANNING | CLINICAL | | INTERNAL ASSESSMENT | TOTAL |
|---|---|---|---|---|---|---|
| | | | Obst. case | Gyne. case | | |
| 15 | 15 | 10 | 25 | 15 | 20 | 100 |

# SECTION 1

# Obstetrics

- History Taking and Clinical Examination — 3
- Obstetric Case Discussions — 16
- Single Best Answers and Multiple Choice Questions — 120
- Labor and Delivery — 165
- Active Management of Labor — 216
- Obstetrics Short Questions — 235
- Operative Obstetrics — 257
- Practical Obstetrics — 279
- Maternal Health: India and Global Scenario — 338
- Drug Therapy, Obstetric Charts, Graphs and Illustrations — 359

# History Taking and Clinical Examination

CHAPTER 1

**Chapter Objectives**

Good knowledge and understanding to demonstrate:
- Clinical skills
- Communication skills
- Review of the physical signs based on physiology/pathology
- Identification of risk factors
- Ability to organize investigations
- Ability to plan the management

| | | |
|---|---|---|
| ❖ | History | 4 |
| ❖ | Examination | 5 |
| ❖ | Obstetric Examination | 8 |
| ❖ | Normal Puerperium | 11 |
| ❖ | Postpartum Exercises | 13 |

## HISTORY

**PATIENT PARTICULARS**

Name: Mrs......................
Age: ............... years          Address: ................................................................
Occupation:                          • Religion:
Educational status:                  • Occupation of the husband:
Duration of marriage:                • Socioeconomic status:
Gravida:                             • Date of admission:
Parity:                              • Date of examination:
Married for (in a case of primigravida):
LMP...............    EDD .................................. Period of gestation in weeks...............

**Chief complaints:** Pain abdomen/headache/vaginal bleeding/urinary problems are to be recorded, in order of priority or according to chronological order of onset of events. Some patients may not have any complaints but have been admitted for observation like raised blood pressure (BP), or for investigations and planning mode of delivery as in a case with Rh-alloimmunization or pregnancy with prior cesarean delivery.

**History of present illness:** Elaboration of the chief complaints as regard to their onset, duration, severity, use of medications, investigations, and progress, is to be made.

**History of present pregnancy:** Important complications of different trimesters of the present pregnancy (if any) are to be recorded carefully. Complications of (i) 1st trimester, (ii) 2nd trimester and (iii) 3rd trimester should be mentioned. Number of antenatal visits (booking status), immunization status, intake of iron and folic acid are to be recorded. Any medication or radiation exposure in early pregnancy or medical/surgical events during pregnancy should be enquired and recorded. Woman's perception of fetal movements may be mentioned.

**Obstetric history (Box 1.1):** Previous obstetric events are to be recorded chronologically. This is relevant in a multigravida. The obstetric history is summed up as:

Gravida..........          Para...........          Miscarriage...........
MTP..........             and Living issue........

**Box 1.1: Obstetric history**

| S. No. | Year and date | Pregnancy events | Labor events | Mode of delivery and the place | Puerperium | Baby |
|---|---|---|---|---|---|---|
| | | | | | | • Weight and sex<br>• Condition at birth (Apgar score)<br>• Breastfeeding<br>• Immunization |
| | | | | | | |
| | | | | | | |

**Menstrual history:** Menarche (age)……..years, cycle 28–30 days, duration 3–4 days; Amount of flow: (average/scanty), dysmenorrhea (if any).

LMP………….. EDD…………. (Naegele's formula); period of gestation………… weeks.

Corrected EDD (in cases with delayed menstruation or pregnancy following IVF):……

*Naegele's formula:*

Due date of delivery = First day of last menstrual cycle + 9 months +7 days

For IVF pregnancy, date of LMP is 14 days prior to date of embryo transfers (266 days)

**Past medical history:** Any relevant past medical illness (malaria and jaundice).

**Past surgical history:** Previous surgery—general (appendicectomy) or gynecological (myomectomy).

**Family history:** Hypertension, diabetes, hemoglobinopathy, twinning or congenital malformation or consanguineous marriage is to be enquired and recorded.

**Personal history:** Contraceptive practice, smoking, chronic medications (corticosteroids), habit forming drugs are to be enquired. Sleep, appetite, bowel and bladder habits are to be mentioned.

## EXAMINATION (FIGS. 1.1 TO 1.9)

- **General physical examination**
  - Build
  - Nutrition
  - Height (Figs. 1.1 and 1.2)
  - Weight (Figs. 1.1 and 1.3)
  - Pallor
  - Jaundice
  - Cyanosis
  - Tongue, teeth, gum and tonsils
  - Neck veins
  - Neck glands
  - Thyroid
  - Breasts
  - Pulse
  - Blood pressure
  - Temperature
  - Respiratory rate
  - Edema legs

- **Mental status**

  To assess whether the individual is alert, conscious and cooperative.

- **Systemic examination**
  - Examination of cardiovascular and respiratory system:
    - Heart
    - Lungs
  - Musculoskeletal system
  - **Examination of abdomen:**
    - Inspection
    - Palpation

  Any tenderness, liver, spleen (any organomegaly)

  - **Obstetric examination:**
    - Inspection
    - Palpation
    - Obstetric grips
    - Percussion (not done)
    - Auscultation for fetal heart sounds

## DIFFERENT GADGETS USED IN THE ANTENATAL CLINIC TO ASSESS MATERNAL HEALTH AND FETAL WELL-BEING

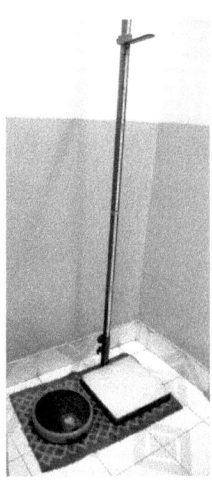

Fig. 1.1: Weight and height measurement tools.

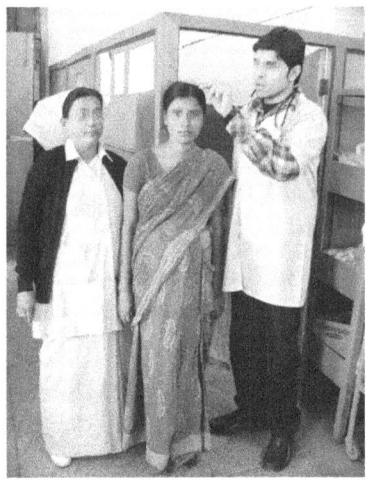

Fig. 1.2: Measurement of height of a pregnant woman.

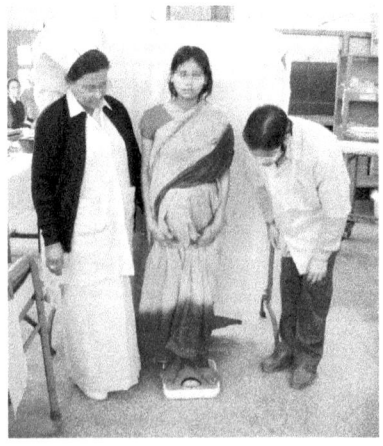

Fig. 1.3: Measurement of weight.

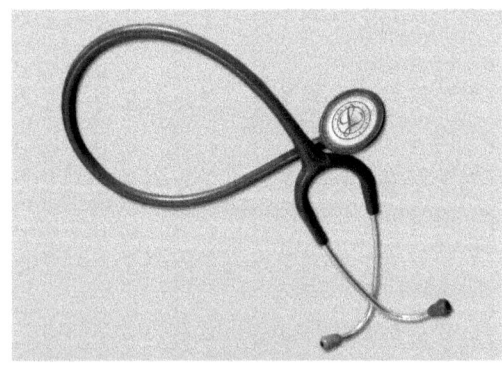

Fig. 1.4: Stethoscope.

## Chapter 1 • History Taking and Clinical Examination

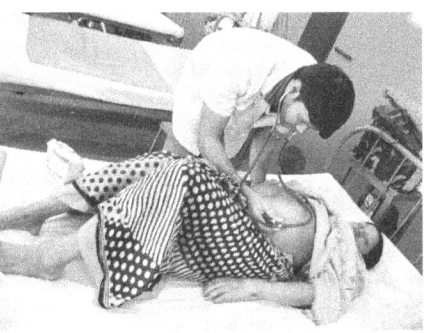

**Fig. 1.5:** Procedure of fetal heart sound auscultation.

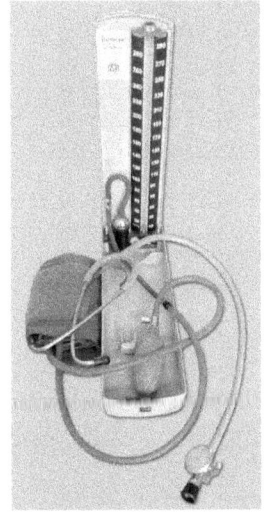

**Fig. 1.6:** BP apparatus.

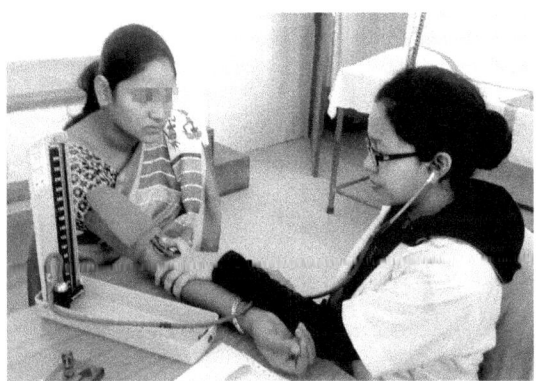

**Fig. 1.7:** Measurement of blood pressure.

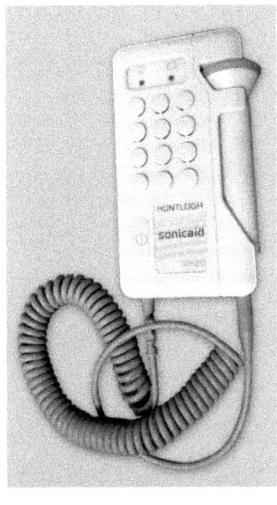

**Fig. 1.8:** Doppler.

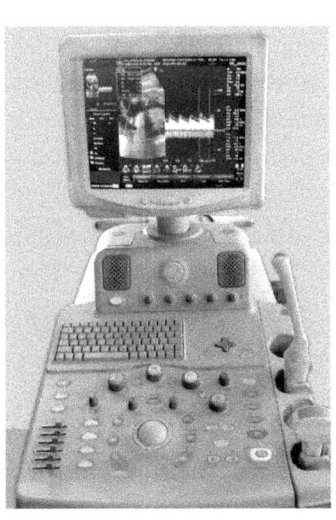

**Fig. 1.9:** USG machine.

## OBSTETRIC EXAMINATION

**Preliminaries:**
(a) Verbal consent from the patient should be taken
(b) Presence of a female attendant
(c) Prior bladder evacuation
(d) Proper exposure of abdomen from xiphisternum to symphysis pubis
(e) Woman in dorsal posture with thighs and knees slightly flexed (Fig. 1.10)
(f) The candidate is to stand on the right side of the patient.
(g) Woman's head should be tilted to the left side.

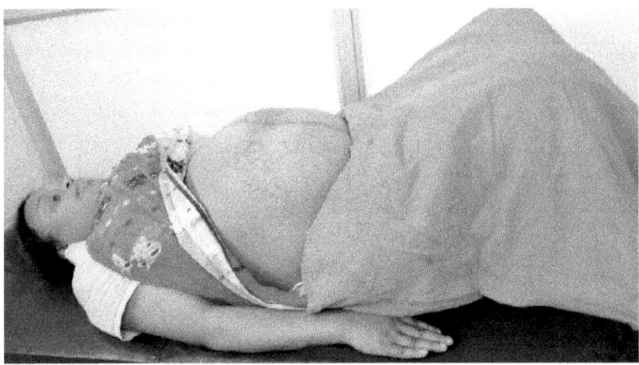

**Fig. 1.10:** Patient's position during obstetric examination.

## EXAMINATION PROPER

**A. Inspection:** Enlargement of the abdomen; uterine shape—ovoid (longitudinal/transverse); contour of uterus—smooth or any fundal notching.

**Skin condition:** Presence of linea nigra (Fig. 1.11), striae gravidarum, umbilicus (everted), presence of any scar mark, infection (scabies, if present) venous prominence, visible fetal movements, etc.

**B. Palpation:** Centralization of the uterus (See Fig. 2.2, p. 21) should be done (Fig. 1.12).

(a) Height of the uterus in terms of weeks (Fig. 1.12)
(b) Symphysis-fundal height in cm (Fig. 1.13)

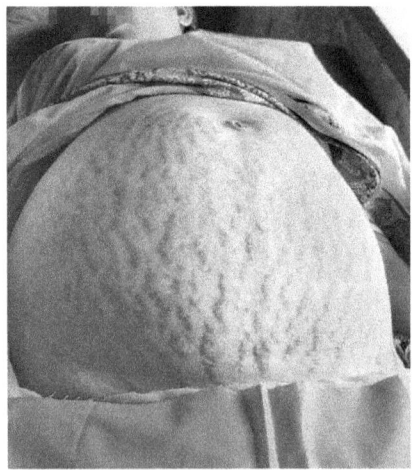

**Fig. 1.11:** Skin changes during pregnancy showing linea nigra and striae gravidarum; inspection of the abdomen shows uniform enlargement of the abdomen.

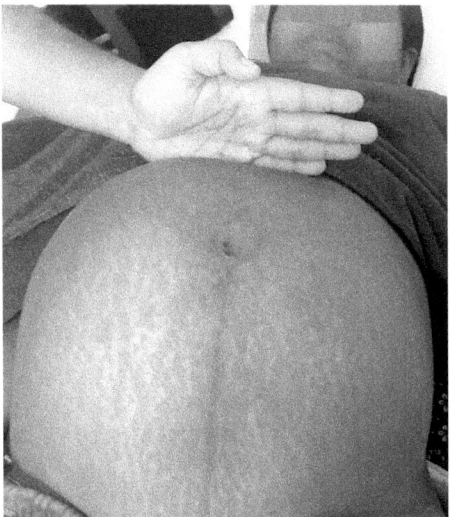

**Fig. 1.12:** Palpation of the height of the (centralized) uterus with the ulnar border of the left hand.

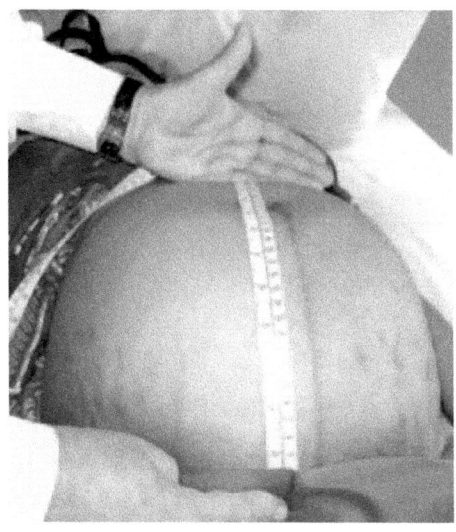

**Fig. 1.13:** Teacher demonstrates Symphysis-fundal height measurement.
[*By Courtesy:* Prof. BN Chakraborty, Director, IRM, Kolkata]

(c) **Obstetric grips** (Leopold's maneuvers):
   (i) First Leopold (fundal grip) (Fig. 1.14)
   (ii) Second Leopold (lateral or umbilical grip) (Fig. 1.15)
   (iii) Third Leopold (Pawlik's grip) (Fig. 1.16)
   (iv) Fourth Leopold (pelvic grip) (Figs. 1.17A and B).

   For methods of examination, observation and inference, See Dutta obs 9/e, p. 71.

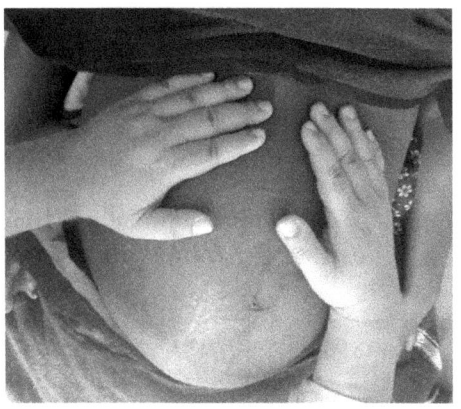

**Fig. 1.14:** Fundal grip (Leopold's first maneuver).

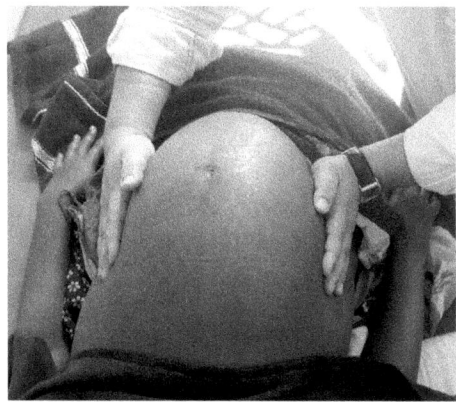

**Fig. 1.15:** Lateral/umbilical grip (Leopold's second maneuver).

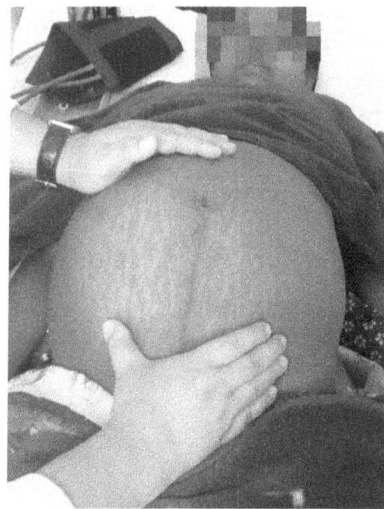

**Fig. 1.16:** Pawlik grip (Leopold's third maneuver).

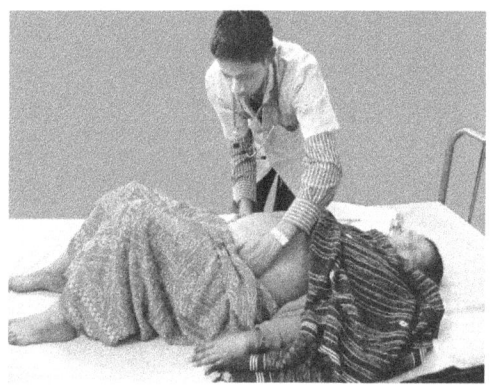
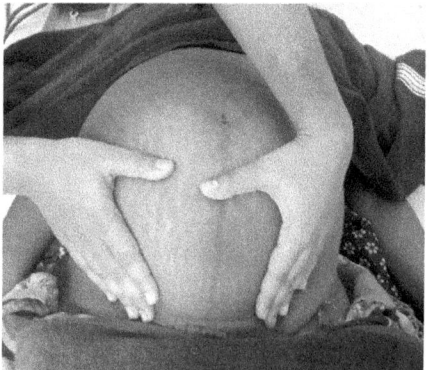

**Figs. 1.17A and B:** Candidate demonstrates obstetric examination by pelvic grip (Leopold fourth maneuver).

**C. Auscultation** of fetal heart sound using a stethoscope (See Fig. 1.5 and Fig. 2.5, p. 22) or Doppler (along the spinoumbilical line in case of cephalic presentation).

Maternal radial pulse to be felt to differentiate the FHS.

**Summary of the case:** A case summary is to be made mentioning the age, parity, period of gestation, highlighting in brief the important and relevant information in the history, general physical examination and obstetric examination (obstetric palpation and auscultation) (See case 1, p. 18).

**Provisional diagnosis:** A provisional diagnosis is to be made and written in few lines mentioning the woman's age, parity, gravida, period of gestation and the complication (if any) in pregnancy.

**Suggested investigations:**
(a) **Routine antenatal investigations:** Blood—Hb%, hematocrit, ABO Rh, blood glucose.
   **Serology:** VDRL, Rubella, HBSAg, HIV (with consent), HCV.

**Ultrasonography:** First trimester scan (TVS), for diagnosis, viability, dating and second trimester scan for anomaly.

**Urine:** Routine and microscopic examination: Protein, sugar, pus cells.

**Cervical Cytology**

**Booking scan at 18-22 weeks.**

(b) **Investigations relevant in the given case for diagnosis and/or management:** Repeat Hb estimation, USG scan, Doppler study.

**Differential diagnosis:** Where applicable.

## NORMAL PUERPERIUM

### HISTORY TAKING AND CLINICAL EXAMINATION

The basic format is more or less same as in an antenatal case.

**Points of difference are:**

(A) Instead of recording the LMP—mention the date and time of childbirth.

(B) Instead of EDD and period of gestation—mention the number of days in puerperium.

(C) Chief complaints should be highlighted; in relation to the problems of puerperium (e.g. pain abdomen, pain perineum, breast problems, urinary problems, etc.) only.

(D) History of present illness: Elaboration of chief complaints since the time of delivery, e.g. pain abdomen starts since the time of delivery. The pain is mild in nature and at times, it is spasmodic. Pain of episiotomy located in the perineum especially over the area of episiotomy. The lochial discharge is normal. It is bright red in color. She changed 3-4 pads in the last 12 hours. Pads are partly soaked. Her pain has improved as she has taken some medicine (analgesic—ibuprofen).

(E) Instead of "History of Present Pregnancy" mention in brief the history of preceeding pregnancy and labor (e.g. Mrs CR was admitted in the hospital last evening at about 7 pm with labor pain following a term pregnancy. She was a booked case in this hospital. Her course in pregnancy in all the trimesters were uneventful. She had a spontaneous vaginal delivery with right mediolateral episiotomy on ................ at.......am/pm. The total duration of labor was 5 hours. She had uneventful third stage of labor.

Rest of history (past, family, obstetric, etc.): Same as that of an antenatal case.

(F) Obstetric history to be described as parity, no need to mention the gravida.

**Examination:**

(A) **General physical examination:** Record of temperature is important, besides the other (BP, pulse, weight) parameters mentioned in an antenatal case (See p. 5).

(B) **Examination of chest:** For **cardiovascular system** and **respiratory system** are same as in an antenatal case.

(C) **Breast examination:** To enquire about breast problems (pain and lactation difficulty) breast examination is needed (in the presence of a female attendant).
(D) **Palpation (abdomen)** for any tenderness and organomegaly (liver/spleen) is done.
(E) **Obstetric palpation:** Preliminaries are same as in an obstetric case.
   (i) Measuring the height of the uterus (bladder should be empty and uterus must be centralized). It is expressed in relation to the level of umbilicus (as the fundus is at the level of the umbilicus or 2 cm below the umbilicus).
   (ii) Symphysis-fundal height measurement (in cm).
   (iii) Palpation of the uterus to note tenderness, surface irregularity, mobility and palpation for any other abdominal mass (ovarian) is done (obstetric grips and auscultation are not applicable here).
(F) **Examination of the perineum to:**
   (i) Inspect the perineum, (ii) Episiotomy wound if any, (iii) Lochial discharge.

## HISTORY AND EXAMINATION OF THE BABY

(A) (i) **Baby:** Date and time of birth, (ii) Apgar score (cried at birth or not), (iii) Weight, (iv) Passage of urine and meconium and (v) Breastfeeding.
(B) **Examination of the baby:** (i) Skin color, (ii) Respiration, (iii) Jaundice, cyanosis, (iv) Head, (v) Oral cavity (fungal infection), (vi) Chest, (vii) Heart (murmers) and lungs, (viii) Abdomen, (ix) Umbilicus (any bleeding, discharge, infection), (x) Genitalia, (xi) Anus, (xii) Any congenital malformation, such as limbs, digits, etc. (xiii) Gestational age (term/preterm), (xiv) Breastfeeding, (xv) Passed urine, meconium, and (xvi) Reflexes.

**Summary of the case:** (Case 3, p. 31).
Mrs ............. 22 years, P1+0+0+1, delivered vaginally in this hospital following a term pregnancy. Live baby boy/girl was born on ............. at ............. Mrs ... has got mild pain in the abdomen and perineum. On examination, she is afebrile, vitals are stable, uterine fundus is at the level of umbilicus (............. cm above the symphysis pubis) and the episiotomy wound is healthy. Lochial discharge is normal. Bladder function is normal (she has passed urine).

Baby cried at birth. Baby on examination is found to be a term one, normal and is on breast milk. Baby has passed uine and meconium.

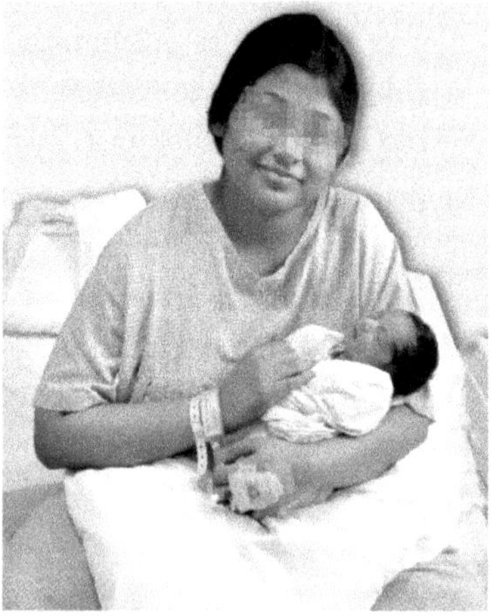

**Fig. 1.18:** Mother in second day of normal puerperium with baby.

**Provisional diagnosis:** Mrs........................, 22 years old, P1+0+0+1 with a term healthy baby girl, 2.7 kg, delivered vaginally on.................... date................... She is on the second day of **normal puerperium** (Fig. 1.18).

**Chapter 1 • History Taking and Clinical Examination** 13

# POSTPARTUM EXERCISES (FIGS. 1.19 TO 1.24)

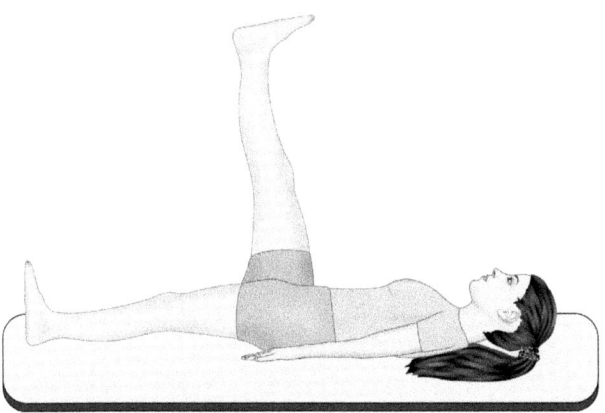

**Fig. 1.19:** Straight leg raising.

To lie on the back and put knees straight and hands by the side. Raise one leg slowly with knee extended and hip (hip at 90° to the upper body). Repeat with the other leg and then with both the legs.

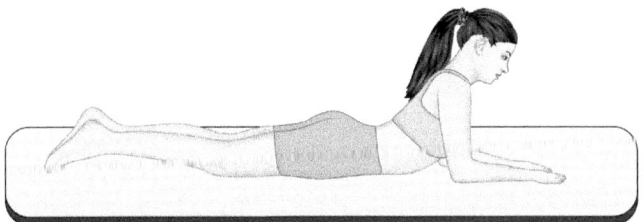

**Fig. 1.20:** Exercise for the back.

To lie on the stomach. Keep the forearms with elbows down on either side of the head on the bed. To raise the head and the shoulders as much as possible with weight on elbows.

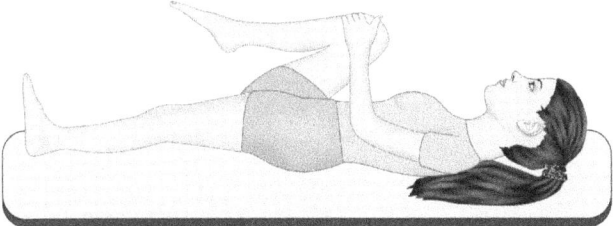

**Fig. 1.21:** Knee chest exercise.

To lie on the back. Slowly lift one leg with knee flexed. With the help of the hands, the knee is pulled over the chest. The other leg to be flat on the bed. Repeat the same with other leg and then with both the legs.

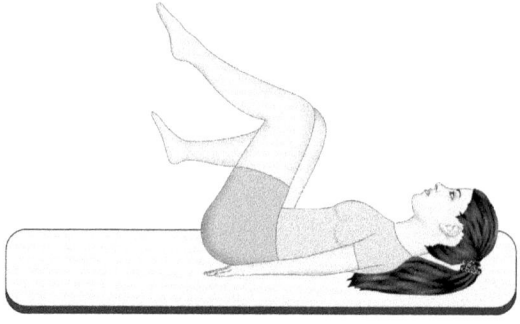

**Fig. 1.22:** Leg cycling exercise.

To lie on the back with hands by the side. In a very relaxed manner get both knees to chest and then stretch the legs out as long and straight as possible. Keep toes pointed. Move the legs in a cycling motion. Movements are made slowly, not in speed.

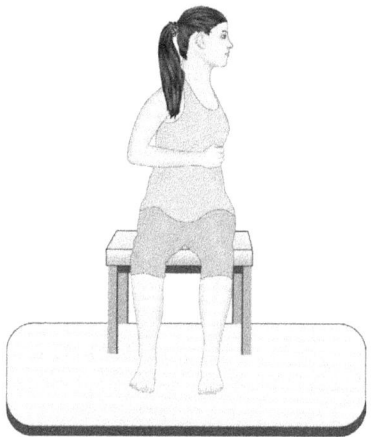

**Fig. 1.23:** Trunk rotation exercise.

To sit on a stool with thighs well supported, and hip and knees at 90°. To rotate the trunk on either side alternately and try to get chest and both elbows rotate to the opposite side.

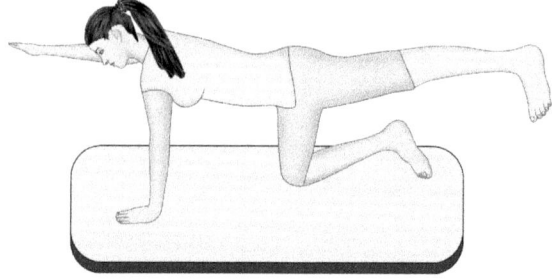

**Fig. 1.24:** Spine and limbs stretching.

To be on fours. To stretch opposite limbs (hand and leg) keeping other limbs (hand and leg) on the ground and to do alternatively.

**SPACE FOR NOTES**

CHAPTER 2

# Obstetric Case Discussions

**Chapter Objectives**
**To demonstrate the knowledge and understanding of:**
- Physiological adaptation in pregnancy (normal pregnancy, normal puerperium)
- Obstetric problems (APH, FGR, alloimmunization in pregnancy, breech presentation, multiple pregnancy, etc.)
- Maternal medicine:
  - Hematological diseases (anemia)
  - Hypertension
  - Seizure disorders
  - Diabetes, etc.
- Maternal and fetal complications
- Puerperium—normal, abnormal
- Miscarriage, Hemorrhage in early Pregnancy, PPH
- Modalities of investigations and interpretation of results
- Management issues

| | | |
|---|---|---|
| ❖ Case–1 | Normal Pregnancy | 18 |
| ❖ Case–2 | Primigravida with Floating (Free) Head at Term | 26 |
| ❖ Case–3 | Normal Puerperium | 31 |
| ❖ Case–4 | Puerperium Normal and Abnormal | 37 |
| ❖ Case–5 | Pregnancy and Labor in a Woman with Prior Cesarean Delivery | 41 |
| ❖ Case–6 | Anemia in Pregnancy | 48 |
| ❖ Case–7 | Diabetes in Pregnancy | 54 |
| ❖ Case–8 | Breech Presentation | 59 |
| ❖ Case–9 | Prolonged Pregnancy (Postterm Pregnancy) | 65 |

## Chapter 2 • Obstetric Case Discussions

- Case–10    Fetal Growth Restriction    68
- Case–11    Pre-Eclampsia and Eclampsia    72
- Case–12    Pregnancy with Maternal Red Cell Alloimmunization    80
- Case–13    Multiple Pregnancy    86
- Case–14    Intrauterine Fetal Death    93
- Case–15    Polyhydramnios    96
- Case–16    Antepartum Hemorrhage (Placenta Previa)    100
- Case–17    Abruptio Placentae (Accidental Hemorrhage)    104
- Case–18    Postpartum Hemorrhage—Prevention and Management    107
- Case–19    Hemorrhage in Early Pregnancy    113
- Case–20    Miscarriage (Spontaneous Abortion)    117

# OBJECTIVE STRUCTURED CLINICAL EXAMINATION (OSCE)

## CASE–1 NORMAL PREGNANCY

### Case Summary

Mrs MR, aged 26 years in her first pregnancy (P0+0+0+0), is admitted at 39 weeks of gestation with pain in the back. She is a booked case and has regular antenatal supervision. She is immunized and has received iron and folic acid supplementation throughout. All the trimesters of her pregnancy were uneventful.

**On General physical examination (GPE),** she is of 156 cm height, 67 kg without any pallor, no edema, BP 120/80 mm Hg and otherwise fit and healthy. She has gained total 11 kg of weight in this pregnancy. **Systemic examination** revealed, normal cardiovascular and respiratory systems. **Obstetric examination** revealed, uterus term size and relaxed, SFH 38 cm. Single fetus, longitudinal lie, cephalic presentation, 3/5th of the head is palpable PA. Fetal back is on the left side. Limbs are on the right side. Liquor volume is adequate. On auscultation FHS is heared on the left spinoumbilical line, 148 beats per minute and is regular.

*Q. What is your provisional diagnosis?*

**Ans.** Mrs MR, aged 26 years, a booked primigravida (P0+0+0+0) at term (39 weeks), in her normal pregnancy.

*Q. How we calculate gestational age?*

**Ans.** Period of gestation is calculated from the first day of the last menstruatrual period. It is important that the woman should have her regular cycle and she should correctly remember her date of last menstruation. Period of gestation is expressed in weeks.

*Example:* Mrs R, had first day of her last menstrual period on 13.1.19. Her expected date of delivery would be on 20.10.19. Her period of gestation as on 10.9.19 would be 34 weeks and 3 days ($34^{3/7}$).

*Q. At what time earliest the urine test becomes positive for pregnancy?*

**Ans.** On the first day of the missed period (for any woman with 28 days cycle).

*Q. What are the other conditions where β-hCG tests are done?*

**Ans.** (a) Trophoblastic disease (hydatidiform moles, choriocarcinoma) for diagnosis, and follow-up after the treatment.
(b) Ectopic pregnancy—diagnosis and follow-up
(c) Problems of miscarriage (threatened/missed/complete); (See p. 113).
(d) To follow-up during early pregnancy, in cases with in vitro fertilization and embryo transfer (IVF-ET).

Serum levels of β-hCG in normal pregnancy doubles by 48 hours. Usually, the rise of serum β-hCG is suboptimal in cases with ectopic pregnancy, or miscarriage.

**Q. How ultrasonograpghy can make early diagnosis of pregnancy?**

**Ans.** Demonstration of the important structures can confirm the diagnosis of pregnancy
  (1) Gestation sac (28–31 days following missed period)
  (2) Yolk sac (with mean sac diameter of 8 mm by TVS)
  (3) Embryonic pole (5.5–6 weeks)
  (4) Measurement of crown rump length
  (5) Transvaginal ultrasonography is helpful in early pregnancy.

**Q. Why do you present her as a case of normal pregnancy?**

**Ans.**
- From history she has no major symptoms except the mild backache which is common in pregnancy.
- On examination she has got no pallor, she is well-nourished, weight gain in pregnancy is normal and she is normotensive.
- On systemic examination there is no abnormality.
- Obstetrical examination revealed no abnormality.

**Q. Why do you call her a booked case?**

**Ans.** Any woman who has been supervised (examined and advised) during pregnancy in an institution at least three times or more.

**Q. What investigations are commonly advised to a pregnant woman in the antenatal clinic?**

**Ans.**
  (i) Blood for Hb%, ABO, Rh grouping, VDRL, and blood glucose estimation is done.
  (ii) Urine for routine and microscopic (protein, sugar, and pus cells) examination.
  (iii) Cervical cytology screening.

**Special investigations:**
  (iv) Serological tests for rubella, hepatitis B virus, and HIV (with consent).
  (v) Maternal serum alpha-fetoprotein (MSAFP), pregnancy associated plasma protein -A (PAPP-A) for prenatal diagnosis of fetal malformation (Dutta Obs 9/e, p. 103).
  (vi) Ultrasound examination in the first trimester and/or routine anomaly scan at 18–20 weeks.

**Q. How often should a woman be examined in the antenatal clinic?**

**Ans.** Generally a pregnant woman is seen at an interval of 4 weeks up to 28 weeks, at interval of 2 weeks up to 36 weeks and thereafter weekly till the expected date of delivery. However, **WHO recommends** at least four visits; **first** around 10–12 weeks, **second** between 24 and 28 weeks, the **third** at 32 weeks and the **fourth** visit at 36 weeks.

**Q. What are the objectives of subsequent visits in the antenatal clinic?**

Ans. To detect any high-risk factor from the history, examination and investigations, each time she attends the clinic. Repeated examinations help to detect any onset of anemia, pre-eclampsia. Assessment of fetal growth and fetal well-being are done. Fetal number, lie, presentation, position and liquor volume are also assessed.

**Q. Name the vaccines which are contraindicated in pregnancy?**

Ans. Live virus vaccines (rubella, measles, mumps, varicella, yellow fever) are contraindicated.

Every pregnant woman should be immunized against tetanus.

**Q. What are the causes of edema in pregnancy? How is physiological edema differentiated from the pathological one?**

Ans. **Causes of edema are:**
   (i) Physiological
   (ii) Pre-eclampsia
   (iii) Anemia, hypoproteinemia
   (iv) Cardiac failure
   (v) Nephrotic syndrome.

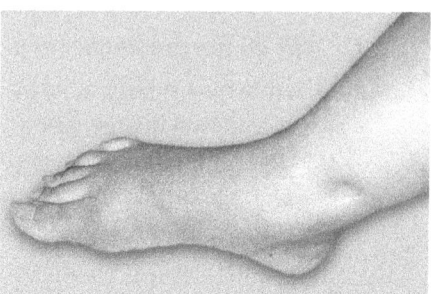

Fig. 2.1: Pitting edema of the leg over the ankle.

**The features of physiological edema are:**
   (i) Usually mild and in one leg (Fig. 2.1).
   (ii) Disappears on rest.
   (iii) Not associated with other features of pre-eclampsia, e.g. hypertension or proteinuria.
   (iv) Not associated with any other pathology (e.g. cardiac, renal or hematological).

**Q. How do you measure symphysis-fundal height and what is its importance?**

Ans. The woman is asked to empty her bladder. The top of the centralized uterine fundus is measured from the superior border of the symphysis pubis with a measuring tape. The symphysis-fundal height (SFH) measured in cm normally corresponds to the period of gestation in weeks. This is applicable after 24 weeks of pregnancy only. It is a good screening method (Figs. 2.2 and 2.3).

**Q. What are the information that can be obtained from the pelvic grips?**

Ans. Pelvic grips are two—Pawlik's grip and pelvic grip. Otherwise these are known as Leopold third and fourth maneuver.

Information obtained are:
   (i) Presentation (cephalic, breech or others)
   (ii) Presenting area (vertex, face, or others)
   (iii) Attitude (flexion or extension) on palpation of the occiput and the sinciput by the pelvic grips.

Chapter 2 • Obstetric Case Discussions 21

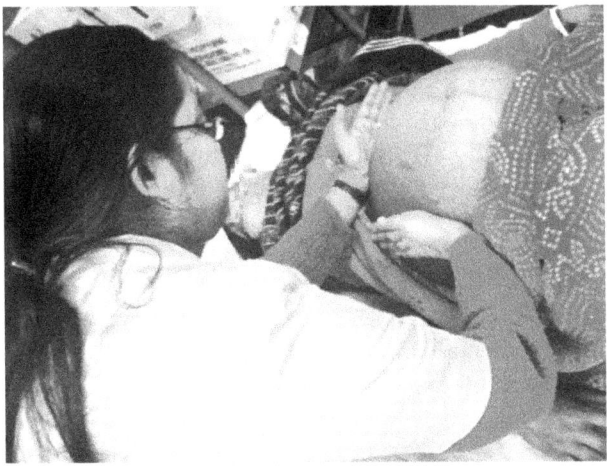

**Fig. 2.2:** Centralization of the uterus and measuring the height of the centralized uterus.

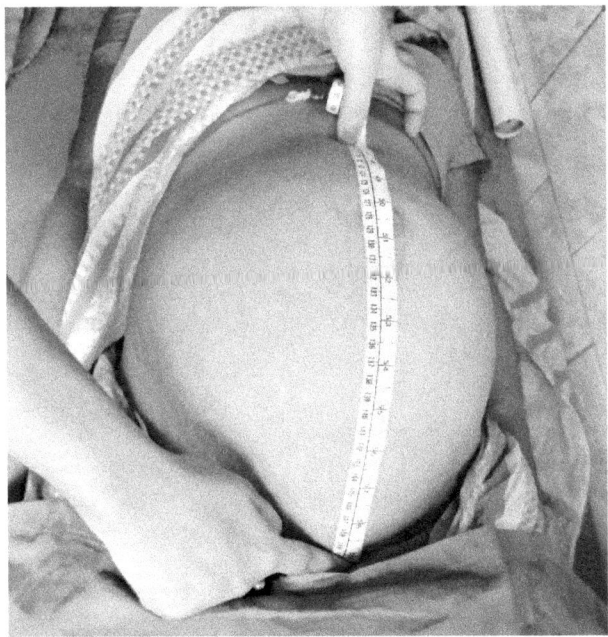

**Fig. 2.3:** Measurement of the symphysis-fundal height with a tape.

 (iv) Engagement (by palpating the sincipital and occipital poles in cephalic presentation).
**Q. What is a booking scan and what are the advantages?**
**Ans.** Ultrasound examination of the fetus at 18–20 weeks has got many advantages. Detailed fetal anatomy, viability, number of fetuses, liquor volume and placental localization can be assessed.

**Q. What investigations are repeated on subsequent antenatal visits?**

**Ans.** Hemoglobin at 28th and 36th weeks. Urine is tested for protein, sugar, and nitrites (dipstick) at every visit (Fig. 2.4). Ultrasonography may be repeated to know the growth profile of the fetus.

**Q. How do you auscultate the fetal heart sound?**

**Ans.** In cephalic presentation, it is heard by placing the fetoscope or the bell of the stethoscope on the spinoumbilical line depending on the side where the fetal back is. In breech presentation fetal heart sound (FHS) is best heard at or above the level of umbilicus. It may be on the right or left depending upon where the fetal back is (Fig. 2.5). In shoulder presentation (transverse lie) FHS is heard either at or below the level of umbilicus in the midline.

In occipitoposterior position, it is more towards the flank and is difficult to locate.

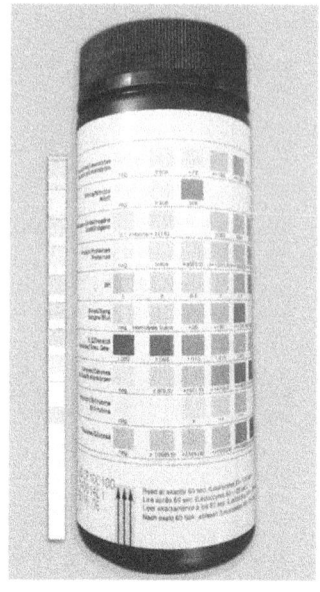

**Fig. 2.4:** Dipstick test.

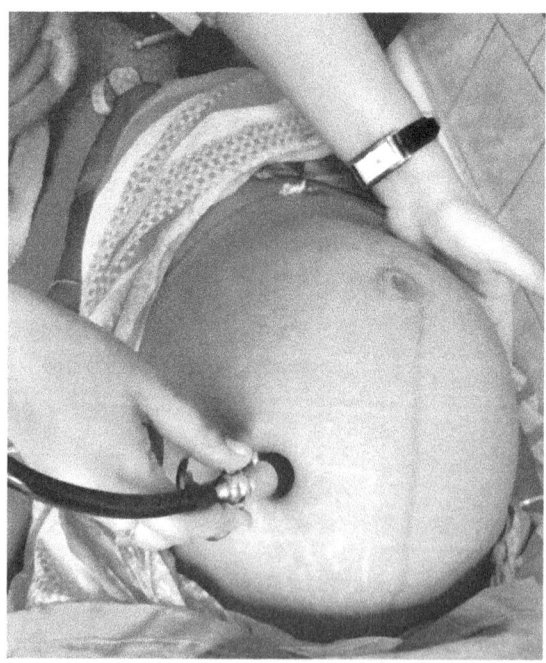

**Fig. 2.5:** Auscultation of the FHS (using a stethoscope) over the right spinoumbilical line.

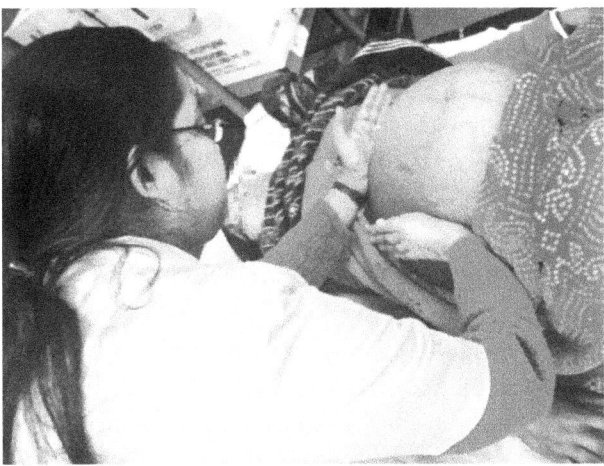

**Fig. 2.2:** Centralization of the uterus and measuring the height of the centralized uterus.

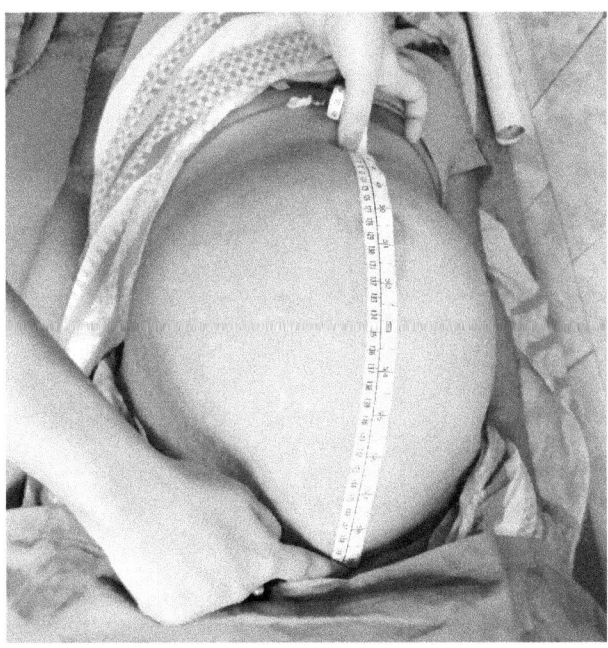

**Fig. 2.3:** Measurement of the symphysis-fundal height with a tape.

(iv) Engagement (by palpating the sinciput and occipital poles in cephalic presentation).

**Q. What is a booking scan and what are the advantages?**

**Ans.** Ultrasound examination of the fetus at 18–20 weeks has got many advantages. Detailed fetal anatomy, viability, number of fetuses, liquor volume and placental localization can be assessed.

**Q. What investigations are repeated on subsequent antenatal visits?**

**Ans.** Hemoglobin at 28th and 36th weeks. Urine is tested for protein, sugar, and nitrites (dipstick) at every visit (Fig. 2.4). Ultrasonography may be repeated to know the growth profile of the fetus.

**Q. How do you auscultate the fetal heart sound?**

**Ans.** In cephalic presentation, it is heard by placing the fetoscope or the bell of the stethoscope on the spinoumbilical line depending on the side where the fetal back is. In breech presentation fetal heart sound (FHS) is best heard at or above the level of umbilicus. It may be on the right or left depending upon where the fetal back is (Fig. 2.5). In shoulder presentation (transverse lie) FHS is heard either at or below the level of umbilicus in the midline.

In occipitoposterior position, it is more towards the flank and is difficult to locate.

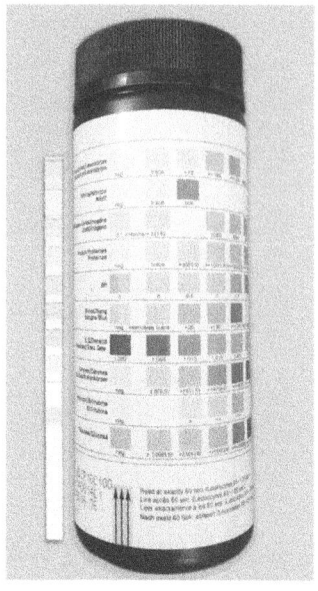

**Fig. 2.4:** Dipstick test.

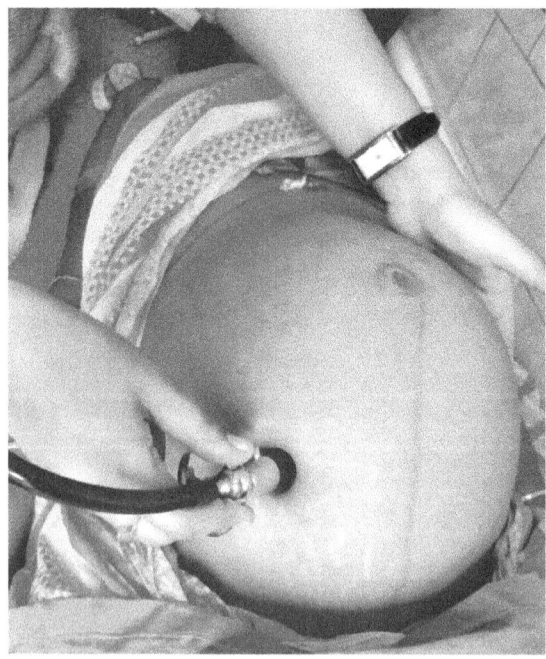

**Fig. 2.5:** Auscultation of the FHS (using a stethoscope) over the right spinoumbilical line.

**Q. Who need routine tests for blood glucose during pregnancy?**

**Ans.** (i) Positive family history of diabetes
   (ii) Previous birth of a baby weighing >4 kg
   (iii) Unexplained intrauterine fetal death in late pregnancy
   (iv) Persistent glycosuria
   (v) Obesity
   (vi) Age over 30 years.

**Q. What are the different methods that can help to estimate the gestational age and predict the expected date of confinement?**

**Ans.** Gestational age is about 280 days calculated from the first day of LMP.
   (i) Naegele's formula— dding 9 calendar months and 7 days to the first day of last normal menstrual period (LMP).
   (ii) Date of fruitful coitus—if this date can be remembered, 266 days are to be added to this date.
   (iii) Date of quickening—to add 22 weeks in a primigravida and 24 weeks in a multipara to this date of quickening.
   (iv) Review of previous antenatal records and to add the required weeks to make it 40 weeks.
      (a) Size of the uterus before 12 weeks (clinical examination).
      (b) Record of positive pregnancy test at first missed period.
      (c) Auscultation of FHS—by stethoscope earliest by 18–20 weeks.
   (v) Height of the uterus above symphysis pubis or measurement of SFH.
   (vi) Sonography:
      (a) First trimester—CRL (variation ± 5 days).
      (b) Second trimester (most accurate between 12 and 20 weeks)—by BPD, AC, HC, and FL (variation 7–10 days).
      (c) Third trimester—less reliable (variation ± 16 days).

**Q. How first trimester ultrasonography can make the correct assessment of gestational age?**

**Ans.** See p. 19.

**Q. How do you assess the well-being of the fetus in this case (late pregnancy)?**

**Ans.** (A) **Clinical**—auscultation of FHS, assessment of fetal growth, liquor volume, and SFH measurement (in cm).
   (B) **Biophysical parameters:**
      (i) **Daily fetal movement count (DFMCR):** Kicks >10 movements in 12 hours is satisfactory (to count 1 hour each in the morning, afternoon and night, then to multiply the total kicks by 4 to get total kicks in 12 hours).
      (ii) **Nonstress test (NST):** Reactive NST—two or more FHR accelerations in 20 minutes observation = Healthy fetus.
      (iii) **Fetal biophysical profile (FBP)** includes: NST, fetal breathing movements, gross body movements, fetal muscle tone and amniotic fluid volume. A FBP score of 8 indicates healthy fetus.

(iv) **Modified biophysical profile** consists of NST and AFI. It is abnormal when NST is nonreactive and/or AFI is <5.
(v) **Ultrasonography:** Serial measurement of BPD, AC, HC, and amniotic fluid volume (AFV) are done to assess fetal growth.
(vi) **Doppler ultrasound:** Doppler velocimetry of the umbilical artery is studied. Reduced, absent or reversed diastolic flow indicates fetal jeopardy.
**Other fetal vessels studied are:** Middle cerebral artery, aortic isthmus, ductus venosus, umbilical vein.

**Q. What is preconceptional counseling and what are its benefits?**

**Ans.** Preconceptional counseling means examination of the woman and counseling her about pregnancy and its outcome before the actual conception occurs.

**Benefits:** Preconceptional counseling can identify the risk factors beforehand. It can also reduce the complications of pregnancy as care (preventive measures) can be provided well ahead.

Anemia, infections, diabetes mellitus can be detected and treated before the actual onset of pregnancy. So the outcome of pregnancy is expected to be improved.

**Q. What is your plan for management of this woman as she has been admitted?**

**Ans.** She is a primigravida at 39 weeks of gestation without any complication. I would wait for spontaneous onset labor. Labor would be monitored closely and with partographic plotting. We except her a successful vaginal delivery.

**Q. Can she be discharged and allowed to go home as she is not in labor?**

**Ans.** She is close to her expected date of delivery (39 weeks). I shall do a pelvic examinations to assess the condition of the cervix. If there is a prospect for her going into labor (ripe cervix) soon, it would be better for her to stay back specially when stays far away from the hospital. Otherwise, she may go home and come back with onset of labor pain for delivery in this institute.

**Q. What do you mean by ripe cervix?**

**Ans.** Ripe cervix means a transition phase of the cervix from the state of pregnancy to labor. Ripe cervix is more soft, shortened (1.5 cm in length), central in position and partly dilated (1.6 cm).

**Q. What is Bishop's score?**

**Ans.** It is a scoring system done during pelvic examination. Five parameters are assessed.
  (1) *Cervix:*
      (a) Effacement
      (b) Dilation (cm)
      (c) Consistency
      (d) Position
  (2) *Fetal head:* Station

**Q. What is the usefulness of the scoring system?**

**Ans.** This scoring system can predict the success of induction of labor. Score marks are: 0, 1, 2, and 3. Total scoring is 13. Score: 6–13 suggests cervix is favorable and success of induction of labor is high. Score: <6 unfavorable for induction of labor.

## CASE–2: PRIMIGRAVIDA WITH FLOATING (FREE) HEAD AT TERM

### Case Summary

Mrs CK, aged 25 years P0+0+0+0, has been admitted at 39 weeks of pregnancy with pain in the back. She is a booked case and had regular antenatal supervision. She is immunized against tetanus and has received iron, calcium and folic acid supplementation throughout.

**On general physical examination (GPE)**, she is of average height 157 cm and weight 65 kg, without any pallor, BP 120/80 mm Hg and otherwise fit and healthy.

**Systemic examination** revealed normal cardiovascular and respiratory systems.

**Obstetric examination** revealed: Uterus term size and relaxed, SFH 38 cm, single fetus, longitudinal lie, cephalic presentation, 5/5th of the head is palpable per abdomen. Fetal back is on the left side. Limbs are on the right side. Liquor volume is adequate. On auscultation FHS is 147 beats per minute and it is regular.

**Provisional diagnosis: Primigravida with floating head at term pregnancy.**

**Q. What are the common causes of floating head at term?**

**Ans.** (i) Normal
(ii) Deflexion of the head
(iii) Occipitoposterior position of the head
(iv) Cephalopelvic disproportion
(v) Placenta previa
(vi) Pelvic tumors (lower segment fibroid, ovarian tumor).

**Q. When the head usually engages?**

**Ans.** In a primigravida, head usually engages after 37 weeks. This is due to increased abdominal muscle tone. However, head may engage even with the onset of labor. Whereas in a multigravida, head usually engages in labor. Overall in 60% of multi and 40% of primi, head do not engage prior to labor.

**Q. How can you exclude the pathologies that hinder or prevent the engagement of a normal head?**

**Ans.** Presence of placenta in the lower uterine segment (placenta previa) usually manifests with episodes of painless vaginal bleeding which is fresh and recurrent. This patient has not got any such history. However, ultrasonography would be helpful to exclude placenta previa or any pelvic tumor.

**Q. How deflexion of the head can cause nonengagement of the head?**

**Ans.** Deflexion of the head brings bigger diameter to the brim of the pelvis. Either suboccipito-frontal (10 cm) or occipitofrontal (11.5 cm) diameter comes on the brim of the pelvis. Occipitoposterior position of the head also causes deflexion and delayed engagement.

**Q. What is a contracted pelvis?**

**Ans.** Alteration in the size and/or shape of the pelvis (due to shortening of pelvic diameters) to sufficient degree so as to alter the normal mechanism of labor for an average-sized baby.

Anatomicaly, when the essential diameters of the pelvis is more than one planes are contracted by 0.5 cm, it is accepted as contracted pelvis.

**Q. What is cephalopelvic disproportion?**

**Ans.** It is the disparity in normal relation between the fetal head and pelvis. Disproportion may be either due to an average-sized baby with a small pelvis or due to a big baby with normal-sized pelvis or due to a combination of both (Fig. 2.6).

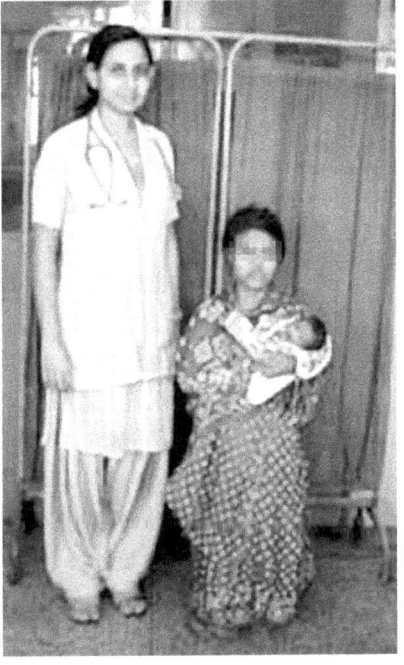

**Fig. 2.6:** Short-statured (3'5") woman delivered by cesarean section due to cephalopelvic disproportion.

**Q. What happens when the woman with occiput-posterior position goes into labor?**

**Ans.** There are some differences in the course of labor compared to occiput-anterior position.
  (i) Engagement of the head is delayed due to deflexion of the head.
  (ii) Membranes rupture early.
  (iii) The first stage of labor is prolonged.
  (iv) Due to long internal rotation of the head, the second stage is delayed.
  (v) Operative interventions (ventouse, forceps or cesarean delivery) are increased.

**Q. What happens as regard to the mechanism of labor in a case with occiput-posterior position?**

**Ans.** (a) **In majority (90%) of cases**, there is favorable outcome as the occiput rotates anteriorly with correction of deflexion.
  (b) **In about 10% of cases**, the outcome is unfavorable as the occiput fails to rotate anteriorly.

The important determinants to this favorable outcome are:
  (i) Shape of the pelvis
  (ii) Force of the uterine contraction
  (iii) Correction of deflexion of the head. Deflection is corrected with good uterine contractions and with an adequate pelvis when the fetus is of average size (<3.5 kg).

**Q. What would be management approach for this case?**

**Ans.** She would be investigated to rule out any cause of floating head (as discussed above) specially placenta previa, pelvic tumor or cephalopelvic disproportion. Ultrasonography is very useful in this regard and also to have an idea about the estimated weight of the fetus (CPD). However, to rule out CPD, we need to wait for spontaneous onset of labor when pelvic assessment could be done.

**Q. How do you make the management decision in the case?**

**Ans.** Once pelvic pathology is ruled out, we would wait for spontaneous onset of labor and by that time the fetal head is expected to be engaged. We would also do the pelvic assessment and rule out cephalopelvic disproportion at that time. There after partographic monitoring of labor will be done for successful vaginal delivery. Augmentation of labor may be done if needed to stimulate uterine contractions. However, in the presence of any abnormality (nonprogress of labor, fetal distress) she would be delivered by cesarean section.

**Q. How cephalopelvic disproportion is diagnosed?**

**Ans.** Cephalopelvic disproportion at the level of the brim is mostly assessed by—
(a) Clinical methods, (b) Imaging pelvimetry.

(a) **Clinical methods**
   (i) Abdominal method: It is done by judging the overriding of the fetal head (parietal bone) over the symphysis pubis when the head is grasped by the left hand and pushed down the pelvic brim. In a case without any disproportion the head usually goes down the brim. It is a good screening method.
   (ii) Abdominovaginal method (Muller-Munro-Kerr method). (Dutta Obs. 9/e, p. 330).

(b) **Imaging pelvimetry**
   (i) **Magnetic resonance imaging (MRI)** can assess the bony pelvis, fetal size and also maternal soft tissues. It is more accurate but expensive.
   (ii) **Computed tomography (CT)** is more informative compared to X-ray pelvimetry. It is done less commonly.
   (iii) **X-ray pelvimetry:** Erect lateral view is generally taken. Antero-posterior view may also be taken. CT and X-ray have got radiation hazards. Imaging studies are rarely done except in a case with fractured pelvis.

   Clinical pelvimetry is only done during the course of labor. The fetal head is the best pelvimeter and is assessed during the course of labor.

**Q. What is clinical pelvimetry and when it is done?**

**Ans.** In vertex presentation pelvic assessment is done at any time beyond 37 weeks but it is better to be done with the onset of labor. The following information are recorded during the pelvic examination.

Assessment is done for the all the levels of the pelvis:
(A) Brim
(B) Cavity
(C) Outlet.

The important landmarks are :
(i) Sacrum—its curvature (well curved sacrum)
(ii) Sacrosciatic notch (wide)
(iii) Ischial spines (not prominent)
(iv) Iliopectineal lines
(v) Side walls (Either parallel or divergent)
(vi) Posterior surface of symphysis pubis (smooth curve)
(vii) Sacrococcygeal joint (mobile)
(viii) Subpubic arch (more rounded)
(ix) Diagonal conjugate (12 cm or more)
(x) Subpubic angle (>85°)
(xi) Transverse diameter of the outlet (TDO) (accomodate 4 knuckles 11 cm).

**Q. What are the different types of pelvis?**

**Ans.** Parent types are four:
(i) Gynecoid (50%)
(ii) Anthropoid (25%)
(iii) Android (20%)
(iv) Platypelloid (5%). More commonly combination of features are found (e.g. 'Gyne-android'— the first part refers the posterior segment and the second part relates the anterior segment). Thus, there are total 14 types of pelvis.

**Q. How do you manage a woman when there is pelvic contraction at the level of the brim?**

**Ans.** We have to ascertain the degree of CPD by clinical examination.
**Minor degree CPD** usually does not give rise to any problem. Such cases are often allowed for spontaneous labor and delivery at term. Women with moderate and severe degree of pelvic contractions are the problem. Usually they are delivered by elective cesarean section.

**Q. What is trial of labor?**

**Ans.** It is the conduction of spontaneous labor in woman with minor degree cephalopelvic disproportion in an institution under supervision for safe vaginal delivery. However, arrangements should be available for operative delivery either vaginal or abdominal, if the condition so arises.

**Q. How do you conduct the "Trial of labor"?**

**Ans.** (i) The labor should preferably be spontaneous in onset.
(ii) The labor progress is carefully monitored (partographic monitoring).

(iii) Augmentation of labor may be done with amniotomy along with oxytocin infusion if needed.
(iv) Trial of labor is continued as long as the progress of labor is satisfactory in terms of dilatation of the cervix, descend of the presenting part and the uterine contractions. Otherwise labor is terminated either by operative vaginal delivery (ventouse or forceps) or by cesarean section.

**Q. How does the trial of labor end?**

**Ans.** Trial of labor ends with any of the following modes of delivery:
(i) Spontaneous vaginal delivery with or without episiotomy (30%).
(ii) Assisted vaginal delivery with ventouse or forceps (30%).
(iii) Cesarean section (40%).

**Q. What are the advantages of successful trial of labor?**

**Ans.** (i) Unnecessary cesarean sections are avoided.
(ii) Successful trial may ensure future good obstetric behavior.

## CASE–3  NORMAL PUERPERIUM

### Case Summary

*Mrs SD, aged 23 years, P1+0+0+1, presents with the complaints of pain in the lower abdomen as well as in the perineum. She had been admitted last night with labor pain at the end of her term pregnancy. She was a booked case. She had spontaneous vaginal delivery with (right) mediolateral episiotomy.*

*On general physical examination, there was no pallor. She was afebrile, normotensive and breasts were normal, pulse 84/min, BP 126/80 mm Hg. Systemic examination (cardiovascular and respiratory system) did not reveal any abnormality. Height of the centralized uterine fundus measured 13 cm above the symphysis pubis with an empty bladder. On perineal examination, lochial discharge (Lochia rubra) was normal. She had changed 3 pads. Episiotomy wound was clean and healthy.*

*A baby girl was born on...... at...... am (last night). The baby weighed 2.7 kg, Apgar score was 8 and 10 (cried at birth). The baby on examination was normal (at term) and healthy. Baby passed meconium and urine. The umbilicus was clean and healthy. There was no obvious congenital abnormality. The baby was on exclusive breastfeeding. See details of history taking and examination methods on p. 11-12.*

**Special features to note in a case of puerperium are:** *(i) Start with the complaints related to puerperium only (not of antecedent pregnancy). (ii) Instead of LMP — mention the date and time of last childbirth. (iii) Instead of EDD and duration of pregnancy (as weeks in antenatal cases), mention the number days in puerperium.*

**Q. What is your diagnosis?**

**Ans.** Mrs SD, 23 years old lady, P1+0+0+1, is in her first day of normal puerperium with her healthy baby.

**Q. What is puerperium?**

**Ans.** It is the period following childbirth during which all the pelvic organs and the body systems revert back to prepregnant state both anatomically and physiologically.

**Q. Why do you consider her as a case of normal puerperium?**

**Ans.** She has got no significant complaints. Slight amount of pain in abdomen is common. This is known as afterpain. She also experienced slight amount of pain in the perineum which is common following vaginal delivery with an episiotomy. Her general physical examination as well as systemic examination did not reveal any abnormality. She is afebrile, her bowel and bladder activities are normal. Involution of the uterus is normal, lochial discharge is normal. Episiotomy wound is healthy and breastfeeding is normal. Baby on examination is normal.

**Q. What is the normal rate of involution of the uterus?**

**Ans.** Following delivery, uterine fundus is about 13 cm above the symphysis pubis and for the first 24 hours the height of the uterus remains unchanged.

Thereafter there is a steady decrease in height by 1.25 cm (1/2") in 24 hours. The uterus becomes a pelvic organ by 14 days' time. It takes about 6 weeks for the uterus to become normal in size.

**Q. What are the causes of subinvolution of the uterus?**

**Ans.** Factors that hinder or delay the involution of the uterus are—overenlargement of the uterus (twins, hydramnios), retained products of conception (blood clots, placental bits), puerperal sepsis following cesarean delivery, uterine fibroid, prolapse uterus and maternal illness (anemia).

**Q. What are the common urinary problems in the puerperium?**

**Ans.** (1) **Urinary tract infection (UTI):** Infection is often contracted during labor and puerperium due to catheterization or due to stasis of urine in puerperium or due to recurrence of previous infection.
(2) **Retention of urine:** Due to pain and spasm following bruising of the paraurethral region and perineal region.
(3) **Incontinence of urine:** Either stress (common) or true incontinence due to fistula formation (rare).

**Q. What is this lower abdominal pain called? How are you going to manage it?**

**Ans.** This is known as afterpain. It is infrequent and spasmodic in nature. It lasts for a variable period of 2–4 days. The pain is either due to retained blood clots and/or placental bits (common in primipara) or due to vigorous spasmodic uterine contractions (common in multipara). Management is to massage the uterus to expel the retained products and to give some analgesics and antispasmodics.

**Q. What are the acute complications (puerperal emergencies) that may arise in puerperium?**

**Ans.** (A) **Immediate:** Postpartum hemorrhage (PPH), shock (hypovolemic or idiopathic), pulmonary embolism, and inversion of the uterus.
(B) **Early** (within 1 week): Urinary complications, puerperal pyrexia, puerperal sepsis, breast complications (engorgement, mastitis, abscess), and puerperal blues.
(C) **Delayed:** Secondary PPH, thromboembolism, and psychosis.

**Q. What are the common causes of puerperal pyrexia?**

**Ans.** (A) Infections of the genital organs (Puerperal sepsis)
(B) Infections of the breast, mastitis, abscess
(C) Urinary tract infection.
(D) Wound infections: Cesarean or episiotomy wound

(E) Septic pelvic thrombophlebitis
(F) Pulmonary infection: Pneumonia.

**Q. What is milk ejection or milk let down reflex?**

**Ans.** Suckling → nipple and areola stimulation → ascending tactile impulse via thoracic sensory nerve (T 4,5,6) → paraventricular and supraoptic nuclei of the hypothalamus → oxytocin release from posterior pituitary → contraction of myoepithelial cells of the alveoli → milk let down. This reflex is inhibited by pain and abnormal psychological condition.

Presence of the infant or even infant's cry can induce let down reflex without suckling.

**Q. What is the relationship between lactation with amenorrhea and ovulation?**

**Ans.** Breastfeeding → increased prolactin level → suppression of FSH and LH levels → less follicular growth and development → hypoestrogenic state (amenorrhea) and anovulation.

Frequency and duration of suckling correlate directly related to the level of prolactin, duration of ovarian suppression and lactational amenorrhea.

**Q. When is she going to resume her menstruation normally?**

**Ans.** It depends on whether she breastfeeds her baby or not. About 70% of the women who are fully breastfeeding may remain amenorrheic for the first 6 months. But a nonlactating woman, may resume her menstruation by 6 weeks time in about 40% cases.

**Q. When she should start contraception in the postpartum phase?**

**Ans.** It depends on whether she is lactating or not. Women who are exclusively breastfeeding, remain anovulatory in 90% of cases. Chance of ovulation is increased if she is not lactating or partially lactating. Recommendation is to start contraception from 3rd postpartum month if she is full breastfeeding and from 3rd postpartum week if she is feeding partially or not breastfeeding.

**Q. What should be the choice of contraception for her?**

**Ans.** It depends on whether she is breastfeeding or not. Combined oral pills should be avoided if she is breastfeeding. However, she can use DMPA 150 mg IM every 3 months (injectable progestin) or progestin only pill (mini pill) orally. Otherwise she can use IUD irrespective of her lactation status. Postplacental IUCD is currently being practised. It is safe and effective. Expulsion rate is higher compared to interval insertion. An especially designed forceps (Kelly's) is used for this purpose (Fig. 2.7).

**Q. Should episiotomy be made a routine procedure?**

**Ans.** Episiotomy has got restricted use. Current recommendation is close intrapartum supervision (to prevent perineal injury) and selective use of episiotomy.

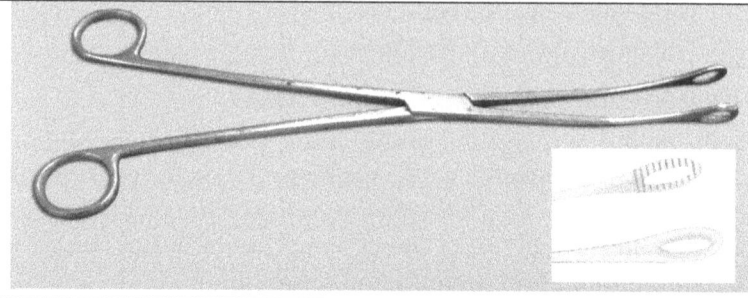

**Fig. 2.7:** Kelly's long forceps.

**Description:** This is a long metallic instrument. It has got a smooth curve close to the blades. The handle has no catch. The blades are fenestrated with transverse serrations on their inner surface.

**Uses:** (1) Postplacental (following delivery of the placenta). Insertion IUCD (Cu T380 A) in the puerperal uterus, (2) As an alternative to ovum forceps for removal of retained placental bits and membranes.

This instrument has got advantages: (1) The length enables it to place the IUCD at the fundus of the puerperal uterus. (2) The transverse serration provides good grip to the IUCD. (3) Absence of catch protects the IUCD from crushing.

**Q. What are the common indications of episiotomy?**

**Ans.** (i) Cases with rigid perineum as in elderly primigravidae; previous perineal scar-like perineorrhaphy.
(ii) Instrumental delivery—forceps and ventouse.
(iii) Malposition (occipito-posterior), malpresentation (breech delivery) or shoulder dystocia.
(iv) Threatened perineal tear.

**Q. When should the baby be put to breast following delivery? What should be the frequency and duration of each feed?**

**Ans.** Following normal delivery, a healthy baby may be put to breast immediately or by 1/2–1 hour. Following cesarean delivery a period of 3–4 hours is sufficient. Initially the frequency should be at 2–3 hours interval. Baby is fed from one breast completely over a period of 5–10 minutes. Baby should get both the foremilk and hindmilk in this way.

**Q. What do you understand by good attachment?**

**Ans.** Good attachment during breastfeeding means infant's mouth is wide open and chin touches the breast. The nipple and areola should be within the baby's mouth between the tongue and palate. This helps effective milk transfer.

**Q. When is she going to be discharged from the hospital?**

Ans. This woman with normal puerperium could be discharged after 24–48 hours.

**Q. What advices do you give her during the discharge?**

Ans. To maintain her general health with good diet and to continue the iron and calcium supplementation.
- To continue breastfeeding exclusively and care of the baby (immunization).
- To take care of her breasts (cleaning the nipples with sterile water before and after each feed).
- Care of the episiotomy wound (cleaning with Savlon swab twice daily and after each act of micturition and defecation). Application of an antibiotic ointment should be done thereafter.
- Family planning guidance (contraceptive advice).
- To come for postnatal check-up after 6 weeks or to report early if she has any problem.
- Postpartum exercises (See p. 13-14).

**Q. What is involution of the uterus?**

Ans. Involution is the process whereby the genital organs revert back approximately to the prepregnancy state.

**Q. What is subinvolution?**

Ans. When the process of normal involution is retarded or impaired it is called subinvolution.

**Q. What are the common causes of subinvolution of the uterus?**

Ans. (i) When the uterus is hugely enlarged as in twins polyhydramnios
(ii) Grand multiparity
(iii) Cesarean section
(iv) Retained products of conceptus
(v) Uterine sepsis
(vi) Uterine prolapse
(vii) Fibroid uterus.

**Q. How can breast engorgement be prevented?**

Ans. Yes, it could be prevented to a large extent. The preventive measures are:
(i) No prelacteal feeds
(ii) To start breastfeeding early and unrestricted
(iii) Exclusive breastfeeding
(iv) Feeding in correct position with proper attachment.

**Q. How do you manage the woman with acute mastitis in puerperium?**

**Ans.** (i) Breast support
(ii) Plenty of oral fluids
(iii) Antibiotic—flucloxacillin
(iv) Analgesic (ibuprofen)
(v) Breastfeeding to be continued.

**Q. She faced difficulty in breastfeeding her baby. How are you going to help her?**

**Ans.** Correct position of the mother, frequent feeding and correct attachment of the baby with the breast can improve the outcome. For any other difficulties, a trained nurse may be helpful.

## CASE-4  PUERPERIUM NORMAL AND ABNORMAL

### Case Summary

Ms CD, 25 years old, P1+0 +0+1, had her spontaneous vaginal delivery 4 days back at home. She was feeling some uneasiness since delivery, and she has developed fever (temperature of 102°F) since yesterday. She also had the problems of burning sensation during passing urine. However, her baby is doing well. She is having normal breastfeeding to her baby.

**Q. How do you define puerperium?**

**Ans.** Puerperium is the period immediately following childbirth and extending up to 6 weeks postpartum.

**Q. What is the usual time period for the involution of the uterus?**

**Ans.** By 2 weeks of puerperium, uterus usually becomes a pelvic organ. However, it takes 6 weeks postpartum for all pelvic organs including uterus to go back to its normal pregravid state.

**Q. What is the cause of amenorrhea in puerperium?**

**Ans.** Women who are breastfeeding remain amenorrheic for a longer period compared to women who are bottle-feeding.

In lactating women, the serum levels of prolactin remain high. High prolactin suppresses both FSH and LH. This causes less follicular growth. There is a hypoestrogenic state and the woman becomes amenorrheic. However, women who are not breastfeeding, menstruation returns by 12th week in majority (80%).

**Q. What is the cause of anovulation in puerperium?**

**Ans.** Suppression of ovulation is related to persistently elevated prolactin levels in a lactating woman. A woman who is exclusively breastfeeding, the contraceptive protection due to anovulation remains up to 6 months postpartum in majority (98%). In a nonlactating woman ovulation may return as early as 4 weeks.

**Q. How do you define puerperal pyrexia?**

**Ans.** A rise in temperature of 100.4°F (38°C) or more on two separate occasions at 24 hours apart (excluding first 24 hours) within first 10 days of following delivery is called puerperal pyrexia.

**Q. What are the common causes of puerperal pyrexia?**

**Ans.** (1) Puerperal sepsis (infections of the genital tract).
(2) Urinary tract infection (cystitis).
(3) Breast infection (mastitis).
(4) Wound infection.
(5) Pulmonary infection (pneumonia and tuberculosis).
(6) Thrombophlebitis.

**Q. What are the common causes of puerperal sepsis?**

**Ans.** (a) Endometritis.
(b) Endomyometritis.
(c) Pelvic cellulitis.

**Q. What are the common predisposing factors for puerperal sepsis?**

**Ans.** (1) **Antenatal factors**
(a) Anemia and malnutrition.
(b) Premature rupture of membranes.
(2) **Intrapartum factors**
(a) Repeated vaginal examination.
(b) Prolonged rupture of membranes >18 hours.
(c) Traumatic instrumental delivery (forceps).
d) Prolonged labor.
(e) Dehydration, ketoacidosis in labor.

**Q. What are the common organisms involved in puerperal sepsis?**

**Ans.** Organisms are often polymicrobial (**aerobic:** Gram-positive and gram-negative, and **anerobic**) in nature.

**Aerobic:**
- Group A *Streptococcus hemolyticus* (GAS)
- *Staphylococcus pyogenes*
  - E.coli
  - Pseudomonas.

**Anerobic:**
- *Streptococcus*
- *Bacteroides* (fragilis), *Clostridia*.

**Q. What investigations do you do in such a case?**

**Ans.** It will depend upon the clinical examination findings.

**Common investigations are:**
(a) High vaginal swab/wound swab for culture and sensitivity.
(b) Midstream urine for culture and sensitivity.
(c) Complete blood count (CBC).
(d) Pelvic ultrasound: To detect any retained bits of tissue inside the uterus or to detect pelvic abscess.
(e) X-ray chest: To detect pathology (pneumonia and Koch's lesion).
(f) Doppler USG study: To detect venous thrombosis.

**Q. What are the conditions when lactation needs to be suppressed?**

**Ans.** Conditions are rare. The situations are:
(a) Stillbirth
(b) Neonatal death

(c) Situations where breastfeeding is contraindicated:
   (i) Maternal acute puerperal illness
   (ii) Puerperal psychosis
   (iii) Mother on high doses of antiepileptic, antithyroid drugs.

**Q. What ate the different breast problems during puerperium?**

**Ans.** Engorgement of breasts, pain in the breast, acute mastitis, breast abscess, cracked nipple, retracted nipple and lactation failure.

**Q. When to start breastfeeding after delivery?**

**Ans.**
- In cases with vaginal delivery, breastfeeding can be started immediately following delivery.
- In case of cesarean delivery it can be started as soon as the mother is fit to feed the baby or within 3-4 hours.

**Q. Will you allow breastfeeding in HIV positive mother?**

**Ans.** Ideally breastfeeding is avoided to minimize the risk of MTCT. However, for the developing countries WHO recommends exclusive breastfeeding to prevent protein-energy malnutrition (PEM).
Neonate is given antiretroviral therapy (Nevirapine syrup) for the first 6 weeks of life.

**Q. If mother is hepatitis B surface antigen positive, what are the risks of the newborn?**

**Ans.** Neonatal transmission occurs mainly at or around the time of delivery. The transplacental risks of transmission to the fetus varies from 10% (first trimester) to 90% (third trimester). The carrier neonate may suffer from cirrhosis of liver or hepatocellular carcinoma as a long-term complication.

**Q. How the baby is managed after delivery?**

**Ans.** The baby is given HBV immunoglobulin within 12 hours of birth. At the same time active immunization with hepatitis B vaccine also given IM at a separate site.

**Q. How is lactation suppressed?**

Methods commonly used are:
(a) To stop breastfeeding
(b) Ice packs to prevent breast engorgement
(c) Analgesics to relieve pain
(d) To use breast support.
Medications to use are bromocriptine or cabergoline.

**Q. How would you diagnose the vulval hematoma?**

**Ans.**
- Symptoms: Pain in the perineum, swelling, sometimes retention of urine.
- General examination: Tachycardia, pallor, hypotension (depending on the severity) may be present.

- Local examination: The swelling feels tense cystic and bluish in color. Tenderness is present. It gradually increases. The swelling may obliterate the vaginal introitus.
- Per rectal examination: Tense tender mass may be palpated in front of rectum.

Ultrasonography may be needed at times to localize it and to determine the extent of the hematoma.

**Q. How will you manage a case of vulval hematoma?**

**Ans.**
- Resuscitation: IV fluids and antibiotics are started. Blood is sent for cross-matching
- Actual management: Small hematoma (<5 cm) could be managed by conservative (cold compress) approach. Antibiotics and analgesics (ibuprofen) are started.
- Large hematoma: Operation—drainage of hematoma under general anesthesia is done. Bleeding points, if any, are secured. Deep mattress sutures are used. The wound is closed with a drain. It is removed after 24 hours.

A *Foley's catheter* is maintained till the tissue edema subsides. Antibiotics are continued for 5 days.

**Q. What is Homan's sign?**

**Ans.** It is the elicitation of pain in calf muscles on sudden dorsiflexion of the foot. It suggests deep vein thrombosis. However, it needs confirmation using the Doppler study of the leg veins.

**Q. How to confirm the diagnosis?**

**Ans.** Confirmation of deep vein thrombosis (DVT) is done by: (a) Venous ultrasonography (femoral vein, popliteal vein and deep veins of the calf), (b) Doppler USG—accurate and (c) with MRI.

## CASE–5 : PREGNANCY AND LABOR IN A WOMAN WITH PRIOR CESAREAN DELIVERY

### Case Summary

*Mrs AR, 24 years old, P1+0+0+1, was admitted at 38 weeks of pregnancy. She had been delivered in her previous pregnancy by LSCS due to fetal distress. She had got no major complaints. On examination, she was not pale. She was otherwise fit and healthy. Her height was 5'3", weight: 61 kg, her BP was 120/80 mm Hg. Obstetric examination revealed—uterus: Term size (SFH 36 cm), single fetus, cephalic presentation, head not engaged. Back on the right side and limbs on the left. Clinically liquor volume average, FHS 142 beats/minute and regular. There was no scar tenderness.*

*Provisional diagnosis (PD)—Mrs AR, 24 years, P1+0+0+1 at 38 weeks of pregnancy with history of prior cesarean delivery.*

**Q. Why had she been admitted?**

**Ans.** To formulate the plan of delivery. Because of her history of previous cesarean delivery, she is a high-risk woman.

**Q. What are the complications that such a woman may have, considering her previous cesarean delivery?**

**Ans.** For such a woman, certain risks are increased in pregnancy and labor.

**Pregnancy:**
(i) Abortion
(ii) Preterm labor
(iii) Normal pregnancy ailments (pain abdomen)
(iv) Placenta previa (APH)
(v) Morbid adherent placenta
(vi) Scar dehiscence
(vii) Scar rupture.

**Labor:**
(i) Scar dehiscence
(ii) Scar rupture
(iii) Retained placenta (placenta accreta)
(iv) Postpartum hemorrhage
(v) Peripartum hysterectomy
(vi) Increased operative intervention.

All these lead to increased **maternal and perinatal** morbidity and mortality.

**Q. What are the different types of uterine scar for cesarean delivery? What type of scar does usually rupture during pregnancy and labor? What type of scar rupture is frequent?**

**Ans.** Lower segment transverse incision is most commonly made in cesarean delivery. Upper segment vertical scar is rare and is either due to classical cesarean delivery or due to hysterotomy.

As regards the rupture of scar, we should consider the following anatomical factors:
(i) Wound apposition
(ii) Healing of the wound following delivery
(iii) The stretching of the wound during subsequent pregnancy and labor.

**Lower segment transverse scar** usually ruptures during labor, whereas classical scar usually ruptures during late pregnancy or in labor.

**Incidence of lower segment transverse scar rupture** is less (about 0.2–1.5%), the risk of lower segment vertical scar rupture is 0.8–1.8%, as compared to classical or T-shaped scar rupture which is common (about 4–9%).

**Q. Why is a lower segment transverse scar more sound than a classical scar?**

**Ans.** (i) Wound margins are perfectly apposed without any pocket formation
(ii) Healing is better as this part remains inert during that time (puerperium)
(iii) In future pregnancy and labor, the wound stretches along the line of the scar. But in classical scar, it is at right angle.

**Q. How do you assess the scar tenderness?**

**Ans.** Commonly lower uterine segment transverse incision is made during cesarean delivery. Therefore, assessment of scar tenderness is done along the transverse length of the scar of the lower segment of the uterus (not the scar of the skin). Pulp of the fingers (using both the hands) is gently rolled up and down over the area above the symphysis pubis to feel any gap in the continuity of vv wall. At the same time we need to look at the face of the woman, to observe any expression of pain. However, there is no single pathognomonic clinical feature to indicate scar dehiscence or rupture (Figs. 2.8 and 2.9).

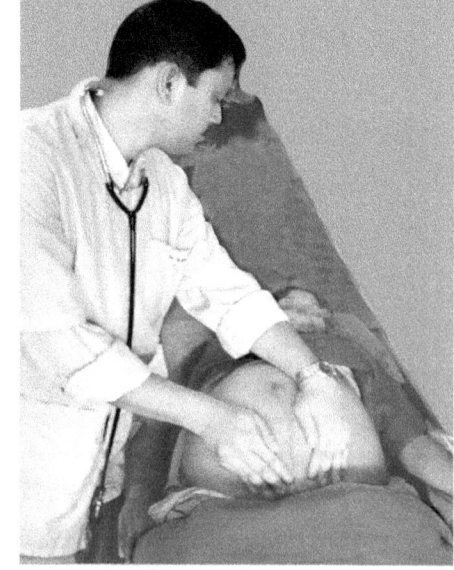

**Fig. 2.8:** Assessment of scar tenderness for a lower segment transverse scar. Pulp of the fingers (using both the hands) are gently rolled up and down over the area above the symphysis pubis, while the examiner looks at the face of the patient.

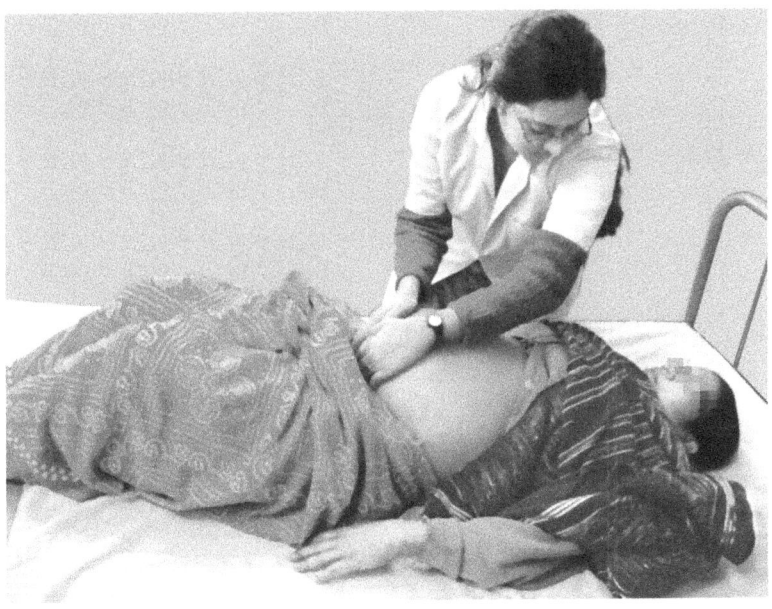

**Fig. 2.9:** Candidate demonstrates assessment of scar tenderness in a woman with history of prior cesarean delivery. Note the candidate's fingers' position and at the same time she looks towards the patient's face for expression of pain (also Fig. 2.8).

*Q. What are the features of impending scar rupture during labor?*

**Ans.** (i) Suprapubic pain
(ii) Vaginal bleeding
(iii) Bladder tenesmus (sometimes hematuria)
(iv) Maternal tachycardia
(v) Falling of blood pressure
(vi) Tenderness over the scar
(vii) Failure in progress of labor
(viii) **Appearance of fetal distress**
(ix) **Abnormal CTG (variable or late deceleration pattern and bradycardia)**
(x) Loss of FHS
(xi) Cessation of uterine contractions
(xii) Loss of uterine contour.

*Q. What is uterine scar dehiscence?*

**Ans.** It is the incomplete disruption of the uterine wall (Fig. 2.10). Usually the uterine serosa, overlying the area of uterine muscular defect remains intact. A dehiscence is described as an uterine window. Uterine dehiscence is usually detected incidentally during the time of cesarean section. Usually, there is either no hemorrhage or minimal hemorrhage. The woman usually remains asymptomatic. However, these two terms (uterine rupture and

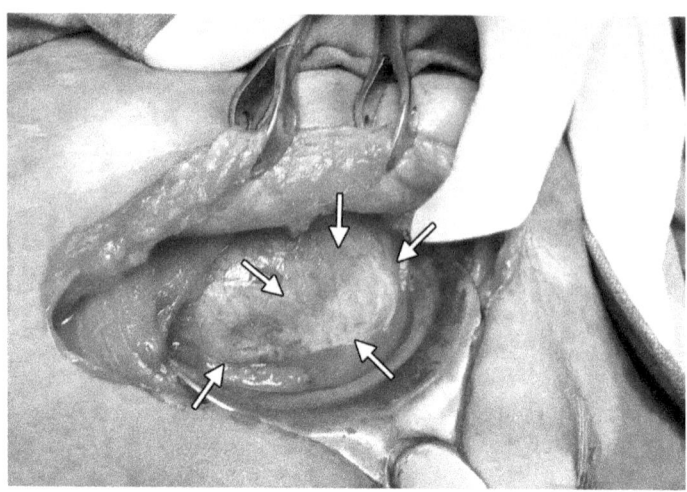

**Fig. 2.10:** Scar dehiscence.
Mrs CR, 2nd gravida, with prior cesarean delivery was admitted at 38 weeks of pregnancy with pain abdomen. Clinical examination revealed vitals were stable with doubtful scar tenderness. Laparotomy for emergency cesarean delivery revealed scar dehiscence (See arrows).

uterine dehiscence) are used frequently interchangeably. But the clinical significance of these two conditions is different.

**Q. What is uterine rupture?**

**Ans.** It is the complete separation of all layers of the uterine wall including serosa. In this situation, uterine cavity and the abdominal cavity are continuous. This is an obstetric emergency putting the fetus and the mother in danger.

**Q. What is the risk of uterine rupture?**

**Ans.** Risk of rupture in a scarred uterus is high compared to an unscarred uterus. Uterine rupture can occur following other operations on the uterus like myomectomy or hysterotomy. The overall risk of uterine rupture with a prior low transverse scar is about 0.1%, with a low vertical scar is 1-7% and with a classical or hysterotomy scar is 4-9%.

**Q. What are complications of uterine rupture?**

**Ans.** (A) **Fetal:** Hypoxia and death.
(B) **Maternal:** Intraperitoneal hemorrhage, shock, urgent need of blood transfusion, laparotomy, hysterectomy or repair of rupture. Risk of maternal and perinatal mortality is high unless managed optimally.

**Q. What is VBAC?**

**Ans.** Vaginal birth after cesarean (VBAC).

**Q. What is TOLAC?**

**Ans.** Trial of labor after cesarean delivery.

**Q. What are the contraindications of VBAC?**

**Ans.** Women with:
   (i) Previous classical cesarean delivery or hysterotomy these women should be delivered by elective cesarean section after 37 completed weeks
   (ii) Woman with history of rupture uterus
   (iii) Women with prior two or more lower segment cesarean section
   (iv) Contracted pelvis or suspected CPD
   (v) Presence of other complications in pregnancy like PIH and malpresentation
   (vi) In a center where facilities for emergency cesarean delivery are not available round the clock
   (vii) Patient refusal.

**Q. Which women are best considered for trial of labor after cesarean section (TOLAC)?**

**Ans.** The woman should fulfill the following criteria:
   (i) Women with singleton pregnancy with cephalic presentation
   (ii) At 37 + weeks of pregnancy
   (iii) With previous single lower segment cesarean delivery
   (iv) A woman for whom indication of primary section was nonrecurrent
   (v) Previous lower segment single transverse scar
   (vi) Pelvis adequate for the fetus
   (vii) Where continued labor monitoring is possible
   (viii) Facilities for emergency cesarean section round the clock are available
   (ix) Facilities for blood transfusion are available
   (x) Patient consent.

**Q. What are the benefits of TOLAC?**

**Ans.**
- If TOLAC is successful, laparotomy for cesarean section can be avoided.
- Recovery following vaginal delivery is quicker compared to that of a cesarean delivery.
- The duration of hospital stay is much less in cases following successful vaginal delivery.
- The associated morbidity due to infections, blood transfusion is also less in VBAC compared to cesarean delivery.
- Above all, the woman's satisfaction is very high.

**Q. What are the risks of VBAC?**

**Ans.** The most important risk of vaginal birth after cesarean (VBAC) is the uterine rupture and its complications mentioned earlier. However, this complication is uncommon (<0.5%) in a well-selected case when labor is monitored carefully in a medical college or a tertiary level center.

**Q. What is the success rate with VBAC?**

**Ans.** Overall success rate is about 72–75%. Success rate is more in women who have delivered vaginally at least once either before or after the index cesarean.

**Q. What is your opinion about "once a cesarean means always a cesarean delivery"?**

**Ans.** See SAQ, p. 246.

**Q. What factors determine the successful success of VBAC?**

**Ans.** The single best predictor for successful VBAC is history of previous vaginal delivery particularly previous VBAC.

**Q. How do you diagnose impending scar rupture?**

**Ans. Appearance of fetal distress is the most consistent sign.** A variable deceleration pattern in CTG changing into late decelerations and bradycardia occurs in about 60% of cases with uterine rupture. In late cases, fetal heart sound may be absent (IUFD).

**Q. When should a woman with previous cesarean section be admitted in pregnancy and why?**

**Ans.** All such cases are considered as "high-risk". Generally women with lower segment scar should be admitted at 38th week and women with classical scar should be admitted at 36th week. This is the plan of elective admission. However, she may be admitted earlier (as an emergency) at any time if she has got any other problem (e.g. pain abdomen and vaginal bleeding).

**Q. How are you going to manage this woman?**

**Ans.** She should be admitted in a tertiary care hospital. Indication of her previous cesarean section was a nonrecurrent one. She has to be examined internally to assess the Bishop's score and also the pelvis. Considering her history and examination, she may be allowed for spontaneous onset of labor and vaginal delivery. However, in that case, she would be monitored carefully during the entire course of labor (FHR, progress of labor and for scar tenderness). Monitoring of labor progress using a partograph and continuous electronic fetal monitoring is needed. Second stage of labor may be cut short with ventouse or forceps. However, if she does not go into spontaneous labor and she crosses her EDC, she should be delivered by planned (elective) cesarean section.

***Q. What is the place of induction of labor for a case with VBAC?***

**Ans** Spontaneous onset of labor is mostly awaited. Induction of labor is not generally done. Induction of labor is associated with 3 to 4 times higher risks of uterine rupture. It also increases the risk of emergency cesarean delivery (1.5 fold). However, if induction is to be done, mechanical methods are preferred. Sweeping of membranes, amniotomy or Foley catheter are associated with a lower risk of uterine rupture, when compared to prostaglandins.

***Q. What is the place for the use of epidural analgesia in a case of VBAC?***

**Ans.** Epidural analgesia is not contraindicated in a planned case of VBAC.

***Q. Would you explore the uterine scar after delivery of the placenta?***

**Ans.** Routine exploration of uterine scar is not done. On clinical examination, if placenta is found complete and the uterus is well-retracted without any significant vaginal bleeding, we generally do not explore the uterine scar as a routine. Otherwise it may be done using two fingers inside to palpate the scar for detection of scar rupture. However, scar separation is difficult to diagnose on digital palpation. Most asymptomatic scar dehiscence heals well.

***Q. How a woman is counseled for VBAC?***

**Ans.** Antenatal counseling should be done. Risks and benefits of of elective repeat cesarean section (ERCS) and that of VBAC are to be discussed. VBAC check lists (leaflets) are to be made and provided. Discussion, informed consent are all documented.

## CASE–6  ANEMIA IN PREGNANCY

### Case Summary

*Mrs BC, a 21 year young primigravida presents with the problem of tiredness, giddiness, and occasional dyspnea while doing her daily household work. She is an unbooked case, admitted at 30 weeks of gestation. On examination, she is severely pale, BP 120/80 mm Hg and with bilateral pedal edema. Her cardiovascular and respiratory systems are normal. Her obstetric examination revealed symphysis-fundal height 30 cm, single fetus, cephalic presentation, FHS 145 beats per minute regular with adequate amount of liquor.*

**Q. What is your provisional diagnosis?**

**Ans.** Severe anemia in pregnancy.

**Q. What would be the possible causes of anemia?**

**Ans.** Deficiency anemia of which iron deficiency anemia (microcytic hypochromic) is common (Fig. 2.11). Other deficiency anemias are— folic acid and vitamin $B_{12}$ (megaloblastic). Dimorphic anemia is due to deficiency of both iron and folic acid or vitamin $B_{12}$ (macrocytic or normocytic and hypochromic or normochromic).

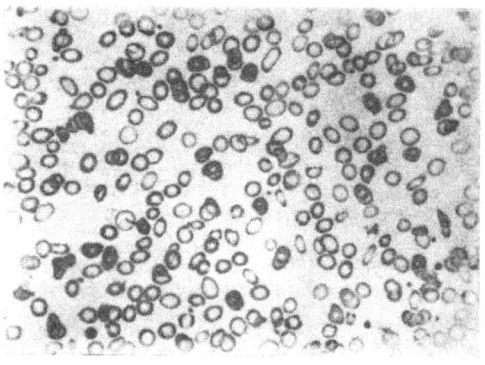

Fig. 2.11: Peripheral blood film showing hypochromic microcytic anemia.

**Other causes of anemia are:** Hemorrhage (APH), hereditary (thalassemia), bone marrow insufficiency, infection (malaria) or chronic disease (renal).

**Q. What do you mean by physiological anemia of pregnancy?**

**Ans.** During pregnancy there is fall of hemoglobin concentration due to hemodilution and negative iron balance. Hemodilution is due to disproportionate rise of plasma volume and RBC volume. Negative iron balance occurs due to excess demand of iron which not replenished even by normal balanced diet.

**Q. Mention the important signs of iron deficiency anemia?**

**Ans.** (1) Pallor (best seen in the tongue, mucosa of the mouth, lower palpebral conjuctiva)
(2) Atrophic glossitis
(3) Koilonichia (spoon shaped nails with longitudinal ridges)
(4) Angular cheilitis: Ulcers at the angle of the mouth
(5) Ankle edema, edema of whole body.

(6) When late: Tachycardia, cardiac mummers, and/or failure may be detected.

**Q. What are the different grades of anemia?**

**Ans.** According to WHO, Normal hemoglobin in a pregnant woman (g/dL): >= 11. Arbitrary gradings with hemoglobin levels done are:

| Anemia | Hemoglobin level |
| --- | --- |
| Mild | 10.0–10.9 g/dL |
| Moderate | 7–8 g/dL |
| Severe | <7 g/dL |
| Very severe | <4 g/dL |

**Q. What investigations are needed to know the cause of anemia?**

**Ans.** Complete hemogram including peripheral blood film.
- If microcytic and hypochromic (MCV <80), serum iron values (serum iron, serum ferritin, serum iron binding capacity) are estimated.
- When serum values of iron and ferritin are low with high serum iron binding capacity—iron deficiency anemia is considered.
- If microcytic but normochromic and serum iron values are normal or high, hemoglobin electrophoresis for detection of hemoglobinopathies is to be done.
- If macrocytic (MCV >94)—serum folic acid and vitamin $B_{12}$ estimation is done. Red cell folate <3 ng/mL (folate deficiency) and serum Vitamin $B_{12}$ level <90 pg/mL (vitamin $B_{12}$ deficiency), indicates megaloblastic anemia.
- If normocytic (MCV: 80–94)—we should think of drugs, infection or bone marrow pathology.

**Q. What test is most reliable for diagnosis of iron deficiency anemia?**

**Ans.** Serum ferritin is the most reliable indicator for iron deficiency in the absence of inflammation and chronic disease.

Serum ferritin levels below 15 ng/mL are consistent with the diagnosis of iron deficiency anemia.

**Q. What are the common gynecological causes of iron deficiency anemia?**

**Ans.** World wide, uterine fibroids (13 most common causes), and women with heavy menstrual bleeding are the major causes of iron deficiency anemia.

**Q. What is Hepcidin?**

**Ans.** Hepcidin is a 25-amino acid, peptide hormone that regulates iron uptake and release from the stores, in response to circulating and tissue requirement of iron.

**Q. What are the complications of untreated anemia in pregnancy?**

**Ans. Maternal**
- **Pregnancy**
  - Infection

- Cardiac failure
- Pre-eclampsia
- Preterm labor
- **Labor:**
  - Cardiac failure
  - Uterine inertia
  - PPH
  - Shock
- **Puerperium:**
  - Puerperal sepsis
  - Subinvolution
  - Venous thrombosis
  - Failing lactation.

**Fetal**
- IUGR
- IUFD
- Preterm baby and its hazards
- Higher perinatal mortality (9 times).

**Q. At what time (pregnancy, labor or puerperium) the risk of cardiac failure is greatest?**

**Ans.** (i) Around 30–32 weeks
(ii) During labor
(iii) Immediately after the delivery
(iv) Any time in puerperium. Risks are mainly due to cardiac failure or infection.

**Q. What treatment you will advise her for the anemia?**

**Ans.** Treatment would be guided according to the cause of anemia, period of gestation, type (discussed here) and severity of the anemia. However, as iron deficiency anemia is common, once she is diagnosed as a case of iron deficiency anemia, she is advised balanced diet rich in protein, iron, folic acid and vitamins.

**Q. How do you prescribe oral iron?**

**Ans.** Fersolate tablet containing 200 mg ferrous sulfate (60 mg of elemental iron) is prescribed 1 tablet 3 times a day. The dose is to be increased depending upon the tolerance (6 tablets a day) till the blood picture is normal. Maintenance dose (1 tablet a day) is continued at least for 100 days following delivery. Drinking of tea should be avoided within an hour of taking iron tablets.

Inorder to increase the absorption of iron, it should be given 1 hour prior to the meal.

**Q. What are the factors that may affect the absorption of iron?**

**Ans.** (A) Inhibiting factors are: Milk, tannins, phytates
(B) Absorption enhancing factors are: Fruit juices, vitamin C,

(C) Side effects of iron may cause poor iron absorption; nausea, vomiting, abdominal discomfort, constipation.

**Q. How do you assess the response of oral iron therapy?**

Ans.
- Improved sense of well-being.
- Increased appetite.
- Rise in hemoglobin level.
- Reticulocytosis.
- Normal hematocrit.

**Q. What different salts of iron can be prescribed?**

Ans. The different salts of iron that can be prescribed are listed in table below:

| Iron contents in different oral iron preparations | | |
|---|---|---|
| **Iron salt** | **Amount** | **Ferrous iron contents** |
| Ferrous fumarate | 200 mg | 65 mg |
| Ferrous gluconate | 300 mg | 35 mg |
| Ferrous sulfate | 300 mg | 60 mg |
| Ferrous sulfate (dried) | 200 mg | 65 mg |

**Q. What are the indications of parenteral iron therapy?**

Ans.
- Patient is intolerant to oral iron (vomiting, diarrhea, and constipation).
- Absorption is unpredictable by oral route (malabsorption).
- Patient seen in her last 8–10 weeks of pregnancy.

**Q. What are the advantages of parenteral iron therapy?**

Ans. Total dose of iron needed to correct the hemoglobin deficit and the amount to build up the iron store is calculated and administered either by IM or IV. Parenteral therapy ensures the certainty of its administration. It avoids the side effects due to gastrointestinal intolerance. However, the rate of rise in hemoglobin is the same with both the methods.

**Q. What are the common preparations available for parenteral iron therapy?**

Ans.
(i) Iron (ferrous) sucrose
(ii) Iron dextran complex
(iii) Iron carboxy maltose
(iv) Iron iso maltose

Iron sucrose and carboxymaltose have similar efficacy.
Iron polymaltose has the advantage of improved gastrointestinal absorption when taken with food.

**Q. What are the side effects of parenteral iron therapy?**

Ans. Side effects are:
(i) Malaise
(ii) Nausea
(iii) Vomiting
(iv) Hypotension

(v) Arthralgia
(vi) Abdominal pain
(vii) Anaphylaxis. Adverse effects are less common with iron sucrose and carboxymaltose compared with iron dextran.

**Ferrous sucrose is safe, effective and has got less side effects (ACOG 2008).** Iron sucrose is given IV 100 mg (at a time) in 100 mL normal saline slowly over 15 minutes.

**Q. What is TDI?**

**Ans.** Total dose infusion (TDI) is the administration of total amount of iron required to correct the deficit. It is given by IV infusion.

**Q. What are the advantages of TDI?**

**Ans.** (i) The woman is given the treatment and discharged on the same day.
(ii) No need of repeated IM injections that are painful.
(iii) It is less costly.

**Q. How do you calculate the total amount of iron for TDI?**

**Ans. Iron sucrose:** 20 mg elemental iron/mL 100 mg/dose, usually one dose daily for 10 days.

**Q. What are the indications of blood transfusion?**

**Ans.**
- Anemia due to blood loss (placenta previa and bleeding piles).
- Severe anemia (Hb <7 g/dL).
- Advanced pregnancy (≥36 weeks).
- Refractory anemia.
- Associated infection.
- Cases of PPH.
- Cases with major obstetric hemorrhage.

**Q. What are the advantages of blood transfusion?**

**Ans.**
- Immediate improvement.
- Increased $O_2$ carrying capacity of blood.
- Stimulates erythropoiesis.
- Supply of blood proteins and antibodies.

**Q. What special precaution should be taken when she goes into labor?**

**Ans.**
- $O_2$ inhalation.
- Strict asepsis.
- Injection oxytocin IM, 10 IU, is given soon following delivery of the baby to prevent PPH.
- May need packed cell transfusion to avoid cardiac overload.

**Q. What are the risks of blood transfusion?**

**Ans.** The adverse effects are:
Fluid overload, anaphylaxis, infections (viral, bacterial, parasitic), allergic reactions, lung injury (TRALI), and febrile reactions.

**Q. What is the overall prevalence of anemia in our country?**

**Ans.** More than 50% of pregnant women in India are anemic, nearly 50% of all adolescent girls (adolescent girls constitute 20% of the total population) suffer from nutritional anemia and nearly 60% of all preschool children (<6 years), suffer from varying degree of anemia.

**Q. What is the major concern with anemia?**

**Ans.** One in five (20%) of all maternal deaths is attributed to anemia in pregnancy. This is the major concern.

**Q. What is the current recommendation (Government of India, WHO) to prevent this complication?**

**Ans.** As a priority:
- **All pregnant and lactating women** must take one iron folic acid (IFA) large tablet per day for a minimum of 100 days (See also SAQ p. 245). She should take this after the first trimester irrespective of her hemoglobin level.
- **All adolescent girls** should take one IFA (large) tablet daily for 100 days since the onset of menstruation.
- **All preschool children** (1–5 years)—should take one IFA (small) tablet daily for 100 days.

## CASE-7  DIABETES IN PREGNANCY

### Case Summary

*Mrs AR, 28 years old, primigravida was admitted at 34 weeks of gestation with complaints of recurrent attacks of vulvovaginitis and urinary tract infection. Her antenatal check-up was otherwise uneventful. Her obstetric examination revealed, single fetus, longitudinal lie, cephalic presentation. FHS was heard 141/minute regular on the left spinoumbilical line. Her investigations revealed fasting plasma glucose level was 110 mg/dL and 2-hour postglucose value was 150 mg/dL. Her plasma glucose values were within normal limits when done before pregnancy.*

**Q. What is your provisional diagnosis?**

**Ans.** Gestational diabetes mellitus (GDM).

**Q. How do you define gestational diabetes mellitus (GDM)?**

**Ans.** GDM is defined as carbohydrate intolerance of variable severity with onset or first recognition during the present pregnancy.

**Q. What are the alterations of carbohydrate metabolism in pregnancy?**

**Ans.** (i) Insulin secretion is increased
(ii) Sensitivity of insulin receptors in tissues is decreased
(iii) Increased peripheral tissue resistance to insulin
(iv) Rise in the levels of contrainsulin factors like estrogens, progesterone, human placental lactogen (hPL) and cortisol. All these make pregnancy a hyperglycemic state.
Pregnancy is a diabetogenic state.

**Q. Classify diabetes in pregnancy?**

**Ans.** • Gestatitional diabetes mellitus.
• Pregestational diabetes mellitus (PGDM) or overt diabetes.

**Q. Who are the high-risk women to develop GDM?**

**Ans.** Women with—
(a) Positive family history of diabetes
(b) Previous baby weight ≥4 kg
(c) Previous stillbirth
(d) Presence of polyhydramnios
(e) Obesity (BMI >30)
(f) Age ≥30 years
(g) Recurrent vaginal candidiasis
(h) Persistent glycosuria—are all considered high-risk women
(i) Ethnic group : East Asia, Pacific Island ancestry.

**Q. When is a woman in pregnancy called diabetic?**

**Ans.** A woman is having fasting plasma glucose >126 mg/dL and 2-hour postglucose (75 g), value exceeds 200 mg/dL is diagnosed in overt diabetes

(ACOG)? Woman with clinical features of diabetes like—polyphasia, polyuria, random. Blood glucose >200 mg/dL or HbA1C >6.5 are considered diabetic.

**Q. What is the prevalence of GDM in India?**

**Ans.** Overall 3.8–21%.

**Q. How do you screen and diagnose GDM?**

**Ans.** According to American Diabetic Association (ADA), screening is done for high-risk women. However, many others recommend universal screening.
**Procedure:**
A 50 g oral glucose challenge test without regard to time of the day or last meal between 24 and 28 weeks of pregnancy is done.

A plasma glucose value >140 mg/dL or that of whole blood 130 mg/dL at 1 hour is considered the cut-off point for doing 100 g (WHO 75 g) oral glucose tolerance test (OGTT). OGTT is done at 0, 1, 2 and 3 hours. GDM is diagnosed (Carpenter and Coustan) if any two values meet or exceed the cut-off value: Fasting >95 mg/dL; postglucose values: 1 hour >180 mg/dL; 2 hours >155 mg/dL and 3 hours >140 mg/dL.

WHO defines GDM with the cut-off value of fasting plasma glucose between 92 mg/dL and 125 mg/dL and 2 hours 75 g postoral glucose value between 153 mg/dL and 199 mg/dL.

According to International Association of Diabetes in Pregnancy Study Group (IADPSG), GDM with cut-off values (following 75 g of oral glucose) are: Fasting—92.3 mg/dL, 1 hour—181 mg/dL, 2 hours—153 mg/dL (one value is sufficient for diagnosis).

**Q. What is the recommendation of Diabetes in Pregnancy Societies of India australasian diabetes in pregnancy societies of india (DPSI) for screening and diagnosis of GDM?**

**Ans.** australasian diabetes in pregnancy societies of india (DPSI) recommends a single test procedure to diagnose GDM in the community.
**Procedure:** In the antenatal clinic, a pregnant woman is given a 75 g oral glucose load without regard to the time of the last meal. A venous blood sample is collected at 2 hours. GDM is diagnosed if 2-hour plasma glucose value is >140 mg/dL.

**Q. What are the effects of diabetes on pregnancy?**

**Ans.** (1) **Effects of diabetes on the mother**
    (A) *During pregnancy:*
        (a) Preterm labor
        (b) Infections (urinary tract, vulvovaginitis)
        (c) Increased risk of pre-eclampsia
        (d) Polyhydramnios (25–50%)
        (e) Diabetic retinopathy, nephropathy.
    (B) *During labor:*
        (a) Shoulder dystocia
        (b) Increased operative delivery (cesarean section).

(2) **Effects on the fetus and neonate**
   (A) *Fetal:*
      (a) Miscarriage
      (b) Fetal macrosomia
      (c) Congenital malformations
      (d) Intrauterine fetal death (IUFD).
   (B) *Neonatal:*
      (a) Hypoglycemia
      (b) Respiratory distress syndrome
      (c) Hyperbilirubinemia
      (d) Hypocalcemia
      (e) Cardiomyopathy.
(3) **During puerperium:**
   (A) Puerperal sepsis
   (B) Fall in the requirement of insulin.

**Q. *What should be the ideal plasma glucose level in woman with diabetes in pregnancy?***

**Ans.** (a) Fasting ≤95 mg/dL
   (b) 2-hour PP ≤120 mg/dL
   (c) Morning (2 am–6 am) ≥60 mg/dL
   (d) Mean plasma glucose should be between 105 and 110 mg/dL.
   (e) Desirable level of HbAIC should be ≤6%.

**Q. *How should the woman be advised as regards diet pattern?***

**Ans.** (a) Diet = 30 kCal/kg for a normal weight woman.
   (b) Carbohydrate = 50%
   (c) Protein = 20%
   (d) Fat = 25–30%

Usually three meal regimen (breakfast 25%, lunch 30% and dinner 30%) of total calorie intake with several snacks in between are advised.

Women are adviced to control diet first and if values are exceeded even on diet, insulin therapy is suggested.

**Q. *What are the different malformations in infants with diabetic mothers?***

**Ans.** (A) CNS : Neural tube defects and microcephaly
   (B) Skeletal system : Sacral agenesis
   (C) Cardiovascular : ASV and VSD
   (D) Renal : Agenesis and horse-shoe kidney
   (E) GI system : Duodenal atresia.

## Chapter 2 • Obstetric Case Discussions

**Q. What are the important issues in the management of a woman with diabetes in pregnancy?**

**Ans.** (a) Preconceptional counseling to maintain optimum glycemic status actually before conception.
(b) Preconceptional folic acid supplementation therapy is to be given.
(c) Prenatal diagnosis to detect fetal congenital malformations including echocardiography.
(d) Dietetic advice to maintain desired glycemic status, if not obtained, to use insulin.
(e) Prevention and early detection of complications.
(f) Close antenatal fetal monitoring (DFMC, NST, BPP and Doppler study as indicated).

**Q. What is the optimum time for delivering such a diabetic woman?**

**Ans.** A woman who is well controlled through pregnancy and fetal monitoring is satisfactory, may be allowed to deliver after 38 completed weeks.

**Q. When will you deliver the baby of GDM?**

**Ans.**
- GDM cases are mostly controlled by diet alone (medical nutrition therapy). In majority of the cases, spontaneous onset of labor is awaited. However, delivery (termination of pregnancy) is done at term (after 38 completed weeks).
- GDM cases on insulin therapy—should be delivered by 38 completed weeks.

In both the situations, spontaneous labor is awaited. However, fetal monitoring and control of glycemic status is maintained.

**Q. What measures are taken for a woman with GDM who is considered for induction of labor?**

**Ans.**
- Induction should be started in the early morning.
- The usual dose of evening insulin is given.
- No breakfast or no morning dose of insulin is given.
- Capillary blood glucose is checked with a glucometer.
- Ringer solution infusion IV is started.
- The goal is to keep the blood glucose level between 80 and 100 mg/dL.
- Induction of labor, when needed, is commonly done by: Intracervical PGE2 gel, and/or ARM. Oxytocin is given when needed.

**Q. When insulin therapy should be started in GDM?**

**Ans:** Human insulin should be started if fasting plasma glucose level exceeds 90 mg/dL and 2 hours postprandial value is greater than 120 mg/dL even on diet control.

**Q. What optimum levels of plasma glucose should be maintained in a case with pregestational diabetes?**

**Ans.** Target plasma glucose levels should be:
  (i) Fasting ≤95 mg/dL
  (ii) Premeal ≤100 mg/dL
  (iii) 2 hours PP value ≤120 mg/dL; and morning (2AM-6AM) value ≥60 mg/dL.

**Q. What are the indications of cesarean delivery for a woman with diabetes in pregnancy?**

**Ans.**
  (a) Fetal macrosomia
  (b) Elderly primigravida
  (c) Diabetes with complications
  (d) Diabetes difficult to control
  (e) Presence of obstetric complications (pre-eclampsia)
  (f) Multigravida with bad obstetric history.

**Q. What are the complications of a woman with GDM?**

**Ans.**
  (1) **Fetal**
    (a) Macrosomia
    (b) Birth trauma
    (c) IUFD
    (d) Increased perinatal morbidity and mortality.
  (2) **Maternal**
    (a) Polyhydramnios
    (b) Recurrence of GDM in subsequent pregnancy
    (c) Development of overt diabetes (50%) by 15–20 years.

**Q. What is the contraceptive advice for such a woman?**

**Ans.** Once blood glucose levels are controlled, many contraceptive options are there:
- Combined oral contraceptive pills (low dose) may be used.
- Barrier method may be used for spacing of birth (failure rate is high).
- Progestin-only pill may be used as an alternative.
- IUCD including LNG- IUCD may be used.
- Sterilization is considered when family is completed.

**Q. What is the significance of measuring HbA1C levels?**

**Ans.**
  (a) Levels of HbA1C are raised in cases where hyperglycemia is present for a long period.
  (b) It reflects the status of glycemic control over the last 3 months.
  (c) Normal level of HbA1C is <6%.
  (d) Levels >6, when measured in early pregnancy, increase the risk of fetal congenital malformations.
  (e) It is not used for diagnosis of GDM, as it reflects the retrospective status.
  (f) Raised value of HbA1C (>6) during pregnancy suggests poor glycemic control and the risks of diabetic complications are high.

## CASE–8  BREECH PRESENTATION

### Case Summary

*Mrs LS, 28 years old, P0+0+1+0 was admitted from the antenatal clinic at 38 weeks of gestation. She did not have any significant complaints. She was advised admission by her physician for the plan of delivery due to the abnormal presentation of the baby. Her general physical examination did not reveal any abnormality. Examination of the CVS and respiratory systems were normal. Obstetric examination revealed, single fetus longitudinal lie, podalic pole on the brim, head at the fundus, back on the right side and limbs are on the left side. FHS was heard above the level of the umbilicus on the right side.*

**Q. What is your provisional diagnosis?**

**Ans.** Mrs LS, 28 years old, P0+0+1+0, admitted at 38 weeks of gestation with clinically diagnosed breech presentation.

**Q. How can you confirm the diagnosis?**

**Ans.** Ultrasound scan.

**Q. What are the different varieties of breech presentation?**

**Ans.** (a) Complete breech (flexed attitude).
   (b) Incomplete breech:
       (1) Breech with extended legs (Frank breech) (Fig. 2.12)
       (2) Footling presentation
       (3) Knee presentation.

   **Clinical varieties are:**
   (a) Uncomplicated breech.
   (b) Complicated breech (associated with placenta previa, pre-eclampsia, etc.).

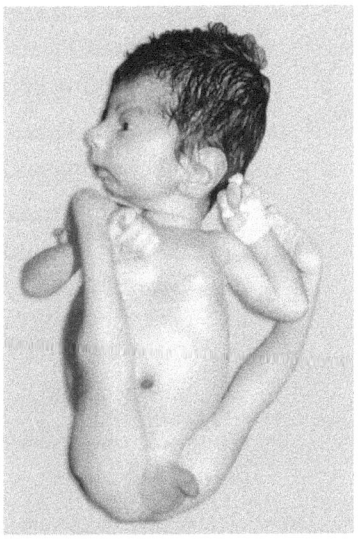

**Fig. 2.12:** Baby delivered as breech with extended legs (Frank breech). Extended position of the legs still maintained.

**Q. What other information can be obtained with sonography besides breech presentation?**

**Ans.** Besides confirmation of the diagnosis of breech presentation, other information that can be obtained with USG are:
   (i) Fetal congenital abnormality
   (ii) Fetal weight
   (iii) Types of breech
   (iv) Attitude of the head (see here)
   (v) Placental localization
   (vi) Uterine anomalies.

**Q. What are the important causes of breech presentation?**

**Ans.** (i) Prematurity—most common
(ii) Breech with extended legs
(iii) Twins
(iv) Short cord
(v) Oligohydramnios
(vi) Polyhydramnios
(vii) Uterine malformations (septate, bicornuate uterus)
(viii) Hydrocephalus
(ix) Placenta previa.

**Q. What are the important areas of breech delivery where the cardinal movements take place?**

**Ans.** (i) **Buttocks**: Engaging diameter—bitrochanteric (4" or 10 cm)
(ii) **Shoulders**: Bisacromial diameters (4¾" or 12 cm)
(iii) **After-coming head**: Suboccipitofrontal diameter (10 cm).

**Q. How do you formulate the management of a case with breech presentation during the antenatal period?**

**Ans.** (i) To identify any complicating factors (e.g. pre-eclampsia, APH) and to continue the antenatal care.
(ii) To perform external cephalic version—if not contraindicated.
(iii) To formulate the management when version fails or is contraindicated (e.g. either to allow assisted vaginal breech delivery or to deliver by elective LSCS).

**Q. What other information are necessary for planning the management of the above woman?**

**Ans.** Type of breech presentation (flexed or Frank breech or footling presentation), attitude of the head (flexed or extended), placental localization, estimated fetal weight, any congenital anomaly of the fetus or of the uterus.

**Q. What are the complications of vaginal breech delivery?**

**Ans Injuries:**
- Birth trauma, spinal cord injury
- Bone injury like fracture of femur, fracture of humerus, clavicle, dislocation of shoulder, dislocation of hip, fracture mandible
- Visceral injuries like injury to testis, liver, spleen, kidney, lungs, trauma to sternomastoid muscle.
  - Nerve injury: Erb's palsy, Klumpkey's palsy
  - Asphyxia: Due to cord prolapse, cord compression, premature attempt at respiration
  - Intracranial hemorrhage: Because of sudden compression followed by decompression during delivery of the after-coming head of breech

**Others:** Intrapartum fetal death, difficulty in delivery of after-coming head.

**Q. What are the contraindications of ECV?**

**Ans.**
- Antepartum hemorrhage.
- Contracted pelvis
- Multiple pregnancy
- Prior cesarean delivery
- Congenital malformation of uterus
- Severe pre-eclampsia
- Fetal factors: Gross congenital anomaly, FGR, IUFD.

**Q. What are the indications of cesarean section in breech presentation?**

**Ans.** Only selected cases are allowed for vaginal delivery (See p. 204)
- Common indications of cesarean delivery are:
- Big baby (>3.5 kg)
- Footing presentation
- Severe IUGR
- Contracted pelvis.

**Q. What are the different methods of vaginal breech delivery?**

**Ans.**
- Assisted vaginal breech delivery
- Spontaneous breech delivery (not preferred)
- Breech extraction (rarely).

**Q. What is the advantage of external cephalic version and what is the chance of success?**

**Ans.** Successful version and delivery as vertex reduces the need for cesarean section significantly. It also reduces the complications of vaginal breech delivery. Use of tocolytis (terbutaline/ritodrine) prior to external cephalic version (ECV) may be done. Success rate of ECV is 70–80%.

**Q. What factors must be considered before proceeding to ECV?**

**Ans.** Case must be evaluated as regards the possibility of success of ECV (adequate liquor volume) and to exclude the contraindications, e.g.
  (i) Diagnosed or suspected placenta previa
  (ii) History of previous cesarean delivery
  (iii) Severe pre-eclampsia
  (iv) Presence of fetal or uterine malformation
  (v) Multiple pregnancy
  (vi) IUFD
  (vii) Abnormal CTG
  (viii) Fetal factors: FGR.

**Q. At what time is ECV appropriate?**

**Ans.** At 37 weeks or thereafter.

**Q. Evaluate critically the place of ECV in the management of breech presentation.**

**Ans.** See SAQ p. 241.

**Q. What factors increases the chance of ECV?**

**Ans.** The favorable factors are:
  (a) Multiparous woman
  (b) Podalic pole not engaged
  (c) Woman not obese
  (d) Adequate liquor.

**Q. What are the complications of ECV?**

**Ans.** Complications are:
  (a) Onset of premature labor
  (b) PROM
  (c) Placental abruption
  (d) Umbilical cord entanglement around the fetal parts
  (e) Fetal distress/death
  (f) Uterine rupture
  (g) Amniotic fluid embolism
  (h) Fetomaternal bleeding
  (i) Alloimmunization.

**Q. What is the place of moxibustion in reducing the incidence of breech presentation?**

**Ans.** Moxibustion a Chinese medicine (dried mugwort), has been used from 32 weeks onwards to promote spontaneous version. It is claimed to be effective when combined with postural management and acupuncture.

**Q. What are the common indications of elective cesarean section in breech?**

**Ans.** (a) Big baby (estimated weight >3.5 kg)
  (b) Hyperextension of the head
  (c) Footling presentation
  (d) Breech with complications (APH and pre-eclampsia)
  (e) Inadequate pelvis
  (f) Absence of expertise for vaginal breech delivery
  (g) Others: Associated complications—FGR, severe pre-eclampsia
  (h) Woman's request for cesarean delivery
  (i) Previous cesarean delivery.

**Q. What important factors must be considered before allowing her for vaginal breech delivery?**

**Ans.** • Size of the baby: Average size (≤3 kg)
  • Pelvic adequacy: Adequate pelvis

- Zatuchni-Andros score >4
- Center having facilities for emergency cesarean section
- No hyperextension of the fetal head
- Good progress in labor
- Experience and skill in vaginal breech delivery is available
- Without any other complications (e.g. severe pre-eclampsia)
- Frank breech is preferred for vaginal delivery
- Consent of the patient.

**Q. What precautionary measures are taken during the process of assisted vaginal breech delivery?**

**Ans. Precautionary measures** are taken beforehand for the availability of:
(i) An anesthetist
(ii) Pediatrician
(iii) Assistant
(iv) Episiotomy set
(v) A pair of obstetric forceps
(vi) Neonatal resuscitation set.

**Q. What principles are followed during the process of assisted vaginal breech delivery?**

**Ans. Principles to follow are:**
(i) Not to be hasty
(ii) Never to pull from below but to push from above
(iii) Always to keep the fetus with the back anterior.

**Q. What are the complications of a vaginal breech delivery?**

**Ans.** *Fetal:*
- Difficulty in delivery of the after-coming head (Fig. 2.13).
- Intracranial hemorrhage.
- Asphyxia.
- Injury: Fracture femur and clavicle.
- Injury to liver and lungs.
- Nerve injury—medullary coning, spinal cord, and brachial plexus.
- Increased perinatal mortality (5-30%).

*Maternal:* Trauma to the genital tract, sepsis and complications due to anesthesia. Maternal morbidity is raised.

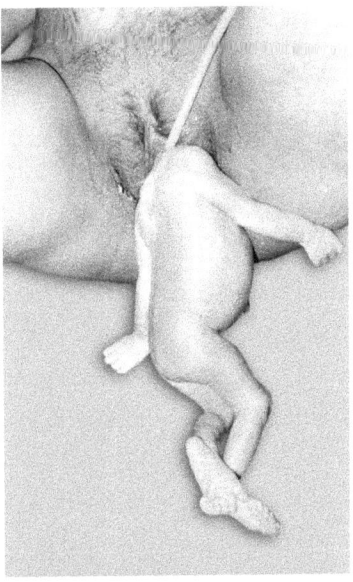

**Fig. 2.13:** Vaginal breech delivery with the after-coming head at the pelvic outlet.

**Q. What are the different methods for the delivery of the after-coming head?**

Ans. (a) **Burns-Marshall method:** Lifting the baby's trunk in an upward and forward direction, holding at the ankles. This is done when the nape of the neck is visible under the pubic arch.

(b) **Forceps delivery** — when the head is in the pelvic cavity. Piper's forceps is specially designed for this. The head is delivered slowly.

(c) **Malar flexion and shoulder traction** (modified Mauriceau Smellie-Veit technique).

Assistant is to give suprapubic pressure during this period to maintain flexion of the head.

**Q. When there is difficulty in delivery of the shoulders, what maneuver is commonly done?**

Ans. Lovset's maneuver is commonly done. Here the fetal trunk is rotated 180°, maintaining a steady downward traction.

With this rotation, the posterior shoulder which was initially below the sacral promontory appears below the symphysis pubis. The process is then repeated in a reverse direction to release the anterior shoulder.

**Q. What is the overall incidence of cesarean section for breech presentation?**

Ans. Overall incidence is 85%, of which 80% is elective.

Currently, the rates for cesarean delivery for breech presentation is rising. This is especially so after the trial "Term Breech Trial–2000". However, PREMODA (French) study (2006) showed no differences in corrected neonatal mortality rates.

Areas of concern are: Medicolegal, training, skill and competence of the birth attendance and the center resources.

## CASE–9   PROLONGED PREGNANCY

### Case Summary

*Mrs VZ, 26 years old, P0+0+0+0, has been admitted in the hospital at 42 weeks and 3 days of gestation. She has no significant complaints. On general physical examination, she is found normotensive. Obstetric examination revealed— single fetus, cephalic presentation, 3/5th palpable per abdomen, adequate liquor. FHR was 148 beats per minute and was regular.*

**Q. What is this clinical situation called?**

**Ans.** Post-term pregnancy

> **Classification of term pregnancy (ACOG-2013)**
> - **Early term:** 37 0/7 weeks through 38 6/7 weeks
> - **Full term:** 39 0/7 weeks through 40 6/7 weeks
> - **Late term:** 41 0/7 weeks through 41 6/7 weeks
> - **Post-term:** 42 0/7 weeks and beyond
> - **Late preterm:** 34 0/7 weeks through 36 6/7 weeks

**Q. What do you understand by post-term pregnancy?**

**Ans.** Pregnancy continuing beyond 2 weeks of the expected date of delivery (>294 days) is called post-term pregnancy (postmaturity).

**Q. How do you assess the well-being of the fetus when pregnancy is postdated?**

**Ans.** (i) Fetal well-being is commonly assessed by: Daily fetal movement counting (kick chart)
(ii) Cardiotocography and nonstress test
(iii) Biophysical profile
(iv) Modified biophysical profile
(v) Doppler study of umbilical artery.

**Q. How do you diagnose postmaturity?**

**Ans.** (i) Menstrual history—is important, provided the woman is very sure of her date and her cycles are regular.
(ii) Weight record—usually it remains stationary.
(iii) Girth of the abdomen—it gradually diminishes.
(iv) Obstetric palpation—uterus is full of fetus.
**Internal examination:** Cervix may be ripe.
**Investigations:**
(i) **Sonography:** Composite biometry (measurement of CRL in first trimester record if available, BPD, FL, AC, and HC) is of value for the assessment of maturity. Ultrasonography record done in the first

trimester is the most accurate method to determine the the expected date of delivery and diagnosis of post-term pregnancy. Early USG scan is more valuable.

(ii) Amniocentesis—the biochemical and cytological parameters are helpful to assess pulmonary maturity of the fetus.

**Q. How do you instruct the woman to maintain the kick chart?**

**Ans.** She is asked to count the number of fetal movements three times a day, each of 1 hour duration (e.g. 1 hour each in the morning (8-9 am), afternoon (3-4 pm) and evening (8-9 pm). The total counts multiplied by 4 gives the total movements in 12 hours. When she feels no movements or less than 10 movements in 12 hours, she must report to her doctor. Absence of fetal movements is commonly followed by disappearance of FHR by next 24 hours.

**Patient observation:** Daily fetal movement counting (kick chart) showed diminished fetal movements (less than 10 in 12 hours).

**Q. What would be your next plan of investigation?**

**Ans.** Fetal monitoring by cardiotocography for nonstress tests.

**Q. What are the risks if she does not go into labor by 42 weeks of pregnancy?**

**Ans.** Risks are mainly to the fetus.

**During pregnancy:** Fetal hypoxia due to placental ageing and insufficiency, oligohydramnios and meconium stained liquor.

**During labor:** Asphyxia, meconium aspiration, shoulder dystocia, brachial plexus injury, birth trauma (due to big baby), intracranial damage (due to nonmoulding of head).

**Following birth:** Chemical pneumonitis (due to meconium aspiration), hypoxia.

**Maternal:** Increased morbidity due to operative delivery (LSCS or instrumental). She may need induction of labor.

**Q. What would be your next course of management if she does not go into labor spontaneously?**

**Ans.** She is assessed clinically and is considered for induction of labor:

(i) **Cervix favorable (Bishop's score >6)** → ARM ± oxytocin → vaginal delivery.

(ii) **Cervix unfavorable** → $PGE_2$ gel (0.5 mg) intracervical → cervix favorable → ARM ± oxytocin → vaginal delivery. Fetal monitoring during the course of labor is essential.

(iii) **Presence of any other obstetric complications preeclampsia, FGR, big baby with unfavorable cervix** → LSCS.

**Q. How should a woman with postmature pregnancy be monitored when she goes into labor?**

**Ans.** Labor should be monitored carefully and partographic plotting is to be maintained. Electronic fetal monitoring (CTG) is preferred. Nonprogress of labor or presence of fetal distress indicates cesarean delivery.

**Q. What is the significance of post-term pregnancy?**

**Ans.** There is significant rise in perinatal mortality when the expected date crosses over 42 weeks. Stillbirth rate is increased from 0.35/1,000 at 37 weeks to 2.12/1,000 at 43 weeks (6-fold). Risks of meconium aspiration, asphyxia, shoulder dystocia and operative delivery (cesarean/operative vaginal—forceps or ventouse) are high.

**Q. How does a postmature baby look after birth?**

**Ans.**
(i) Skin is wrinkled
(ii) There is absence of vernix caseosa
(iii) Nails are protruding beyond the nail beds
(iv) Baby may be stained greenish-yellow (meconium).
(v) Liquor is often meconium stained
(vi) Placenta shows areas of calcification and infarction
(vii) Umbilical cord is thin due to lack of Wharton's jelly.

## CASE–10 FETAL GROWTH RESTRICTION

### Case Summary

*Mrs LM, 27 years old, P0+0+0+0, was seen in the antenatal clinic at 36 weeks of gestation. On general physical examination, she weighed 47 kg (her weight remained the same for last three visits), mild pallor and her BP measured 144/96 mm Hg. Obstetric examination revealed : Uterus 32 weeks size, SFH measured 32 cm, single fetus, cephalic presentation, 3/5th of the head is palpable per abdomen. Liquor volume is reduced. On auscultation, FHS is 146 beats/minute and it is regular.*

**Q. What is the most likely clinical diagnosis?**

**Ans.** Small for gestational age, probably due to intrauterine growth restriction (Fig. 2.14).

**Q. How do you diagnose IUGR clinically?**

**Ans.** (i) Obstetric palpation—fundal height is less, liquor volume is reduced and fetal mass is less when compared to the gestational age.
(ii) Symphysis-fundal height (SFH) is less by 4 cm or more.
(iii) Maternal weight gain—is either stationary or falling.
(iv) Measurement of the abdominal girth—either remains the same or may be less.

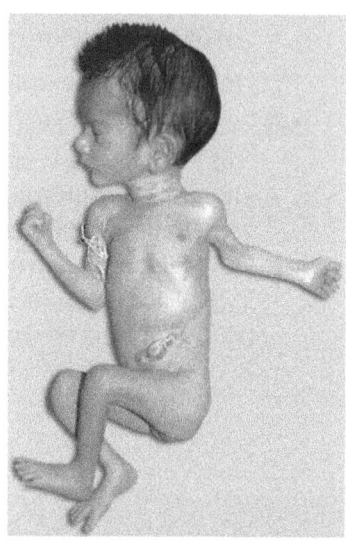

**Fig. 2.14:** Neonate with the features of intrauterine growth restriction.

**Q. How do you confirm the diagnosis?**

**Ans.** Sonography is extremely useful. Fetal parameters measured are:
(i) BPD, HC, AC, and FL for fetal biometry; estimated fetal weight.
(ii) *HC and AC ratio:* Normally, HC/AC is <1 after 34 weeks of gestation. In asymmetric IUGR, it is >1.
(iii) *Amniotic fluid volume:* AFI<5 indicates oligohydramnios. This is common in IUGR.
(iv) *Doppler velocimetry:* Reduced, absent or reversed diastolic flow in the umbilical artery indicates fetal jeopardy. This is due to chronic placental insufficiency (*see* Fig. 2.15).

**Q. How should the fetus be monitored?**

**Ans.** • Daily fetal movement counting (kick chart)—normally, it is >10 in 12 hours but in a case with FGR, fetal movements are reduced.
• Cardiotocography—for nonstress test (normally, it is reassuring pattern).

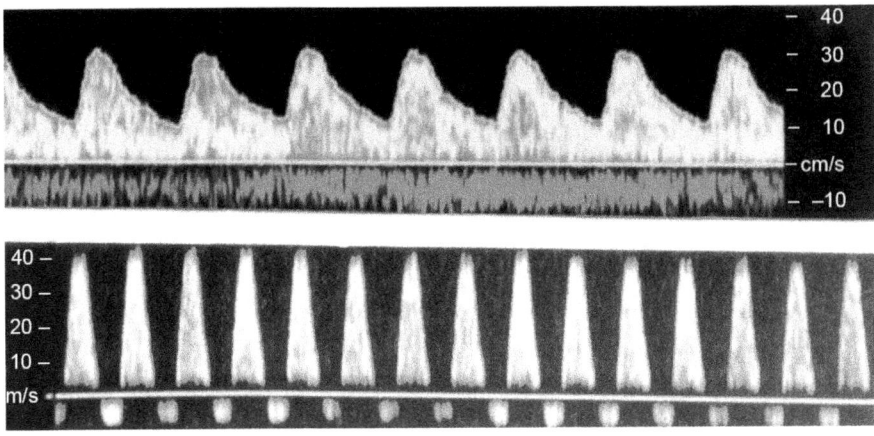

**Fig. 2.15:** Flow velocity waveform (Doppler velocimetry) of the umbilical artery showing normal forward flow (above) and reversed end diastolic flow (below).

- Ultrasound scan—in a case with FGR, the liquor pocket is reduced for liquor volume (more than one vertical pool depth >2 cm is normal).
- Ultrasound is also done to rule out fetal structural anomalies which is a cause for IUGR.
- Biophysical profile—especially the nonstress test and amniotic fluid volume are done. In a case with FGR, the biophysical profile (BPP) score is reduced.
- **Doppler flow study** of the umbilical artery and middle cerebral artery. Appearance of reversed end-diastolic flow velocity may lead to IUFD. Abnormal venous waveforms (pulsations in ductus venosus, IVC) indicates incipient cardiac failure. Increased peak systolic flow velocity in middle cerebral artery indicates redistribution of blood flow (brain sparing effect in hypoxia).

*Q. How frequently we need to assess the well-being of a FGR baby?*

**Ans.** It depends on the severity of the FGR.

**Generally**
- Clinical examination—daily
- DFMC counting—daily
- CTG—on alternate day
- USG—at an interval of 10-14 days.
- Doppler velocimetry—weekly.

*Q. What are the common causes of fetal growth restriction?*

**Ans.**
- *Maternal*—severe pre-eclampsia, nutritional deprivation, smoking and heart disease.
- *Fetal*—chromosomal abnormality structural anomalies and infection.
- *Placental*—infarction, placenta previa or chronic abruption.
- *Idiopathic*—in majority.

**Q. How do you manage a woman with IUGR?**

**Ans.** *General management includes:* Adequate rest and balanced diet. Treatment of the etiological factor, if any (smoking, tobacco, correction of maltrition), is to be done. Low dose aspirin therapy (50 mg daily) in a selected case with pre-eclampsia or with recurrent IUGR may be started. Increased fluid intake is recommended.

At present, there is no effective intervention to improve FGR except delivery. Delivery is to be done in an appropriate time.

Regarding delivery the following factors are considered:
(i) Duration of pregnancy
(ii) Degree of growth restriction
(iii) Presence of any complicating factor (pre-eclampsia)
(iv) The result of fetal monitoring as mentioned above. Doppler studies of umbilical artery (UA), ductus venosus (DV) and middle cerebral artery (MCA) are also done. Diastolic flow in the UA when reduced, absent or even reversed indicates fetal compromise. Increased blood flow in the MCA suggests vasodilatation (brain sparing effect). Abnormal MCA PI indicates fetal compromise. Doppler ultrasound parameters studied done to make the decision of delivery.

**Q. What should be the guideline to deliver such a patient?**

**Ans.** It depends on the individual case. Factors to be considered here are duration of pregnancy, severity of IUGR, presence of other obstetric complications and result of the monitoring parameters.
- Pregnancy >37 weeks: Delivery.
- Pregnancy <37 weeks: Fetal monitoring (fetal well-being assessment).

(1) No fetal compromise → continue till 37 weeks → with monitoring → delivery.
(2) Fetal compromise detected on Doppler study (UA, DV and middle cerebral artery) before 37 completed weeks → delivery in a tertiary care center having the facilities of NICU. Pregnancy <37 weeks → injection betamethasone/dexamethasone to the mother to accelerate fetal lung maturation. The neonatologist should be involved.

**Q. What should be the method of delivery?**

**Ans.** It depends on the severity of IUGR and the Bishop's score (vaginal examination).
(i) Bishop's score ≥6 = Induction of labor with $PGE_2$ gel followed by artificial rupture of membranes (ARM) and syntocinon augmentation if needed. Fetal monitoring (clinical and preferably electronic) during labor is essential.

(ii) Cervix unfavorable and/or gross IUGR or IUGR with fetal compromise as revealed with Doppler study → elective cesarean delivery.

**Q. What are the perinatal complications in such a pregnancy?**

**Ans.** Asphyxia, meconium aspiration, intrauterine fetal death, neonatal hypoglycemia, necrotizing enterocolitis, polycythemia, pulmonary hemorrhage.

**Q. How on clinical examination does a neonate appear?**

**Ans.** The important physical features are of the neonate with IUGR are: Skin is dry and wrinkled due to less subcutaneous fat. Abdomen is scaphoid. Umbilical cord is thin and may be stained with meconium. Plantar creases are well-developed. All these features give the baby an "old man look".

**Q. What is pondral index (PI)?**

**Ans.** It is a measure to evaluate the neonatal nutritional status. It is a ratio of fetal weight to body length.
PI = [Fetal weight (g)/Crown − heel length in cm$^3$]: × 100
Normal value 8.3, whereas less than 7 indicates malnutrition.

**Q. What is the difference between small for gestation age (SGA) and low birth weight and FGR fetuses?**

**Ans.**
- Low birth weight (LBW) is defined as birth weight less than 2.5 kg. These neonates suffer from the problems of preterm births (See p. 191).
- Small for gestational age (SGA) infants may not be pathologically growth restricted, they are the constitutionally small babies. They are small but healthy babies.
- In FGR, the fetus has not met the genetic growth potential due to the particular pathological process which operates to reduce it growth rate.

**Q. What are the types of FGR?**

**Ans.**
- Early onset: <34 weeks (Symmetrical)
- Late onset: After 34 weeks (Asymmetrical).

## CASE–11 | PRE-ECLAMPSIA AND ECLAMPSIA

### Case Summary

*Mrs MR, 26 years old, was admitted in her first pregnancy at 34 weeks of gestation with BP of 150/96 mm Hg and protein in the urine (+++). She was recorded normotensive (BP: 110/70 mm Hg) and nonproteinuric in her early visits in the antenatal clinic. She had no symptoms. On general physical examination, there was no pallor but mild pedal edema was present. Her cardiovascular and respiratory systems were normal. Obstetric examination revealed: Uterus 34 weeks, SFH 34 cm, single fetus, cephalic presentation, free, fetal back on the left, limbs on the right side. Liquor volume was adequate. On auscultation, FHS was 146 beats per minute and was regular.*

**Q. What is the clinical diagnosis?**

**Ans.** Pre-eclampsia.

**Q. What other important symptoms she may have?**

**Ans.** Edema over the ankles, vulva (Fig. 2.16), abdominal wall and face. There may be headache, epigastric or right hypochondriac pain, oliguria or blurring of vision.

**Q. Suggest few important investigations for her.**

**Ans.** (i) Complete hemogram, urea and electrolytes.
(ii) Urine for 24 hours protein.
(iii) *Coagulation profile:* Serum fibrinogen level, PT and APTT.
(iv) *LFTs:* Serum AST, ALT and bilirubin.
(v) Serum uric acid (normal <4 mg/dL).

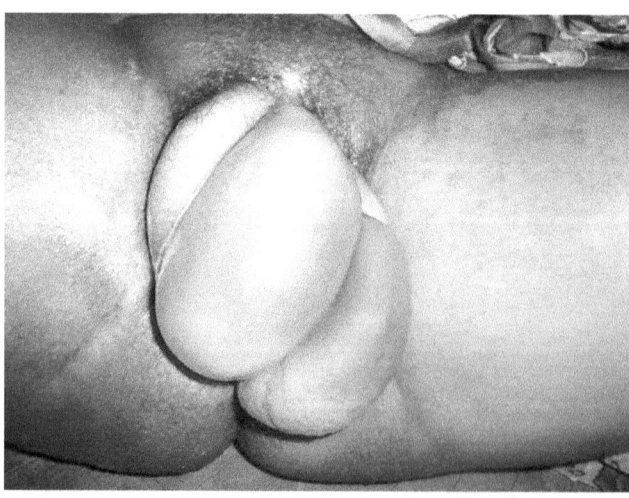

**Fig. 2.16:** Massive vulval edema in pregnancy with pre-eclampsia.

(vi) Serum creatinine (normal <1 mg/dL).
(vii) Platelet count (normal >1.5 lacs/mm³).
(viii) Ophthalmoscopic examination to detect any retinal edema, constriction of the arterioles, exudate or hemorrhage.
(ix) Fetal monitoring: DFMC, USG for fetal growth, liquor pockets, nonstress test and biophysical profile depending upon the situation.

**Q. Mention few important hematological abnormalities of the patient.**

**Ans.** Thrombocytopenia (platelet count is <100,000/mm³), hemolysis, hemoconcentration and DIC.

**Q. What is the basic pathology of this clinical problem?**

**Ans.** Endothelial cell dysfunction and vasospasm.

**Q. What are the risk factors for the development of pre-eclampsia?**

**Ans.**
(i) Primigravida (first-time exposure to chorionic villi)
(ii) Positive family history
(iii) Exposure to superabundance of chorionic villi (twins and molar pregnancy)
(iv) Genetic (polygenic disorder)
(v) Pre-existing vascular or renal disease
(vi) Thrombophilia
(vii) Immunological maladaptation
(viii) New paternity.

**Q. What is severe pre-eclampsia?**

**Ans.** (i) Level of blood pressure systolic >160 mm Hg and/or diastolic >110 mm Hg (Fig. 2.17).

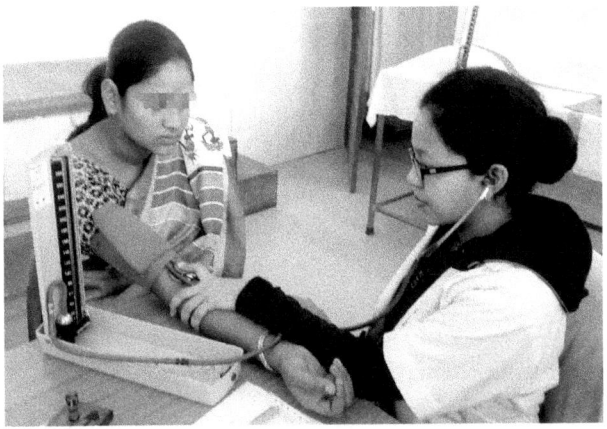

Fig. 2.17: Measurement of blood pressure of a pregnant woman is a routine in each antenatal examination.

(ii) Headache
(iii) Visual disturbances
- Convulsion (eclampsia)
- Gestational age: Early
  However, this classification is misleading and it is important to note that a case with nonsevere disease may rapidly become a severe one.
(iv) Persistent epigastric pain
(v) Oliguria (urine volume <400 mL in 24 hours)
(vi) Proteinuria (>5 g/day or ≥3+)
(vii) Low platelet count (<100,000/mm$^3$)
(viii) HELLP syndrome
(ix) Retinal pathology—hemorrhage, exudate
(x) Fetal growth restriction (FGR)
(xi) Cases without these features are considered as nonsevere
(xii) Pulmonary edema
(xiii) Serum creatinine: >1.1 mg/dL
(xiv) Convulsions.

**Q. What are the complications of pre-eclampsia?**

**Ans.** Complications are both to the mother and the fetus.

| Maternal | Fetal |
| --- | --- |
| • Eclampsia | • IUGR |
| • Cerebrovascular accident (cerebral hemorrhage, infarction) | • Preterm delivery and prematurity |
| | • Asphyxia |
| • Abruptio placentae | • IUFD |
| • DIC | • Oligohydramnios |
| • Oliguria, anuria and renal failure | • Increased perinatal death |
| • Pulmonary edema | |
| • HELLP syndrome | |
| • Hepatic failure | |
| • Blurring of vision and blindness | |
| • Preterm labor | |
| • PPH | |
| • Death | |

| Long-term sequelae of Pre-eclampsia syndrome | |
| --- | --- |
| • Chronic hypertension | • Dyslipidemia |
| • Ischemic heart disease | • Metabolic syndrome |
| • Cardiomyopathy | • Renal dysfunction |
| • Stroke | |

**Q. How do you manage a case of pre-eclampsia?**

**Ans.** (i) To control blood pressure—antihypertensive (labetalol, nifedipine or hydralazine), methyldopa.

(ii) Fetal monitoring and other investigations (mentioned earlier).

(iii) Blood pressure controlled → to continue pregnancy till 37 completed weeks → termination of pregnancy (either by induction of labor or by cesarean section).

(iv) Blood pressure not controlled or rising → termination of pregnancy irrespective of duration of pregnancy.
(Termination may be done either by induction of labor when Bishop's score is favorable or by cesarean section).

(v) Presence of ominous symptoms like headache, blurring of vision, epigastric or right hypochondriac pain, falling platelet count, rising blood pressure and in spite of medical therapy.

**Urgent delivery inspective of gestational age.**

In such a situation, patient should be given:

(A) Betamethasone or dexamethasone to accelerate pulmonary maturity when the gestational age is 37 weeks.

(B) Antiseizure prophylaxis—$MgSO_4$ is to be started (IM or IV regimen) in a woman with severe pre-eclampsia.

**Q.** *What is eclampsia?*

**Ans.** Woman with pre-eclampsia when complicated with convulsions and/or coma is called eclampsia.

**Q.** *What are the different types of eclampsia?*

**Ans.** (i) Antepartum (majority 50%)
(ii) Intrapartum (30%)
(iii) Postpartum (20%).

**Q.** *What are the different stages of convulsion in eclampsia?*

**Ans.** (i) Premonitory stage, (ii) tonic stage, (iii) clonic stage, and (iv) stage of coma.

**Q.** *What are the maternal complications of eclampsia?*

**Ans.** (i) *Pulmonary:* Edema, pneumonia, ARDS
(ii) *Cardiac:* LVF
(iii) *Renal:* Oliguria, anuria and renal failure
(iv) *Hepatic:* Subcapsular hematoma, hepatic cell necrosis and jaundice
(v) *Eyes:* Retinal detachment and blindness
(vi) *Cerebral:* Encephalomalacia, hemorrhage, edema: PRES
(vii) Injuries: Tongue bite (Fig. 2.18), injuries from fall, bedsore.
**Postpartum:** • Sepsis • Psychosis • Shock.
**Fetal:** • Prematurity • IUGR • Asphyxia • IUD • Increased perinatal morbidity and mortality.

**Q. What anticonvulsant regime is commonly used for the management?**

**Ans.** Magnesium sulfate ($MgSO_4$, 7 $H_2O$) is the drug of choice. It has got excellent result. Maternal mortality is of 0.4%. It is to be continued for 24 hours after last seizure or delivery, whichever is later. The woman is monitored clinically by presence of knee jerks, urine output (p. 335) (>30 mL/hour) and respiration rate (>16/minute). Monitoring is done so that toxicity is avoided. $MgSO_4$ is recommended for the cases with severe pre-eclampsia (ACOG Task Force 2013). Presently, it is not recommended for the nonsevere cases though there is uncertainty about the indicators of severity.

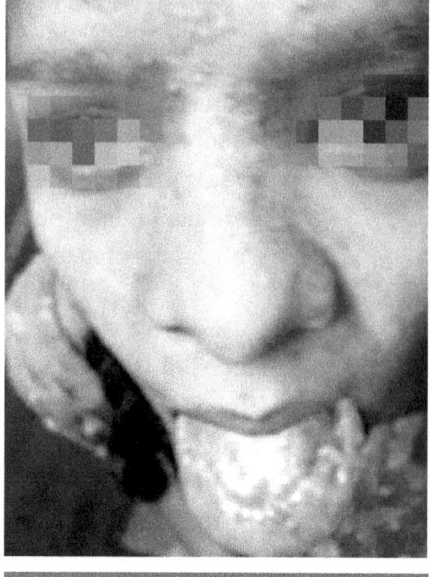

Fig. 2.18 : Extensive bite of the entire tongue following repeated eclamptic convulsions in labor. This patient suffered tuberous sclerosis. Cutaneous angiofibromas are seen.

**Q. What are the common causes of maternal death in eclampsia?**

**Ans.**
(i) Cardiac failure
(ii) Pulmonary edema
(iii) Aspiration
(iv) Cerebral hemorrhage
(v) Renal failure
(vi) Postpartum shock
(vii) Puerperal sepsis.

**Q. What are poor prognostic factors of eclampsia?**

**Ans.**
(i) Late referral (delay in start of treatment)
(ii) Number of fits >10
(iii) Coma in between fits
(iv) Temperature >102°F, pulse >120/minute
(v) Prolonged admission delivery interval
(vi) Pulmonary edema
(vii) Blood pressure >200 mm Hg systolic
(viii) Oliguria
(ix) Proteinuria >5 g/24 hours
(x) Poor response to treatment
(xi) Appearance of jaundice.

**Case discussion continued:**

The same patient as discussed on p. 72, was seen after 4 days, her BP record was 160/120 mm Hg and proteinuria persisted. She complained of right upper abdominal pain.

**Q. What is the possible diagnosis?**
Ans. Severe pre-eclampsia.

**Q. What complications might she develop if left untreated?**
Ans. Eclampsia, abruptio placentae, renal failure, HELLP syndrome, and cerebrovascular accident.

**Q. What immediate management should she have?**
Ans. (i) *Control of blood pressure:* Antihypertensive drug to be started. Labetalol (IV), injection hydralazine (IV), or Ca-channel blocker.
(ii) *To prevent fits:* Prophylactic anticonvulsive therapy—magnesium sulfate (IM/IV regimen).
(iii) To administer steroid to accelerate fetal lung maturity (pregnancy <37 weeks).
(iv) To monitor the fetus and to organize delivery once the maternal condition is stable.

**Q. What are the possible fetal complications in this condition?**
Ans. IUGR, IUFD and problems of prematurity, if delivered before term.

**Q. What is HELLP syndrome?**
Ans. HELLP is an acronym for a syndrome of **H**emolysis, **E**levated **L**iver enzymes and **L**ow **P**latelet count. It is considered as the severe variety of pre-eclampsia.
H = Hemolysis (abnormal peripheral blood smear)
EL = Elevated liver enzymes (SGOT >121 U/l; LDH >600 U/L)
LP = Low platelet count (<100,000/mm$^3$).

**Q. What are the maternal complications of HELLP syndrome?**
Ans.
- Pulmonary edema
- Acute renal failure
- DIC
- Abruptio placenta
- *Liver*
  - Infarction; hepatic rupture
  - Subcapsular liver hematoma
- ARDS
- Stroke
- Sepsis
- Maternal mortality rate is 1%.

**Q. What are the laboratory observations in HELLP syndrome?**
Ans.
- *Hemolysis in HELLP is characterized by:*
  - Peripheral smear (schistocytes, burr cells)
  - Severe anemia not due to blood loss
- *Elevated liver enzymes:*
  - AST
  - ALT    Levels ≥ twice the normal
  - LDH
- *Low platelets:* <100,000/mm$^3$.

**Q. What is the management of HELLP syndrome?**

Ans.
- Urgent hospitalization
- Tertiary care center (preferred)
- Investigations to organize as in severe pre-eclampsia
- Antiseizure prophylaxis: $MgSO_4$
- Antihypertensive drug
- *Delivery:* Corticosteroids—when pregnancy <37 weeks.

**Q. What are the important medical management HELLP syndromes?**

Ans. Plasma volume expansion:
- IV infusion—crystalloids
- Colloids—albumin (5%)
- Antithrombotic agent—heparin
- Fresh frozen plasma
- *Platelet transfusion:*
  - Platelet count <20,000/mm$^3$
  - Presence of bleeding (bleeding gums).

**Q. Is there any risk of recurrence of pre-eclampsia in subsequent pregnancy?**

Ans. Yes. Risk of recurrence in next pregnancy is about 25%.

**Q. Classify the hypertensive disorders complicating pregnancy.**

Ans. (1) **Gestational Hypertension:**
  - Systolic BP ≥140 or diastolic ≥90 mm Hg, detected first time during pregnancy after 20 weeks in a woman who was normotensive previously
  - No proteinuria.

(2) **Pre-eclampsia:**

| **Nonsevere Pre-eclampsia** Minimum criteria: | *Severe pre-eclampsia* |
|---|---|
| - BP ≥140/90 mm Hg after 20 weeks gestation | - Persistently BP: Systolic ≥160 and Diastolic ≥110 mm Hg |
| - Proteinuria ≥300 mg/24 hours or ≥1 + dipstick | - Proteinuria >2 g/ 24 hours or ≥ 2+ dipstick (degrees of proteinuria is disregarded for classification) |
| - Urine protein : Creatinine ratio ≥3 or | - Serum creatinine >1.1 mg/dL |
| - Urine dipstick test: 1+ persistent | - Platelets <100,000/mL |
| | - Increased LDH |
| | - Elevated ALT or AST |
| | - Persistent headache or cerebral or visual disturbances |
| | - Persistent epigastric pain |
| | - Pulmonary edema |

(3) **Superimposed pre-eclampsia on chronic Hypertension:** New onset of proteinuria ≥ 300 mg/24 hours in a hypertensive woman who was earlier nonproteinuric.

(4) **Chronic hypertension:**
- BP ≥140/90 mm Hg before pregnancy or diagnosed before 20 weeks of gestation
- Hypertension first diagnosed after 20 weeks gestation and persistent after 12 weeks postpartum.

**Q. What is heat test and acetic acid test?**

Ans. Heat test and acetic acid test is a qualitative test by which the presence of protein is detected in the urine.

Urine is taken in a test tube. The upper ¾ part of urine is heated. The heated part may become cloudy. Then 5 drops of 10% acetic acid is added to it. Disappearance of turbidity indicates presence of phosphate and if the turbidity persists it indicates presence of protein (albumin).

**Q. How one can predict the onset of pre-eclampsia by USG Doppler study?**

Ans. In Doppler velocimetry presence of notching on maternal uterine artery flow at 22-24 weeks of gestation is thought to have high predictive value.

**Q. What is Pritchard's regimen using $MgSO_4$ in eclampsia?**

Ans. Loading dose followed by intermittent intramuscular dose is the most popular regimen.
The dose schedule is as follows: Loading dose 20 cc, 20% $MgSO_4$ (4 g) is given intravenously slowly over 4-5 minutes time. This is followed by 20 cc 50% $MgSO_4$ (10 g) deep intramuscular injection, given half (5 g, i.e. 10 cc 50%) in each buttock. Maintenance dose is continued : 10 cc 50% (5 g) 1M 4 hourly on alternative buttock for 24 hours after the last seizure or delivery which is later.

*For IV use, $MgSO_4$ concentration should be 20%. One part of 50% $MgSO_4$ injection is diluted with 1.5 parts of water for injection to make it 20%. It is then given IV slowly.*

**Q. What is Zuspan regimen?**

Ans. Intravenous regimen of $MgSO_4$ therapy in eclampsia is known as Zuspan's regimen.
Dose schedule: 4 to 6 g is given slowly IV over 15 to 20 minutes. This is followed by maintenance dose of 1 to 2 g/hour IV infusion.

**Q. What is the therapeutic level of $MgSO_4$?**

Ans. 4-7 mEq/L

**Q. What is the side effect of $MgSO_4$ on the kidneys?**

Ans. No significant effect. The only route of excretion of $MgSO_4$ is through kidneys, that is why measurement of urine volume is required.

## CASE-12: PREGNANCY WITH MATERNAL RED CELL ALLOIMMUNIZATION

### Case Summary

*Mrs GT, P0+0+0+0, at 36 weeks of gestation was seen in the antenatal clinic. Her obstetric examinations were within normal limits. Investigation reports revealed that her blood group was Group A, rhesus negative while her husband was group B, rhesus positive.*

**Q. What is the basic underlying pathology of rhesus isoimmunization?**

**Ans.** When Rh-positive red cells of the fetus enter into the maternal circulation, they generate antigenic response to produce antibodies by the reticuloendothelial system. At least 0.1 mL of fetal blood and about 6 months are required to produce detectable antibodies. These antibodies (IgG), when they enter the fetal circulation (crossing the placental barrier), agglutinate the fetal red cells, which are ultimately removed by the reticuloendothelial cells. Fetal affection depends upon the degree of agglutination and destruction of fetal red cells.

**Q. What is the chance that this baby will be affected due to rhesus problem?**

**Ans.** In a primigravida, who is otherwise uncomplicated, it is unlikely that the baby would be affected due to rhesus problem (for reasons see below).

**Q. Under what circumstances may even the mother in her first pregnancy be sensitized?**

**Ans.** History of amniocentesis, chorionic villus sampling, antepartum hemorrhage, threatened miscarriage, external cephalic version, blood transfusion with rhesus positive red cells.

**Q. What test should be done to detect isoimmunization status?**

**Ans.** Detection of antibodies in maternal blood by indirect Coombs' test (ICT).

**Q. How is the immune response of a Rh-negative woman to RhD positive red cells?**

**Ans.** The response may vary in an individual. The response may be any of the following three varieties.
  (1) **Responders (60–70%):** Who develop an antibody to a small volume of red cells.
  (2) **Hyperresponders (few):** Who develop antibodies even with a very small volume of red cells.
  (3) **Poor responders (10–20%):** Who respond to develop antibodies with a very large volume of red cells.
  (4) **Nonresponders (10–20%):** Individuals who do not respond to any amount of red cell transfer.
  The time taken to develop anti-D antibody following a sensitizing event is 5 to 16 weeks.

## Chapter 2 • Obstetric Case Discussions

**Q. What is the critical titer?**

**Ans.** A critical titer is the anti-red cell antibody titer that is associated with significant risk of hydrops fetalis. In most center, a critical titer for anti-D antibody is 16 (dilution of 1:16 is equivalent to a titer of 16).

**Q. If the ICT is positive, what should be the next course of action?**

**Ans.**
- Quantitative estimation of antibody (IgG type) at weekly interval.
- Antibody titer 1/16th is considered critical titer (some center) or antibody level <4 IU/mL (automated measurement) is considered safe.
- Genotype of the husband.
  Husband → homozygous → fetus is likely to be affected.
  Husband → heterozygous → fetus is affected only in 50% cases.

**Q. How could the severity of the disease be assessed?**

**Ans.** Amniocentesis or by fetal blood sampling (cordocentesis) or middle cerebral artery (MCA), Doppler velocimetry.

**Amniocentesis:** Optical density (OD) difference of **amniotic fluid** at 450 nm is assessed. In presence of bilirubin, there is a 'deviation bulge' (Figs. 2.19A and B). Higher the bulge, more severe is the fetal affection. The spectrophotometric "deviation bulge" at Δ OD450 is plotted in Liley's chart and accordingly the management is formulated.

**Zone A:** Fetus is unlikely to be affected — to continue pregnancy to term (Hb >11.0 g/dL).

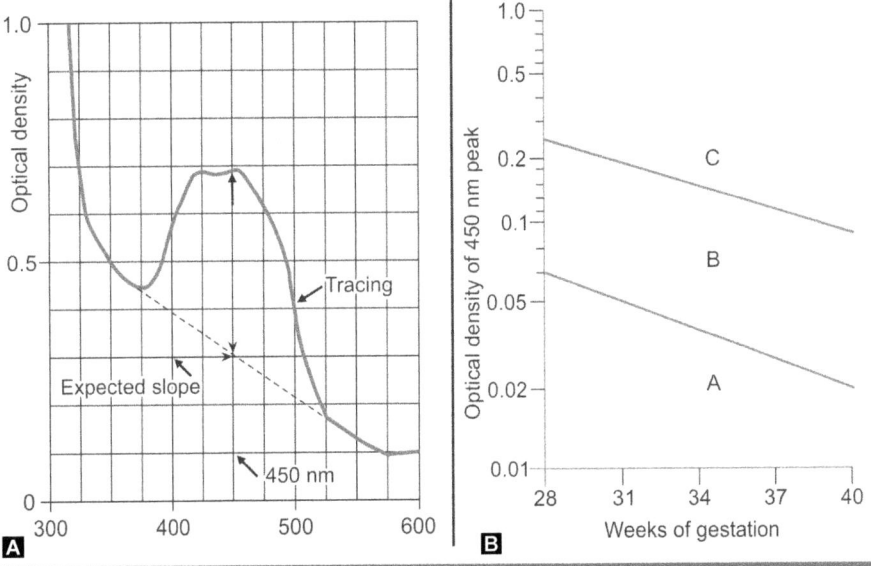

**Figs. 2.19A and B:** (A) Spectrophotometric analysis of amniotic fluid showing optical density difference at 450 nm wavelength with "deviation bulge" in Rh hemolytic disease; (B) Plotting of the "deviation bulge" in Liley's prediction chart at different periods of gestation. Currently Liley's graph is modified (Queenan – 1993) that begins at 14 weeks of pregnancy.

**Zone B**: Fetal anemia; pregnancy termination after 34 weeks (Hb 8.0–10.9 g/dL).

**Zone C**: Severe anemia; severe fetal affection (Hb <8.0 g/dL).
- Pregnancy >34 weeks — delivery.
- Pregnancy <34 weeks → Cordocentesis and intrauterine fetal transfusion (when hematocrit <30%). Repeat transfusion may be needed, pregnancy to continue till 34 weeks and then delivery.

**Middle cerebral artery (MCA)-peak systolic velocity (PSV):** Presently MCA-PSV is the main stay of fetal surveillance in a case with Rh-alloimmunization. Doppler ultrasound study of MCA PSV >1.5 MoM for the corresponding gestational age predicts moderate to severe anemia. Serial study with MCA-PSV has replaced amniocentesis for ΔOD450. It is more accurate than amniocentesis.

**Cordocentesis**—It can assess the degree of fetal affection more correctly compared to amniocentesis. A fetus with hemoglobin deficit 2 g/dL or more from the mean value of the corresponding gestational age (hematocrit <30%) should be transfused.

Intrauterine fetal transfusion may be either by—(a) Intraperitoneal or (b) intravascular (umbilical vein) route.

**Q. What are the benefits and the risks of cordocentesis in the management?**

**Ans.** Benefits of cordocentesis or funipuncture:
- Fetal ABO blood group Rh type, hematocrit, direct Coombs' test, reticulocyte count and total bilirubin level can be determined.
- *Risks*: Cordocentesis has got the risk of fetal loss (1–2%) and fetomaternal hemorrhage in 50% of cases. For this reason, it is done only in patients with elevated peak MCA Doppler velocities.

**Q. What are the sonographic findings in a fetus that is affected due to rhesus alloimmunization?**

**Ans.** *Serial ultrasound scan reveals:* Increased amniotic fluid volume, hepatosplenomegaly, placental thickness >4 cm, echogenic bowel, scalp edema, cardiomegaly with increased cardiac chambers, pericardial effusion, ascites, umbilical vein dilation and fetal edema (hydrops). Scalp edema, presence of hydrops indicates severe fetal anemia.

**Q. What is the significance of middle cerebral artery Doppler ultrasound?**

**Ans.** Peak velocity of systolic blood flow in the MCA is increased (preferential redistribution) when the fetus is anemic due to rhesus alloimmunization. MCA Doppler flow velocity is used as a noninvasive method to detect fetuses with moderate to severe affection. Value of MCA peak systolic velocity >1.5 MoM, suggests fetal anemia. Cordocentesis and intrauterine fetal transfusion may be needed depending upon the severity of anemia.

**Q. What are the fetal complications that may occur when mother is immunized?**

**Ans. Hemolytic disease of the fetus and newborn (HDFN)** depends upon the severity of the pathological process. It may cause:
   (a) **Hydrops fetalis:** It is severe form of the hemolytic disease. Either there is intrauterine fetal death or early neonatal death due to cardiac failure.
   (b) **Icterus gravis neonatorum:** It is less severe form of the fetal hemolysis. Baby develops jaundice soon following birth.
   (c) **Congenital anemia of the newborn:** It is the mild form of the disease.
   The underlying pathology of the hemolytic disease:
   Hemolytic anemia → tissue (organ) hypoxemia.
   Liver damage → hypoproteinemia → cardiac failure → fetal hydrops → IUFD.

**Q. What neonatal complications may occur after the delivery?**

**Ans.** Icterus gravis neonatorum, congenital anemia of the newborn, neonatal jaundice and kernicterus.

**Q. What treatment might the fetus/neonate need if found affected?**

**Ans.** • Intrauterine fetal transfusion either intraperitoneal or intravascular.
   • Exchange blood transfusion of the neonate.
   *The blood should be group O and Rh-negative.*

**Q. What special investigations would be done for this baby following birth?**

**Ans.** Cord blood sample to be taken.
   *Cord blood investigations*: Hb%, hematocrit, reticulocyte count, ABO grouping, Rh typing, direct Coombs' test and serum bilirubin.

**Q. What measure should be taken to prevent active immunization of the mother?**

**Ans.** If the baby is rhesus positive, anti-D gamma globulin 300 µg IM is given to the mother within 72 hours of delivery.

**Q. What is the best way to assess the dose of anti-D?**

**Ans.** By measuring extent of fetomaternal hemorrhage by performing 'Kleihauer count' (acid elution test). The dose of Rh immunoglobulin calculated is 10 µg for 1 mL of fetal blood when fetomaternal hemorrhage is >30 mL.

**Q. What could be the reason that the first pregnancy is often not affected?**

**Ans.** In majority of cases, fetomaternal hemorrhage occurs predominantly during the course of labor and delivery. Detectable antibodies usually develop 2-4 months after the episode of fetomaternal bleed. Thus, the first pregnancy is not generally affected. However, antepartum sensitization may occur in small percentage of cases (1-2%).

**Q. What are the conditions where prophylactic anti-D is needed to prevent Rh-alloimmunization even in the first pregnancy?**

Ans. Causes of fetomaternal hemorrhage during pregnancy are:
  (A) **Prior history of or in the present pregnancy:**
      (i) Miscarriage
      (ii) MTP
      (iii) Ectopic pregnancy
      (iv) Molar pregnancy.
  (B) **Procedures:**
      (i) CVS
      (ii) Genetic amniocentesis
      (iii) Cordocentesis.
  (C) **Others:**
      (i) External cephalic version
      (ii) Manual removal of placenta
      (iii) Placental abruption.

**Q. What could be the reason that anti-D prophylaxis is not needed for such a mother?**

Ans. If the baby is rhesus negative.

**Q. Is there any place of prophylactic anti-D therapy during pregnancy?**

Ans. Yes. To combat any fetomaternal hemorrhage during pregnancy. It is currently recommended to give 300 µg anti-D immune globulin at around 28 weeks of pregnancy. However, after birth, it is again given 300 µg within 72 hours.

**Q. Why are not all the babies born following Rh incompatibility affected?**

Ans. (i) Inborn inability to respond to the Rh antigenic stimulus.
  (ii) The particular woman may be immunologic nonresponder.
  (iii) There may be associated ABO incompatibility.
  (iv) Variability of Rh antigenic stimulus depending upon the genotype of the fetus.
  (v) Less volume of fetal blood entering into the maternal circulation. Minimal volume required is 0.1 mL.
  (vi) Fetal response to maternal antibodies varies on fetal sex. Rh-D positive male fetuses run the higher risk of severe hemolysis and death, compared to a female fetus.

**Q. What care during delivery can minimize the risk of fetomaternal hemorrhage?**

**Ans.** (a) **During labor:**
  (i) Not to give prophylactic ergometrine during second stage of labor.
  (ii) Gentle handling of the uterus during the third stage.
(b) **During cesarean delivery:**
  (i) To avoid blood spillage into the peritoneal cavity.
  (ii) To avoid routine manual removal of the placenta.
(c) **Early cord clamping.**

**Q. What are the indications of exchange transfusion in the newborn?**

**Ans.** Rh-positive with direct Coombs' test positive babies having:
  (i) Cord blood bilirubin level >4 mg/dL and hemoglobin level is <11 g/dL.
  (ii) Rising rate of bilirubin over 1 mg/dL/hour despite phototherapy.
  (iii) Total bilirubin level is 20 mg/dL or more.

**Q. What are the objectives of exchange transfusion?**

**Ans.** (i) To correct anemia and to prevent cardiac failure.
(ii) To remove the circulatory antibodies.
(iii) To remove the circulatory bilirubin.

**Q. What is the type, nature and amount of blood to be transfused?**

**Ans.** (i) Rh negative, whole blood with the same blood group to that of the baby or with group 'O'.
(II) It should be relatively fresh.
(iii) The amount is about 160 mL/kg body weight of the baby.

**Q. Can the mother breastfeed the baby?**

**Ans.** Yes, there is no contraindication to breastfeeding.

**Q. What is "Grand Mother's theory"?**

**Ans:**

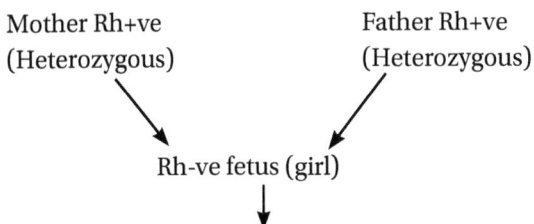

May get immunized with her mother's Rh+ve blood cells before birth
↓

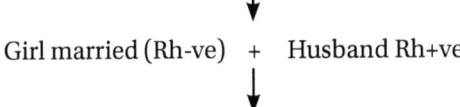

When the girl becomes a mother herself and exposed to a new load of D antigen from her fetus (hence the grandmother connection) the immune memory is recalled and a secondary immune response occur.

## CASE–13 | MULTIPLE PREGNANCY

### Case Summary

*Mrs YM, P0+0+0+0, 27 years old, pregnancy following induction of ovulation, was admitted at 36 weeks of gestation with occasional dyspnea due to huge enlargement of the abdomen. On clinical examination, she had mild pedal edema; BP 140/94 mm Hg. Her cardiovascular and respiratory system examination was normal. Obstetric examination revealed symphysis-fundal height of 40 cm and abdominal girth at the level of umbilicus was 120 cm. Difficulties were faced in palpating the fetal parts. Too many fetal parts were felt. On auscultation, two fetal heart sounds could be heard at two different sites. One over the right spinoumbilical line and the other over the left spinoumbilical line at a higher level.*

**Q. What is the likely diagnosis?**

**Ans.** Multiple pregnancy and/or polyhydramnios.

**Q. How can you confirm the diagnosis?**

**Ans.** Ultrasound scan of the gravid uterus.
The USG scan is shown in Figure 2.20.

**Q. What is the diagnosis?**

**Ans.** Twin pregnancy.

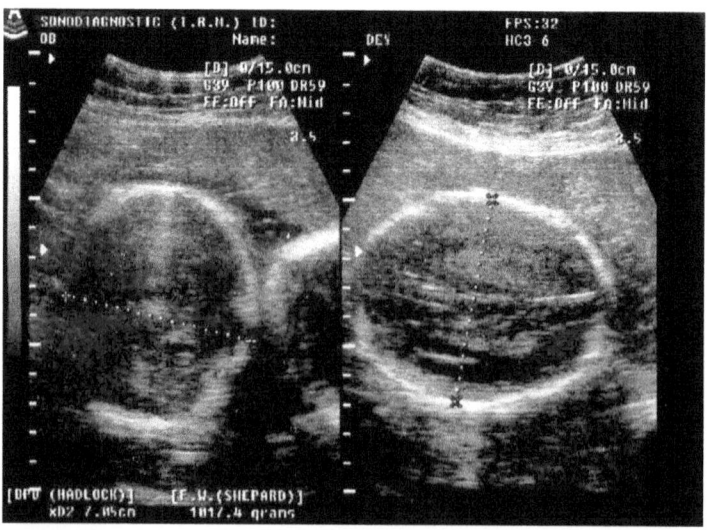

Fig. 2.20: Ultrasonography of a twin pregnancy showing two fetal heads. [*Courtesy*—Dr (Mrs) S Ghosh and Prof BN Chakravorty, Director, IRM, Kolkata].

**Q. How can you suspect the diagnosis of twin pregnancy clinically?**

Ans. (a) **From the history:** (i) Use of ovulation inducing drugs and (ii) Family history of twinning.

(b) **Symptoms:** Increased nausea, vomiting, cardiorespiratory embarrassment, pedal edema, unusual enlargement of the abdomen.

(c) **Signs:**
  (i) Unusual weight gain
  (ii) Pre-eclampsia—early onset.
  (iii) Fundal height more than the period of amenorrhea.
  (iv) Abdominal girth (at umbilicus) is more than 100 cm.
  (v) Palpation of too many fetal parts.
  (vi) Findings of two fetal heads or three fetal poles of the uterus.

(d) **Auscultation:** Two distinct fetal heart sounds heard at two separate sites by two observers with a difference in heart rates by at least 10 beats/minute.

**Q. What additional information can be obtained on ultrasonography besides the presence of two fetuses?**

Ans. (i) Number and viability of the fetuses.
(ii) Chorionicity (lambda or twin peak sign).
(iii) Gestational age and weight of the fetuses.
(iv) Fetal malformations.
(v) Presentation and lie of the fetuses.
(vi) Twin transfusion.
(vii) Placental localization.
(viii) Amniotic fluid volume.

**Q. What are the common maternal complications during pregnancy?**

Ans.

| | |
|---|---|
| • Nausea, vomiting | • Anemia |
| • PIH and pre-eclampsia | • Polyhydramnios/oligohydramnios |
| • Preterm labor | • Malpresentation |
| • Antepartum hemorrhage | • Mechanical distress (dyspnea, palpitation) |
| • Prolonged labor | • Operative interference |
| • Postpartum hemorrhage | • (↑) Postnatal support |

**Q. What are the different combinations of twin presentations?**

Ans. The following combinations are in the descending order of frequency:
(i) Both cephalic (most common 40% and most favorable)
(ii) First cephalic, second breech (26%)
(iii) Both breech (10%)
(iv) Cephalic and transverse lie (8%)
(v) Breech and transverse lie
(vi) Both transverse lie.

**Q. What are the common fetal complications? Why is twin pregnancy considered high-risk?**

**Ans.** Common complications are listed below: (also *see* SAQ, p. 242).

- Miscarriage
- Preterm birth
- Discordant growth
- Twin-twin transfusion syndrome
- Locked twins
- (↑) Perinatal mortality (complications are more in monochorionic twins)
- Vanishing twin
- Fetus papyraceus (Fig. 2.21)
- Fetal anomalies (Figs. 2.22 and 2.23)
- Intrauterine death of one fetus
- Cord prolapse

**Q. How would you organize the management of the woman during her antenatal period?**

**Ans.** Considering the number of complications both to the mother and fetus—**twin pregnancy is a high-risk one**. The antenatal management protocol should be:

(i) Diet—increased dietary supplementation (additional 300 kcal/day).
(ii) Increased rest at home and early cessation of work.
(iii) Increased supplement therapy of iron (100–200 mg/day), folic acid, calcium and vitamins.
(iv) Regular antenatal visit—sometimes, it may be frequent at an interval of 2–3 weeks.
(v) Fetal monitoring—clinical and by serial sonography at 3–4 weeks interval.

**Hospitalization:** Routine hospital admission for bed rest is not essential. Early cessation of work and rest at home is helpful. Emergency admission for any complication (e.g. preterm labor) may be needed any time during pregnancy.

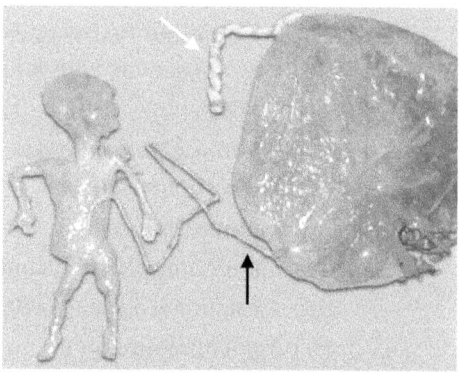

**Fig. 2.21:** Fetus papyraceus, umbilical cord of the live fetus (red arrow) and that of the lead (blue arrow) are seen.

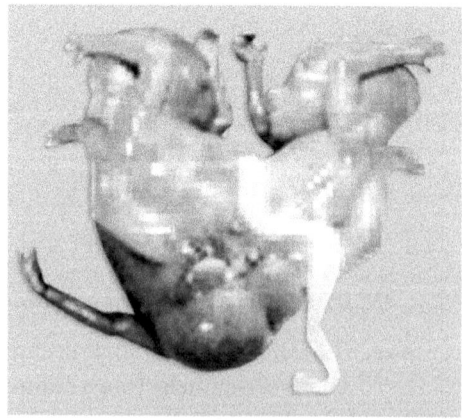

**Fig. 2.22:** Conjoint twins—showing pyopagus (joined from umbilicus to the buttocks). [*Courtesy:* Prof BN Chakravorty, Director, IRM, Kolkata].

***Q. What is fetus papyraceus or compressus?***

**Ans.** This is a situation where one fetus dies in early pregnancy. The dead fetus is flattened, mummified and compressed between the membranes of the living fetus and the uterine wall. It is detected by sonography or seen after delivery.

***Q. What precautionary measures should be taken when she goes into labor?***

**Ans.** Twin pregnancy is a high-risk one. Women with twins should be delivered preferably at an equipped center having an intensive neonatal care unit. An intravenous line with Ringer's solution is started. Arrangement is made for availability of one unit of cross-matched blood to ensure the availability of the senior obstetrician, the anesthetist and the neonatologist.

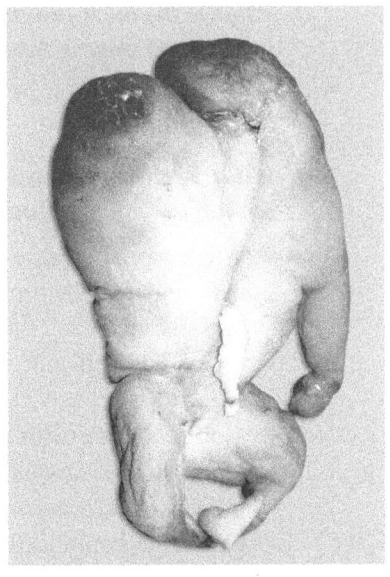

**Fig. 2.23:** Acephalus, acardiac fetus in a twin pregnancy.
[*Courtesy*: Dr A Mukherjee, Gynecologist, Purulia Hospital, West Bengal, India].

***Q. What would be the steps of management following birth of the first baby?***

**Ans.** • Twin A → vertex → deliver vaginally.
↓ **No methergin**
- Twin B → vertex → ARM ± oxytocin → deliver vaginally
- Twin B → breech → ARM ± oxytocin → assisted breech delivery
- Twin B → transverse → external cephalic version (ECV) → ARM ± oxytocin → vaginal delivery.
    If external cephalic version fails → internal podalic version (IPV) → followed by breech extraction.
- Average delivery interval between Twin A and Twin B is 15–20 minutes.
- Injection methergin 0.2 mg IV is given soon following the birth of the second baby. To continue IV oxytocin infusion after delivery of the placenta.
- **Twin A** → nonvertex → cesarean delivery.

***Q. What are the second stage complications of twin pregnancy?***

**Ans.** • Cord prolapse of the twin B.
- Placental abruption after delivery of twin A.
- Retention of twin B due to premature closure of the cervix.
- Intrapartum hemorrhage.
- Locked twins (rarely) (Fig. 2.24).

**Q. What is the most common complication in the third stage of labor?**

**Ans.** Primary postpartum hemorrhage due to uterine atony.

**Q. What are the indications of cesarean section in twin pregnancy?**

**Ans.**
- When both the twins or the first twin is with noncephalic presentation (breech or transverse).
- Twins with estimated weight 2,000 g or less.
- Monoamniotic twins.
- Monochorionic twins with twin-to-twin transfusion syndrome (TTTS).
- Pregnancy complications — severe pre-eclampsia, previous cesarean section (obstetric indications).
- Conjoint twin (See Fig. 2.22).

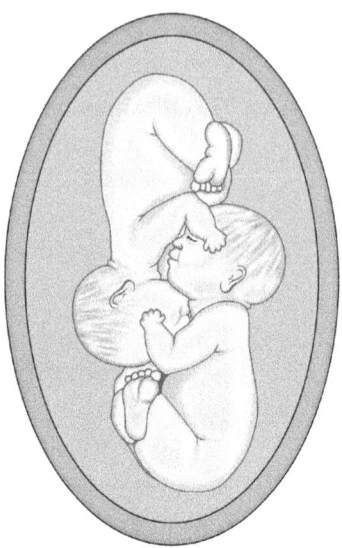

**Fig. 2.24:** Interlocking of twins between the after-coming head of first baby with the forecoming head of the second baby.

**Q. Which type of twins are associated with higher rate of complications?**

**Ans.** Monochorionic twins.

**Q. What are the complications of monochorionic twins?**

**Ans.**
- Congenital fetal malformations
- Twin-to-twin transfusion syndrome
- Polyhydramnios
- IUGR
- Dead fetus syndrome
- Conjoint twin
- Twin reversed arterial perfusion or acardiac twin (*see* Fig. 2.23)
- Increased perinatal mortality.

**Q. What is the membrane status of dizygotic twins?**

**Ans.** Dizygotic (DZ) twins are always dichorionic and diamniotic as they result from fertilization of two different ova.

**Q. What is the membrane status in monozygotic twins?**

**Ans.** It depends upon the time of twining division following fertilization. The possibilities are:
(a) Division <72 hours: Diamniotic dichorionic (D/D)
(b) Division between 4th day and 8th day: Diamniotic monochorionic (D/M)
(c) Division >8 days: Monoamniotic monochorionic (M/M)
(d) Division >2 weeks: Conjoint twins.

## Q. What is meant by vanishing twin and selective fetal reduction?

**Ans.**
- Intrauterine death of one fetus before 14 weeks usually results in complete resorption, as if the fetus has vanished.
- To improve fetal survival in multifetal pregnancy (especially following assisted reproductive technique), selective fetal reduction is done when there are 4 or more fetuses. Generally two fetuses are allowed to grow and the rest are destroyed.

## Q. How can you diagnose chorionicity of twin pregnancy and what is its significance?

**Ans.** Ultrasound scan around 10-12 weeks can identify "twin peaks" or "Lambda" sign a projection of placental tissue that grows into the interchorionic space of the two placentas. Presence of "twin peaks" sign indicates dichorionic placenta. Thickening of the intervening membrane >2 mm indicates dichorionic and diamniotic twins (Figs. 2.25 and 2.26A and B). It is the **"chorionicity"** not the "Zygosity" which is related to the degree of complications. This is the clinical significance.

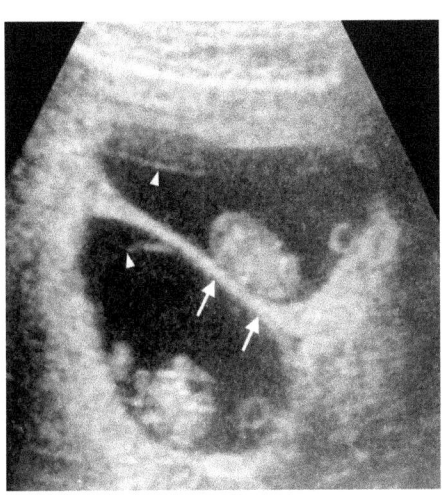

**Fig. 2.25:** Dichorionic, diamniotic twin gestation—"twin peak sign". Thick intertwin membrane confirms dichorionicity (arrows).

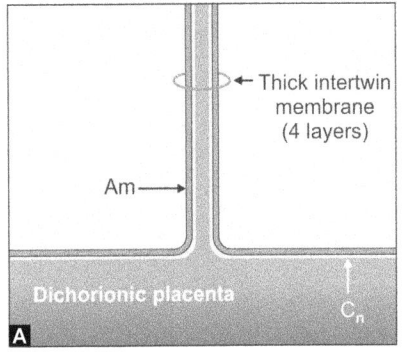
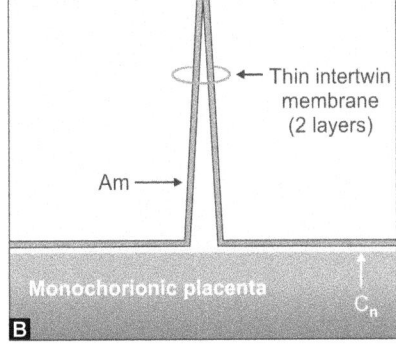

**Figs. 2.26A and B:** (A) Diagram of the "twin peak" sign. In dichorionic diamniotic twin gestations, the chorion and amnion for each twin reflect away from the fused placenta to form the intertwin membrane. A potential space exists in the intertwin membrane which is filled by proliferating placental villi giving rise to the twin peak sign. Twin peak sign appears as a triangle with the base at the chorionic surface and the apex in the intertwin membrane; (B) In monochorionic, diamniotic twins, the intertwin membrane is composed of two amnions only (Am, amnion; Cn, Chorion).

**Q. What is the pathology of twin-to-twin transfusion?**

**Ans.** It is seen in monozygotic twins (10–15%). One twin bleeds into the other twin through some kind of placental vascular anastomosis. As a result the donor twin is smaller, hypovolemic, anemic, hypotensive, with oligohydramnios. On the other hand the recipient twin is larger with hydramnios, polycythemic, plethoric, hypertensive and hypervolemic. This leads to anemia—polycythemia (Oli-Poly) syndrome.

**Q. What are the complications of TTTS?**

**Ans.** Death of one or both the fetuses depending upon the severity of twin-to-twin transfusion.

**Q. How can you manage a pregnancy with twin-to-twin transfusion?**

**Ans.**
- **Repeated amnio reduction** in the recipient twin to control polyhydramnios.
- **Laser photocoagulation** of the anastomotic vessels or laser division of the placenta.
- **Septostomy** of the intertwin membrane to make a hole between the two sacs. Septostomy equalizes the amniotic fluid pressure between the two sacs.
- **Selective feticide** by occlusion of the umbilical cord of the worse affected fetus to prevent exsanguination into the dead twin and placenta.

## CASE–14 | INTRAUTERINE FETAL DEATH

### Case Summary

*Mrs CM, 23 years old, P0 + 0 + 0 + 0, is admitted at 36 weeks pregnancy with the complaints of loss of fetal movements for the last 2 days. She had irregular antenatal supervision in the pregnancy. On examination, she is pale (mild), BP is 150/94 mm Hg with pedal edema. Obstetric examination revealed: Uterus 36 weeks size, uterus felt flaccid, single fetus, cephalic presentation. Clinically, liquor volume appeared to be reduced, FHS could not be localized on repeated examination using a stethoscope and also with a hand-held Doppler.*

**Q. What is your provisional diagnosis?**

**Ans.** The mother could not feel fetal movements for the last 2 days and the FHS could not be localized by repeated auscultation with a stethoscope or a hand-held Doppler. This raises the clinical suspicion of intrauterine demise of the fetus. However, the diagnosis needs to be confirmed by other investigations.

**Q. What other investigations do you recommend to confirm the diagnosis?**

**Ans.** Earliest diagnosis can be made by ultrasonography. Real time sonography is essential for accurate diagnosis of IUFD (RCOG-2011). Absence of fetal cardiac motion (real time) and all other body movements for a period of 5–10 minutes of careful observation with real time sonography is a presumptive evidence of fetal death.

Auscultation of FHR by stethoscope (Pinard) or Doppler is not accurate for diagnosis.

Other secondary features (on radiology) might be seen.

Spalding sign—irregular overlapping of cranial bones

(i) Hyperflexion of the spine

(ii) Crowding of the ribs

(iii) Appearance of gas shadow in the heart chambers and blood vessels (Robert's sign)

Usually these features take sometime (7–10 days) to appear, expect the Robert's sign (12 hours)

**Q. What are the common causes of IUFD?**

**Ans.** The fetal deaths are due to complications in pregnancy related to the mother, fetus or placenta. The important causes are:

**(A) Maternal (5–10%)**
- Hypertensive disorders
- Diabetes (Fig. 2.27)
- Maternal infections (malaria)

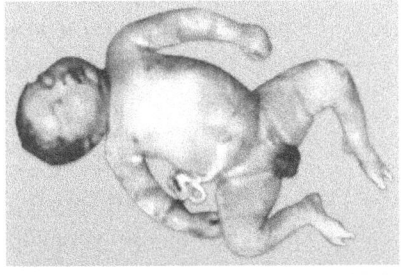

**Fig. 2.27:** Stillborn baby weighing 5.1 kg (macrosomic) of an uncontrolled diabetic mother.

- Severe anemia
- Hyperpyrexia
- Antiphospholipid syndrome.

**(B) Fetal (25–40%)**
- Chromosomal abnormalities
- Infections (rubella and CMV)
- Rh-incompatibility
- Birth defects (Fig. 2.28)

**(C) Placental (25–35%)**
- Antepartum hemorrhage
- Cord accident (true knot)
- Placental insufficiency

**(D) Unexplained (10–35%)**

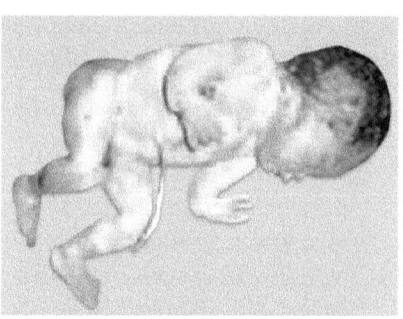

**Fig. 2.28:** IUFD due to multiple congenital (skeletal and visceral) malformations.

**Q. What are the clinical features suggestive of IUFD?**

**Ans. Symptoms:** Absence of fetal movements as noted by the mother.
**Signs:** Per abdomen:
(a) Regression of fundal height
(b) Uterine tone diminished
(c) Fetal movements not felt during palpation
(d) FHS is absent.
**Investigations:** Absence of cardiac motion on ultrasonography using **real time** is a strong presumptive evidence of fetal death.

**Q. What are the complications that may arise due to IUFD?**

**Ans.** (i) Psychological upset of the woman, (ii) onset of infection, (iii) blood coagulation disorders (rare), (iv) during labor—uterine inertia, retained placenta and postpartum hemorrhage.

**Q. How are you going to manage the woman with the IUFD?**

**Ans.** In about 80% of cases spontaneous expulsion occurs within 10–14 days of the fetal death. In certain cases, interference is needed. Termination of pregnancy when required should always be done by medical induction (oxytocin or/and prostaglandin).

**Methods of induction are:** Clinical examination of the woman including pelvic examination is done.

(A) Cervix favorable → Oxytocin infusion (IV)
Few cases may need repeat oxytocin (IV).

(B) Cervix unfavorable → $PGE_2$ gel intracervical or $PGE_1$ tab 25 µg–50 µg vaginally (may be repeated after 6–8 hours).
Tablet Mifepristone (200 mg) orally followed by vaginal $PGE_1$, has been found very effective. This regimen may be used as the first line choice.
Few patients may need oxytocin infusion in addition to vaginal prostaglandins.

(C) Once delivery occurs—evaluation of the stillbirth infant is to be done and bereavement management is also to be arranged.

**Q. What are the indications of early interference?**

Ans. Indications of early interference are:
   (a) Psychological upset of the woman (common)
   (b) Failure of expulsion of the dead fetus by 7–10 days
   (c) Evidence of uterine infection
   (d) Falling fibrinogen level.

**Q. What is the place of cesarean section in a case with IUFD?**

Ans. Very rare. The indications are:
   (a) Central placenta previa
   (b) previous cesarean scar (two or more).

**Q. What is the evaluation protocol of the stillborn?**

Ans. **Infant examination:** Malformations, maceration; **umbilical cord:** Entanglement of cord, number of cord vessels, cord prolapse, true knot (Fig. 2.29); **placenta:** Abnormalities and meconium staining.

**Q. What are the investigations protocol in a case with IUFD?**

Ans. To find out the cause of fetal death, the following investigations are commonly done:
   **Hematological:** Maternal blood for ABO, Rh, Kleihauer-Betke, VDRL, thyroid profile, blood sugar, HbAIC, anticardiolipin antibodies.
   Autopsy and cytogenetic study of the stillborn.

**Q. What bereavement care does the woman or the couple need?**

Ans. The bereaved couple is provided with all the support and sympathy. They are allowed to see the baby, if desired. The couple should be seen in the postpartum clinic after 6 weeks with the investigation reports. They are also counseled for future pregnancy. Their questions are answered in simple terms.

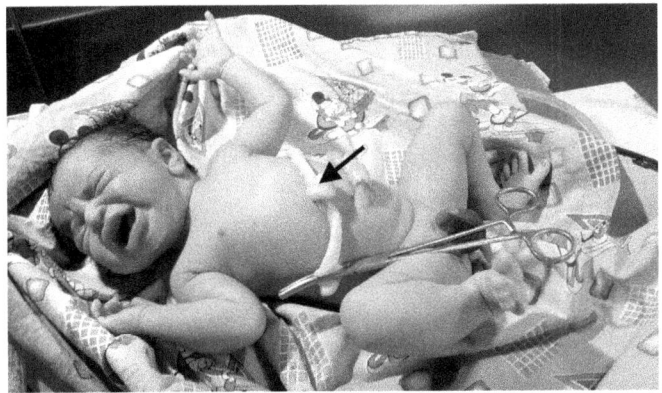

Fig. 2.29: True knot in the umbilical cord

**Q. In which condition, repeated induction may fail?**

Ans: Abdominal pregnancy.

## CASE-15 POLYHYDRAMNIOS

### Case Summary

*Mrs AC, 27 years old, para-1, gravida-2, miscarriage-0, living-1 (P1+0+0+1), admitted at 34 weeks of gestation with dyspnea, difficulty to walk and lie down due to huge enlargement of the abdomen. Clinical examination revealed: On inspection huge abdominal enlargement from symphysis pubis to xiphisternum. Maximum enlargement is observed at the level of the umbilicus. Symphysis-fundal height measured was 41 cm and the abdominal girth measured at the level of umbilicus was 122 cm. Palpation of fetal parts was difficult. Fluid thrill could be elicited. Clinically amount of liquor appeared more than normal. FHS could not be heard.*

**Q. What is your provisional diagnosis?**

**Ans.** Polyhydramnios/hydramnios (Fig. 2.30).

**Q. Mention the differential diagnosis of excessive uterine enlargement.**

**Ans.** The different causes for disproportionate enlargement of the uterus are:
(1) Wrong date
(2) Multiple pregnancy
(3) Big baby
(4) Pregnancy with pelvic tumors (fibroid or ovarian) and
(5) Maternal ascites.

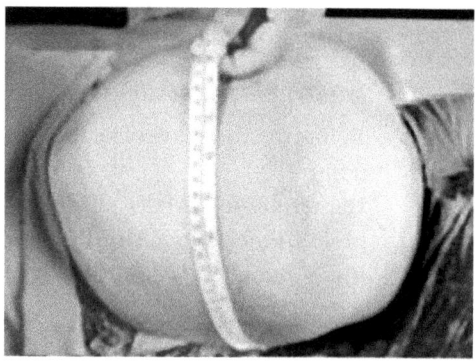

**Fig. 2.30:** Hugely enlarged abdomen (excess measurement of the girth of the abdomen around the umbilicus) due to polyhydramnios.

**Q. How do you define polyhydramnios?**

**Ans. Clinically:** Excessive volume of liquor causing discomfort to the patient and/or causing difficulties to the clinical diagnosis of the lie and presentation of the fetus.

**Anatomically:** When liquor amnii is >2,000 mL.

**Sonographically:** When the amniotic fluid index (AFI) is >24 cm (>95th percentile for gestational age) and a single deepest liquor pocket is >8 cm.

**Q. How can you confirm the diagnosis of polyhydramnios in your case?**

**Ans.** Clinically, it is suggested but ultrasonographic assessment would be the best way to confirm the diagnosis.

**Q. What are the common causes of polyhydramnios?**

Ans. (i) Fetal congenital malformations (20%): Anencephaly, open spina bifida, esophageal or duodenal atresia and fetal hydrops
(ii) Multiple pregnancy
(iii) Maternal diabetes
(iv) Idiopathic
(v) Chorioangioma of placenta.

**Q. What are the different fetal congenital anomalies seen with polyhydramnios?**

Ans. The major anomalies include anencephaly, open spina bifida, esophageal or duodenal atresia, diaphragmatic hernia, fetal hydrops and cardiac anomalies. Karyotyping would be worthwhile in some selected cases.

**Q. What are the different investigations that you plan to do in your case besides the routine ones?**

Ans. **Ultrasonography:** Confirms the diagnosis. It has also got other benefits:
(i) To exclude multiple pregnancy
(ii) To note the lie and presentation of the fetus
(iii) To diagnose fetal congenital malformations (mentioned above)
(iv) Placental localization.
**Blood:** Maternal blood glucose, ABO, Rh group (rhesus-alloimmunization).
**Amniocentesis:** Amniotic fluid for α-fetoprotein estimation. Fetuses with open neural tube defects have elevated AFP levels. Karyotyping would also be worthwhile.

**Q. What are the common obstetric complications in a case with polyhydramnios?**

Ans. **Maternal:**
(i) Pre-eclampsia
(ii) malpresentation
(iii) Premature rupture of membranes
(iv) Preterm labor
(v) Placental abruption
(vi) Cord prolapse
(vii) Uterine atony
(viii) Postpartum hemorrhage.

**Puerperium:**
(i) Subinvolution
(ii) Increased risk of infection and puerperal morbidity.

**Fetal:** Increased perinatal mortality (50%) due to congenital malformations and prematurity.

**Q. What could be the underlying basic pathology of polyhydramnios?**

Ans. Fetal urine and the amniotic epithelium secretion are the major sources of amniotic fluid and fetal swallowing is the major mode of absorption. Therefore either excessive production or deficient absorption is the basic underlying pathology. However, in about 60% of cases the etiopathology is unknown.

**Q. What is your plan of management in this case?**

Ans. Usually, **cases with mild degree of polyhydramnios do not require any active intervention.** But cases with severe degree polyhydramnios, the woman needs to be admitted. My plan is to do the investigations as early as possible. Aim of investigations is to look for any cause of polyhydramnios like fetal congenital malformation, maternal diabetes, rhesus isoimmunization, etc. Subsequent management would be according to the pathology:

(a) **When fetal congenital malformation is present**—delivery is an option with counseling. In that case, cervical ripening may be done by using $PGE_2$ gel intracervically.

(b) **When fetal malformation is absent**—pregnancy may be continued till 37 weeks (as she is <37 week of gestation now). Management will be done if any complicating factor (diabetes mellitus) is detected. As this woman is having cardiorespiratory embarrassment, amnioreduction (1-1.5 liters) may be done slowly under ultrasonographic guidance to relieve her symptoms. Once she reaches ≥37 weeks, delivery is to be planned.

Cervical ripening may be done using intracervical $PGE_2$ gel followed by controlled artificial rupture of membranes. Oxytocin infusion may be started if contractions are poor.

**Q. What complication may arise in such a case during the third stage of labor and how do you prevent it?**

Ans. Atonic postpartum hemorrhage is a significant complication. To prevent this complication, active management of third stage of labor should be done. For this reason she should be delivered in an equipped center.

## OLIGOHYDRAMNIOS

**Q. What are the functions of the amniotic fluid?**

Ans. **During pregnancy:**
  (A) **Physical functions are:**
   (a) Maintain the temperature around the fetus
   (b) Allows fetal movements
   (c) Allows fetal breathing movements and prevents pulmonary hypoplasia
   (d) Swallowing allows movements of the digestive tract
   (e) It allow functions of the urinary tract (formation of urine)

(f) Protects against fetal injury
(g) Nutritive value is less.

**(B) During labor:**
(a) Helps dilation of the cervix by forming the bag of forewater
(b) Flushes the birth canal before delivery at the end of first stage of labor
(c) It has bacteriocidal action and protects the fetus against infection
(d) Study of amniotic fluid is done for well being of the fetus and the maturity of the fetus also.

**Q. What is amniotic fluid index and what is its significance?**

**Ans.** Maternal abdomen is divided into quadrants taking the umbilicus, symphysis pubis and the fundus as the reference points. With ultrasound, the largest vertical pocket in each quadrant is measured. The sum of the four measurements (cm) is the amniotic fluid index (AFI). It is measured to diagnose the clinical condition of polyhydramnios or oligohydramnios, respectively.

**Q. What is oligohydramnios?**

**Ans.** Clinically when the liquor volume is deficient (<200 mL at term) and the AFI is <5 (<10th percentile) or maximum vertical liquor pool is <2 cm.

**Q. What are the common causes of oligohydramnios?**

**Ans.** Common causes:
(A) **Fetal:** (i) Fetal chromosomal anomalies, (ii) fetal malformations (renal agenesis, obstruction of the urinary tract).
(B) **Maternal:** Hypertension in pregnancy.
(C) **Others:** (i) Placental insufficiency (IUGR), (ii) drugs (ACE inhibitor), (iii) postmaturity, and (iv) intrauterine infection.
(D) **Idiopathic**

**Q. Mention the fetal complications due to oligohydramnios.**

**Ans.**
(i) Increased risk of miscarriage or preterm delivery
(ii) Fetal deformity (club foot, skull deformity)
(iii) Fetal pulmonary hypoplasia
(iv) Cord compression
(v) Meconium-stained liquor
(vi) Increased risks of fetal distress in labor, stillbirth, and neonatal death
(vii) High neonatal complications.

**Q. How do you manage a case of oligohydramnios?**

**Ans.** (A) Presence of fetal congenital malformations: Couple counseling and delivery.
(B) Isolated and late onset oligohydramnios: This may be managed conservatively with careful monitoring. Increase in oral fluids intake, amniofusion have been tried to improve the outcome. Delivery is done with completion of 37 weeks.
(C) Women with oligohydramnios and abnormal Doppler ultrasound: This indicates placental insufficiency and needs urgent delivery.

## CASE–16  ANTEPARTUM HEMORRHAGE (PLACENTA PREVIA)

**Q. What are the causes of vaginal bleeding in later months of pregnancy?**

**Ans.** (a) **Placental bleeding (70%):** (i) Placenta previa (Fig. 2.37) and (ii) Abruptio placentae.
(b) **Extraplacental bleeding (5%):** Cervical polyp, ectopy, cervical carcinoma and local trauma.
(c) **Unexplained (25%).**

**Q. Define antepartum hemorrhage.**

**Ans.** It is the bleeding from or within the genital tract after 28th week of pregnancy but before the birth of the baby.

## PLACENTA PREVIA

### Case Summary

*Mrs CR, 26 years old, was P1+0+0+1 was admitted at 35 weeks of gestation with painless recurrent, fresh vaginal bleeding. Her general physical examination revealed: Pulse—96/min, BP—110/70 mm Hg, and mild pallor. Her cardiovascular and respiratory systems were normal. Obstetric examination revealed: Uterus 36 weeks, relaxed, SFH 36 cm, single fetus, cephalic presentation free, liquor adequate and FHS was 146 beats/minute and was regular. On vulval inspection, slight fresh bleeding per vaginam was still present.*

**Q. What is the clinical diagnosis?**

**Ans.** Antepartum hemorrhage, most likely placenta previa.

**Q. How do you define placenta previa?**

**Ans.** When the placenta is implanted partially or completely over the lower uterine segment it is cell placenta previa.

**From management point of view it is classified as:**
(A) **Low lying placenta:** When placental edge lies in the lower uterine segment within 20 mm of the internal os but does not cover the internal os. It is diagnosed using either transabdominal or transvaginal sonography after 16 weeks of pregnancy (RCOG 2018).
(B) **Placenta previa:** When the placenta covers the internal os directly and completely.

**Q. What are the types of placenta previa?**

**Ans.** (1) **Marginal:** Edge of the placenta near the internal os, but does not cover it.
(2) **Partial:** Placenta covers the internal os partially.
(3) **Complete:** Placenta covers the internal os completely.

**Q. What is the cause of bleeding in placenta previa?**

**Ans.** The inelastic placenta is separated from the wall of the lower uterine segment as it progressively enlarges in later months. This leads to opening up of the uteroplacental vessels and leads to bleeding.

**Q. What are the complications of placenta previa?**

**Ans.** Complications are both to the mother and fetus.

| Maternal complications | Fetal complications |
|---|---|
| • Severe antepartum hemorrhage may lead to shock | • Low birth weight babies |
| • Preterm labor | • Asphyxia, fetal growth restriction |
| • Hemorrhage during labor (intrapartum) | • Intrauterine fetal death |
| • Increased risk cesarean delivery | • Birth injuries |
| • Increased risk of retained placenta → placenta accreta → requiring hysterectomy | • Congenital malformations |
| • Postpartum hemorrhage | • Fetal anemia |
| • Postpartum sepsis | • Fetal exsanguination |
| • Increased maternal mortality<br>• Increased need of blood transfusion | • Increased perinatal mortality |

**Q. How does a woman with placenta previa present?**

**Ans.** Painless, sudden onset, apparently causeless and recurrent vaginal bleeding is the hallmark of diagnosis of placenta previa. Bleeding is fresh and without any uterine contractions.

**Q. How should a case of placenta previa be diagnosed?**

**Ans.** Vaginal examination is contraindicated in a case with placenta previa. It may cause further bleeding. **Ultrasonography** is the mainstay of diagnosis. Transabdominal ultrasonography (TAS) is accurate in about 98% of cases (Fig. 2.31). Transvaginal sonography (TVS) is more accurate than TAS.

**Magnetic resonance imaging (MRI)** is a noninvasive method. It is superior to USG in the diagnosis. It is especially helpful in cases with placenta previa accreta, or placenta previa percreta with bladder invasion.

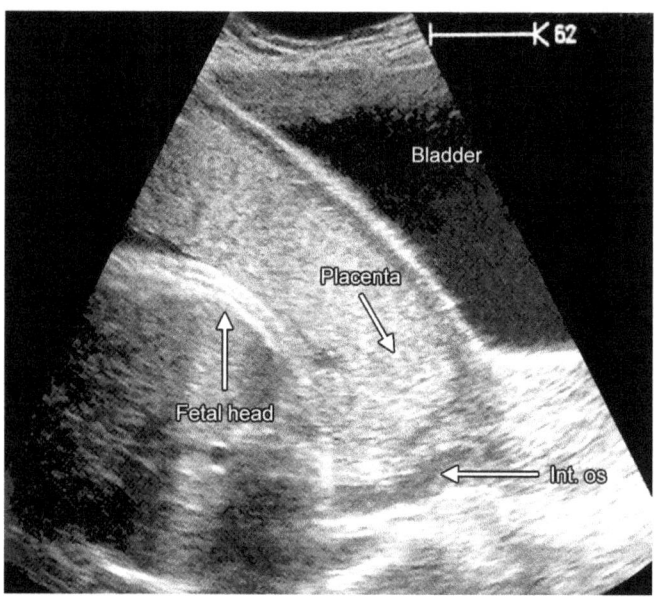

**Fig. 2.31:** Transabdominal sonogram showing anterior placenta previa (Type-II).

**Q. What are the benefits of USG and MRI in a case with placenta previa?**

**Ans.** USG and MRI (i) reduce the need of unnecessary vaginal examination and the risk of bleeding, (ii) can make the diagnosis of placenta accreta and percreta. (iii) help to make the plan of delivery accordingly.

**Q. How is case of placenta previa managed?**

**Ans.** All cases with APH are to be admitted. Maternal and fetal conditions are evaluated. USG is done for placental localization and fetoplacental unit. Large bore IV cannula is sited. Blood is sent for complete hemogram, ABO, Rh grouping, coagulation profile and cross-matching. Maternal hemodynamic stabilization is done with aggressive crystalloids and blood replacement when needed. A large bore IV canmula is sited. Actual management is:

(a) **Active interference:** This is done in cases when:
- Vaginal bleeding continues
- Pregnancy ≥37 weeks
- Patient in labor
- Fetus is dead
- Fetus is congenitally malformed

Steriod (betamethasone therapy is given to accelerate pulmonary maturity when pregnancy is <37 weeks)

(b) **Expectant management:** Mcafee regimen—this is done in cases when:
- No active vaginal bleeding
- Pregnancy is <37 weeks
- Patient is hemodynamically stable and with CTG-reactive fetus.

Aim is to continue pregnancy to 37 weeks or at least to 34 weeks.

Mode of delivery in either of the mentioned here two groups may be:
(a) **Cesarean section** when placenta is Type II (posterior) Type III or IV. **However, all cases of placenta previa, where placenta encroaches within 2 cm of the internal os, cesarean section is recommended (RCOG 2008).**
(b) **Vaginal delivery** in cases with minor degree placenta previa and with spontaneous onset of labor may be allowed. Induction may be done with ARM ± oxytocin (in cases with Type I or II anterior placenta
   However, all cases considered for vaginal delivery need close monitoring. Such a case may need cesarean section if there is any obstetric indication (vaginal bleeding).
   **Woman should be given steroid therapy if pregnancy at the time of delivery is <37 weeks.**

**Q. Is there any special arrangement for cesarean delivery in such a case?**

Ans. Yes, cesarean delivery in this patient needs a special arrangement to be organized beforehand. Operation should preferably be done by a senior obstetrician. Prior blood arrangement is essential. Type of uterine incision depends upon the type of placenta previa. Patient should be counseled as regard to the risk of morbid adherent placenta and the need of emergency hysterectomy.

**Q. What is the relationship between previous cesarean section and incidence of placenta accreta?**

Ans. The risk increases with number of prior cesarean delivery. Risk of placenta accreta is around 11% when the women has got one previous cesarean delivery. It rises to 61% when she has got prior three cesarean delivery.

**Q. What is the risk of recurrence for placenta previa?**

Ans. Overall incidence of placenta previa is 0.3%. Recurrence risk is about 2.4% (8-fold increase).

**Q. What is the place of tocolytic drugs in the management of placenta previa?**

Ans. Tocolytic drugs are not commonly used specially when the decision for termination of pregnancy (delivery) has been made. Tocolysis can be used when time of 48 hours is needed for the steroid therapy to be effectively completed.

**Q. Is there a place for cervical cerclage in women with placenta previa or a low-lying placenta?**

Ans. Use of cervical cerclage in the management for the purpose of controlling the bleeding and/or prolonging pregnancy has not been found effective.

**Q. How do you differentiate placenta previa from abruptio placenta?**

Ans. Placental abruption is characterized by the followings: Association of pain abdomen, pre-eclampsia, blood is of dark color and not bright red. On examination: Uterus is tender, tense and rigid. Fundal height is increased. FHS may be absent. On USG, the placenta is situated in the upper segment of the uterus. Retroplacental blood clot may be seen.

## CASE–17 | ABRUPTIO PLACENTAE (Accidental Hemorrhage)

### Case Summary

*Mrs AR, 34 years old (P3+0+0+3) was admitted at 34 weeks of gestation with the complaints of abdominal pain and vaginal bleeding. She was hemodynamically stable. On general physical examination: Pulse—100/minute and BP—140/90 mm Hg, marked pallor and mild pedal edema. Her cardiovascular and respiratory systems were normal. Obstetric examination revealed: Uterus 36 weeks size, tense, tender and rigid. SFH 37 cm, single fetus, cephalic presentation, FHS could not be localized. On vulval inspection, slight vaginal bleeding was present. It looked dark in color.*

**Q. What is your clinical diagnosis?**

**Ans.** Antepartum hemorrhage, most likely abruptio placentae.

**Q. Why do you say so?**

**Ans.** This multiparous woman presents with abdominal pain and vaginal bleeding. She is hypertensive. Her uterus is tense, tender and rigid. SFH is more than the period of amenorrhea. FHS could not be localized. The vaginal bleeding is dark in color. All these suggests the clinical diagnosis of abruptio placentae.

**Q. What is placental abruption?**

**Ans.** It is the premature separation of a normally implanted placenta before delivery of the fetus. It may be:
(i) **Revealed type:** When the bleeding comes out of the cervical canal and is visible externally (90%), (ii) **Concealed type:** When the hemorrhage is concealed (10%) and (iii) **Mixed type.**

**Q. What are the complications of abruptio placentae?**

**Ans.** Complications occur both in the mother and fetus.

| Maternal | Fetal |
| --- | --- |
| ♦ Hemorrhage (antepartum) | ♦ Prematurity |
| ♦ Disseminated intravascular coagulation (DIC) | ♦ Fetal death |
| ♦ Shock | ♦ Hypoxia |
| ♦ Oliguria and anuria—renal failure | ♦ Fetal anemia |
| ♦ Hemorrhage (postpartum) | ♦ Intrauterine growth restriction |
| ♦ Puerperal sepsis | ♦ Low birth weight |
| ♦ Increased maternal mortality | ♦ Increase perinatal mortality |

**Q. What are the common causes of abruptio placentae?**

**Ans.**  (i) Hypertension in pregnancy
(ii) Increasing parity
(iii) Increasing maternal age
(iv) Smoking

(v) Short cord
(vi) Folic acid deficiency
(vii) Thrombophilias, and
(viii) Placental abnormalities (circumvallate placenta).

**Q. How clinically is a case of placental abruption suspected?**

**Ans.** Woman presents with vaginal bleeding in second or third trimester of pregnancy (90%). It is associated with abdominal pain, uterine tenderness and often with a dead fetus.

**Q. Is ultrasound helpful to confirm the diagnosis?**

**Ans.** Ultrasonography is useful to exclude the diagnosis of placenta previa. But it can neither confirm nor can exclude the diagnosis of abruptio placentae.

**Q. How do you differentiate placental abruption from placenta previa?**

**Ans: Placental abruption** is differentiated from **placenta previa** mainly with clinical presentation.

**Diagnostic clinical features in a case with placental abruptions (Fig. 2.32) are:**

(a) Vaginal bleeding is associated with **abdominal pain**. Whereas in a case with placenta previa the bleeding **is painless**.
(b) Often it is associated with **pre-eclampsia**.
(c) The blood is of **dark in color**. In a case with placenta previa the bleeding is fresh and red.

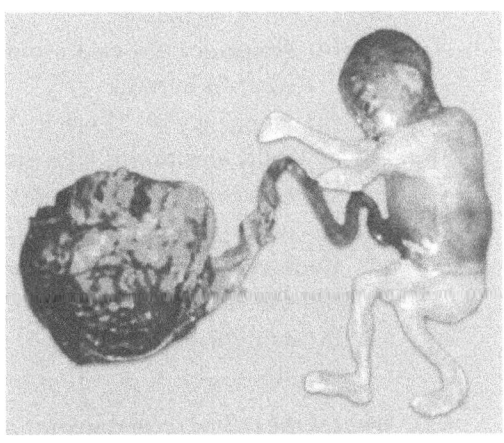

Fig. 2.32: Fetal death due to placental abruption. Retroplacental clots are seen.

(d) The **height of the uterus is increased** (concealed variety).
(e) The uterus feels **tense, rigid and tender**. In placenta previa the uterus is soft and relaxed.
(f) Fetal heart sound **may be absent** (as there is fetal death in majority of the cases).
(g) Sonography—placenta is in the upper segment whereas in a case with placenta previa, placenta is seen in the lower uterine segment.

**Q. What is the source of bleeding in placental abruption?**

**Ans.** It is mainly the maternal bleeding. But it may be either maternal or fetal in origin.

**Q. How should a case of abruptio placentae be managed?**

**Ans.** All cases of abruptio placentae are to be admitted. Maternal and fetal conditions are evaluated. A wide bore cannula is sited. Blood is sent for complete hemogram, coagulation profile, ABO, Rh grouping and cross-matching. Resuscitation is started with IV crystalloid solutions, cross-match, blood transfusion and $O_2$ administration. An urinary catheter is placed and urine output is monitored hourly. Fetal evaluation is done with USG and CTG.

*Actual Management*

(A) **Concealed variety with increase in symphysis-fundal height**

**Delivery**
  (i) Patient in labor → ARM ± oxytocin (it is commonly done)
  (ii) Patient not in labor and/or unfavorable cervix → cesarean delivery.

(B) **Revealed variety:**
  (i) Patient is in labor → delivery
  (ii) Patient is not in labor:
    (a) Pregnancy ≥34 weeks → delivery either by ARM ± oxytocin or by cesarean section;
    (b) Pregnancy is <34 weeks: Bleeding stops, fetus remote from term, mild abruption, CTG reactive fetus → may be considered for expectant management to get the benefit of steroid therapy. She is given steroid therapy if pregnancy is <37 weeks.

  **Conservative management of placental abruption is an exception, not the rule.** The patient is closely monitored while admitted, only to attain the fetal maturity or to buy time to get the benefit of steroid therapy.

**Q. What is the risk of recurrence for placental abruption?**

**Ans.** The overall risk of recurrence is 6–17% in subsequent pregnancy.

**Q. What is a Couvelaire uterus?**

**Ans.** It is a pathological condition of the uterus seen in a woman during laparotomy following massive placental abruption. There is widespread extravasation of blood into uterine musculature up to the serosa. The uterus appears bluish in color.

**Q. Is Couvelaire uterus an indication of hysterectomy?**

**Ans.** Generally the condition does not interfere with the uterine myometrial contractions. Usually this condition does not lead to postpartum hemorrhage. Couvelaire uterus is not an indication of hysterectomy.

# OBSTETRIC COMPLICATIONS

## CASE–18 | POSTPARTUM HEMORRHAGE—PREVENTION AND MANAGEMENT

Obstetric hemorrhage (mainly antepartum and/or postpartum) is a leading cause of maternal death in both developed and developing countries (*see* p. 340). Primary postpartum hemorrhage (PPH) is most common.

**Q. How do you define PPH?**

**Ans.** Amount of blood loss 500 mL or more following birth of the baby is defined as PPH (WHO). The clinical definition states "any amount of bleeding from or within the genital tract following birth of the baby up to the end of puerperium which adversely affects the general condition of the mother as evidenced by rise in pulse rate or falling in blood pressure is called post-partum hemorrhage".

**Q. How do you define primary PPH?**

**Ans.** Primary postpartum hemorrhage is defined as the hemorrhage that occurs within 24 hours following birth of the baby. It may be before (third stage hemorrhage) or after (true PPH) expulsion of the placenta.

Depending upon the amount of blood loss PPH can be: (A) Minor (<1 L), (B) major (>1 L) or (C) severe (>2 L). Estimation of blood loss by inspection only is often underestimated. Accurate methods are blood collected in drapes and weighing the swabs.

## Case Summary

*Mrs Balamma, 30 years old (P3-G4-A1-L3) had her vaginal delivery at home with the SBA. She started bleeding following delivery of the placenta. Placenta was found complete on examination. She was rushed to the hospital and was admitted as an emergency.*

**Q. What is this clinical condition called?**

**Ans.** Primary postpartum hemorrhage (true).

**Q. What are the important causes of PPH?**

**Ans.** Causes can be divided under the heads of **'four Ts'**:
(1) Tone (atonic uterus)
(2) Trauma (genital tract)
(3) Tissue (retained products of conception)
(4) Thrombin (coagulopathy).
**The most common cause of primary PPH is atonic uterus (80%).**

**Q. What is the major concern about PPH?**

**Ans.** Obstetric hemorrhage is the major cause of maternal deaths in both developed and developing countries. PPH is the lead cause of maternal mortality in India. However, maternal mortality due to PPH is a preventable condition.

**Q. What are the high-risk factors of PPH?**

**Ans.** High-risk factors of PPH are:
  (a) Grand multipara
  (b) Overenlargement of uterus—multiple pregnancy and hydramnios
  (c) Anemia
  (d) Antepartum hemorrhage
  (e) Prolonged labor
  (f) Morbidly adherent placenta
  (g) Genital tract trauma.

**Q. What should you do immediately to manage a case of major primary PPH?**

**Ans.**
- To alert obstetric and anesthetic seniors and the on-duty midwife (call for help).
- To start IV infusion with crystalloids (Ringer's solution) putting two large bore (14-gauge) cannulas (up to 2 liters).
- To send blood for ABO, Rh grouping, cross-matching and to ask for at least 2 units of blood.
- To give $O_2$ by face mask at 10–15 liters/minute, keeping the patient flat.
- To start 40 units of oxytocin in 1 liter of normal saline, IV at the rate of 60 drops/minute.
- Continuous catheterization (Foley catheter), to monitor hourly urine output.
- To transfuse blood as soon as available.

**Q. What is the other medical management available for atonic PPH?**

**Ans.**
- To massage the uterus (fundus) to simulate uterine contractions
- To start oxytocin infusion (discussed above)
- Use of other oxytocics:
  (a) Injection methergin 0.2 mg IV
  (b) Injection carboprost ($PGF_{2\alpha}$) 250 μg IM may be repeated at intervals (>15 minutes), maximum 8 doses. Injection carboprost 250 μg intramyometrial may be given.
  (c) Misoprostol ($PGE_1$) 1,000 mg can be given rectally.

**Q. Besides atonic hemorrhage, what other conditions must be excluded?**

**Ans.**
- Retained products of conception (placenta, clots and membranes).
- Genital tract injury (cervix, vagina and perineum).
- Broad ligament hematoma.
- Ruptured uterus.
- Coagulation failure (rare).

**Q. What are the different surgical measures that can be taken to control the hemorrhage?**

**Ans.**
- **Exploration** of the uterus under general anesthesia.
- **To repair** any injury of the genital tract (cervix, vagina, perineum).
- **Compression of the aorta:**
  - The abdominal aorta may be compressed against the spine (Fig. 2.33) this may reduce the bleeding.
- **Uterine tamponade:**
  - Balloon tamponade is **ideal and is the first line surgical management for atonic PPH.** It is done by using different types of hydrostatic balloon catheter (Foley catheter, Bakri balloon (Fig. 2.34), Condom catheter, Sangstaken-Blakemore esophageal catheter). Balloon is inflated with 200–500 mL saline. This is effective and can avoid hysterectomy in 78% cases. The balloon tamponade is kept 4–6 hours for hemostasis. Balloon is deflated before it is removed.
  - Tight intrauterine packing.
  - Bimanual compression.
  - Compression of the aorta may be a temporary but effective measure to allow sometime for resuscitation.
- **Uterine compression sutures**
  - Uterine compression sutures are found to be effective in cases with atonic PPH. External compression sutures have been popularized by Dr B Lynch and Cho. With these methods uterus could be preserved. Large absorbable sutures (such as Catgut No. 2) are used to bind the uterus and force compression of the bleeding sinuses. In B-Lynch

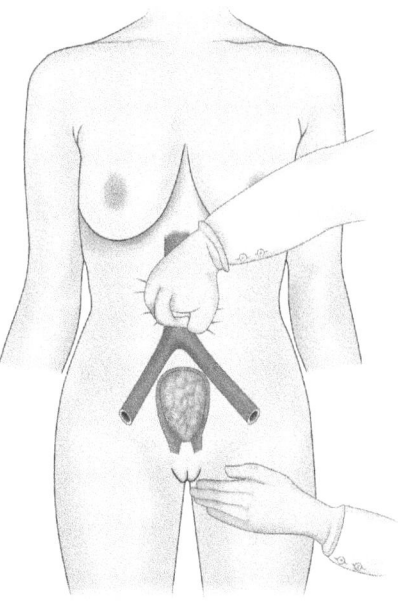

Fig. 2.33: Compression of the aorta.

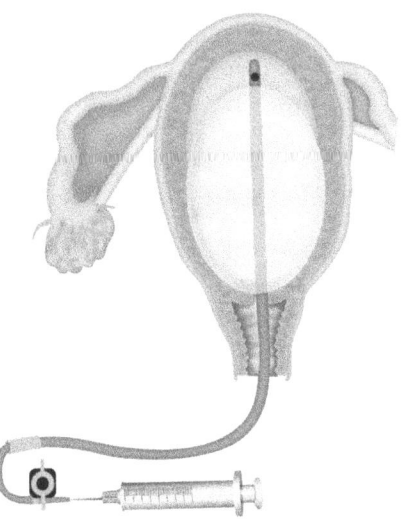

Fig. 2.34: Balloon temponade.

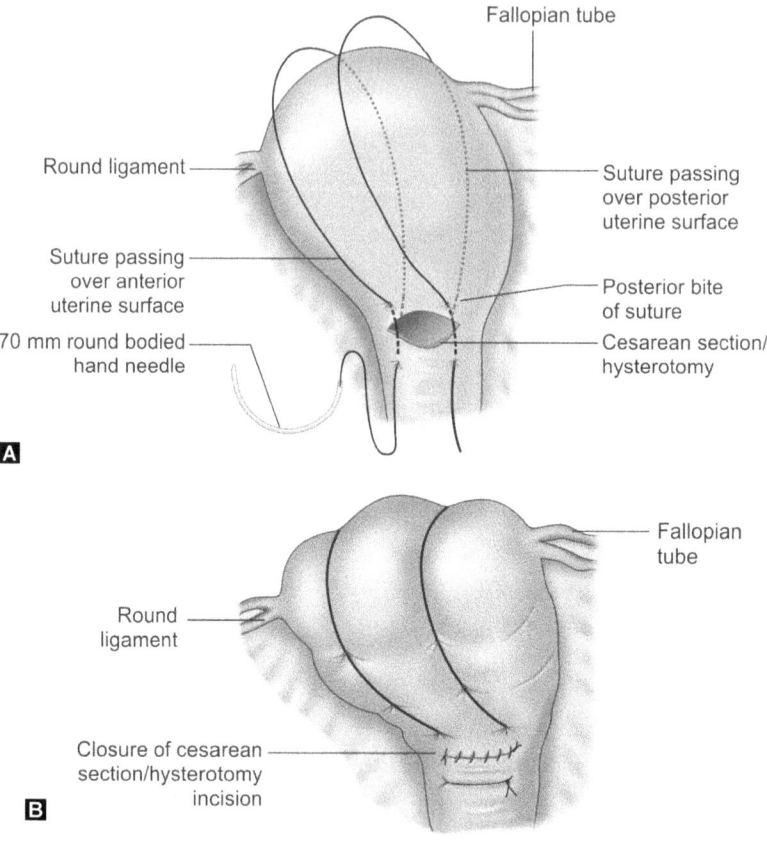

**Figs. 2.35A and B:** Application of the B-Lynch technique.

technique whole of the uterus is compressed (Figs. 2.35A and B). In the Cho "square Sutures" technique, areas of posterior and anterior myometrium are sutured together to force compression (Fig. 2.36).

- Hemostatic brace (compression) suture (B-Lynch, 1997 or its modifications—successful in 81% cases). Hemostatic suture techniques are effective in controlling severe PPH. This can reduce the need of hysterectomy.
- Procedure of B-Lynch suture (Christopher B-Lynch, 1997):
  (1) The suture commonly used is No. 2 chronic catgut on round bodied needle (70–80 mm)
  (2) The suture is passed 3 cm below the lower incision margin on the left side.
  (3) It is passed through the uterine cavity and taken out 3 cm above the upper cut margin. Both these points are about 4 cm medial to the lateral border of the uterus.

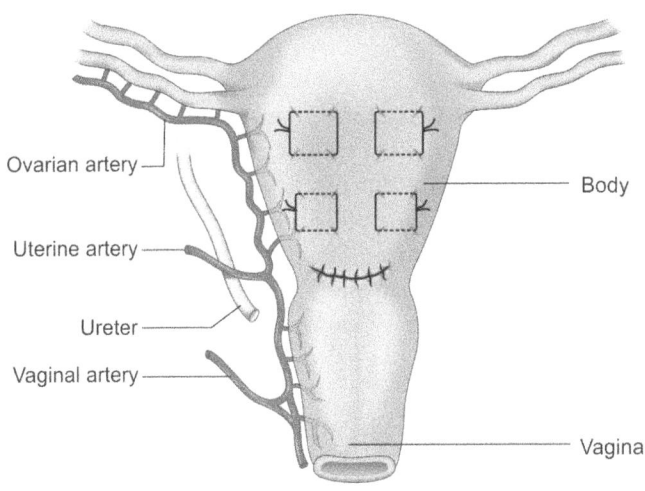

**Fig. 2.36:** Cho "Square sutures" technique.

(4) The suture is passed over the posterior surface of the uterus and over the uterine fundus (4 cm medical to the uterine cornua).
- **Uterine devascularization procedures:** Bilateral ligation of uterine or utero-ovarian vessels.
- **Internal iliac artery ligation:** Bilateral is an effective method to control PPH. However, balloon tamponade and hemostatic suturing methods are simpler and much easier to perform.
- **Selective arterial embolization or occlusion** has been found successful in 97% of cases of PPH. However, it needs the equipment and an interventional radiologist. Arterial embolization for control of PPH does not impair subsequent menstruation and fertility.
- **Hysterectomy** (sooner than later). A second consultant/senior obstetrician should be involved in decision-making.
- Once bleeding is controlled, patient is observed in an ICU or in high dependency unit.

**Q.** *Mention the different preventive measures for PPH?*

**Ans.** Preventive measures may be there in the antenatal and in the intrapartum period.
However, most cases of PPH have no identifiable risk factors.
(A) **Antenatal preventive measures:**
- Improvement of anemia
- Blood group and Rh typing for all women
- Localization of placenta by ultrasonography in women with prior cesarean delivery.

(B) **Intrapartum preventive measures:**
- Active management of third stage of labor
- Prophylactic oxytocic for women with high-risk factors for PPH (oxytocin 5 IU, IM) in the third stage of labor is the drug of choice.

**Q. Considering the importance of PPH management, how should the labor ward staff be trained?**

**Ans.** Important issues are:
- (A) **Regular drill of PPH management** should be organized to improve the skill and competence of labor ward staff.
- (B) **Accurate documentation** of sequence of events is very important. Time of onset of events, time of start of treatment to record the category of staff involved, clinical condition of the patient, monitoring parameters, management issues are all docuemented. Careful documentation can avoid many litigation problems.

## CASE–19 HEMORRHAGE IN EARLY PREGNANCY

### Case Summary

*Mrs AR, A 30-year-old lady was admitted due to the problems of recurrent episodes of vaginal bleeding for last one week. Her last menstrual period was 8 weeks back. Urine pregnancy was positive when done 2 weeks ago. She perceived some amount of pain in the lower abdomen also.*

**Q. What is your provisional diagnosis?**

**Ans.** She may be a case of threatened miscarriage.

**Q. What are the common causes of hemorrhage in early pregnancy?**

**Ans.** The causes are divided into two groups:
- (A) **Related to pregnancy:** (i) Abortion (95%), (ii) ectopic pregnancy, (iii) hydatidiform mole, and sometimes (iv) implantation bleeding.
- (B) **Other causes not related to pregnancy:** (i) Cervical pathology—cervical ectopy, polyp or malignancy.

**Q. What are the different types of abortions?**

**Ans.** Abortion may be: (A) Spontaneous (miscarriage), or (B) induced.
- (A) Spontaneous abortion or miscarriage may be further classified into: (a) Threatened, (b) inevitable, (c) complete, (d) incomplete, (e) missed and (f) septic.
  Spontaneous abortion may again be: (1) Isolated, or (2) recurrent.
- (B) Induced abortion may be: (1) Legal (MTP), and (2) illegal, criminal or unsafe.

**Q. What is a threatened miscarriage?**

**Ans.** When the process of miscarriage has started but continuation of pregnancy is still possible.

**Q. How clinically is a threatened miscarriage diagnosed?**

**Ans.** Clinically the patient presents with (a) bleeding per vaginum, (b) pain in the lower abdomen, (c) on speculum examination, slight bleeding from the external os and (d) on pelvic examination, uterine size corresponds to the period of amenorrhea.

**Q. How do you confirm the diagnosis?**

**Ans.** Transvaginal sonography (TVS) reveals a well-defined gestational sac within the uterine cavity. Depending on the gestational age, gestational sac diameter, fetal node (CRL measurement), yolk sac, cardiac motion and fetal outline may be seen.

**Q. What is an anembryoinic pregnancy (silent miscarriage)?**

**Ans.** It is a sonographic diagnosis of a pregnancy without a fetus.

**Q. How is anembryonic pregnancy diagnosed?**

**Ans.** Clinically, uterine size is less than the period of amenorrhea. There is lack of uterine growth. On ultrasound (TVS), there is absence of fetal pole within the gestational sac even with a diameter of 3 cm or more (Fig. 2.37). There is discrepancy between gestational sac development and the embryonic development.

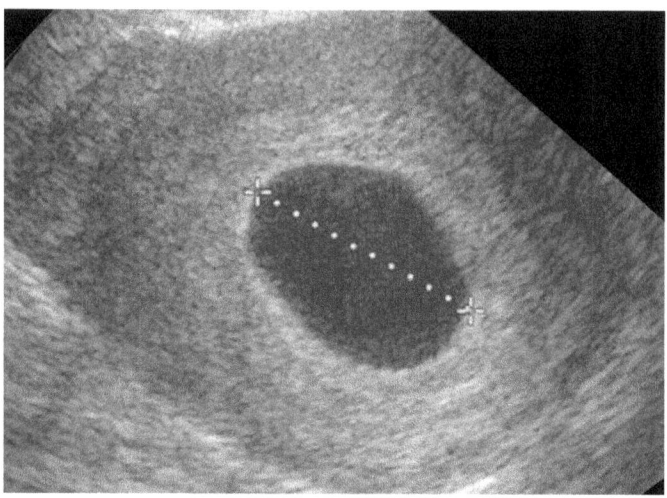

Fig. 2.37: Blighted ovum.

**Q. What is the management outline for a case with anembryonic pregnancy?**

**Ans.** Suction evacuation or dilation and evacuation is done. Alternatively, medical methods can be used to terminate the pregnancy.

**Q. What is an inevitable miscarriage?**

**Ans.** It is a clinical type of miscarriage where the abortion process has progressed to a state wherefrom continuation of pregnancy is impossible. Sometimes products of conception may be seen to come out through the external os.

**Q. How can you make the diagnosis clinically?**

**Ans.** Clinically the patient presents with (a) increased vaginal bleeding, (b) increased lower abdominal pain, (c) on internal examination: Internal os is dilated through which the products of conception can be felt. Same observation is made while sonography is done (*See* p. 118).

**Q. How do you manage a case of inevitable abortion?**

**Ans.** Abortion process is to be expedited.
  (a) Pregnancy is ≤12 weeks: Suction evacuation or dilation and evacuation followed by curettage is done under general anesthesia.
  (b) Pregnancy is >12 weeks: Oxytocin drip IV is started. This is followed by evacuation of the uterus.

**Q. What is a complete miscarriage?**

**Ans.** When the products of conception are expelled completely, it is called complete miscarriage.

**Q. What is a missed miscarriage?**

**Ans.** When the fetus is dead and is retained inside the uterus for a variable period of time. It is also known as early fetal demise.

**Q. What is a septic abortion?**

**Ans.** Any abortion process when complicated with features of infection (sepsis) of its contents either local (uterus) or systemic is called septic abortion. Sepsis may be so severe as to cause death of the woman.

**Q. What is a recurrent miscarriage?**

**Ans.** Three or more consecutive miscarriages (spontaneous abortions) before 20 weeks of pregnancy in a woman is defined as recurrent miscarriage.

**Q. How a case of ectopic pregnancy could be suggested?**

**Ans.** Ultrasonography is the mainstay in the diagnosis of an ectopic pregnancy. In an early intrauterine pregnancy, early pregnancy failure, or ectopic pregnancy, it is not always possible to identify the gestational sac.
  (1) Negative serum β-hCG excludes a live pregnancy by all means.
  (2) Ectopic pregnancy is mostly excluded with the demonstration of an intrauterine pregnancy (IUP) which reduces the risk of co-existent ectopic pregnancy (1 in 7,000)
  (3) When there is no sonographic evidence of an IUP, the pregnant patient is more likely to have an extrauterine gestation.
  (4) The sonographic demonstration of a live embryo in the adnexa is specific for the diagnosis of ectopic pregnancy.
  (5) Doppler ultrasound and in particular color flow Doppler imaging may further help to distinguish a gestational sac from pseudosac.

**Q. How do you diagnose a ectopic pregnancy by USG?**

**Ans.** TVS is the gold standard. The diagnostic features are:
  (a) Absence of an intrauterine pregnancy (IUP) with a positive pregnancy test.
  (b) Fluid (echogenic) in the pouch of Douglas.
  (c) Adnexal mass seen clearly separated from the ovary (Blob sign)
  (d) Rarely cardiac motion may be seen in an unruptured tubal ectopic Pregnancy
Doppler USG shows peritrophoblastic flow.

***Q. What are the diagnostic features of pregnancy of unknown viability on TVS?***

**Ans.** The diagnostic features of pregnancy of unknown viability (NICE, RCOG, ACR, RANZCOG) are:
  (a) Intrauterine gestational sac (IUGS) with MSD ≤ 25 mm without visible yolk sac/embryonic pole.
  (b) IUGS containing an embryo with CRL ≤ 7 mm but no cardiac activity.
  (c) Intrauterine gestation sac of ≤ 25 mm with presence of yolk sac but no embryonic pole (Power Doppler sonography to be used).

For any doubt USG to be repeated at an interval of 10-14 days.

***Q. What are the conservative surgical measures for tubal ectopic pregnancy?***

**Ans:** (a) Salpingotomy
  (b) Salpingostomy
  (c) Segmental resection of the tube and anastomosis.

## CASE–20 | MISCARRIAGE (SPONTANEOUS ABORTION)

### Case Summary

Mrs CK, a 27-year-old woman was seen for the problem of three previous miscarriages. All the miscarriages occurred between 14 and 20 weeks of gestation. She seeks advice as she is planning for the next pregnancy.

**Q. What is her problem?**

**Ans.** She is a case of recurrent miscarriage.

**Q. How do you define recurrent miscarriage?**

**Ans.** Three or more consecutive spontaneous abortions (miscarriages) before 20 weeks are defined as recurrent miscarriage.

**Q. What are the common causes of recurrent miscarriage?**

**Ans.** (A) **Genetic causes**
- Trisomy (trisomy 21, 18, 13)
- Aneuploidy
- Polyploidy
- Translocations (balanced/reciprocal).

(B) **Endocrine causes**
- Uncontrolled thyroid dysfunction (hypo-hyperthyroidism)
- Diabetes mellitus (uncontrolled)
- Luteal phase defect
- Polycystic ovarian syndrome.

(C) **Anatomical causes**
- Uterine anomalies: Septate uterus, subseptate uterus
- Uterine synechiae
- Leiomyoma
- Cervical incompetence.

(D) **Infections:** Chlamydia, bacterial vaginosis, genital tuberculosis.

(E) **Immunological:** Antiphospholipid syndrome, SLE.

(F) **Thrombophilias** (inherited or acquired).

(G) **Toxins:** Smoking, alcohol, radiation.

(H) **Drugs:** Misoprostol, quinine.

**Q. What percentages of genetic abnormalities are responsible for miscarriages?**

**Ans.** About 50–70% of all miscarriages are due to genetic abnormalities. In the first trimester, about 70% and about 30% in the second trimester, and only 3% of stillbirths are due to fetal chromosomal abnormalities.

**Q. What are the different types of miscarriages? Outline the important diagnostic features and management issues for each of them.**

Ans. Refer Table 2.1.

Table 2.1: Types of miscarriages and the management issues.

| Type | Definition | Management option(s) |
|---|---|---|
| Complete abortion | Spontaneous expulsion of all the products of conception from the uterus | No further management is required if certain on clinical examination or on ultrasonography (USG) that uterus is empty |
| Threatened abortion | Uterine bleeding is continuing (slight). There is no cervical dilation or effacement | USG to confirm fetal viability. Rest is adviced till bleeding stops (as fetus is live). Progesterone therapy (vaginal/oral) may be given |
| Incomplete abortion | Partial expulsion of fetal or placental tissues (products of conception) | USG confirmation of products of conception left inside the uterus. IV line is sited to start infusion of crystalloids/cross-matched blood depending upon the hemorrhage. Evacuation of the uterus as early as possible is done to remove the retained products of conception |
| Missed abortion | Fetus is dead and is retained inside the uterus for a variable period of time | Suction evacuation or dilatation and evacuation of the uterus. Cervix may need to soften with the use of $PGE_1$ (misoprostol) 4–6 hours prior to evacuation |
| Inevitable abortion | Process of abortion is associated with cervical dilatation and effacement. The products of conception can be seen (on speculum examination) | Resuscitation of the patient, as it is associated with bleeding. Evacuation of the uterus with surgical or medical (oxytocin infusion) methods |
| Septic abortion | Patient presents with features of sepsis: Abnormal foul-smelling vaginal discharge, bleeding, rise in temperature and tachycardia | Control of sepsis with appropriate antibiotics (IV) following septic screen. USG to exclude foreign body. Evacuation of the uterus to eliminate the source of infection. May need laparotomy |

**Q. What is the most common type of chromosomal anomaly found in the aborted fetuses?**

**Ans.** Autosomal trisomies are the most common of abnormalities found in the aborted fetuses. However, monosomy X or 45, XO is the singlemost common (10–20%) karyotype seen in aborted fetuses.

**Q. What percentage of pregnancies does end in miscarriages?**

**Ans.** About 15–20% of all clinically diagnosed pregnancies end in a miscarriage. But loss of subclinical pregnancy loss is about 40%. Combining together clinical and subclinical, about 50% of all pregnancies end in miscarriage.

**Q. What is the place of anti-D immunoglobulin for patients with miscarriage?**

**Ans.** All Rh-negative women with vaginal bleeding in early pregnancy (miscarriage or ectopic pregnancy) should receive anti-D immunoglobulin. When pregnancy is ≤12 weeks, 50 µg IM is given and after 12 weeks, full dose—300 µg IM is given.

**Q. What are the common causes of abdominal pain during pregnancy?**

**Ans.** The common causes of abdominal pain during pregnancy are listed in the table below:

| Pregnancy | Medical and surgical | Gynecological |
|---|---|---|
| **Early pregnancy** | **Medical** | • Torsion of ovarian cyst |
| • Miscarriage | • Pyelitis | • Red degeneration of fibroid |
| • Disturbed tubal ectopic | • Cystitis | |
| • Hydatidiform mole | • Hepatitis | |
| | • Peptic ulcer | |
| **Late pregnancy** | **Surgical** | |
| • Preterm labor | • Acute appendicitis | |
| • Abruptio placentae | • Cholecystitis | |
| • Labor pain | • Renal calculi | |
| • Acute severe pre-eclampsia | • HELLP syndrome | |

CHAPTER 3

# Single Best Answers and Multiple Choice Questions

**Chapter Objectives**
- **Single Best Answers (SBAs)**
- **Multiple Choice Questions (MCQs)**

  Total **209** SBAs and MCQs in Obstetrics are there for comprehensive revision of the subject with added explanations
- It is a good practice area to test an individual's level of knowledge
- To detect area weakness and to make it up

❖ Single Best Answers (SBA)     121

❖ Multiple Choice Questions (MCQs)     121

Chapter 3 • Single Best Answers and Multiple Choice Questions

# 1. FUNDAMENTALS OF REPRODUCTION

## QUESTIONS

In this section, textbook page reference is given for explanation of the SBAs and MCQs.

**Q.01** *Fetal blood is returned to the umbilical arteries and the placenta through the:*
- (a) Hypogastric arteries
- (b) Ductus venosus
- (c) Ductus arteriosus
- (d) Foramen ovale

**Q.02** *A fully mature ovum measures about:*
- (a) 100 microns
- (b) 130 microns
- (c) 170 microns
- (d) 180 microns

**Q.03** *Morula (12–16 cell stage) enters the uterine cavity on:*
- (a) 2nd day
- (b) 3rd day
- (c) 4th day
- (d) 6th day

**Q.04** *Regarding time division, all the statements are correct, except:*
- (a) Ovular period lasts for 2 weeks following ovulation
- (b) Embryonic period begins at 3rd week following ovulation
- (c) Fetal period begins at 8th week
- (d) Fetal embryonic age is commonly used

**Q.05** *After ovulation, primitive fetal circulation is established by the following days:*
- (a) 7
- (b) 14
- (c) 21
- (d) 28

## ANSWERS

**Ans 01.** (a) Dutta Obs 9/e, p. 39
**Ans 02.** (b) Ovum measures about 130 microns.
**Ans 03.** (c)
**Ans 04.** (d) Menstrual age is commonly used.
**Ans 05.** (c) Dutta Obs 9/e, p. 27

## QUESTIONS

**Q.06** *The following changes occur in the vascular system of the newborn after birth:*
(a) Distal parts of the obliterated umbilical arteries form superior vesical arteries
(b) Umbilical vein becomes ligamentum venosum
(c) Ductus venosus becomes ligamentum teres
(d) Functional closure of the ductus arteriosus occurs soon after birth

**Q.07** *In embryonic development, primitive chorionic villi is formed in the stage of:*
(a) Zygote  (b) Morula
(c) Blastocyst  (d) Embryo

**Q.08** *Fetal hematopoiesis first occurs in:*
(a) Yolk sac  (b) Fetal spleen
(c) Fetal liver  (d) Fetal bone marrow

**Q.09** *Embryonic period commences at:*
(a) Fertilization  (b) Third week after fertilization
(c) Sixth week after fertilization  (d) Eighth week after fertilization

**Q.10** *Fertilized ovum is embedded in the endometrium at about which day after fertilization:*
(a) 2nd day  (b) 4th day
(c) 6th day  (d) 10th day

**Q.11** *False statement regarding hCG is:*
(a) It is a glycoprotein hormone
(b) The level peaks at term
(c) Doubling time is longer in ectopic pregnancy than in normal pregnancy
(d) Subunit cross reacts with subunit of LH

## ANSWERS

**Ans 06.** (d) The distal parts of obliterated umbilical arteries become lateral umbilical ligaments. Umbilical vein becomes ligamentum teres. Ductus venosus becomes ligamentum venosum. (Dutta Obs 9/e, p. 40)

**Ans 07.** (c)

**Ans 08.** (a)

**Ans 09.** (b) Dutta Obs 9/e, p. 37

**Ans 10.** (c)

**Ans 11.** (b) Dutta Obs 9/e, p. 54

## 2. PLACENTA, AMNIOTIC FLUID

### QUESTIONS

**Q.12** The following placental hormones are protein hormones, except:
(a) Human chorionic gonadotropin (hCG)
(b) Human placental lactogen (HPL)
(c) Progesterone
(d) Pregnancy-specific β-1 glycoprotein (PSBG)

**Q.13** The greenish color of meconium is due to:
(a) Bile pigment
(b) Altered blood
(c) Bile salts
(d) Desquamated epithelial cells

**Q.14** Placenta with umbilical cord attached to its margin is called:
(a) Battledore placenta
(b) Circumvallate placenta
(c) Succenturiate placenta
(d) Velamentous placenta

**Q.15** Human placenta develops predominantly from:
(a) Chorion frondosum
(b) Decidua basalis
(c) Decidua capsularis
(d) Decidua parietalis

**Q.16** Volume of blood in a mature placenta approximates:
(a) 300 mL
(b) 500 mL
(c) 700 mL
(d) 1000 mL

**Q.17** The amniotic fluid is completely changed and replaced in every:
(a) 2 hours
(b) 3 hours
(c) 4 hours
(d) 5 hours

### ANSWERS

**Ans 12.** (c)
**Ans 13.** (a)
**Ans 14.** (a) Dutta Obs 9/e, p. 204
**Ans 15.** (a)
**Ans 16.** (b)
**Ans 17.** (b)

## QUESTIONS

**Q.18** *The decidua is a source of:*
- (a) Human placental lactogen
- (b) Prolactin
- (c) Chorionic gonadotropin
- (d) Thyrotropin

**Q.19** *Umbilical cord contains:*
- (a) Two arteries and two veins
- (b) Two veins and one artery
- (c) Two arteries and one vein
- (d) One artery and one vein

**Q.20** *Localization of placenta is best done by:*
- (a) Displacement radiography
- (b) Isotopic scanning
- (c) Ultrasonography
- (d) Clinical methods

**Q.21** *Amount of liquor volume is highest at which time of pregnancy?*
- (a) 34 weeks
- (b) 37 weeks
- (c) 40 weeks
- (d) 42 weeks

**Q.22** *The following is true about amniotic fluid index:*
- (a) The largest vertical pocket is measured
- (b) Four quadrants are measured
- (c) Sum of the measurements (cm), is the amniotic fluid index (AFI)
- (d) Measurement is most accurate with computed tomography (CT)

## ANSWERS

**Ans 18.** (b)
**Ans 19.** (c) Dutta Obs 9/e, p. 35
**Ans 20.** (c)
**Ans 21.** (b) Dutta Obs 9/e, p. 34
**Ans 22.** (a), (b), (c)

## 3. THE FETUS, MATERNAL PELVIS, FETAL SKULL

### QUESTIONS

**Q.23** Pick up the correct statement:
(a) Umbilical arteries carry pure blood from placenta to fetus
(b) Umbilical vein carries impure blood from fetus to placenta
(c) Umbilical arteries carry pure blood from fetus to placenta
(d) Umbilical vein carries pure blood from placenta to fetus

**Q.24** In android type of pelvis, the sacrosciatic notch is:
(a) Narrow and shallow  (b) Narrow and deep
(c) Wide and deep  (d) Very wide and shallow

**Q.25** In markedly deflexed vertex, the engaging diameter of fetal head is:
(a) Suboccipitobregmatic  (b) Suboccipitofrontal
(c) Occipitofrontal  (d) Mentovertical

**Q.26** In vertex LOT position, caput succedaneum is found over:
(a) Left parietal bone  (b) Right parietal bone
(c) Occipital bone  (d) Frontal bone

**Q.27** Submentobregmatic diameter of a mature fetus averages:
(a) 8.5 cm  (b) 9.5 cm
(c) 10.5 cm  (d) 11.5 cm

### ANSWERS

**Ans 23.** (d)
**Ans 24.** (b)
**Ans 25.** (c)
**Ans 26.** (b)
**Ans 27.** (b)

## QUESTIONS

**Q.28** *In platypelloid pelvis, head engages in:*
(a) Transverse diameter
(b) Oblique diameter
(c) Obstetric conjugate
(d) Sacrocotyloid diameter

**Q.29** *Method of pelvic assessment in a gravid woman is generally:*
(a) Clinical
(b) Radiological
(c) Ultrasonic
(d) CT scanning

**Q.30** *Pelvis should be assessed in a primigravida at:*
(a) 32 weeks
(b) 35 weeks
(c) 37 weeks
(d) Onset of labor

**Q.31** *True conjugate diameter of the pelvic brim measures:*
(a) 10 cm
(b) 11 cm
(c) 12 cm
(d) 13 cm

**Q.32** *Engaging diameter in fully flexed vertex presentation is:*
(a) Suboccipitobregmatic
(b) Suboccipitofrontal
(c) Occipitofrontal
(d) Mentovertical

**Q.33** *The parameters measured by USG to assess the gestational age of the fetus are all, except:*
(a) Biparietal diameter
(b) Femur length
(c) Crown rump length
(d) Fetal weight

**Q.34** *Longest anteroposterior diameter of the pelvic inlet is seen in:*
(a) Anthropoid pelvis
(b) Android pelvis
(c) Platypelloid pelvis
(d) Gynecoid pelvis

## ANSWERS

Ans 28. (a)
Ans 29. (a)
Ans 30. (d)
Ans 31. (b)
Ans 32. (a)
Ans 33. (c)
Ans 34. (a)

## QUESTIONS

**Q.35** All the diameters are 9.4 cm, except:
(a) Biparietal
(b) Suboccipitobregmatic
(c) Suboccipitofrontal
(d) Submentobregmatic

**Q.36** The upper boundary of the obstetric outlet is formed by the:
(a) Plane of inlet
(b) Midpelvic plane
(c) Plane of least pelvic dimension
(d) Plane of the anatomical outlet

**Q.37** Shortest diameter of pelvic inlet in gynecoid pelvis is:
(a) True conjugate
(b) Obstetric conjugate
(c) Transverse diameter
(d) Oblique diameter

**Q.38** Relationship between different parts of fetus with one another is called:
(a) Lie
(b) Presentation
(c) Attitude
(d) Position

**Q.39** The largest presenting diameter in cephalic presentation is:
(a) Biparietal diameter
(b) Mentovertical
(c) Suboccipitobregmatic
(d) Submentobregmatic

**Q.40** Engaging diameter in face presentation:
(a) Submentobregmatic
(b) Submentovertical
(c) Occipitofrontal
(d) Mentovertical

## ANSWERS

**Ans 35.** (c)
**Ans 36.** (c)
**Ans 37.** (b)
**Ans 38.** (c)
**Ans 39.** (b)
**Ans 40.** (a)

## QUESTIONS

**Q.41 Shortest diameter of inlet in female pelvis:**
(a) True conjugate
(b) Obstetric conjugate
(c) Diagonal conjugate
(d) Left oblique diameter

**Q.42 Subpubic angle is narrow in:**
(a) Gynecoid pelvis
(b) Anthropoid pelvis
(c) Android pelvis
(d) Platypelloid pelvis

**Q.43 Shortest diameter of fetal skull is:**
(a) Suboccipitobregmatic
(b) Bitemporal
(c) Suboccipitofrontal
(d) Biparietal

**Q.44 Estimated uteroplacental blood flow at term:**
(a) 100–200 mL
(b) 600–750 mL
(c) 1,000 mL
(d) None

**Q.45 The following is true about fetal hemoglobin (HbF):**
(a) It is less resistant than adult Hb to denaturation by acid
(b) It has higher binding to 2,3-DPG
(c) Accounts for 90% of all fetal Hb at 20 weeks of gestation
(d) Consists of two delta and two alpha chains

## ANSWERS

**Ans 41.** (b)
**Ans 42.** (c) Dutta Obs 9/e, p. 325
**Ans 43.** (b)
**Ans 44.** (b) Dutta Obs 9/e, p. 28
**Ans 45.** (c) Dutta Obs 9/e, p. 38

## 4. PHYSIOLOGICAL CHANGES IN PREGNANCY

### QUESTIONS

**Q.46** *Amount of water retained during normal pregnancy at term is approximately:*
  (a) 4.5 liters
  (b) 6.5 liters
  (c) 8.5 liters
  (d) 10 liters

**Q.47** *The uterine musculature during pregnancy is arranged in the following layers:*
  (a) Inner longitudinal
  (b) Intermediate interlacing
  (c) Outer-circular
  (d) Interlacing all the layers

**Q.48** *Principal blood values during pregnancy are all except:*
  (a) Blood volume — rise by 40%
  (b) Plasma volume — rise by 50%
  (c) Red cell volume — rise by 20%
  (d) Hematocrit — rise by 10%

**Q.49** *The following changes occur in blood coagulation factors in pregnancy, except:*
  (a) Fibrinogen level is very much elevated
  (b) Fibrinolytic activity is enhanced
  (c) Platelet count remains static or there is slight fall
  (d) Factor II is increased

**Q.50** *The following are the hemodynamic changes at term in normal pregnancy, except:*
  (a) Cardiac output is increased by 30%
  (b) Stroke volume is decreased in lateral position
  (c) Pulse rate is increased
  (d) Blood viscosity is decreased

### ANSWERS

Ans 46. (b)
Ans 47. (b) The muscles are arranged as inner circular, outer longitudinal and intermediate interlacing one.
Ans 48. (d) There is slight fall in hematocrit.
Ans 49. (b) The fibrinolytic activity is depressed during pregnancy.
Ans 50. (b) Stroke volume is increased from 65 mL to 75 mL during pregnancy.

## QUESTIONS

**Q.51** *The following changes occur in the respiratory system at term in normal pregnancy, except:*
   (a) Vital capacity remains unaffected
   (b) Tidal volume is increased by 40%
   (c) Residual volume is increased by 20%
   (d) Respiratory rate remains unaffected

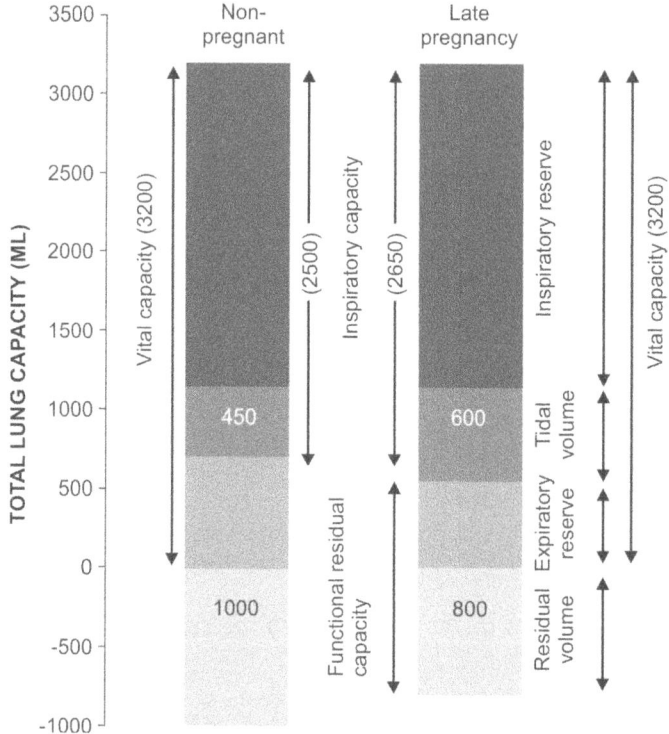

**Fig. 3.1:** Lung volumes in non-pregnant and pregnant women. [TLC: total lung capacity (4200 is same for non-pregnant and pregnant conditions); VC: vital capacity; IC: inspiratory capacity; FRC: functional residual capacity; IRV: inspiratory reserve volume; TV: tidal volume; ERV: expiratory reserve volume, RV: residual volume. Values of TLC and VC remains unaltered in both the conditions].

## ANSWERS

**Ans 51.** (c) Residual volume is decreased by 20% (Fig. 3.1).

Chapter 3 • Single Best Answers and Multiple Choice Questions

## QUESTIONS

**Q.52** *The following are the physiological changes during late pregnancy, except:*
(a) Blood volume is increased
(b) Cardiac output is increased
(c) Arterial $PO_2$ is decreased
(d) Tidal volume is increased

**Q.53** *As regards supine hypotension syndrome, true statement is:*
(a) Observed in about 1% of cases
(b) Commonly seen in early pregnancy
(c) Measurement of brachial artery pressure reflects the pressure in the uterine artery
(d) It is relieved by turning the woman on her side

**Q.54** *Expected date of delivery (EDD) is calculated by the following methods, except:*
(a) By adding 9 calendar months and 7 days to the first day of LMP
(b) By adding 9 calendar months and 7 days to the last day of LMP
(c) By adding 22 weeks to the date of quickening in primigravida
(d) By adding 30 weeks since the documentation of fetal heart tones by Doppler ultrasound.

**Q.55** *Peak levels of hCG in the urine during pregnancy is seen around:*
(a) 30 days
(b) 45 days
(c) 70 days
(d) 120 days

**Q.56** *Fundal height of uterus is more than the period of gestation in all, except:*
(a) Multifetal gestation
(b) Anencephaly
(c) Hydatidiform mole
(d) Intrauterine fetal death

## ANSWERS

**Ans 52.** (c) Arterial $PO_2$ is increased.
**Ans 53.** (d) Observed in 10% of cases in late pregnancy. Uterine artery pressure is lower than that of brachial artery.
**Ans 54.** (b)
**Ans 55.** (c)
**Ans 56.** (d)

## QUESTIONS

**Q.57** *Best diagnosis of early pregnancy could be done by:*
(a) Plasma progesterone update level
(b) Urine for pregnancy test
(c) TVS
(d) Presence of corpus luteum (CL) of pregnancy

**Q.58** *Changes in heart and circulation in a normal pregnancy are all, except:*
(a) Cardiac output is increased
(b) Pulse rate is increased
(c) Blood viscosity is increased
(d) Venous pressure is increased

**Q.59** *All of the following rises physiologically in pregnancy, except:*
(a) Heart rate
(b) Cardiac output
(c) Blood volume
(d) Blood pressure

**Q.60** *Daily folic acid requirement during pregnancy:*
(a) 50–100 μ
(b) 100–200 μ
(c) 300–500 μ
(d) 1000–1200 μ

**Q.61.** *Fetal structures and gestational age as calculated by transvaginal Sonography:*
(a) Gestational sac by 4.5 weeks
(b) Yolk sac by 5 weeks
(c) Fetal pole by 6 weeks
(d) Fetal cardiac activity by 7.5 weeks

## ANSWERS

**Ans 57.** (c) *See* p. 19, 369
**Ans 58.** (c) Dutta Obs 9/e, p. 48
**Ans 59.** (d) Dutta Obs 9/e, p. 48
**Ans 60.** (c) Dutta Obs 9/e, p. 90
**Ans 61.** (a), (b), (c) *See* p. 369

# 5. ANTENATAL CARE

## QUESTIONS

**Q.62** *Number of antenatal visits in an uncomplicated pregnancy should be minimum:*
- (a) 4 times
- (b) 8 times
- (c) 12 times
- (d) 16 times

**Q.63** *Gestational age is evaluated from:*
- (a) Calculation from LMP
- (b) Height of the uterus
- (c) Counting from the date of ovulation
- (d) Counting from the date of fertilization

**Q.64** *Absolute (positive) signs of pregnancy are:*
- (a) Abdominal enlargement
- (b) Braxton-Hicks contraction
- (c) Ballottement
- (d) Audible FHS

**Q.65** *The following is related to gravida and parity, except:*
- (a) A nulligravida is one who is not pregnant now but may have had a pregnancy before
- (b) Gravida and para refer to pregnancies and not to babies
- (c) A nullipara is one who has never completed a pregnancy to the stage viability
- (d) Gravida denotes a pregnant state, both present and past, irrespective of period of gestation

## ANSWERS

**Ans 62.** (a) Timings are : 16, 24–28, 32 and 36 weeks (technical working group, WHO).
**Ans 63.** (a)
**Ans 64.** (d)
**Ans 65.** (a) A nulligravida is one who is not now and never has been pregnant.

## QUESTIONS

**Q.66** *Preventive vaccination in pregnancy is contraindicated in the following except:*
- (a) Chickenpox
- (b) Mumps
- (c) Influenza
- (d) Measles

**Q.67** *In transverse lie Pawlik grip is:*
- (a) Full
- (b) Empty
- (c) Podalic pole
- (d) Head on one side

**Q.68** *Folic acid deficiency in pregnancy is manifested by:*
- (a) Hypersegmentation of neutrophils
- (b) Angular stomatitis
- (c) Microcytes
- (d) Anemia

**Q.69** *Post-term pregnancy is defined as (ACOG 2013):*
- (a) 37 0/7 weeks through 38 6/7 weeks
- (b) 39 0/7 weeks through 40 6/7 weeks
- (c) 41 0/7 weeks through 41 6/7 weeks
- (d) 42 0/7 weeks and beyond

## ANSWERS

**Ans 66.** (c) Dutta Obs 9/e, p. 281
**Ans 67.** (b)
**Ans 68.** (a) and (d)
**Ans 69.** (d)

## 6. ANTENATAL ASSESSMENT OF FETAL WELL-BEING

### QUESTIONS

Q.70 *Chorionic villus sampling is done in all, except:*
 (a) Thalassemia
 (b) Phenylketonuria
 (c) Down's syndrome
 (d) Neural tube defect

Q.71 *Manning scoring system (fetal biophysical profile) includes assessment of all, except:*
 (a) Fetal urine production
 (b) Fetal breathing movement
 (c) Amniotic fluid volume
 (d) Fetal movement

Q.72 *For cordocentesis umbilical vein is punctured at which part of umbilical cord:*
 (a) Anywhere
 (b) At the middle
 (c) Near its insertion at placenta
 (d) Near its insertion at umbilicus

Q.73 *The following are ultrasonographic markers for increased chromosomal abnormality, except:*
 (a) Nuchal translucency >3 mm
 (b) Short femur
 (c) Rocker bottom foot
 (d) Jejunal atresia

### ANSWERS

**Ans 70.** (d)
**Ans 71.** (a) Dutta Obs 9/e, p. 98
**Ans 72.** (c) Dutta Obs 9/e, p. 105
**Ans 73.** (d) Dutta Obs 9/e, p. 604

# 7. EARLY PREGNANCY

## QUESTIONS

**Q.74** First trimester MTP is best achieved by:
(a) Suction evacuation
(b) Prostaglandins
(c) Oral mifepristone (RU 486) only
(d) Mifepristone and misoprostol ($PGE_1$)

**Q.75** The diagnosis of ruptured tubal ectopic pregnancy is principally made by:
(a) History and examination of the patient
(b) Sonography
(c) Laparoscopy
(d) Culdocentesis

**Q.76** The best method of management of molar pregnancy of uterine size 20 weeks in a woman aged 20:
(a) Suction evacuation with or without oxytocin infusion
(b) Dilatation and evacuation
(c) Hysterotomy
(d) Episiotomy

**Q.77** The commonest complication of hydatidiform mole is:
(a) Hemorrhage
(b) Pulmonary embolism
(c) Hyperemesis
(d) Choriocarcinoma

**Q.78** Vomiting is a common feature of the following, except:
(a) Missed miscarriage
(b) Hydatidiform mole
(c) Multiple pregnancy
(d) First pregnancy

## ANSWERS

**Ans 74.** (d) Dutta Obs 9/e, p. 165
**Ans 75.** (a)
**Ans 76.** (a)
**Ans 77.** (a)
**Ans 78.** (a)

## QUESTIONS

**Q.79** *Most common chromosomal pattern in hydatidiform mole is:*
- (a) 46 XX
- (b) 45 XO
- (c) 69 XXY
- (d) 69 XXX

**Q.80** *Ultrasonography at 10 weeks can diagnose:*
- (a) Hydrocephalus
- (b) Microcephalus
- (c) Anencephaly
- (d) Abruptio placentae

**Q.81** *Chorionic villus sampling is done in all, except:*
- (a) Thalassemia
- (b) Phenylketonuria
- (c) Down's syndrome
- (d) Neural tube defect

**Q.82** *Snow-storm appearance in USG is seen in:*
- (a) Ectopic pregnancy
- (b) Hydatidiform mole
- (c) Hydramnios
- (d) Hydrocephalus

**Q.83** *Most constant symptom in disturbed ectopic pregnancy is:*
- (a) Amenorrhea
- (b) Bleeding PV
- (c) Pain in lower abdomen
- (d) Passage of decidual cast

**Q.84** *Threatened miscarriage is diagnosed by all, except:*
- (a) Abdominal pain with slight vaginal bleeding
- (b) Uterine size is normal
- (c) Fetus is alive on USG examination
- (d) Retroplacental hemorrhage may be present

## ANSWERS

**Ans 79.** (a)
**Ans 80.** (c)
**Ans 81.** (d)
**Ans 82.** (b)
**Ans 83.** (c)
**Ans 84.** (b) Dutta Obs 9/e, Table 16.1 p. 159.

## QUESTIONS

**Q.85** *Ultrasonic recognition of gestation is possible as early as (post-conceptional):*
  (a) 2nd to 3rd week
  (b) 4th to 5th week
  (c) 6th to 7th week
  (d) 8th to 10th week

**Q.86** *Real-time sonography can demonstrate fetal cardiac activity as early as (postconception):*
  (a) 4th week
  (b) 6th week
  (c) 8th week
  (d) 10th week

**Q.87** *Gestational age of the fetus is best assessed by:*
  (a) Calculation from the correct menstrual date
  (b) Ultrasonographic assesment of the parameters in the first trimester
  (c) Bimanual examination in the first trimester
  (d) Ultrasonographic measurements of BPD, FL, AC and HC carefully.

## ANSWERS

**Ans 85.** (b)
**Ans 86.** (b)
**Ans 87.** (b) See p. 369.

Chapter 3 • Single Best Answers and Multiple Choice Questions

## 8. LABOR: NORMAL AND COMPLICATED

### QUESTIONS

**Q.88** The average blood loss during normal delivery is approximately:
(a) >700 mL
(b) <500 mL
(c) >250 mL
(d) <100 mL

**Q.89** Important features of true labor pain are all, except:
(a) Lightening
(b) Show
(c) Dilatation and effacement of the cervix
(d) Bulging of the membrane during uterine contraction

**Q.90** The following are the events during labor, except:
(a) In primigravida, dilatation precedes effacement of the cervix
(b) In multipara, both occur simultaneously
(c) During contraction, the transverse diameter of the uterus is reduced but the longitudinal diameter increases
(d) Membranes usually rupture with full cervical dilatation

**Q.91** The first stage of labor is said to be completed:
(a) When the membrane ruptures
(b) When the cervix fully dilates (10 cm)
(c) When active phase of labor begins
(d) With the appearance of bearing down efforts

**Q.92** To be of value FHR is to be auscultated:
(a) During uterine contraction
(b) Before and during uterine contraction
(c) Immediately following uterine contraction
(d) During uterine relaxation

### ANSWERS

**Ans 88.** (b) Dutta Obs 9/e, p. 385.
**Ans 89.** (a)
**Ans 90.** (a) In primigravida, effacement precedes dilatation of the cervix.
**Ans 91.** (b)
**Ans 92.** (c)

## QUESTIONS

**Q.93** *Following the delivery of a healthy baby, which one is the first to be done?*
(a) To place the baby on a tray with head slightly downwards
(b) To clear the air passage
(c) Apgar rating
(d) Clamping the umbilical cord

**Q.94** *The first stage of labor:*
(a) Begins when the membrane ruptures
(b) Normal duration is 20 hours
(c) Can be shortened by use of oxytocin
(d) Can be shortened by use of forceps

**Q.95** *Early clamping of the umbilical cord is indicated in all, except:*
(a) Rh-incompatibility
(b) Asphyxiated baby
(c) During CS when the baby is delivered by cutting through the placenta
(d) Postmature baby

**Q.96** *The following are related to molding of the head, except:*
(a) During normal delivery, molding is inevitable
(b) In labor, parietal bones overlap the adjacent bones
(c) In grade-I, the bones touch but do not overlap
(d) Molding takes few days to disappear

**Q.97** *The official time of birth in normal delivery is the moment when:*
(a) Head is out
(b) Whole of the baby is out of the mother's body
(c) As soon as umbilical cord is cut
(d) As soon as baby cries

## ANSWERS

**Ans 93.** (b)
**Ans 94.** (c)
**Ans 95.** (d)
**Ans 96.** (d) It takes few hours to disappear.
**Ans 97.** (b)

## QUESTIONS

**Q.98** The engaging diameter of the after-coming head in breech is:
(a) Suboccipitobregmatic
(b) Suboccipitofrontal
(c) Occipitofrontal
(d) Submentovertical

**Q.99** Intrauterine pressure is highest in:
(a) First stage of labor
(b) Second stage of labor
(c) Third stage of labor
(d) Fourth stage of labor

**Q.100** Placental separation and descent in third stage of labor is due to:
(a) Contraction of uterus
(b) Retraction of uterus
(c) Controlled cord traction
(d) Contraction superadded on maximum retraction

**Q.101** Which layer of the musculature of pregnant uterus forms figure of 8 and acts as living ligature during the 3rd stage of labor?
(a) External
(b) Internal
(c) Middle
(d) Neither of these

**Q.102** Which of the following statements is false in connection with Caput succedaneum?
(a) It is due to venolymphatic stasis of scalp
(b) It is not limited to suture lines
(c) It occurs beneath the girdle of contact
(d) It disappears over a week

**Q.103** The diameter of cervical canal of the full dilatation during labor is:
(a) 6 cm
(b) 8 cm
(c) 10 cm
(d) 12 cm

## ANSWERS

**Ans 98.** (b)
**Ans 99.** (b)
**Ans 100.** (d)
**Ans 101.** (c) Dutta Obs 9/e, p. 42
**Ans 102.** (d)
**Ans 103.** (c)

## QUESTIONS

**Q.104** *Diagnosis of 2nd stage of labor:*
- (a) Rupture of bag of water
- (b) 10 cm dilatation of cervix
- (c) Bearing down pain
- (d) Meconium-stained liquor

**Q.105** *From which layer placenta gets separated:*
- (a) Basal layer
- (b) Spongy layer
- (c) Superficial layer
- (d) Compact layer

**Q.106** *Crowning is known to occur when:*
- (a) head is at inlet
- (b) head is at perineum
- (c) head is at ischial spine
- (d) head is at perineum and there is no recession

**Q.107** *Mechanism of central separation of placenta is known as:*
- (a) Matthews Duncan
- (b) Schultze
- (c) Letymen
- (d) Naegele's

## ANSWERS

**Ans 104.** (b)
**Ans 105.** (b)
**Ans 106.** (d) Dutta Obs 9/e, p. 119
**Ans 107.** (b)

## 9. PUERPERIUM—NORMAL AND ABNORMAL

### QUESTIONS

**Q.108** The normal lochia discharge at the end of second week is called:
(a) Lochia rubra
(b) Lochia serosa
(c) Lochia alba
(d) Lochia mixed

**Q.109** The most common cause of retained placenta:
(a) Uterine atonicity
(b) Hour-glass contraction
(c) Placenta accreta
(d) Placenta increta

**Q.110** Composition of human milk (g%) is as below, except:
(a) Sugar—7
(b) Fat—3.5
(c) Protein—3.4
(d) Minerals—0.4

**Q.111** As regards breastfeeding, true statement is:
(a) Hindmilk gives more energy to the infant
(b) Baby should be changed to each breast at every 2-3 minutes
(c) Early and exclusive breastfeeding for 3-4 months
(d) Good attachment means baby should always be with the mother

**Q.112** In relation to breastfeeding, match the following:
(a) Baby after vaginal birth      1. 5-10 minutes
(b) Baby after cesarean birth     2. 2-3 hours
(c) Duration of feed              3. 2-3 hours
(d) Frequency of feed             4. Soon after birth

### ANSWERS

**Ans 108.** (c)
**Ans 109.** (a) Dutta Obs 9/e, p. 393
**Ans 110.** (c) Protein content is 1.2 g%. (Dutta Obs 9/e, p. 425)
**Ans 111.** (a) Q. (c): It should be 4-6 months.
**Ans 112.** (a) = 4; (b) = 3; (c) = 1; (d) = 2.

## QUESTIONS

**Q.113** *Commonest cause of retained placenta is:*
(a) Nonseparated placenta in atonic uterus
(b) Separated placenta in atonic uterus
(c) Constriction ring
(d) Placenta accreta

**Q.114** *Commonest cause of puerperal pyrexia is:*
(a) Genital infection
(b) Urinary infection
(c) Mastitis
(d) Thrombophlebitis

**Q.115** *Puerperal pyrexia is the fever lasting for 24 hours or more after child birth if temperature is more than:*
(a) 99°F
(b) 99.5°F
(c) 100°F
(d) 100.4°F

**Q.116** *Breastfeeding should be started:*
(a) Immediately after birth
(b) 6 hours after birth
(c) 12 hours after birth
(d) 24 hours after birth

## ANSWERS

**Ans 113.** (b)
**Ans 114.** (a)
**Ans 115.** (d)
**Ans 116.** (a)

## Chapter 3 • Single Best Answers and Multiple Choice Questions

### QUESTIONS

**Q.117** Suppression of lactation is best achieved by:
(a) Estrogen
(b) Estrogen + Testosterone
(c) Vitamin $B_6$
(d) Bromocriptine

**Q.118** The following is true about lactation:
(a) Progesterone promotes growth of ducts rather than alveoli
(b) An intact nerve supply is needed for growth of mammary glands
(c) Prolactin causes milk ejection
(d) Maintenance of lactation needs suckling

**Q.119** The most common cause of postpartum hemorrhage is:
(a) Atonicity of the uterus
(b) Trauma to the genital tract
(c) Forceps delivery
(d) Blood coagulopathy

**Q.120** In a neonate born to a Rh-negative mother, the cord blood of the neonate is sent for the following investigations:
(a) Hemoglobin
(b) Serum bilirubin
(c) Blood group and Rh type
(d) Indirect Coomb test

### ANSWERS

**Ans 117.** (d) Dutta Obs 9/e, p. 474
**Ans 118.** (d) Dutta Obs 9/e, p. 58
**Ans 119.** (a) Dutta Obs 9/e, p. 385
**Ans 120.** (a), (b) and (c)

## 10. COMPLICATED PREGNANCY

### QUESTIONS

**Q.121** Type of eclampsia common in India is:
(a) Antepartum
(b) Intrapartum
(c) Postpartum
(d) Mixed variety

**Q.122** The following are related to the diagnosis of iron deficiency anemia, except:
(a) Low serum iron
(b) MCH is the most sensitive index
(c) MCV is less than 80 μm$^3$
(d) Low serum ferritin

**Q.123** Best way to diagnose postmaturity is:
(a) Ultrasonography in late pregnancy
(b) Serial sonographic fetal biometry
(c) Amniocentesis
(d) Clinical examination

**Q.124** Conclusive early evidence of intrauterine fetal death is:
(a) Spalding sign
(b) Hyperflexion of the spine
(c) Appearance of gas shadow in the chambers of the heart and great vessel
(d) Doppler USG: Absence of cardiac motion

**Q.125** The commonest indication for termination of IUFD is:
(a) Uterine infection
(b) Falling fibrinogen level
(c) Psychological upset of the mother
(d) Request by the husband

### ANSWERS

**Ans 121.** (a)
**Ans 122.** (b) MCHC is the most sensitive index to diagnose iron deficiency anemia and not MCH.
**Ans 123.** (b)
**Ans 124.** (d)
**Ans 125.** (c)

## QUESTIONS

**Q.126** To prevent active immunization of Rh-negative mother, Rh anti-D immunoglobulin is administered intramuscularly to all mothers, except:
(a) Within 72 hours following delivery, or after abortion or ectopic
(b) Following external cephalic version or amniocentesis
(c) Each time following subsequent delivery
(d) When the neonate is Rhesus-negative

**Q.127** The following statements are related to the mechanism of labor in breech, except:
(a) The engaging diameter of the buttocks is bitrochanteric—10 cm
(b) The engaging diameter of the shoulders is bisacromial—11 cm
(c) The engaging diameter of the head is suboccipitofrontal—10 cm
(d) The after-coming head is born by flexion

**Q.128** In transverse lie — match the following:
(a) Lie may change and the fetus becomes vertex:      1. Evolution
(b) Lie may change and the fetus becomes breech:      2. Version
(c) Delivery in doubled up fashion:                   3. Rectification
(d) Delivery of breech followed by the head:          4. Expulsion

**Q.129** Macrosomia is occasionally related to all, except:
(a) Maternal obesity
(b) Gestational diabetes
(c) Prolonged pregnancy
(d) Maternal hypertension

**Q.130** Induction is less likely to be successful in all except:
(a) Delivery before term
(b) Elderly primigravida
(c) Cases with prolonged retention of dead fetus
(d) Bishop's score >6

## ANSWERS

**Ans 126.** (d) No antigenic stimulus, when the neonate is Rh-negative.
**Ans 127.** (b) Bisacromial diameter measures 12 cm.
**Ans 128.** (a) = 3; (b) = 2; (c) = 4; (d) = 1.
**Ans 129.** (d)
**Ans 130.** (d)

## QUESTIONS

**Q.131** The most common complication of eclampsia is:
(a) Renal failure
(b) Pulmonary edema
(c) Cerebral hemorrhage
(d) Psychosis

**Q.132** Source of hemorrhage in placenta praevia is:
(a) Torn fetal blood vessels
(b) Torn maternal blood vessels
(c) Torn both maternal and fetal blood vessels
(d) Tear of lower uterine segment

**Q.133** Which one of the following pairs is not correctly matched?
(a) Anemia in pregnancy — preterm labor
(b) Diabetes in pregnancy — fetal macrosomia
(c) Rheumatic heart disease — unexplained stillbirth
(d) Hypertension in pregnancy — IUGR

**Q.134** The lower limit of hemoglobin below which a pregnant lady is called anemic is:
(a) 8 g%
(b) 9 g%
(c) 11 g%
(d) 12 g%

**Q.135** Deep transverse arrest is common in:
(a) Gynecoid pelvis
(b) Android pelvis
(c) Anthropoid pelvis
(d) Flat pelvis

**Q.136** The most common cause of nonengaged head at term is:
(a) Hydrocephalus
(b) Cephalopelvic disproportion
(c) Deflexion of head
(d) Hydramnios

## ANSWERS

Ans 131. (b)
Ans 132. (b)
Ans 133. (c)
Ans 134. (c)
Ans 135. (b)
Ans 136. (c)

# Chapter 3 • Single Best Answers and Multiple Choice Questions

## QUESTIONS

**Q.137** *The commonest cause of transverse lie is:*
(a) Multiparity
(b) Placenta previa
(c) Contracted pelvis
(d) Congenital malformation of uterus

**Q.138** *All of the following are associated with polyhydramnios, except:*
(a) Anencephaly
(b) Diabetes in pregnancy
(c) Renal agenesis (bilateral)
(d) Esophageal atresia

**Q.139** *DIC in pregnancy is seen in following conditions, except:*
(a) Amniotic fluid embolism
(b) Abruptio placentae
(c) Intrauterine death
(d) Threatened abortion

**Q.140** *Lovset's maneuver is done for:*
(a) Delivery of after-coming head
(b) Delivery of legs
(c) Delivery of arms
(d) Delivery of placenta

**Q.141** *Causes of intrauterine fetal death are all, except:*
(a) Rh-isoimmunization in pregnancy
(b) Severe pregnancy-induced hypertension
(c) Pregnancy with syphilis
(d) Physiological anemia of pregnancy

**Q.142** *Treatment of choice in a case of IUFD:*
(a) Immediate delivery
(b) Surgical: LSCS
(c) Induction with ARM
(d) Medical induction

## ANSWERS

**Ans 137.** (d)
**Ans 138.** (c)
**Ans 139.** (d)
**Ans 140.** (c)
**Ans 141.** (d)
**Ans 142.** (d)

## QUESTIONS

**Q.143** *All belong to gestational trophoblastic tumor, except:*
(a) Hydatidiform mole
(b) Choriocarcinoma
(c) Placental site trophoblastic tumor
(d) Tubal mole

**Q.144** *All may be the causes of nonimmune hydrops fetalis, except:*
(a) Rh-isoimmunization
(b) Diabetes in pregnancy
(c) Syphilis
(d) Fetal cardiac malformation

**Q.145** *Characteristics of placenta previa are all, except:*
(a) Painless and causeless bleeding
(b) Uterus is large, hard and tender
(c) Fetal parts easily felt
(d) Presenting part high up

**Q.146** *Constriction ring is associated with all, except:*
(a) Injudicious use of oxytocics
(b) Premature rupture of membranes
(c) Obstructed labor
(d) Premature instrumentation

**Q.147** *Causes of hydramnios are all, except:*
(a) Anencephaly
(b) Spina bifida
(c) Diabetes mellitus
(d) Hypothyroidism

## ANSWERS

**Ans 143.** (d)
**Ans 144.** (a)
**Ans 145.** (b)
**Ans 146.** (c) Dutta Obs 9/e, p. 338
**Ans 147.** (d)

Chapter 3 • Single Best Answers and Multiple Choice Questions

## QUESTIONS

**Q.148** Dose of anti-D gammaglobulin following 22 weeks of abortion is:
(a) 300 µg
(b) 150 µg
(c) 100 µg
(d) 50 µg

**Q.149** Renal agenesis is associated with:
(a) Oligohydramnios
(b) Hydramnios
(c) Anencephaly
(d) Tracheoesophageal fistula

**Q.150** Indications for induction of labor are all, except:
(a) Postmaturity
(b) Transverse lie
(c) Pre-eclampsia
(d) Intrauterine fetal death

**Q.151** Regarding anemia in pregnancy, all are correct, except:
(a) Hemoglobin level is usually less than 10 g/dL
(b) Hemorrhage is the commonest cause
(c) Iron supplementation is a must
(d) Blood transfusion may be needed

**Q.152** APH is defined as hemorrhage from or within the genital tract at any time of pregnancy from 28 weeks to:
(a) Onset of labor
(b) End of first stage
(c) End of second stage
(d) End of third stage

## ANSWERS

**Ans 148.** (a) Dutta Obs 9/e, p. 314
**Ans 149.** (a)
**Ans 150.** (b) Dutta Obs 9/e, p. 484
**Ans 151.** (b) Dutta Obs 9/e, p. 245
**Ans 152.** (c) Dutta Obs 9/e, p. 228

## QUESTIONS

**Q.153** Which type of pelvis is associated with higher incidence of face to pubis delivery?
(a) Gynecoid
(b) Anthropoid
(c) Platypelloid
(d) Android

**Q.154** All the following are indications for immediate termination of pregnancy in placenta previa, except:
(a) Pregnancy beyond 37 weeks of gestation
(b) Transverse lie
(c) Patient in labor
(d) Continuous bleeding

**Q.155** The following is true about characteristics of shock:
(a) Hypovolemic shock occurs after loss of 10% of normal blood volume
(b) Tissue hypoxia leads to metabolic alkalosis
(c) The circulation in the adrenal gland is spared unless the condition is extreme
(d) Endotoxic shock is caused by protein toxins

**Q.156** The following are related to the diagnosis of iron deficiency anemia, except:
(a) Low serum iron
(b) MCH is the most sensitive index
(c) MCV is less than 80 mm$^3$
(d) Low serum ferritin

## ANSWERS

**Ans 153.** (b)
**Ans 154.** (b)
**Ans 155.** (c) Dutta Obs 9/e, p. 575
**Ans 156.** (b) Dutta Obs 9/e, p. 248

## 11. MEDICAL AND SURGICAL ILLNESS DURING PREGNANCY

### QUESTIONS

Q.157 Malaria in pregnancy:
  (a) Causes fetal abnormalities
  (b) Quinine is contraindicated
  (c) Congenital malaria is frequent
  (d) Pregnancy complications are more with *P. falciparum* infection

Q.158 The most common fetal hazard in diabetes mellitus is:
  (a) Macrosomia           (b) Congenital malformations
  (c) Intrauterine fetal death    (d) Birth injuries

Q.159 Antimalarial drug of choice during pregnancy is:
  (a) Chloroquine          (b) Quinine
  (c) Pyrimethamine        (d) Spiramycin

Q.160 Perinatal transmission of virus in an HIV-positive woman is mostly:
  (a) Transplacental
  (b) Contamination during vaginal delivery
  (c) Breast milk
  (d) Body contact after birth

Q.161 Commonest degeneration in a fibroid uterus during pregnancy:
  (a) Hyaline              (b) Fatty
  (c) Cystic               (d) Red degeneration

### ANSWERS

Ans 157. (d) Congenital malaria is <5%. (Dutta Obs 9/e, p. 277)
Ans 158. (a) Dutta Obs 9/e, p. 264
Ans 159. (a) Dutta Obs 9/e, p. 278
Ans 160. (b) Dutta Obs 9/e, p. 282
Ans 161. (d) Dutta Obs 9/e, p. 289

## QUESTIONS

**Q.162** *Common benign ovarian tumor with potentiality of torsion in pregnancy:*
   (a) Dermoid cyst
   (b) Pseudomucinous cyst adenoma
   (c) Corpus luteum of pregnancy
   (d) Papilliferous cyst

**Q.163** *Retention of urine in a pregnant woman with a retroverted uterus usually occurs at:*
   (a) 6–10 weeks
   (b) 12–16 weeks
   (c) 20–24 weeks
   (d) 28–32 weeks

**Q.164** *A pregnant woman presents with red degeneration of fibroid management. This is called:*
   (a) Myomectomy
   (b) Hysterectomy
   (c) Termination of pregnancy
   (d) Conservative

**Q.165** *The following is true about Swine flu in Pregnancy:*
   (a) It is due to the flu virus H1N1
   (b) It is a mosquito born disease
   (c) Flu vaccines are contraindicated in pregnancy
   (d) Oseltamivir, the antiviral drug, is safe in pregnancy

## ANSWERS

**Ans 162.** (a) Dutta Obs 9/e, p. 290
**Ans 163.** (b) Dutta Obs 9/e, p. 291
**Ans 164.** (d) Dutta Obs 9/e, p. 288
**Ans 165.** (a) and (d)

## 12. NEWBORN INFANT

### QUESTIONS

Q.166 The neonatal complications of a growth-restricted fetus are all, except:
 (a) Cerebral hemorrhage
 (b) Hypoglycemia
 (c) Meconium aspiration pneumonia
 (d) DIC

Q.167 The causes of neonatal respiratory distress are all except:
 (a) Maternal diabetes
 (b) Prematurity
 (c) Cesarean birth
 (d) Hyperbilirubinemia

Q.168 The causes of physiological jaundice in the newborn are all, except:
 (a) Increased red cell destruction
 (b) Defective conjugation due to decreased UDPGT activity
 (c) Decreased RBC survival (90 days vs. 120 days)
 (d) Enhanced conversion of bilirubin to urobilinoids by intestinal flora

Q.169 Fetal renal agenesis is commonly associated with all, except:
 (a) Polyhydramnios
 (b) Fetal growth restriction
 (c) Pulmonary hypoplasia
 (d) Fetal deformity

### ANSWERS

Ans 166. (a) Cerebral hemorrhage is common in preterm baby.
Ans 167. (d)
Ans 168. (d) It should be reduced conversion Uridine diphosphate glucuronyltransferase (UDPGT).
Ans 169. (a)

## QUESTIONS

**Q.170** *The neonatal complications of premature babies are all, except:*
   (a) Hypothermia
   (b) Infection
   (c) Meconium aspiration pneumonia
   (d) Anemia

**Q.171** *Regarding respiratory distress syndrome of the newborn, all are correct, except:*
   (a) It is common with preterm birth
   (b) Hyperthermia is a precipitating factor
   (c) It may be associated with cesarean delivery
   (d) It is common in a newborn of a diabetic mother

**Q.172** *The following is true regarding lactation:*
   (a) Progesterone promotes growth of the ducts and alveoli
   (b) Prolactin causes milk ejection
   (c) Cry of the baby can initiate milk let down reflex
   (d) Pyridoxin therapy enhances milk production

## ANSWERS

**Ans 170.** (c)
**Ans 171.** (b) Dutta Obs 9/e, p. 443
**Ans 172.** (c)

## 13. PHARMACO THERAPY IN OBSTETRICS

### QUESTIONS

Q.173 *The biological half-life of oxytocin is:*
(a) 1-2 minutes
(b) 3-4 minutes
(c) 5-6 minutes
(d) 7-8 minutes

Q.174 *The following are related to ergot derivatives, except:*
(a) It acts directly on the myometrium
(b) It initiates uterine contraction with increasing intensity
(c) It can effectively be used for induction of abortion
(d) It is highly effective in hemostasis following delivery

Q.175 *The following drugs cross the placental barrier to the fetus, except:*
(a) Warfarin
(b) Heparin
(c) Digoxin
(d) Aspirin

Q.176 *IV ergometrine during third stage of labor should not be given in these cases, except:*
(a) Cardiac disease
(b) Pre-eclampsia
(c) Rhesus-negative
(d) Fibroid uterus

Q.177 *Match the onset of action for the following oxytocics:*
(a) IV Methergin        1. 1/2 minute
(b) IV Oxytocin         2. 1 minute
(c) IV Ergometrine      3. 1.5 minutes
(d) IM Syntometrine     4. 2.5 minutes

### ANSWERS

**Ans 173.** (b)
**Ans 174.** (c) It is absolutely ineffective in induction of abortion.
**Ans 175.** (b)
**Ans 176.** (d)
**Ans 177.** (a) = 3; (b) = 1; (c) = 2; (d) = 4.

## QUESTIONS

**Q.178** Drugs contraindicated in breastfeeding:
(a) Warfarin
(b) Metronidazole
(c) Carbamazepine
(d) None of the above

**Q.179** Most common of the following fetal malformations is:
(a) Cardiac defect
(b) Spina bifida
(c) Cleft palate
(d) Renal defect

**Q.180** Preferred drugs to treat urinary tract infection during pregnancy are the following, except:
(a) Ampicillin
(b) Amoxicillin
(c) Cephalosporins
(d) Ciprofloxacin

**Q.181** Anticoagulant which does not cross placental barrier:
(a) Warfarin
(b) Heparin
(c) Both of the above
(d) None of the above

**Q.182** The following are used in obstetrics as tocolytic agents, except:
(a) Isoxsuprine hydrochloride
(b) Salbutamol
(c) Aspirin
(d) Carbetocin

**Q.183** Which antihypertensive drug is contraindicated in pregnancy:
(a) Methyldopa
(b) Hydralazine
(c) ACE inhibitors
(d) Nifedipine

## ANSWERS

**Ans 178.** (d)
**Ans 179.** (b)
**Ans 180.** (d)
**Ans 181.** (b)
**Ans 182.** (d)
**Ans 183.** (c)

# Chapter 3 • Single Best Answers and Multiple Choice Questions

## QUESTIONS

**Q.184** *Contraindications of oxytocin in labor are all, except:*
- (a) Multigravida
- (b) Malpresentation
- (c) Heart disease
- (d) Diabetes

**Q.185** *All are true about drugs affecting myometrial contraction, except:*
- (a) Oxytocin acts via receptors on the cell surface
- (b) $PGF_{2\alpha}$ produces sustained uterine contraction
- (c) Ergometrine acts by 40–60 seconds of IV injection
- (d) Half-life of oxytocin is 5–10 minutes

**Q.186** *Oxytocin infusion is contraindicated in all, except:*
- (a) Obstructed labor
- (b) Grand multipara
- (c) Augmentation of labor
- (d) Malpresentation

**Q.187** *Which one does not cross through placenta?*
- (a) Warfarin
- (b) Heparin
- (c) Morphine
- (d) Naloxone

## ANSWERS

**Ans 184.** (d)
**Ans 185.** (d) Dutta Obs 9/e, p. 464
**Ans 186.** (c) Dutta Obs 9/e, p. 465
**Ans 187.** (b) Dutta Obs 9/e, p. 473

## 14. MANEUVERS AND OPERATIVE OBSTETRICS

### QUESTIONS

**Q.188** In suction evacuation for MTP, the pressure of the suction is raised to:
(a) 100-200 mm Hg
(b) 200-300 mm Hg
(c) 400-600 mm Hg
(d) 700-900 mm Hg

**Q.189** The following statements related to episiotomy are all correct, except:
(a) It is a routine procedure in all cases
(b) It is a deliberate incision made on the perineum during the second stage
(c) It is in fact an inflicted second degree perineal injury
(d) It is the most common obstetric operation

**Q.190** As regards the induction of labor — true statement is:
(a) Induction and augmentation are synonymous
(b) Preinduction Bishop's scoring can predict the success of induction
(c) In Bishop's cervical scoring system, total score is 10
(d) There is no extra benefit of combining medical and surgical methods

**Q.191** The optimum interval between uterine incision and delivery during cesarean section should be:
(a) Less than 90 seconds
(b) Between 90 and 180 seconds
(c) Between 180 and 210 seconds
(d) Between 210 and 240 seconds

### ANSWERS

**Ans 188.** (c)

**Ans 189.** (a) It should be made selectively.

**Ans 190.** (b) Q. (a): Augmentation accelerates already initiated labor. Q. (c): Total score 13. Q. (d): Combined method increases efficiency by reducing induction-delivery interval.

**Ans 191.** (a) Incision and manipulation of the uterus cause reflex uterine vasoconstriction resulting in fetal asphyxia. Interval >90 seconds are associated with significant lowering of Apgar scores.

## QUESTIONS

**Q.192** Optimum negative pressure to form a stable chignon in ventouse delivery is:
(a) 0.2 kg/sq cm
(b) 0.4 kg/sq cm
(c) 0.6 kg/sq cm
(d) 0.8 kg/sq cm

**Q.193** Muscles cut in mediolateral episiotomy are:
(a) Levator ani only
(b) Levator ani and transverse perineal muscles
(c) Levator ani, transverse perineal muscles and bulbospongiosus
(d) Levator ani and sphincter ani externus

**Q.194** Common indications of primary cesarean section in our country are the following, except:
(a) Cephalopelvic disproportion
(b) Fetal distress in first stage of labor
(c) Eclampsia, pre-eclampsia
(d) Previous cesarean delivery

**Q.195** Amniocentesis is the best diagnostic if done:
(a) 8-10 weeks
(b) 12-14 weeks
(c) 16-18 weeks
(d) 20-22 weeks

**Q.196** Criteria for application of forceps are all, except:
(a) Head must be engaged
(b) Pelvis must be adequate
(c) Cervix should be at least 8 cm dilated
(d) Membrane should be ruptured

## ANSWERS

**Ans 192.** (d) Dutta Obs 9/e, p. 540
**Ans 193.** (c)
**Ans 194.** (d)
**Ans 195.** (c)
**Ans 196.** (c) Dutta Obs 9/e, p. 533

## QUESTIONS

**Q.197** *Match the following:*

(a) Craniotomy  1. Division of clavicle(s)
(b) Evisceration  2. Fetal head is severed from trunk
(c) Decapitation  3. Removal of viscera in piece meal
(d) Cleidotomy  4. Perforation of fetal head

**Q.198** *White's classification of diabetes mellitus in pregnancy is based on all, except:*

(a) Onset of diabetes (age)   (b) Duration of diabetes
(c) Level of hyperglycemia   (d) Need of insulin

**Q.199** *External cephalic version is more likely to be successful in all conditions, except:*

(a) Presenting part not engaged   (b) Adequate liquor
(c) Patient not obese   (d) Fetal back placed posteriorly

**Q.200** *Regarding cesarean section, all are correct, except:*

(a) Cephalopelvic disproportion is a common indication
(b) Lower segment scar heals better than the classical scar
(c) Lower segment transverse incision is commonly done
(d) Fetal head is delivered commonly by the forceps

**Q.201** *Match the following:*

(a) Genital tubercle  1. Labia minora
(b) Urogenital sinus  2. Clitoris
(c) Müllerian ducts  3. Lower third of vagina
(d) Urethral folds  4. Fallopian tubes

## ANSWERS

**Ans 197.** (a) = 4; (b) = 3; (c) = 2; (d) = 1. (Dutta Obs 9/e, p. 543)
**Ans 198.** (c) Dutta Obs 9/e, p. 264
**Ans 199.** (d) Dutta Obs 9/e, p. 356
**Ans 200.** (d) Dutta Obs 9/e, p. 552
**Ans 201.** (a) = 2; (b) = 3; (c) = 4; (d) = 1.

## 15. CONTROL OF CONCEPTION

### QUESTIONS

**Q.202** *Pearl index is related with:*
(a) Degree of contracted pelvis
(b) Cervical scoring prior to induction
(c) Assessment of high-risk pregnancy
(d) Contraceptive effectiveness

**Q.203** *Pregnancy failure rate per HWY in IUCD (CuT):*
(a) 1.5    (b) 2
(c) 4.5    (d) 6

**Q.204** *The condom is suitable in all cases, except:*
(a) Known cases of sexually transmitted disease
(b) Missing 'oral pills' in consecutive 2 days in a cycle
(c) Coital act is infrequent
(d) Following tubectomy operation

**Q.205** *The failure rate of Pomeroy's technique is:*
(a) 0.01%    (b) 0.1%
(c) 0.5%     (d) 1%

### ANSWERS

**Ans 202.** (d)
**Ans 203.** (b) 3rd generation IUDs (CuT 380A) have got lesser failure rate (0.6) than CuT.
**Ans 204.** (d) It should be following vasectomy operation.
**Ans 205.** (b)

## 16. SAFE MOTHORHOOD

### QUESTIONS

**Q.206** The following are the direct obstetric cause of maternal death, except:
(a) Abortion
(b) Hemorrhage
(c) Anemia
(d) Eclampsia

**Q.207** Leading causes of maternal mortality in our country are the following, except:
(a) Sepsis
(b) Hemorrhage
(c) Pre-eclampsia and eclampsia
(d) Thromboembolism

**Q.208** Some of the leading causes of stillbirth in our country are the following, except:
(a) Antepartum hemorrhage
(b) Pregnancy-induced hypertension
(c) Prolonged and obstructed labor
(d) Severe anemia

**Q.209** The following is true about maternal health in India and Globally:
(a) SDG targets MMR reduction ≤70 per 100,000 LB
(b) Target for NMR, it is ≤ 12 per 1000 LB
(c) Hemorrhage is the lead cause of maternal death globally
(d) The target year for the SDG goals to achieve is 2020

### ANSWERS

**Ans 206.** (c) Anemia is an indirect cause of death.
**Ans 207.** (d)
**Ans 208.** (d)
**Ans 209.** (a), (b), (c) (See p. 344 )

# CHAPTER 4

# Labor and Delivery

**Chapter Objectives**

Candidate should have the knowledge and understanding of:
- Physiology of labor
- Myometrial contractions
- Assessment of fetal well-being
- Labor monitoring
- Management of normal labor
- Labor: Induction, augmentation
- Malposition, malpresentations
- Abnormal labor: Prolonged labor, obstructed labor

| | |
|---|---|
| ❖ Maternal Pelvis | 166 |
| ❖ Fetal Skull | 174 |
| ❖ Mechanism of Labor | 176 |
|     ➤ Mechanism of Normal Labor | 176 |
| ❖ Labor-Normal, Vaginal Delivery and Management | 180 |
|     ➤ Preterm Labor and Delivery | 191 |
|     ➤ Prelabor Rupture of Membranes (PROM) | 197 |
| ❖ Labor-Abnormal | 198 |
| ❖ Malposition and Malpresentation | 198 |
|     ➤ Occiput Posterior Position (OP) | 198 |
|     ➤ Breech Presentation | 202 |
|     ➤ Face Presentation | 206 |
|     ➤ Brow Presentation | 209 |
|     ➤ Transverse Lie | 209 |
|     ➤ Cord Prolapse | 210 |
|     ➤ Compound Presentation | 211 |
|     ➤ Unstable Lie | 212 |
| ❖ Prolonged (Protracted) Labor | 212 |
| ❖ Obstructed Labor | 214 |

# MATERNAL PELVIS

Study of bony pelvis is essential from obstetric point of view (Fig. 4.1). Architecture of maternal bony pelvis is extremely important to understand the mechanism of labor and to assess the success of the vaginal delivery. Articulated pelvis is composed of four bones—innominate bones-2, the sacrum and the coccyx. There are four joints that unite the four bones—sacroiliac joints-2, symphysis pubis in front and the sacrococcygeal joint posteriorly and inferiorly.

Anatomically the pelvis is divided into:

**False pelvis:** The part that lies above the pelvic brim.

**True pelvis:** The part that lies below the brim.

**Brim of the pelvis (inlet):** The important landmarks on the brim of the pelvis from anterior to posterior on each side are (Fig. 4.2):

(1) Upper border of the symphysis pubis
(2) Pubic crest
(3) Pubic tubercle
(4) Pectineal line
(5) Iliopubic eminence
(6) Iliopectineal line
(7) Sacroiliac articulation
(8) Anterior border of ala of the sacrum
(9) Sacral promontory
(10) To be continued with similar borders on the opposite side

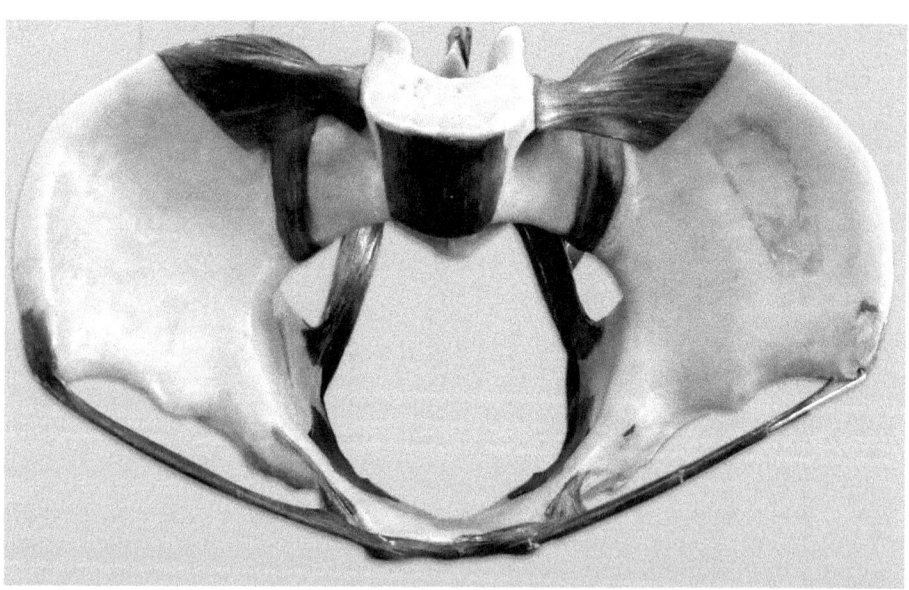

**Fig. 4.1: Female pelvis:** Anatomically pelvis is held with slight forward tilt, bringing the anterior superior iliac spine and the pubic symphysis in one coronal plane. This will also make the angle of inclination 55° with the horizon (Also see Figs. 4.5A and B).

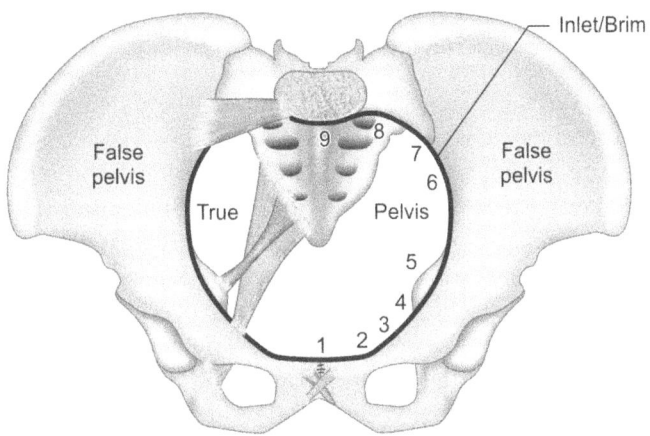

**Fig. 4.2:** Bony landmarks on the brim of the pelvis separating the true from the false pelvis; 1—symphysis pubis, 2—pubic crest, 3—pubic tubercle, 4—pectineal line, 5—iliopubic eminence, 6—iliopectineal line, 7—sacroiliac articulation, 8—anterior border of the ala of sacrum and 9—sacral promontory.

**True pelvis:** It is bounded anteriorly by symphysis pubis. It measures 4 cm (1½ inches). Posteriorly, it is bounded by the sacrum and coccyx. It measures 11.5 cm (4½ inches). True pelvis is divided into:

    A. Inlet    B. Cavity    C. Outlet

**Q. What are the different areas of the pelvis?**

**Ans.** Two main areas are:
  (1) False pelvis above. It has no obstetric significance.
  (2) True pelvis below.
  The boundary line between the two is the brim of the pelvis or inlet of the pelvis.

**Q. What are the different parts of the true pelvis?**

**Ans.** There are three parts:
  (1) Inlet or brim of the pelvis
  (2) Cavity of the pelvis
  (3) Outlet of the pelvis

**Q. What are the different boundary lines that divide the false pelvis, from the true pelvis?**

**Ans.** The division between the false and true pelvis is made by the brim or inlet of the pelvis (Fig. 4.2).

**Q What is the boundary line between the cavity and outlet?**

**Ans.** The division between the cavity and outlet of the pelvis is made by the plane of least pelvic dimension (Fig. 4.3)

**Q. What are the different planes of the pelvis?**

**Ans.** There are four planes of the pelvis (Fig. 4.3):
- (A) **Plane of the inlet:** It an imaginary plane bounded by the points on the brim of the pelvis (mentioned earliers).
- (B) **Plane of the cavity:** This plane extends from the mid point of the posterior surface of the symphysis pubis to junction of the second and third sacral vertebra. It is called plane of **greatest pelvic dimension**.
- (C) **Plane of least pelvic dimension:** This plane extends from the lower border of the symphysis pubis to the tip of ischial spine and posteriorly it extends up to the tip of 5th sacral vertebra.
- (D) **Plane of the outlet (anatomical outlet):** It is formed by a line joining the lower border of symphysis pubis to the tip of the coccyx.

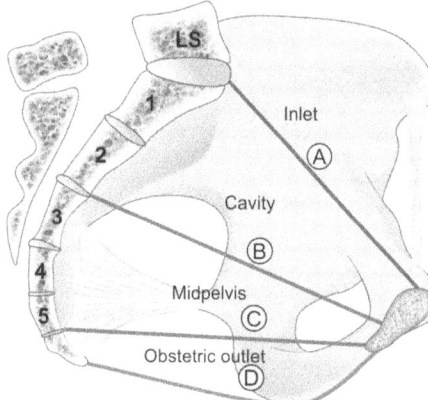

Ⓐ Plane of the inlet
Ⓑ Plane of cavity/plane of greatest pelvic dimension
Ⓒ Mild pelvic plane/plane of least pelvic dimension
Ⓓ Plane of the outlet (anatomical outlet)

**Fig. 4.3:** Planes of the pelvis.

**Q. Mention the different diameters at the brim of the pelvis.**

**Ans.** (1) *Anteroposterior diameters (Fig. 4.4A):*
  - (a) True conjugate, anatomical conjugate or conjugate vera: 11cm
  - (b) Obstetric conjugate : 10 cm
  - (c) Diagonal conjugate : 12 cm

(2) *Transverse diameters (Fig. 4.4B).*
  - (a) Anatomical transverse diameter 13 cm
  - (b) Obstetrical transverse diameter ($\leq$13 cm)

(3) *Oblique diameters—12 cm (Fig. 4.4B):*
  It starts from one sacroiliac joint and ends with the opposite iliopubic eminence. They are:
  - (a) Left
  - (b) Right
  - (c) Sacrocotyloid diameters (9.5 cm): It is the distance between the mid point of the sacral promontory to the iliopubic eminence. It is useful in flat pelvis where biparietal diameter lies during labor.

(4) *Posterior sagittal diameters:*
   (a) Cavity: Distance between the tip of the sacrum to the midpoint of bispinous diameter. It measures 5 cm.
   (b) Outlet: It is the anteroposterior diameter extending between the sacrococcygeal joint and the midpoint of the transverse diameter of the outlet (anterior margin of the anus). It measures 8.5 cm.

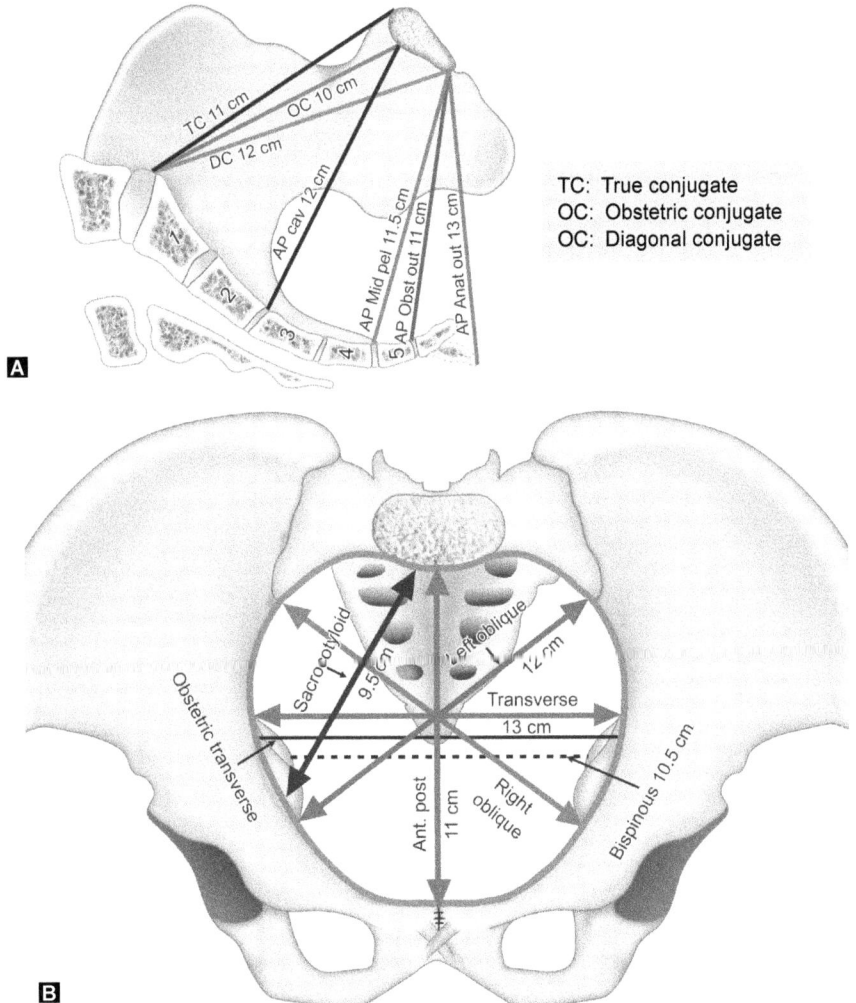

**Figs. 4.4A and B:** (A) Anteroposterior diameters of the pelvis; (B) Diameters of the inlet.

**Q. What is the significance of the plane of least pelvic dimension?**
**Ans.** (1) It is the **narrowest plane** in the pelvis.
   (2) This plane corresponds to the **origin of levator ani muscle**. This is known as **pelvic floor**.
   (3) During the course of mechanism of labor, **internal rotation of the fetal head** takes place at this plane.
   (4) This level marks the beginning of the **forward curve of the pelvic axis**.

(5) Pudendal nerve hooks around the dorsal surface of the ischial spine and enters the perineal pouch. It is a landmark used for **pudendal nerve block analgesia**.
(6) Bispinous diameter (10.5 cm): The distance between the tips of two ischial spines is in this plane. **Station of the presenting part** is expressed in either (above) – or (below) + in relation to this plane
(7) Deep transverse arrest (DTA) usually occurs at this plane.

**Q. What are the different axes of the pelvis?**

**Ans.** There are two axes:
(a) **Anatomical pelvic axis (curve of Carus):** It is an uniformly curved line fitting with the concavity of the sacrum. It is formed by joining the axes of the inlet, cavity and outlet. Fetus does not traverse through this path (Fig. 4.5A).
(b) **Obstetric pelvic axis:** Fetal head negotiates through the obstetric pelvic axis. It is directed first downwards and backwards from the brim up to the level of ischial spine, then abruptly forwards (Fig. 4.5B).

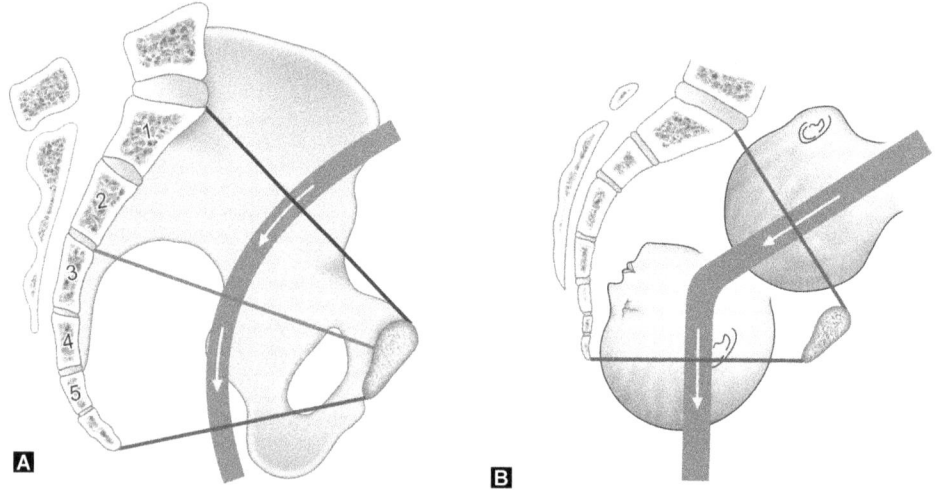

**Figs. 4.5A and B:** (A) Anatomical pelvic axis; (B) Obstetric pelvic axis.

**Q. What are the different bones that constitute the pelvis?**

**Ans.** The bones are four. These are:
(1) Innominate bones—2 (on one either side)
(2) Sacrum—1
(3) Coccyx—1

**Q. What are the different joints in the pelvis?**

**Ans.** Joints are total four:
(1) Sacroiliac joints—2: One on either side: These are synovial joints
(2) Symphysis pubis: Fibrocartilaginous joints
(3) Sacrococcygeal joints: Synovial hinge joint.

**Q. What are the different types of female pelvis?**

**Ans.** On the basis of the shape of the inlet, female pelvis is divided into four parent types:

(A) Gynecoid (50%)  (B) Anthropoid (25%)
(C) Android (20%)   (D) Platypelloid (5%)

However, in majority of cases, combination of features is found.

**Q. What are the important differences in the four types of parent pelvis?**

**Ans.** Differences between four types of pelvis have been described below in tabular form:

| Pelvis type | Inlet | Midcavity | Outlet: Subpubic angle |
|---|---|---|---|
| A. Gynecoid | Round | Divergent sidewalls, Ischial spines (IS): Not prominent | Wide (85°) TDO: 11 cm |
| B. Anthropoid | Anteroposteriorly oval | Straight or divergent Sidewalls, Ischial spines: Prominent | Slightly narrow (medium) TDO: 11 cm |
| C. Android | Triangular | Convergent sidewalls, IS: Prominent | Narrow TDO: <11 cm |
| D. Platypelloid | Transversely oval | Divergent sidewalls, IS: Not prominent | Very wide >90° TDO: 11 cm |

*Note:* Different diameters of the female bony pelvis have been measured by X-ray pelvimetry and computed tomography (CT). However, CT and X-ray pelvimetry are rarely used for pelvic assessment in labor. **Clinical pelvimetry is the only method of assessing the pelvis in labor. Fetal head is the best pelvimeter.**

**Q. What is diagonal conjugate?**

**Ans.** It is the distance between the lower border of the symphysis pubis and the midpoint on the sacral promontory. It measures 12 cm (4¾ inches).

**Q. How do you measure the diagonal conjugate?**

**Ans.** Steps of assessment (Fig. 4.6):

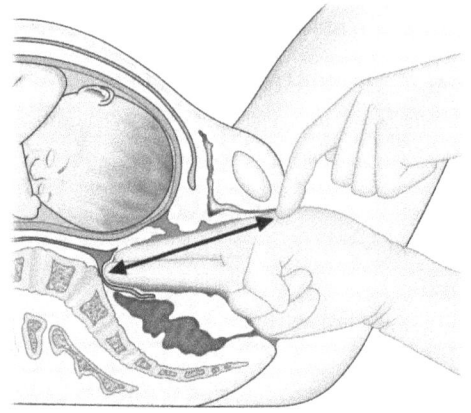

**Diagonal conjugate:**
Two fingers of gloved right hand are introduced into the vagina along the sacral curvature to reach the sacral promontory. In a normal pelvis, it is usually not felt. The point where the bone recedes from the fingers is the sacral promontory. The radial border of the fingers are then mobilized underneath the symphysis pubis and a mark is made over the gloved index finger. The distance between the marking and the tip of the middle finger is the measurement of diagonal conjugate.

**Fig. 4.6:** Measurement of diagonal conjugate.

**Q. What is angle of pelvic inclination?**

**Ans.** See Fig. 4.7.

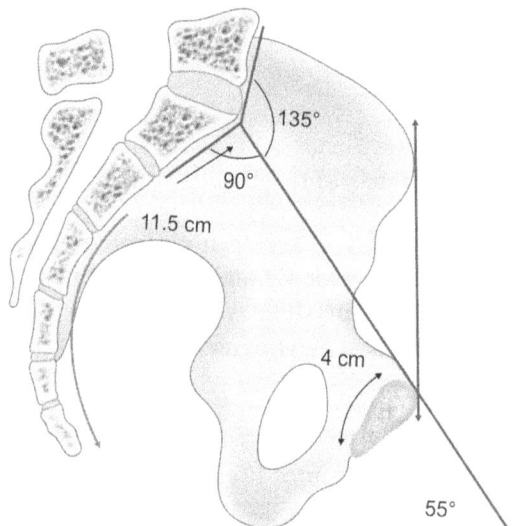

**Angle of pelvic inclination:**
Angle of pelvic inclination is the angle subtended by the plane of pelvic inlet with the horizon, when the plane of pelvic inlet is extended downwards to meet the ground. It is measured when the woman is in upright standing position. The anterior superior iliac spine and the pubic tubercle are in the same vertical plane. The angle measures about 55°.

**Fig. 4.7:** Angle of inclination.

**Q. What is the bony pelvic outlet?**

**Ans.** See Fig. 4.8.

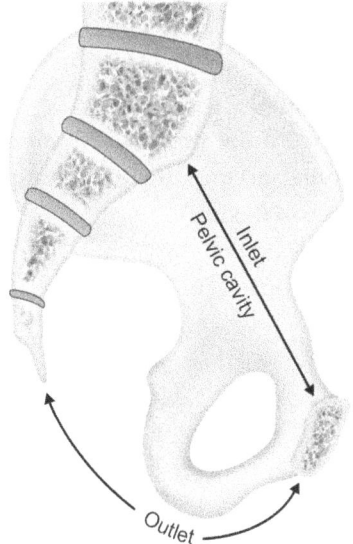

**Bony pelvic outlet or anatomical pelvic outlet:** It is bounded anteriorly by the under surface of the symphysis pubis, laterally by the conjoint ischiopubic rami, ischial tuberosity and sacrotuberous ligament and posteriorly by the tip of the coccyx. (*See* also Fig. 4.7)

**Fig. 4.8:** Pelvic outlet.

**Q. What is meant by transverse diameter of the outlet?**

**Ans.** See Fig. 4.9.

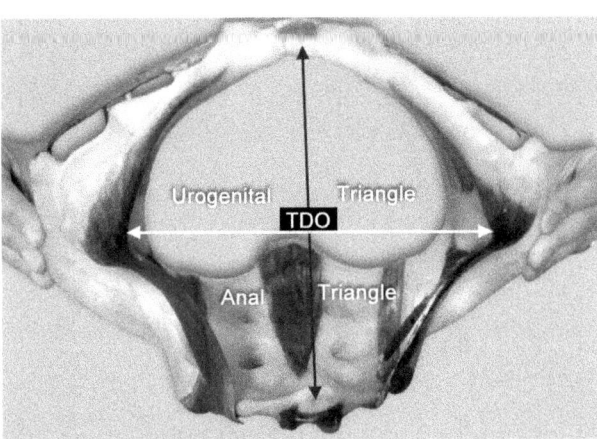

**Fig. 4.9:** Bony pelvic outlet. (TDO is shown).

**Transverse diameter of the Outlet (TDO):** It is the distance between the inner margin of the two ischial tuberosities. It measures 11 cm. Clinically, it is measured by placing the four knuckles of the clinched fist placed between the two ischial tuberosities. TDO forms the common base for the two triangular planes. The apex of the anterior triangle (urogenital) is formed by the inferior border of the pubic arch. The apex of the posterior triangle (anal) is formed by the sacrococcygeal joint.

## FETAL SKULL

Fetal skull is arbitrarily divided into several zones of obstetric significance (Fig. 4.10).
These are: ♦ Vertex ♦ Brow ♦ Face ♦ Sinciput ♦ Occiput ♦ Fontanelles.

(1) Fontanelle:  Anterior (Bregma)
 Posterior (Lamda)
(2) Sutures:  Sagital (between the two parietal bones)
 parietal, frontal, occipital (lamdoid suture)

**(3) Anteroposterior diameters (Varies with degree of flexion):**

(i) Complete flexion (when chin touches chest)
 Suboccipitobregmatic diameter : 9.5 cm
(ii) Incomplete flexion:
 Suboccipitofrontal diameter : 10 cm
(iii) Markedly deflexed:
 Occipitofrontal diamerter : 11.5 cm
(iv) Partial extension
 Mentovertical diameter : 14 cm
(v) Incomplete extension
 Submentovertical diameter : 11.5 cm
(vi) Complete extension
 Submentobregmatic diameter : 9.5 cm

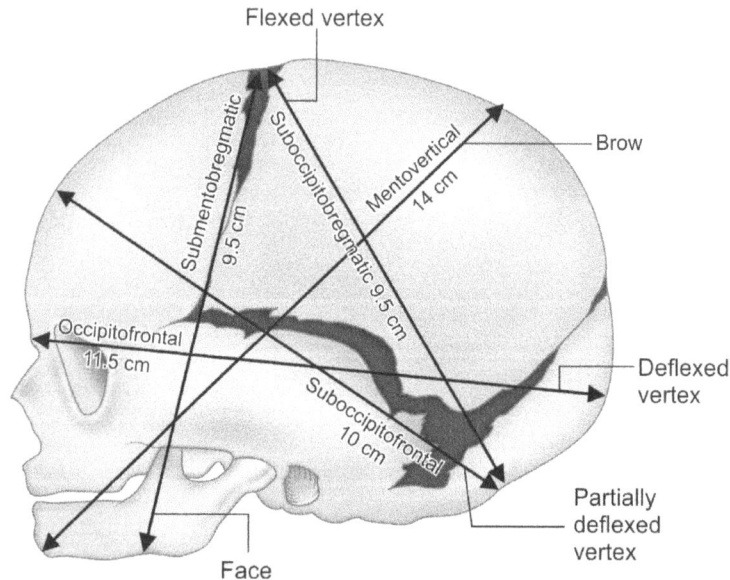

**Fig. 4.10:** Important landmarks of fetal skull.

**(4) Transverse diameters of the fetal skull:**
 (i) Biparietal diameter : 9.5 cm
 (ii) Super-subparietal diameter : 8.5 cm
  (Asynclitism)
 (iii) Bitemporal diameter : 8 cm
 (iv) Bimastoid diameter : 7.5 cm
 (Not compressible even after doing craniotomy.

**Q. Mention the different engaging diameters of the skull that come into play from the attitude of complete flexion to complete extension.**

**Ans.** (*See* Table below)

|   | Diameters | Measurement in cm (inches) | Attitude of the head | Presentation |
|---|---|---|---|---|
| 1. | *Suboccipitobregmatic*—extends from the nape of the neck to the center of the bregma | 9.5 cm (3¾") | Complete flexion | Vertex |
| 2. | *Suboccipitofrontal*—extends from the nape of the neck to the anterior end of the anterior fontanelle or center of the sinciput | 10 cm (4") | Incomplete flexion | Vertex |
| 3. | *Occipitofrontal*—extends from the occipital eminence to the root of the nose (glabella) | 11.5 cm (4½") | Marked deflexion | Vertex |
| 4. | *Mentovertical*—extends from the midpoint of the chin to the highest point on the sagittal suture | 14 cm (5½") | Partial extension | Brow |
| 5. | *Submentovertical*—extends from junction of floor of the mouth and neck to the highest point on the sagittal suture | 11.5 cm (4½") | Incomplete extension | Face |
| 6. | *Submentobregmatic*—extends from junction of floor of the mouth and neck to the center of the bregma | 9.5 cm (3¾") | Complete extension | Face |

# MECHANISM OF LABOR

## MECHANISM OF NORMAL LABOR

**Q. What do you understand by the mechanism of labor?**

**Ans.** It is the series of movements that occur in the fetal head in the process of adaptation during its journey through the pelvis.

**Q. What are the principal movements that occur on the fetal head during the course of labor (mechanism of labor)?**

**Ans.** The cardinal movements are: Here, it is described as in left occiput posterior position (Fig. 4.11).

(1) **Engagement:** Biparietal diameter passes through the pelvic brim. In a primigravida, engagement usually occurs before the onset of labor, whereas in a multigravida the same may occur during the course of labor.

(2) **Descent:** It is a continuous process throughout the course of labor.

(3) **Flexion:** Flexion is achieved when the head meets the resistance of the birth canal (pelvic floor muscles, cervix, pelvic walls) during descent. Flexion brings lesser diameter in the pelvis.

(4) **Internal rotation:** It is mainly due to:
   (i) Gutter-shaped arrangement of the levator ani muscles (two halves)
   (ii) Pelvic shape having the long anterior-posterior diameter of the outlet to accommodate the long diameter of the fetal head.

(5) **Crowning:** The biparietal diameter stretches the vulval outlet and there is no recession of the head even when the contractions are over.

(6) **Extension:** It is the result of final driving force that expels the fetal head out. The uterine contraction force is directed downward and the forces exerted by the pelvic and perineal floor muscles are upward and forward. The resultant force drives the head downward and upward (extension).

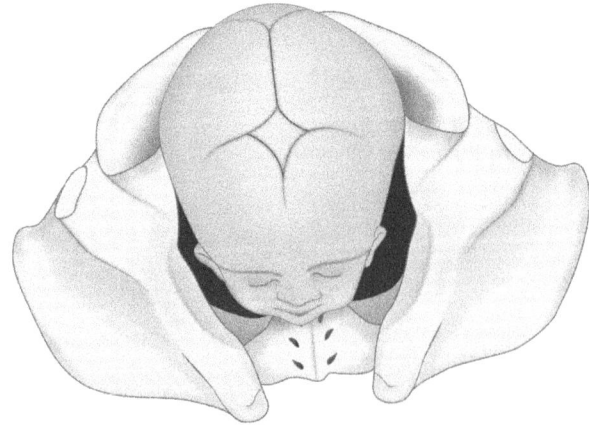

**Fig. 4.11:** Extension of the fetal head during normal delivery.

(7) **Restitution:** It is the rotation of the head (45°) due to untwisting of the neck that occurred during internal rotation.

(8) **External rotation:** It is due to internal rotation of the shoulder.

(9) **Delivery of the shoulders:** The shoulders are placed in the anteroposterior diameter of the outlet. With further descent, the anterior shoulder is pushed below the symphysis pubis and is born first. Posterior shoulder then sweeps over the perineum by lateral flexion.

(10) **Delivery of the trunk:** It occurs by lateral flexion.

*Q. What do you understand by asynclitism? What is its significance?*

**Ans.** See p. 186.

# STEPS FOR THE DEMONSTRATION OF MECHANISM OF LABOR

## METHOD OF HOLDING THE MATERNAL BONY PELVIS ANATOMICALLY AND TO DEMONSTRATE THE PELVIC DIAMETERS AND MECHANISM OF LABOR

The bony pelvis is held with the fingers of the left hand. The left-sided ischium bone of the maternal bony pelvis is held with the fingers of the left hand keeping the symphysis pubis in front and the sacrum behind (Fig. 4.12). It is convenient to hold the ischium bone by the index, and middle fingers passing through the obturator foramen. The thumb is placed behind the ischium. A firm grip is made with pressure using the fingers as described earlier. Now the pelvis is held with a forward tilt to maintain the other points in relation to the anatomical position (*See* description Fig. 4.1, p. 166 and Fig. 4.7, p. 172). The right hand fingers are free for demonstration.

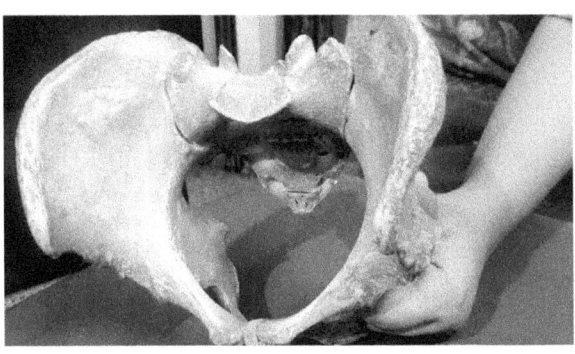

**Fig. 4.12:** Anatomical position of the pelvis.

### Q. How to hold the fetal skull?

**Ans.** The index finger of the right hand is introduced through the foramen magnum (Fig. 4.13A) and the skull is hold by the thumb and the middle fingers placed over the parietal eminence one on either side. The occiput is directed anteriorly and the vault of the skull directed below (Fig. 4.13B). The occiput is tilled downwards so as to put the mentum at a higher level. This suggests attitude of flexion of the head.

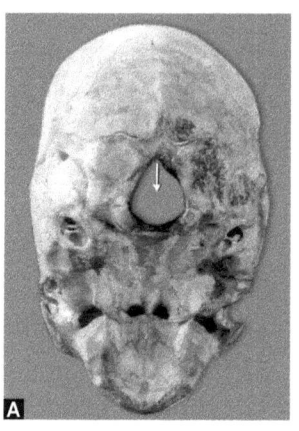
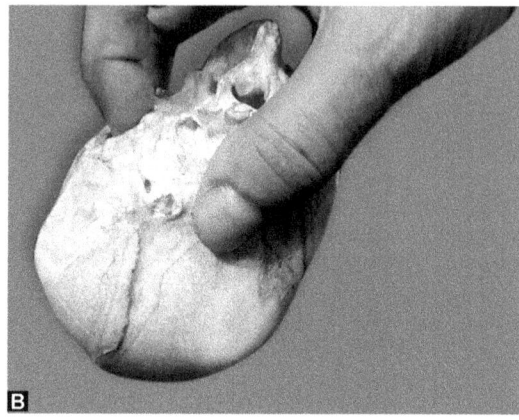

**Figs. 4.13A and B:** (A) Base of skull showing foramen magnum; (B) Demonstration of holding fetal skull is shown. Index finger is placed within the foramen magnum and the thumb and the middle finger are placed over the parietal eminence one on either side.

## PROCEDURES TO DEMONSTRATE THE POSITION OF FETAL HEAD IN RELATION TO THE QUADRANT OF THE PELVIS

### Q. Show the left occiput anterior position?

**Ans.** The maternal bony pelvis and the fetal skull are held as described in Fig. 4.14. Now the candidate is needed to direct the occiput of the fetal skull towards the left iliopubic eminence of the maternal bony pelvis (Fig. 4.15).

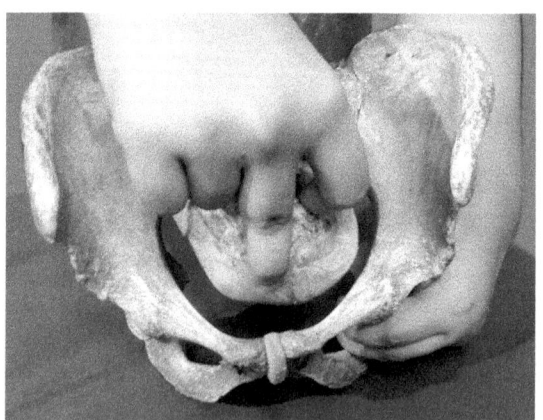

**Fig. 4.14:** Demonstration of the position of fetal head in relation to the Quadrant of the pelvis. Maternal pelvis (left hand) and fetal skull (right hand) is held and the position of left occiput anterior position is demonstrated.

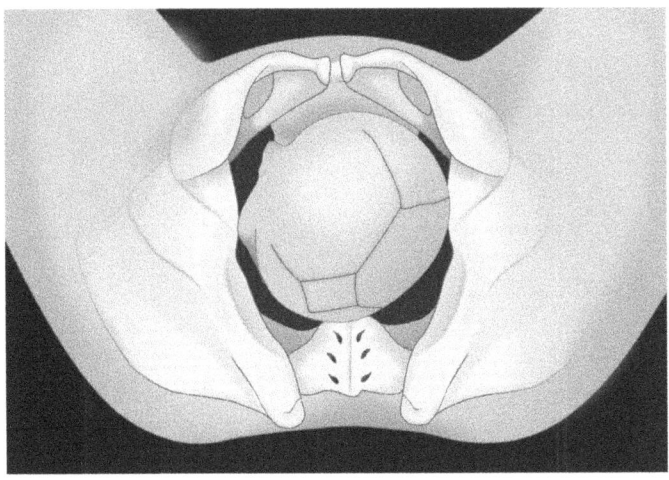

**Fig. 4. 15:** Left occiput anterior (LOA) (viewed from below).

**Q. Show the left occiput transverse position of the fetal skull?**

**Ans.** The candidate needs to direct the occiput towards left end of the obstetric transverse diameter of the pelvis (Fig. 4.16).

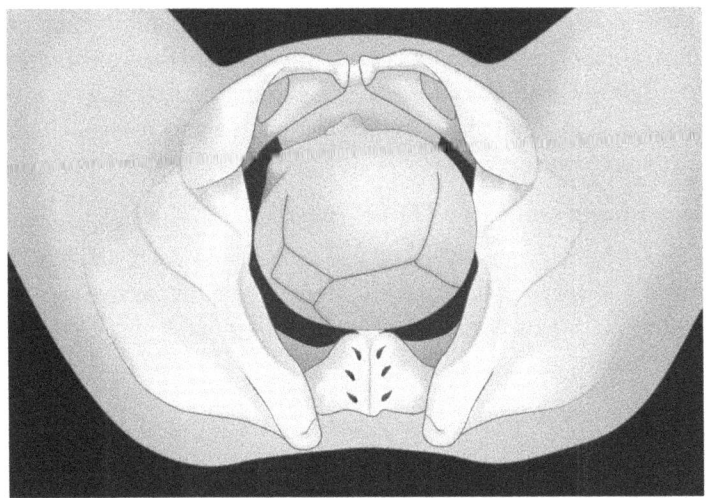

**Fig. 4.16:** Left occiput transverse (LOT) (viewed from below).

**Q. Show the right occiput transverse position of the fetal skull?**

**Ans.** The candidate needs to direct the occiput towards right end of the obstetric transverse diameter of the pelvis (Fig. 4.17).

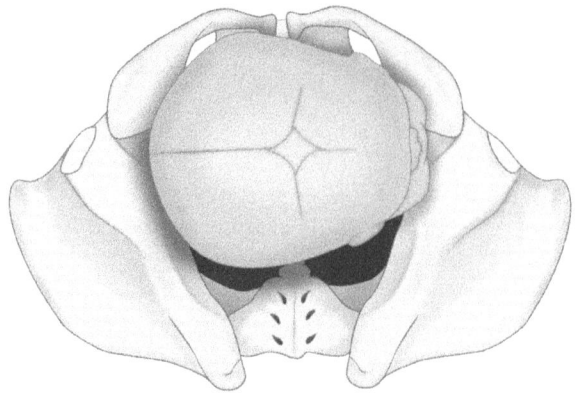

**Fig. 4.17:** Right occiput transverse position (ROT) (viewed from below).

## LABOR–NORMAL, VAGINAL DELIVERY AND MANAGEMENT

**Q. How do you define labor?**

**Ans. Labor** is the series of changes that take place in the genital organs in an effort to expel the viable fetus from the womb to the outside world through the vagina. Labor begins when the uterine contractions are of sufficient frequency, intensity and duration to cause progressive effacement and dilatation of the cervix.

**Q. What do you understand by delivery?**

**Ans.** Delivery is the process of expulsion or extraction of a viable fetus out of the womb. Delivery can take place without labor as in elective cesarean delivery (abdominal). However, delivery may be vaginal also (forceps or ventouse delivery).

**Q. What is normal labor?**

**Ans.** Normal labor fulfills the following criteria:
(1) Fetus with vertex presentation
(2) Spontaneous onset of term
(3) Without undue prolongation of labor
(4) Spontaneous delivery with minimal aids
(5) Without any complications.

**Q. What are the clinical stages of labor?**

**Ans.** Stages of labor are total three:
**First stage** begins with onset of true labor pains and ends with full dilatation of the cervix (10 cm). Its duration is 12 hours in a primigravida and 6 hours in a multigravida.

**Second stage** begins with full dilatation of the cervix and ends with delivery of the fetus—duration is 2 hours in a primigravida and 30 minutes in a multigravida.

**Third stage** begins after the delivery of the fetus and ends with the delivery of the placenta and the membranes. Average duration is 15 minutes in both primi-and multigravida.

Q. *What is "show"?*

Ans. It is the vaginal discharge of cervical mucus mixed with blood seen with the onset of labor.

Q. *What are the important characteristics of uterine contractions during labor?*

Ans. In a normal labor, the **uterine contractions** should have **adequate:**
  (a) Frequency (3-4 contractions every 10 minutes)
  (b) Duration (30-40 seconds for each contraction)
  (c) Intensity to increase intrauterine pressure. Intensity is considered good when clinically uterine wall cannot be indented by the fingers.

Q. *What are the clinical phases of the first stage of labor?*

Ans. The first stage is divided into two phases:
  (a) **Latent phase:** It is of variable duration during which cervix becomes pliable and effaced. It ends when cervix is 3-5 cm dilated. Duration of latent phase has minimum effect on the subsequent course of labor.
  (b) **Active phase:** It begins when the cervix is 3-5 cm dilated in the presence of uterine contractions. In the active phase, cervix dilates at the rate of 1 cm/hour in a primigravida and 1.5 cm/hour in a multigravida. During the active phase, the uterine contractions become regular in terms of frequency, intensity and duration.

Q. *What are the different phases of parturition?*

Ans. Arbitrarily, there are four phases since conception:
  **Phase 1:** Uterine—quiescence till the end of pregnancy due to the effects of progesterone, prostacyclin and relaxin.
  **Phase 2**—preparation for labor.
  **Phase 3**—active labor process (3 clinical stages).
  **Phase 4**—involution (puerperium).

Q. *What are the major changes (events) in the first stage of labor?*

Ans. Three major changes (events) are:
  (i) Effacement of the cervix
  (ii) Dilatation of the cervix
  (iii) Formation of the lower uterine segment.

**Q. What are the predisposing factors for the effacement and dilatation of the cervix?**

Ans. (a) Increased vascularity of the cervix
(b) Fibromuscular glandular hypertrophy and hyperplasia of the cervix
(c) Fluid accumulation in between the collagen fibers
(d) Breaking down of collagen fibers by collagenase and elastase enzymes
(e) Changes in various glycosaminoglycans in the matrix of the cervix.
(f) Softening of the cervix.

**Q. What factors are actually responsible for the changes as mentioned above?**

Ans. (i) **Uterine contractions and retractions** are important. Changes are due to the attachment of the longitudinal muscle fibers of the uterus to the circular muscle fibers of the lower uterine segment and upper part of the cervix. Progressive contractions and retractions result in effacement and dilatation of the cervix as the circular muscle fibers are pulled up over the presenting part by the longitudinal muscle fibers.

(ii) **Fetal axis pressure:** In labor with fetal longitudinal lie, and with well applied fetal head, strong uterine contractions pushes the fetus down. The well-fitted fetal head causes mechanical stretching of the lower segment and dilatation of the cervix. With progressive uterine contractions and retractions the upper uterine segment becomes thicker and the lower segment becomes thinner. The cervical canal starts dilating.

(iii) **Formation of the bag of forewater** when the girdle of contact of the fetal head with the lower uterine segment occurs. The uterine contractions and retractions generate hydrostatic pressure in the forewater. This forwater pressure acts as a wedge and causes dilatation of the cervix.

(iv) **There is progressive mechanical stretching** of the lower uterine segment and the cervical canal by the presenting part. The strong contraction force of the uterine fundus is transmitted through the fetal podalic pole and the vertebral column to the well applied fetal head. This causes effacement and dilatation of the cervix.

**Q. What is the clinical significance of lower uterine segment?**

Ans. During labor, lower uterine segment forms a complete birth canal when the cervix is fully dilated. The other clinical importances are:
(a) Implantation of placenta in the lower segment is known as placenta previa.
(b) Lower segment cesarean section is done here.
(c) Once placenta is implanted here, the risk of morbid adherent placenta is high.

In obstructed labor, this segment becomes thin and maximally stretched. Ultimately uterus ruptures through segment.

**Q. What is bearing down (pushing effort) during labor?**

**Ans.** It is the additional voluntary expulsive effort of the mother in the second stage of labor. Along with uterine contraction, there is maternal voluntary pushing effort to shorten the duration of second stage of labor.

**Q. How do you differentiate true labor pain from false labor pain?**

**Ans.**

| True labor | False labor |
| --- | --- |
| 1. Pain at regular interval | 1. Pain at irregular interval |
| 2. Pain is associated with hardening of the uterus | 2. No such |
| 3. Frequency of contractions gradually increase | 3. No such, it is inconsistent |
| 4. Duration and intensity of pains gradually increase | 4. No change |
| 5. Pain starts in the back and gradually moves to lower abdomen | 5. Pain in the lower abdomen, groin |
| 6. Pain is associated with show | 6. No such |
| 7. Cervix is effaced and dilated | 7. No such |
| 8. Presenting part descends | 8. No descent of presenting part |
| 9. Pain is not relieved by analgesics and/or enema | 9. Relieved by analgesics or enema |

**Q. How do you assess the separation of placenta in the third stage of labor?**

**Ans. Abdominal examination:**
 (a) Uterus becomes globular, firm and ballotable.
 (b) The fundal height is raised.
 (c) There is bulging of the suprapubic region as the placenta occupies the lower uterine segment.

**Vaginal examination:**
 (a) There is a gush of vaginal bleeding.
 (b) Permanent lengthening of the umbilical cord (there is no indrawing of the cord on suprapubic pressure).

**Q. What are the important phases of the second stage of labor?**

**Ans.** (i) **Propulsive**—from full dilatation of the cervix to the time when head has reached the pelvic floor.
 (ii) **Expulsive**—since the mother has the irresistible desire of "**bearing down**" or "**pushing down**" till the baby is delivered. Here both the forces of uterine contractions and the voluntary contractions of abdominal muscles are combined.
 (iii) Delivery of the fetus.

**Q. What are the important events in the third stage of labor?**

Ans. (i) Separation of the placenta
(ii) Expulsion of the placenta.

**Q. How is the uterine bleeding controlled after the placenta is normally separated?**

Ans. (i) The bleeding sinuses are occluded by the interlacing muscle fibers of the uterus as these fibers undergo complete retraction. **These interlacing myometrial fibers act as living ligatures**.
(ii) Formation of thrombus as there is the hypercoagulable state in pregnancy.
(iii) Myotamponade action of the uterine walls.

**Q. What are the cardinal movements of the fetal head during labor?**

Ans. The cardinal movements are the series of movements that occur on the head in the process of adaptation during its journey through the pelvis. Cardinal movements, though we consider it separately for our understanding, consists of a combination of movements simultaneously.
**These are:** (a) **Engagement** → (b) **Descent** → (c) **Flexion** → (d) **Internal rotation** → (e) **Extension** → (f) **Restitution** → (g) **External rotation** and → (h) **Delivery of the shoulder** and **trunk**.

**Q. What is a partograph?**

Ans. It is a composite graphical record of cervical dilatation and descent of the head and FHR against the duration of labor with time.

**Q. How can abdominal examination help to assess the progress of labor?**

Ans. The amount of fetal head felt suprapubically (in finger breadth) is assessed by placing the fingers above the symphysis pubis. **This is the Crichton fifth formula ("fifths of the fetal head felt above the maternal pubic symphysis")**.
The basovertical (fetal skull) distance is 9-10 cm and the width of the obstetrician's finger is about 1.6-2 cm. With this, **no more than two finger breadths of fetal skull should be palpable above the symphysis pubis when the lower pole of the fetal skull is at zero station (level of ischial spines)**. If three finger breadths are palpable above, the fetal head is not engaged. This is true even if a portion of fetal head is palpable below the level of ischial spine (Figs. 4.18A and B).

**Q. What is station of the fetal head?**

Ans. It is the relationship of the lower pole of the fetal head (presenting part) to that of the plane of the ischial spines. When the lower pole lies at the level of ischial spines, it is known as station zero. The levels above are known as minus (-1 cm, -2 cm, -3 cm, -4 cm and -5 cm) station and the levels below are known as plus (+1 cm, +2 cm, +3 cm, +4 cm and +5 cm) station.

**Q. What important information is recorded following an abdominal examination when the woman is in labor?**

**Ans.** (a) **Palpation:**
  (i) Uterine contractions—frequency (number of contractions in 10 minutes' time), intensity and duration (in seconds)
  (ii) Pelvic grip—gradual disappearance of poles of the fetal head (sinciput and occiput). Assessment of fetal head above symphysis pubis by Crichton fifth formula (Figs. 4.18A and B).
(b) **Auscultation:** Fetal heart rate (FHR)—in beats per minute (bpm). Normal 100–160 bpm, rhythm and intensity.

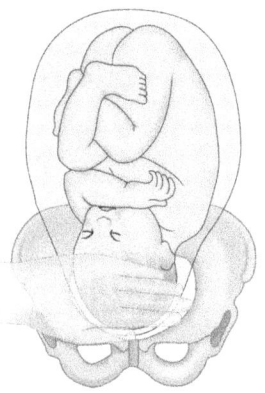
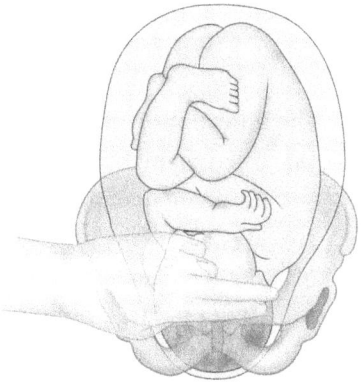

**Fig. 4.18A:** Head is palpable 5/5th above the symphysis pubis. Head is mobile, free and not engaged.

**Fig. 4.18B:** Head is palpable 2/5th above the brim and the rest 3/5th is gone down the brim. Head is engaged.

**Q. In the management of first stage of labor, when should vaginal examination be done?**

**Ans.** In the management of labor, vaginal examination should be restricted to a minimum possible extent. The examination is uncomfortable for the woman, but the main risk is the introduction of infection with each examination. However, the common indications of vaginal examination are:
  (1) **At the onset of labor** to detect the cervical changes in association with uterine contractions felt per abdomen. Pelvic assessment especially in primigravida is done at the same time.
  (2) **To assess the progress of labor** by noting cervical dilatation, effacement and descent of the head in relation to ischial spines (station).
  (3) Once the membrane ruptures, **to exclude cord prolapse**.
  (4) **To confirm the onset of second stage** when the woman starts bearing down efforts.

**Q. What important information is recorded following a vaginal examination when the woman is in labor?**

**Ans.** Vaginal examination is done aseptically with the woman in dorsal position (Fig. 4.19). Gloved middle and index fingers of the right hand are introduced inside the vagina.

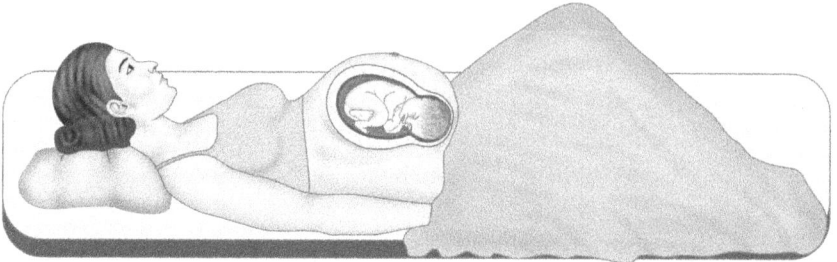

**Fig. 4.19:** Position of the woman during obstetric examination.

**The information obtained is as follows:**
(a) Dilation of the cervix (cm)
(b) Effacement of the cervix (%)
(c) Position of the presenting part (head)
(d) Station of the presenting part
(e) Status of the membranes
(f) Color of the liquor if the membranes are ruptured
(g) Caput or molding of the head
(h) Assessment of the pelvis.

**Q. What is meant by deflexion?**

**Ans.** It is the attitude of the fetal head within the uterus. Usually in a flexed head, the occiput lies at a lower level than the sinciput. When the sinciput remains at or slightly below the level of occiput it is called deflexion.

**Q. What is asynclitism?**

**Ans.** It is the failure of the sagittal suture of the fetal head to descent along with the available (obstetric) transverse diameter of the pelvic inlet.

The sagittal suture may either be deflected anteriorly toward the symphysis pubis or posteriorly toward the sacral promontory. When sagittal suture lies anteriorly, the posterior parietal bone becomes the leading presenting part. **This is known as posterior asynclitism or posterior parietal presentation.** This is observed more in primigravida.

In others, the sagittal suture lies more posteriorly when the anterior parietal bone becomes the leading presenting part. **This is known as anterior asynclitism or anterior parietal presentation.** This is common in multipara.

Mild degrees of asynclitism are common. **Severe degrees of asynclitism indicate cephalopelvic disproportion. Presence of molding or caput** makes detection of asynclitism difficult. This is important during forceps applications.

**Q. When the cervix is considered as fully dilated?**

**Ans.** The measurement of 10 cm is considered the full dilatation. It is approximately the diameter of the fetal head at term.

**Q. What is Ritgen maneuver?**

**Ans.** This maneuver is done for controlled delivery of the head in between the uterine contractions. The right hand covered with a sterile towel is placed over the anococcygeal region. The chin is pushed with the fingers of the right hand. The left hand simultaneously exerts counter-pressure on the occiput. The purpose is to deliver the head with its smallest diameters while passing through the introitus and perineum. This prevents perineal injuries.

**Q. What are the clinical features to suggest the onset of second stage of labor?**

**Ans.** (a) Uterine contractions are found with increased intensity and duration.
(b) Appearance of maternal bearing down efforts (pushing efforts).
(c) Urge to defecate with descent of the presenting part.
However, vaginal examination is to be done to confirm the diagnosis.

**Q. How do you deliver the fetal head?**

**Ans.**
- Mother is encouraged to push down (bearing down efforts) in the second stage of labor
- Following crowning, with further contractions, perineum is bulged and thinned out. Episiotomy (selective) may be made at this time
- Head is allowed to deliver slowly in between the contractions with the use of **Ritgen maneuver**
- Flexion of the head is maintained during contractions by pushing down the occiput backward using the thumb and index fingers of the left hand
- Care following delivery of the head:
  (a) Mucus and blood from the mouth
  (b) Face and eyes are wiped off by sterile cotton swabs
- Neck is then palpated to exclude any loop of cord and, if found, it may be slipped over the head. When it is found tight, cord is cut in between two clamped Kocher's forceps.

**Q. How do you deliver the shoulders and trunk?**

**Ans.** There is no rush to deliver the shoulders. One should wait for the next uterine contractions when anterior shoulder is born underneath the symphysis pubis.

Anterior shoulder may be released from underneath the pubis by grasping the head with both the palms and gently drawing posteriorly. Similarly, the posterior shoulder is released by drawing the head gently upward.

Trunk is delivered by lateral flexion.

**Q. What immediate care of the newborn is done?**

**Ans.**
- Baby is placed in a tray covered with dry linen (to keep baby warm) with head slightly downward (15°)
- Mucus in the air passage (mouth and oropharynx) is cleared off mucus by gentle suction
- Apgar scoring is done at 1 and 5 minutes
- Clamping of the umbilical cord is done.

The cord is clamped by two Kocher's forceps. The cord is cut in between. The Kocher's forceps are replaced by cord clamps or cotton cord ligatures. Quick examination of the baby is done to detect any problem or abnormality. Baby is wrapped with a dry warm towel. Identification tag (disc number) is tied on the wrist of both the baby and mother.

**Q. What is the procedure of cord clamping?**

**Ans.** The cord is clamped by two Kocher's forceps. The near one is placed 5 cm away from the umbilicus and the cord is cut in between. Presence of any abnormality in cord vessels is checked. The Kocher's forceps on the baby's side is replaced by cord clamp (disposable), placed 2.5 cm away from the umbilicus or with two separate cord ligatures of cotton threads.

**Delay in cord clamping** for 2-3 minutes or till cessation of cord pulsation helps transfer of 80-100 mL of blood from the placenta to the baby. This procedure may not be recommended as a routine due to the risk of polycythemia and hyperbilirubinemia in a normal neonate. **Early cord clamping** is done in cases with:
(a) Rh-incompatibility
(b) Birth asphyxia
(c) Preterm baby
(d) Baby of a diabetic mother.

**Q. How do you manage the third stage of labor?**

**Ans.** Third stage is managed either by:
(i) Expectant method
(ii) Active management: Active management of third stage of labor is preferred (*See* SAQ p. 237).

**Q. How to differentiate caput succedaneum from cephalhematoma?**

| Caput succedaneum | Cephalhematoma |
|---|---|
| **Appearance**: At birth | Hours after birth |
| **Feel**: Soft, and compressible | Soft but incompressible |
| **Extent**: Diffuse, spreads over the suture lines | Limited to a bone, does not cross the suture lines |
| **Position:** Changes and moves to the dependant part | Does not change, fixed to one site |
| **With observation:** Gradually reduces in size and disappears within few hours | It increases in size with time. Disappears only after weeks or months |
| **Definition:** Localized swelling on the scalp due to effusion of serum | It is the hemorrhage under the periosteum of bone(s) of the skull |
| **Etiology:** Pressure by the dilating cervix (Cervical ring) causing obstruction to the venous and lymphatic return resulting in scalp edema | It is following trauma to the skull due to (a) prolonged pressure on head during labor, (b) forceps/ventouse delivery. Often associated with the fracture of the skull bone(s) |

Women those are delivered at home, she should be given tablet misoprostol 600 µg orally or rectally (WHO—2012). This tablet may be administered by a community health worker or a SBA.

**Q. How do you manage the third stage of labor?**

**Ans.** Third stage is the most crucial stage of labor, as the complications are more serious in nature. The woman is kept under constant observation. One palm is placed over the fundus of the uterus to note:
(1) Signs of separation of placenta
(2) To feel the tone of the uterus
(3) To detect any early evidence of uterine inversion.

**Q. How do you understand the separation of the placenta?**

**Ans.** After separation of the placenta the following changes are observed:
**Per abdomen:**
(a) Uterus becomes globular and firm
(b) Fundal height is slightly raised
(c) Bulging of the suprapubic region.

**Per vaginum**
(a) Gush of vaginal bleeding
(b) Permanent lengthening of the cord and there is no in drawing or receding of the cord on suprapubic pressure.

**Q. How do you deliver the separated placenta?**

**Ans.** (A) Placenta may be expelled spontaneously with uterine contraction and with bearing down efforts. When the placenta is seen to come down at the introitus, it is grasped by both the palms and is twisted round with gentle traction. Complete delivery of the placenta could be done with this method.

(B) Otherwise placenta is delivered by **assisted expulsion or controlled cord traction (Fig. 4.20)** (modified Brandt Andrew method) method. The palmer surface of the left hand is placed over the suprapubic region and the uterus is pushed upward and backward towards the umbilicus. The right hand exerts a steady traction over the umbilical cord holding the clamp, until the placenta comes out of the introitus. The rest of the procedure is as discussed above.

Thereafter the placenta, membranes and the cord are examined thoroughly under running tap water to detect its completeness. The cord is examined for any abnormalities.

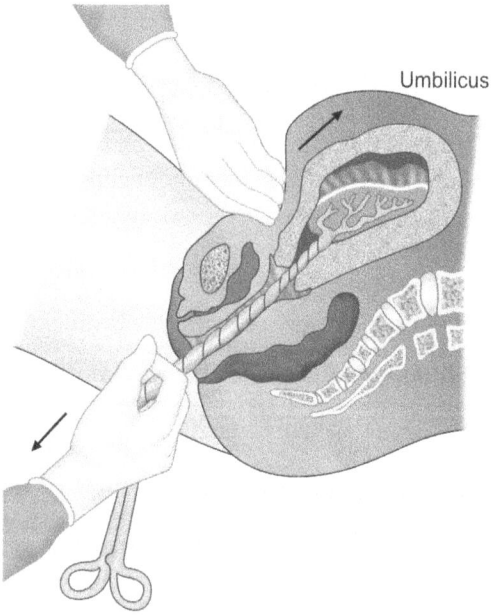

**Fig. 4.20:** Expression of the placenta by controlled cord traction method.

## PRETERM LABOR AND DELIVERY

**Q. What is a preterm baby?**

**Ans.** As per World Health Organization (WHO), a preterm baby is defined as a baby who is born before 37 completed weeks of gestation. The rate of preterm birth ranges from 5-18%.

**Q. What is the signicicance of pretrem birth and prematurity?**

**Ans.** Neonatal deaths due to prematurity are significantly high. Preterm babies that they survive often face a lifetime of disability including learning, hearing and visual disabilities. Preterm birth is a risk factor in at least 50% of all neonatal deaths and is the second most common cause of death after pneumonia among children under the age of five.

**Q. How the preterm neonates are classified?**

**Ans.** Preterm newborns are classified on the basis of completed gestation period as:
- Extremely preterm—less than 28 weeks
- Very preterm—28–<32 weeks
- Moderate preterm—32–<34 weeks
- Late preterm—34–<37 weeks.

The relative proportion of these groups is 5%, 10% and combined moderate and late is 85%, respectively. The mortality rate among preterm newborns increases with decreasing gestational age. It may be noted that even the moderate and late preterm neonates have an increased mortality risk as compared to those born at term gestation.

Extremely preterm babies require neonatal intensive care for survival.

**Q. What are the major concerns for the preterm babies?**

**Ans.** Preterm babies have numerous challenges:
 (a) Feeding
 (b) Maintaining body temperature (hypothermia)
 (c) Increased susceptibility to infections
 (d) Other serious complications which can develop are: Necrotizing enterocolitis and intraventricular hemorrhage
 (e) However, the most common cause of death among preterm babies less than 34 weeks is respiratory distress syndrome (RDS).

This is an acute lung disease due to surfactant deficiency in the lungs which leads to atelectasis and subsequent failure of gas exchange.

Fortunately, RDS can be largely prevented by administering injection corticosteroids to the pregnant woman as soon as she is diagnosed with preterm labor.

**Q. What is the place of antenatal corticosteroid therapy to the mother with preterm labor?**

**Ans.** Injection corticosteroids (dexamethasone or betamethasone) when administered to the pregnant woman antenatally, cross the placenta and reach the fetal lung and stimulate surfactant synthesis and maturation of other system.

Following corticosteroid therapy the baby will have a low risk of developing RDS and therefore, much higher chance of surviving with supportive care.

**Q. What other benefits could be obtained with antenatal corticosteroid therapy?**

**Ans.** Use of antenatal corticosteroids in a mother with preterm labor (<34 weeks) has the following advantages:
- 34% reduction in respiratory distress syndrome
- 46% reduction in intraventricular hemorrhage (IVH)
- 54% reduction in necrotising enterocolitis (NEC)
- 31% reduction in mortality
- Reduction in the incidence of PDA
- Reduction in systemic infections
- Decreased need for respiratory support and therefore
- Reduced length of hospital stay
- Low rate of intensive care admissions and finally
- Low cost of care.

**Q. When should corticosteroid therapy should be given to get the benefit of therapy?**

**Ans.** Antenatal corticosteroid therapy has maximal effect if the fetus is delivered 24 hours after the last dose and up to 7 days thereafter. Thus, even if the delivery occurs in the course of treatment regimen, there are clinically some benefits. Therefore, there are good reasons to initiate antenatal corticosteroids as soon as preterm labor in diagnosed.

**Q. Is there any adverse effect of the therapy on long-term follow-up basis?**

**Ans.** Long-term follow-up of survivors from randomized trials of antenatal corticosteroids therapy through childhood to adulthood (up to 20 years of age) showed no adverse effects.

**Q. What is the current recommendation of the Government of India as regard the corticosteroid therapy?**

**Ans.** Government of India recommends the administration of antenatal corticosteroids in preterm labor:

Single course of injection of dexamethasone to be administered to women with preterm labour (between 24 and 34 weeks of gestation) at all levels.

(1) **To empower auxiliary nurse midwives (ANMs)** to administer intramuscular injection **Dexamethasone**, as a pre-referral dose to a pregnant woman in preterm labor (between 24 and 34 weeks of gestation) and appropriate referral to health facility utilizing the free referral transport. In case the referral is delayed, refused, or referral is

not possible, ANM may complete the full course of treatment (4 doses 12 hour apart).

(2) Appropriate and timely in-utero referral of pregnant women with preterm labor to facilities with provision of cesarean section and special care newborn units.

### Preference of Injection Dexamethasone over Betamethasone

Dexamethasone sodium phosphate and Betamethasone acetate and phosphate are the two corticosteroids that are effective and safe to be used during antenatal period. Both these drugs are identical in biologic activity and readily cross the placenta.

**Dexamethasone** is listed in the WHO essential medicines list. It is inexpensive and widely available in facilities for multiple indications.

Betamethasone acetate and phosphate which requires only two doses at 12 hourly interval is not available. The available salt in India is Betamethasone phosphate which is short acting and requires more frequent administration as compared to the former. Further, Betamethasone is more costly and less stable than Dexamethasone at high temperature. However, in individual cases where injection Dexamethasone is not available the service provider may use injection Betamethasone phosphate to give the advantage of corticosteroids to the newborn.

- **Preparation:** Injection Dexamethasone sodium phosphate is available in 4 mg/mL.

| Dose and Route of Administration of Injection Dexamethasone | |
|---|---|
| Dose | 6 mg each |
| No. of injections | 4 |
| Interval between injections | 12 hours |
| Route of administration | Deep intramuscular |
| Site of administration | Preferably anterolateral aspect of high |
| Complete course | Four doses (equivalent to 24 mg total) |
| Storage | No need to refrigerate |

| Indications and Contraindications for using Corticosteroids in Antenatal Period | |
|---|---|
| Indications | Contraindications |
| 1. True preterm labor<br>2. Any condition that lead to imminent preterm delivery:<br>• Antepartum hemorrhage<br>• Preterm premature rupture of membrane<br>• Severe pre-eclampsia | 1. Frank chorioamnionitis corticosteroids<br>2. History of fever and lower abdominal pain<br>3. On examination: Foul smelling vaginal discharge,<br>4. Tachychardia and uterine tenderness<br>5. Fetal tachycardia |

Maternal diabetes, pre-eclampsia and hypertension are not contraindications for using injection corticosteroid in pregnant women. Dexamethasone can be administered if otherwise indicated with a careful watch on blood sugar and blood pressure. If chorioamnionitis is suspected, consider delivering the baby.

The pregnant woman and her family should be counseled by ANM/Asha for birth preparedness, danger signs and to opt for institutional delivery.

***Role of ANM:*** This guideline enables ANM to give the prereferral dose of corticosteroid, to pregnant women with preterm labor between 24 to 34 weeks of gestation. To avoid the misuse/overuse of the drug, ANM needs to assess correctly the gestational age and true labor pains (*See* p. 192).

Once the ANM confirms the diagnosis of true preterm labor between 24 and 34 weeks she will follow the instructions given in the box below:

(1) If the mother is in true labor (*See* p. 193), give the recommended dose of Dexamethasone.
(2) Refer the pregnant women to higher center where neonatal resuscitation facilities exist under *Janani Shishu Suraksha Karyakram (JSSK)* Scheme.
(3) In case the referral is not possible, complete the course of antenatal steroid and contact the nearest health facility.
(4) In case the delivery is imminent, prepare for delivery and resuscitation of the baby.
(5) Refer neonate to the nearest ANCU after appropriate stabilization with a duly filled referral slip. Ensure that the temperature of the newborn is maintained during transportation.

## Case Summary

Mrs LC, 25 years old, G2, P0, A1, (P0+0+1+0) admitted at 32 weeks of gestation due to recurrent episodes of pain abdomen associated with the hardening of the uterus. On general physical examination, she weighed 45 kg, mild pollor, and her BP measured 130/80 mm Hg, temperature was normal. Obstetric examination revealed: Uterus was 32 weeks size, Symphysis-fundal height measured 32 cm, single fetus, cephalic presentation. The head was free, uterine contraction were mild and were present 2 to 3/10 minutes lasting for 10 to 15 seconds, on auscultation FHS was 147 beats/minute of it was regular.

**Pelvic examination** on inspection slight mucoid vaginal discharge was seen. Speculum examination revealed: Cervix is shortened <2 cm in length. OS is dilated by 2 cm. Show is present. High vaginal swab is taken for culture sensitivity.

> **Q. *What is the provisional diagnosis?***
>
> **Ans.** This 25 years old second gravida with one previous miscarriage, presently at 32 weeks of gestation with preterm labor.
>
> **Q. *What is threatened preterm labor?***
>
> **Ans.** Presence of uterine contractions without any evidence of cervical change is called threatened preterm labor (PTL).

**Q. How do you define preterm labor?**

**Ans.** When labor starts before 37 completed weeks (<259 days), counting from the first day of last menstrual period. Lower limit of gestation vary from 20 weeks (developed world) or it may be from 28 weeks depending on the country.

**Q. What is the total duration of pregnancy in human?**

**Ans.** It is 9 calendar months and 7 days or 280 days or 40 weeks. This duration is calculated from the first day of the last menstrual period.

**Q. What is a term pregnancy?**

**Ans.** Any pregnancy after completed 37 weeks (>259 days) but before 42 completed (294 days) weeks is called a term pregnancy.

**Q. What is postdated or prolonged pregnancy?**

**Ans.** Any pregnancy that has crossed the expected day of delivery is called postdated or prolonged pregnancy.

**Q. What are the etiological factors for preterm labor?**

**Ans.** It is often multifactorial.
  (A) **History of previous preterm delivery** is an important risk factor.
  (B) **Others are**: Pregnancy complications like:
   - Pre-eclampsia,
   - APH
   - PROM
   - Polyhydramnios
   - Multiple pregnancy
   - Genital tract infection (bacterial vaginosis)
   - Iatrogenic
   - Unexplained (50%).

**Q. How to diagnose PTL?**

**Ans.** (1) Regular uterine contractions (at least one in every 10 minutes)
  (2) Cervical dilatation (≥2 cm) and effacement (80%)
  (3) Cervical length <2.5 cm as measured by TVS
  (4) Pelvic pressure, vaginal discharge and bleeding.

**Q. What is the major concern for preterm birth (PTB)?**

**Ans.** Preterm neonates suffer many complications. These are:
  (a) Hypoxia
  (b) Asphyxia
  (c) Hypothermia

(d) Pulmonary syndrome
(e) RDS is the major cause of death due to deficiency of surfactant.
(f) Cerebral hemorrhage
(g) Hypoglycemia
(h) Infection (pneumonia)
(i) Jaundice.

**Some long-term complications are:**
(a) Attention deficit disorder
(b) Cerebral palsy.

All these lead to high perinatal mortality and morbidity.

*Q. What is the biochemical predictor of PTL?*

**Ans.** Presence of fetal fibronectin (a glycoprotein) in the cervicovaginal discharge of a pregnant woman between 24 weeks and 34 weeks is thought to be predictor of preterm labor.

*Q. How do you manage case of PTL?*

**Ans.** Management includes:
(A) **Prevention**—by reducing the high-risk factors like infection
(B) **To arrest PTL** with the following measures:
- Bed rest
- Adequate hydration
- Use of tocolytics (nifedipine, progesterone, $MgSO_4$) for short-term use.

(C) **Glucocorticoid therapy** to accelerate fetal lung maturation
(D) **Magnesium sulfate** is a neuroprotector to reduce neonatal cerebral palsy.

*Q. How labor is managed in such a woman?*

**Ans.** Management of labor is done to avoid birth asphyxia and birth trauma. Mothers should be shifted to a hospital with the facilities of intensive care unit (NICU).
- Mother: To administer oxygen by face mask
- Pain is relieved by epidural analgesia
- EFM should be done for labor monitoring.
- Cesarean delivery is for obstetric indications only
- Baby need to be shifted to the neonatal intensive care unit.

## PRELABOR RUPTURE OF MEMBRANES (PROM)

**Q. What are the etiological factors for PROM?**

**Ans.** In majority, the causes are not known. The possible causes are:
(1) Friability of membranes
(2) Decreased tensile strength of the membranes
(3) Uterine over enlargement as in:
   (a) Polyhydramnios
   (b) Multiple pregnancy
(4) Cervical incompetence
(5) Infection: Chorioamnionitis, UTI, lower genital tract infections
(6) Cervical length <2.5 cm
(7) History of prior preterm labor.

**Q. What are the molecular changes in the membranes to cause PROM?**

**Ans.** The molecular changes in PROM are:
(1) Increased fetal membrane cells apoptosis
(2) Increased degradation of amniotic membrane collagens by specific proteases
(3) Matrix metalloproteinase (MMP) enzymes
(4) Inflammation with release of cytokines, 1L-1β, TNFa, leukocyte activation and proliferation.

**Q. What are the important changes in the molecular level for the pathogenesis of PROM?**

**Ans.** Several factors are involved to explain the pathogenesis of:
(a) Increased membrane friability
(b) Decreased tensile strength of the membranes. The molecular basis of pathogenesis are:
   (1) Increased apoptosis of the fetal amniotic membrane cells.
   (2) Incased degradation of amniotic membrane collagens by specific proteases
   (3) Increased activity of the matrix metalloproteinase (MMP) family of enzymes (MMP-1,2,3 and 9) to cause membrane collagen degradation.
   (4) Infection and Inflammation—cause release of cytokines, 1L-1β, leukocyte proliferation and activation.
All these ultimately lead to: (A) decreased tensile strength and (B) increased friability of the membranes.

**Q. What is the overall prevalence of preterm birth (PTB)?**

**Ans.** It ranges between 10 and 15%.

**Q. Is there any change in the prevalence of PTB?**

**Ans.** Currently, there is some decline in the incidence of spontaneous preterm birth when compared to the past. This is mainly due to actual assessment of gestational age by USG. However, there is some rise in the incidence medically and obstetrically indicated preterm birth (iatrogenic). However, PTB is more attributed to race, ethnicity and socioeconomic status.

# LABOR-ABNORMAL

## MALPOSITION AND MALPRESENTATION

### OCCIPUT POSTERIOR POSITION

***Q. What do you understand by occiput posterior (OP) position?***

**Ans.** In vertex presentation, occiput lies posteriorly over the sacroiliac joint or directly over the sacrum. It may occur either on the left side, left occiput posterior (LOP) (Fig. 4.21) or on the right side as right occiput posterior (ROP) (Fig. 4.22). It is an abnormal position of the vertex presentation.

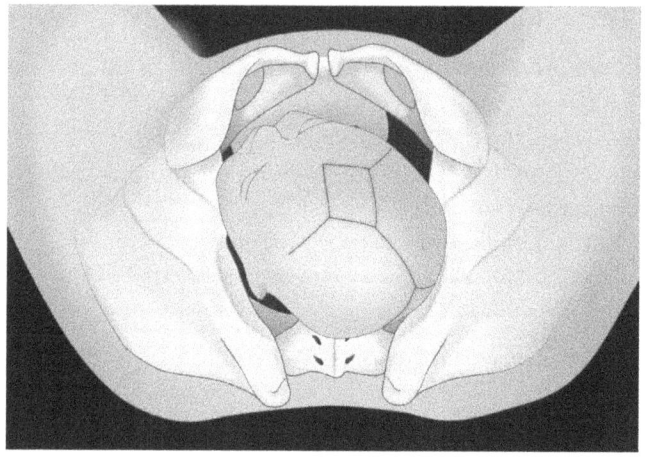

**Fig. 4.21:** Left occiput posterior (LOP).

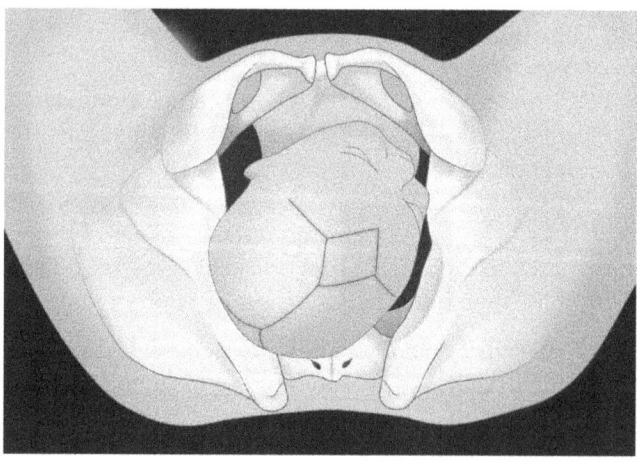

**Fig. 4.22:** Right occiput posterior (ROP).

**Q. What are the important factors that favor successful vaginal delivery in a case with OP?**

**Ans.** There are four important issues that are taken into consideration in predicting the successful outcome. The favorable factors are:
  (1) Adequacy of the pelvis
  (2) Good uterine contractions
  (3) Good flexion of the fetal head
  (4) Average size of the fetus

**Q. How can the outcome of labor be predicted in a case with OP?**

**Ans.** (A) Woman having all the above favorable factors including good flexion, 90% have the chance of successful vaginal delivery symbol. There is long anterior rotation of the occiput (3/8 of a circle) spontaneous or assisted vaginal delivery.
  (B) In unfavorable circumstances, the chance of vaginal delivery is less (10%).

**Q. What are different outcomes of labor with unfavorable circumstances?**

**Ans.** Depending upon the degree of flexion of the fetal head, uterine contractions, pelvic adequacy and with size of the baby, the occiput may fail to rotate complete anteriorly. This results in any of the following outcomes:
  (1) **In a case with mild deflexion: Incomplete anterior rotation**—it may result in **deep transverse arrest (Fig. 4.23)**.
  (2) **In a case with severe deflexion: Nonrotation**—oblique occiput posterior position may result in arrest.
  (3) **In a case with severe deflexion: Malrotation**—occipitosacral position. In this position, vaginal delivery is possible as **face to pubis**, provided the baby is of average size, there are good uterine contractions and the pelvis is adequate (anthropoid or gynecoid). Otherwise labor process may get arrested as in **occipito-sacral arrest**.

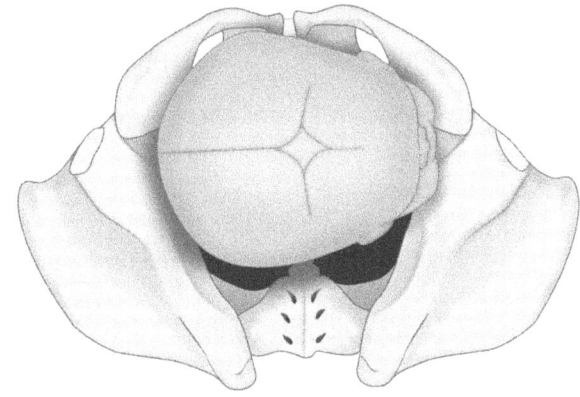

**Fig. 4.23:** Sagittal suture in the transverse diameter of the pelvis.

**Q. What do you understand by persistent occipitoposterior position?**

**Ans.** Commonly **occiput-sacral position** is described as **persistent occiput posterior position**. However, in a wider sense, keeping in mind the management issues, the other two arrested posterior positions (deep transverse arrest and the oblique posterior arrest) are also included as persistent occiput posterior position (POP).

**Q. Give an outline in the management of a case with occiput posterior position.**

**Ans.** (1) Early diagnosis
(2) Careful monitoring of labor:
  (A) Early cesarean delivery:
    (a) Inadequate pelvis
    (b) Presence of complications
  (B) Oxytocin augmentation if needed—anterior rotation—vaginal delivery.
  (C) Persistent occiput posterior position:
    (a) Pelvis adequate: Ventouse, or forceps
    (b) Pelvis Inadequate: Cesarean delivery.

*(Note: Occiput posterior—occiput lies in relation to the left or right sacroiliac joint. The occiput lies in the posterior quadrant (either left or right) of the pelvis. Accordingly it is named as Left OP (LOP) or right OP (ROP). It is the vertex presentation).*

**Q. What are the common causes of the OP position?**

**Ans.** (A) **Pelvic factors:** Shape of the pelvic inlet OP position is more common with an android or anthropoid type of pelvis.
(B) **Fetal factors:** Marked deflexion of the fetal head.
  - **Causes of deflexion are:**
    (a) High pelvic inclination
    (b) Anterior placenta
    (c) Brachycephaly
    (d) Big baby.
(C) **Uterine factors:** Weak or abnormal uterine contractions.

**Q. How occiput posterior position could be diagnosed clinically?**

**Ans. Abdominal examination** (obstetric grips):
(a) Suprapubic flattening
(b) Fetal back lies far away from the midline
(c) Pelvic grips: The head is not engaged. The cephalic prominence is not felt
(d) FHS—is heard (commonly) on the flank.

**Vaginal examination**
(a) The sagittal suture is felt in any of the oblique diameters
(b) Posterior fontanel is felt near the sacroiliac joint
(c) The anterior fontanel is felt easily due to deflexion.

**Q. Discuss the mechanism of labor in a case with occiput posterior position.**

**Ans.** See Dutta Obs 9/e, p. 345.

**Q. What are the adverse outcomes for a woman with occiput posterior position in labor?**

**Ans.** (1) Delayed engagement due to persistent deflexion of the fetal head
 (2) Early rupture of the membranes—risk of infection, cord prolapse
 (3) Uterine contractions are either inadequate or abnormal due to the ill-fitting of fetal head to the lower uterine segment
 (4) Delay in the first stage of labor
 (5) Delay in the second stage of labor due to long anterior rotation (3/8th of a circle)
 (6) Posterior rotation or nonrotation or short anterior rotation of the head may end in prolonged or obstructed labor.
 (7) Increased incidence of operative delivery: Either operative vaginal (ventouse/forceps) or abnormal delivery (cesarean section). Maternal morbidity is also high.
 (8) Perinatal mortality and morbidity are also increased due to birth asphyxia and birth trauma.

**Q. What is deep transverse arrest (DTA)?**

**Ans.** It is defined and explained as:
 (1) **Deep:** Head is deep into the pelvis **(engaged)**
 (2) **Transverse:** The sagittal suture is in the **transverse (bispinous) diameter** of the pelvis (Fig. 4.23).
 (3) **Arrest:** There is no progress of labor **(arrest of labor)** in descent of the head for 1 hour (primi) or ½ hour (multi).
 (4) **Full dilatation** of the cervix.

**Q. Outline the management issues for a case with DTA.**

**Ans.** The woman is assessed as regard:
 (a) Any complication in pregnancy (obstetrics or medical)
 (b) Fetal condition
 (c) Pelvic adequacy
 (d) Uterine contractions
 (e) Degree of deflexion of the fetal head
 (f) Estimated fetal weight
 (g) Presence of any associated complications in labor (fetal distress).
 **Options for the management:**
 (A) **Vaginal delivery not safe**
  Cesarean delivery:
  (a) Pelvic inadequacy
  (b) Big baby
  (c) Fetal compromise.
 (B) **Vaginal delivery safe:** Oxytocin augmentation of labor in the presence of weak uterine contractions.
 (C) **Ventouse delivery** for autorotation and delivery
 (D) Manual rotation and application of forceps for delivery in a selected case
  *In majority of the cases with DTA cesarean delivery is done.*

## BREECH PRESENTATION

**Q. What are the important sites where essential movements occur as a part of mechanism of labor in vaginal breech delivery?**

**Ans.** (A) **Buttocks:** Diameter of engagement—Bitrochanteric (4" or 10 cm).

(B) **Shoulders:** Diameter of engagement: Bisacromial diameter (4³/4" or 12 cm).

(C) **Head:** Diameter of engagement: Suboccipitofrontal (10 cm).

**Q. What is breech extraction and what are the indications?**

**Ans.** When the fetus is extracted out of the uterus by the obstetrician in a situation of emergency. It is rarely done nowadays.

**Indications are:**
(a) Delivery of the second twin after internal podalic version (IPV).
(b) Cord prolapse during labor.
(c) Intrapartum hemorrhage.
(d) Extended legs arrested at the outlet.

**Q. What are the principles of conduction of vaginal breech delivery?**

**Ans.** (1) Never to rush and not to be hasty in delivery process

(2) Never to pull from below but push from above

(3) To keep the back of the fetus always anterior.

**Q. What are different methods used to deliver the after-coming head of the fetus in assisting vaginal breech delivery?**

**Ans.** Delivery of the after-coming head is a very crucial stage. The procedure whatever used, must be safe, gentle and without any prolongation. The commonly employed methods are (Dutta Obs 9/e, p. 359):

(a) **Malar flexion and shoulder traction** (modified Mauriceau-Smellie-Veit technique)
(b) **Forceps delivery**
(c) **Burns-Marshall method**

**Q. What is breech presentation?**

**Ans.** When the podalic pole of the fetus presents at the pelvic brim it is called breech presentation. Here the lie is longitudinal. It is the commonest malpresentation.

**Q. How do you make the diagnosis of breech presentation clinically?**

**Ans.** (A) Abdominal examination:
(a) Fundal grip: The hard globular head
(b) Lateral grip: The back on one side and the limbs on the other side
(c) Pelvic grips: Broad, soft, irregular mass—podalic pole
(d) Auscultation: FHS at a higher level around the umbilicus.

(B) Vaginal examination: Palpation of soft and hard irregular parts, (buttocks, sacrum, ischial tuberosities, foot) are suggestive. Anal opening could be felt.

***Q. How ultrasonography is helpful in the diagnosis and management?***

**Ans.** *Benefits of USG are many:*
  (a) Confirmation of diagnosis
  (b) Detection of any congenital malformation
  (c) Type of breech presentation (complete/incomplete)
  (d) Placental localization
  (e) Assessment of liquor volume (as regard the place of ECV)
  (f) Estimated fetal weight
  (g) Attitude of fetal head (as regard the mode of delivery).

***Q. As regard the mechanism of labor what is the denominator in breech presentation?***

**Ans.** It is the sacrum (bone) (Figs. 4.24 and 4.25).

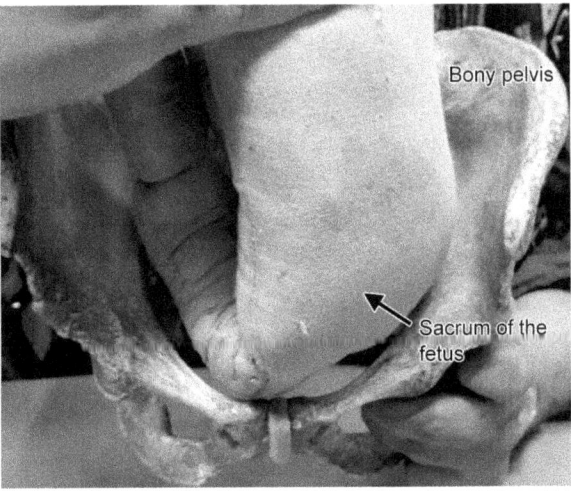

**Fig. 4.24:** Breech presentation showing sacrum as the denominator. This is the left sacroanterior position of breech presentation.

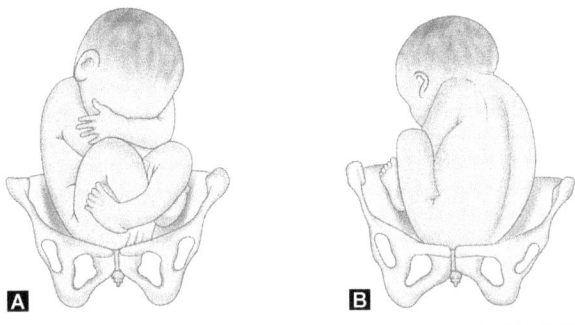

**Figs. 4.25A and B:** (A) Right sacroposterior position of breech presentation; (B) Left sacroanterior position of breech presentation.

**Q. What are the complications to the baby following vaginal breech delivery?**

**Ans.** (1) Birth asphyxia due to cord prolapse, delay in delivery especially the after-coming head.
(2) Injury to the brain (intracranial hemorrhage) and the skull (fracture).
(3) Intrapartum fetal death due to birth asphyxia.
(4) Birth injuries:
  (a) Hematoma formation
  (b) Fractures: Femur, humerus
  (c) Visceral injury: Rupture of liver, kidney, testicles
  (d) Nerve: Spinal cord, medulla.
(5) Long-term neurological morbidity.
(6) Congenital malformations.

**Q. What are the principles of management in the antenatal clinic?**

**Ans.** (1) Identification of complicating factors
(2) External cephalic version (ECV) if not contraindicated
(3) To plan the management for the delivery.

**Q. What are the benefits of ECV?**

**Ans.** (a) Mainly, it reduces the incidence of cesarean delivery. In a case with successful ECV, vaginal delivery with vertex presentation may be possible.
(b) It reduces the risk of vaginal breech delivery and the associated complications.

**Q. What are the contraindicators of ECV?**

**Ans.** (a) Antepartum hemorrhage
(b) PROM
(c) Large fetus (>3.5 kg)
d) Prior cesarean delivery
(e) Known uterine malformation
(f) Oligohydramnios
(g) Inadequate pelvis
(h) Multiple pregnancy
(i) Fetal distress/death.

**Q. When ECV should preferably be done?**

**Ans.** From 37 weeks onwards.

**Q. Where ECV should be done?**

**Ans.** It is usually done in the antenatal clinic. However, arrangement/facilities should be made available for emergency cesarean delivery when there is any urgent need due to the complications of the ECV. (*see* complications of ECV).

**Q. What are the complications of ECV?**

Ans. (a) Premature onset of labor
 (b) Placental abruption
 (c) Cord entanglement around the fetal parts
 (d) Rupture of membranes
 (e) Fetal distress
 (f) Uterine rupture (rare).

**Q. What are the important causes of breech presentation?**

Ans. (a) **Prematurity** is the commonest cause
 (b) **Uterus:** Congenital malformations—septate/bicornuate uterus
 (c) **Umbilical cord:** Short
 (d) **Placenta previa**, cornu-fundal attachment
 (e) **Excess mobility of the fetus**, polyhydramnios, multiparity
 (f) **Restricted mobility** of the fetus, oligohydramnios.

**Q. What are the different varieties of breech presentation and their clinical associations?**

Ans.

| Type | Common association | Labor outcome |
| --- | --- | --- |
| **Complete breech** | Multigravida | Prospect of vaginal delivery: Good |
| **Frank breech** | Primigravida | Effective cervical dilator outcome: Good |
| **Footling presentation** | Multigravida | Increased risk of operative delivery. Risk of cord prolapse: More often has poor outcome |

**Q. What is the place of cesarean delivery for breech presentation?**

Ans. Based on the review of current studies (Hannah and Hannah 2000, ACOG 2006), it is considered that the route of delivery for term singleton breech should be by cesarean section. Vaginal delivery may be allowed in a very selected situation.

**Q. What criteria should be fulfilled for allowing vaginal breech delivery?**

Ans. (a) Average fetal weight (between 1.5 and 3.5 kg)
 (b) Flexed fetal head
 (c) Adequate pelvis
 (d) Without any complications (medial/obstetric)
 (e) Availability of facilities for emergency cesarean section
 (f) Facilities for continuous fetal monitoring (electronic preferred)
 (g) Presence of an obstetrician experienced with vaginal breech delivery
 (h) Informed consent
 (i) Frank breech is preferred.

**Q. What could be the reason for the difficulties of delivery for the shoulders?**

**Ans.** It occurs when one or both the arms are fully stretched along the side of the head or lies behind the neck (extension of arms).

**Q. How breech with extended arms could be managed during delivery?**

**Ans. Lovset's maneuver** is widely practiced. It is based on the principle that due to the curved birth canal, when the anterior shoulder is above the symphysis pubis the posterior shoulder is below the sacral promontory. Shoulders are thereby delivered by rotating the trunk. The baby is hold with the femoro-pelvic grip and the trunk is rotated through 180° to bring the posterior shoulder under the pubic arch. It is then hooked out. Thereafter, the trunk is rotated in the reverse direction to release the anterior shoulder underneath the symphysis pubis.

## FACE PRESENTATION

**Q. What is the engaging diameter of the fetal head in face presentation?**

**Ans.** It is commonly the submentobregmatic 9.5 cm (fully-extended head) or the submentovertical diameter 11.5 cm (partially extended head) (Fig. 4.26).

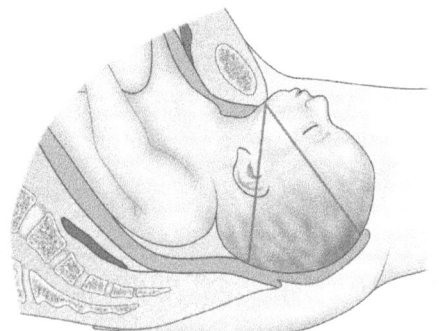

Fig. 4.26: Engaging diameter of the fetal head showing submentobregmatic and submentovertical diameter.

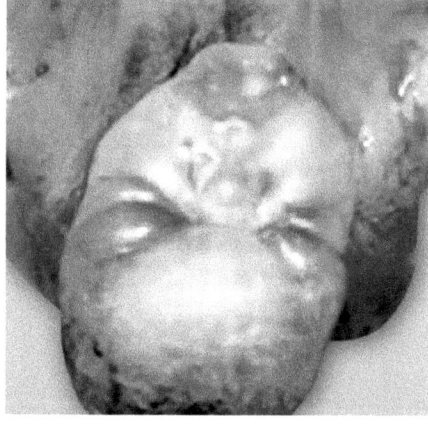

Fig. 4.27: Vaginal delivery in a case with face presentation. Mentum is seen behind the symphysis pubis. The face appears markedly swollen and congested.
[*Courtesy*: Dr Subrata Bhattacharya, *Silchar*]

**Q. Could there be any possibility of vaginal delivery in a woman in labor with face presentation of the fetus?**

**Ans.** Successful vaginal delivery is possible in a case with mento-anterior face presentation (Fig. 4.27) rather than mentoposterior one. However, engagement is delayed (Dutta Obs 9/e, p. 357).

*Q. What is the presenting area?*
**Ans.** It is the area of face (Fig. 4.28).

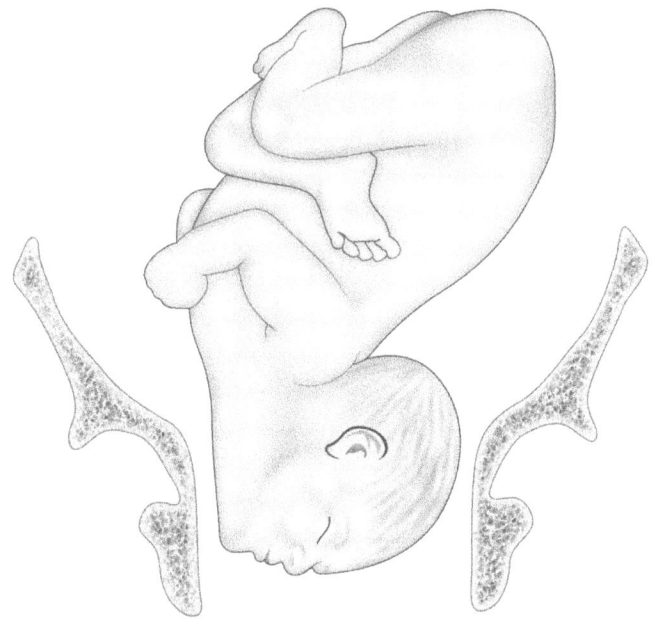

**Fig. 4.28:** Face presentation.

*Q. What is the denominator of face presentation?*
**Ans.** It is the mentum (chin).

*Q. What is the attitude of the head?*
**Ans.** It is the attitude of extension.

*Q. What are the different positions of face presentation?*
**Ans.** There are four positions which are follows:
 (1) Left mentoanterior—LMA
 (2) Right mentoanterior—RMA
 (3) Right mentoposterior—RMP
 (4) Left mentoposterior—LMP
 Left mentoanterior (LMA) is the most common position.

*Q. What are the causes of face presentation?*
**Ans.** • **Maternal:**
 (a) Multiparity
 (b) Contracted pelvis
 (c) Pelvic tumors
 • **Fetal:**
 (a) Anencephaly
 (b) Dolichocephalic head.

**Q. How the diagnosis of face presentation is made clinically?**

**Ans.** Clinically, it is difficult to make the diagnosis on abdominal examination and even by vaginal examination in early labor. The diagnostic features on vaginal examination during labor are: Palpation of the mouth, nose, malar eminences and mentum. It is often confused with breech presentation.

**Q. How one can differentiate face presentation from breech presentation in labor?**

**Ans:**

| Face presentation | Breech presentation |
|---|---|
| 1. Mouth and malar eminences (triangular in position) not in one line | 1. The anus and ischial tuberosities are all in one line |
| 2. Sucking effect of mouth with fingers | 2. Anal sphincteric grip effect |
| 3. Hard alveolar margins felt | 3. No such |
| 4. No meconium staining of the examining finger | 4. Meconium staining of the finger |

**Q. What are the adverse effects that may arise when a women goes into labor within such presentation?**

**Ans.** The clinical course of labor with *face presentation* is adversely affected though the engaging transverse diameter is the biparietal (9.5 cm) in both the presentations (flexed vertex and extended face).

**The reasons for adverse outcomes are:**
(a) Irregular area of face fits partially to the lower uterine segment.
(b) Risks of cord prolapse is more.
(c) *Delay in labor is due to:*
   (i) Delayed engagement as the distance of biparietal plane from the chin in 7 cm.
   (ii) Late internal rotation,
   (iii) Arrest of labor may occur due to mentoposterior face presentation.
   (iv) Risks of perineal injury is high as the wide biparietal diameter stretches the perineum.
   (v) Risks of postpartum hemorrhage is high due to uterine atonicity and genital tract injury (both traumatic and atonic)
   (vi) Maternal morbidity is increased specially in mentoposterior face presentation.
   (vii) Fetal and neonatal outcome are also adversely affected due to:
      (a) Cord prolapse, (b) Infection, (c) Increase operative delivery.

**Q. Which variety of face presentation has got better prospect of vaginal delivery?**

**Ans.** In an uncomplicated case with mentoanterior face presentation has got better prospect of vaginal delivery either spontaneous or with forceps.

## BROW PRESENTATION

**Q. How frequent is the brow presentation? What is the denominator?**

Ans. Brow is the rarest cephalic presentation. Incidence is 1 in 1,000 births.

**Q. What is the attitude of the head?**

Ans. Attitude of the head is incomplete extension.

**Q. What is the denominator of brow presentation?**

Ans. The denominator is the forehead (frontum: Fr).

**Q. What is the diameter of engagement of the fetal head in brow presentation?**

Ans. It is the mentovertical diameter (14 cm).

**Q. Could there be any mechanism of labor in brow presentation?**

Ans. There is no diameter in the bony pelvis measuring 14 cm (maximum being 13 cm). As such there is no mechanism of labor unless the fetus is small and true pelvis is roomy with good uterine contractions.

**Q. What would be the course of labor and the prognosis?**

Ans. In a case with persistent brow presentation, there is risk of obstructed labor if left unattended. It ultimately leads to rupture of the uterus.

**Q. What should be the mode of delivery?**

Ans. Cases with persistent brow presentation are delivered by elective cesarean section.

The diameter of engagement is the mentovertical which is 14 cm. The maximum diameter in the brim of the pelvis is 13 cm. Therefore, the head cannot pass through the brim. Therefore no mechanism of labor is possible.

## TRANSVERSE LIE

**Q. What is the presentation in a case with transverse lie?**

Ans. Shoulder presentation.

**Q. What is this denominator in shoulder presentation?**

Ans. It is the acromion.

**Q. Give an outline of the clinical course of labor in transverse lie when left uncared for.**

Ans. The major complications are—premature rupture of membranes, unfavorable outcome is common. Rarely, the fetus may be delivered as breech following spontaneous version or as vertex following spontaneous rectification. This is seen when the fetus is small and the mother is a multipara.

**Unfavorable outcomes are:** PROM—drainage of liquor, hand prolapse/cord prolapse, fetal death, onset of infection, obstructed labor, maternal sepsis, dehydration, ketoacidosis, rupture of uterus, even maternal death when she is left uncared for maternal death.

**Q. Give an outline of the management protocol in a case with transverse lie.**

**Ans.** (1) External cephalic version is done at or beyond 35 weeks provided there is no contraindication (*See* p. 204).

(2) When version fails or is contraindicated:
   (a) Patient is admitted at 37 weeks or earlier and elective cesarean section is the preferred method of delivery.
   (b) Vaginal delivery may be allowed in small size fetus which is congenitally malformed or dead.

## CORD PROLAPSE

**Q. What is cord prolapse?**

**Ans.** Cord is lying inside the vagina or outside the vulva following rupture of the membranes (Figs. 4.29 and 4.30).

**Q. What is cord presentation?**

**Ans.** When the cord is slipped down below the presenting part and the membranes are intact.

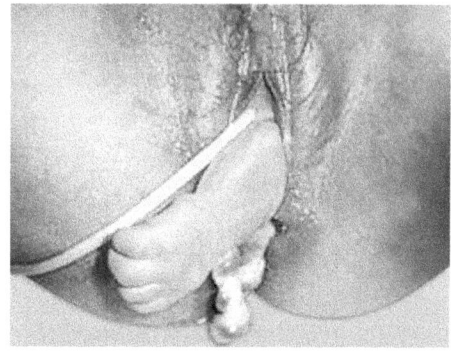

**Fig. 4.29:** Woman in labor with hand prolapse and cord prolapse.
[*Courtesy*: Dr Subrata Bhattacharya, Silchar]

**Q. Outline the management of case with cord prolapse.**

**Ans.** The management protocol depends upon following factors:
(a) Baby alive or dead to verify with cord pulsation (cord pulsation)
(b) Maturity of the baby
(c) Degree of cervical dilatation
The fetal heart sounds should be auscultated before performing cesarean section. The umbilical cord pulsation can be felt if the fetus is alive.
   (A) Baby living: Cesarean delivery is the best option when the baby is sufficiently mature to survive.
   (B) Baby dead: Vaginal delivery is allowed.

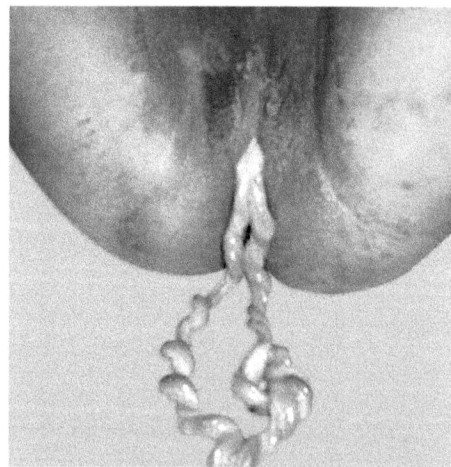

**Fig. 4.30:** Woman in labor with cord prolapse with true knot.
[*Courtesy*: Dr Subrata Bhattacharya, Silchar]

(C) Baby living and safe vaginal delivery is possible: Delivery may be contemplated by forceps when the presenting part (head) is engaged and the cervix is fully dilated.

**Q. What are the temporary measures that could be taken to minimize pressure on the cord?**

Ans. The followings are temporary measures that can minimize pressure on the cord till baby is delivered:
(1) Filling of the bladder with normal saline
(2) Postural treatment: Sim's left lateral position with a pillow under the hip
(3) Trendelenburg or knee-chest position.

**Q. What are the common causes of cord prolapse?**

Ans. (a) Malpresentation (transverse lie)
(b) Contracted pelvis
(c) Prematurity
(d) Twins
(e) Polyhydramnios
(f) Iatrogenic (version, low rupture of the membranes).

**Q. What are the complications of cord prolapse?**

Ans. (A) **Fetal**:
(i) Fetal hypoxia or anoxia due to umbilical cord compression as blood flow is compromised
(ii) High perinatal mortality.
(B) **Maternal** risks are due to increase the risk of operative delivery (cesarean section), anesthesia, blood loss and infection.

**Q. Give an outline of management of a case with cord prolapse.**

Ans. (A) Baby living: Cesarean delivery is done when the baby is viable.
(B) Baby dead: To allow vaginal delivery.

## COMPOUND PRESENTATION

**Q. What is a compound presentation?**

Ans. When more than one fetal presenting part overlies the lower pole (internal os) of the uterus it is called compound presentation.

**Q. What are the common varieties of compound presentation?**

Ans. • Cephalic with hand or foot
• Breech with hand(s).

**Q. How the case is managed during labor?**

Ans. **Cesarean delivery:** A term living fetus associated with inadequate pelvis or any other complicating factors (cord prolapse) is delivered by cesarean section. Expectant management may be done with the progressive descent of the presenting part, in a selected case with careful monitoring of labor.

## UNSTABLE LIE

**Q. What is an unstable lie?**

**Ans.** It is a condition where the presentation of the fetus constantly changes even beyond 36th week of pregnancy when it should have been stabilized.

## PROLONGED (PROTRACTED) LABOR

**Q. What are the different abnormal labor patterns?**

**Ans.** (a) **Prolonged labor:** When total duration of labor (combined duration of 1st stage and 2nd stage) is >20 hours in a primigravida and >14 hours in a multigravida it is called prolonged labor.

(b) **Protracted labor (ACOG) (Fig. 4.31):** (1) Protracted dilatation—when the rate of cervical dilatation is <1.2 cm/hour in a primigravida and <1.5 cm/hour in a multigravida, (2) protracted descent—when rate of descent of the head <1.0 cm/hour in a primigravida and <2.0 cm/hour in a multigravida.

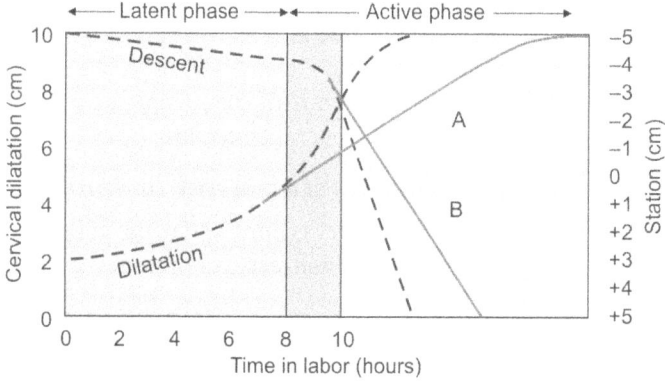

**Fig. 4.31:** Protraction disorders in the active phase of labor. (A) Protracted dilatation pattern; (B) Protracted descent pattern. The normal dilatation and descent curves are shown with (dotted) lines.

(c) **Arrest disorder** in labor (ACOG) (Fig. 4.32):
  (1) Secondary arrest of dilation—when there is no dilation of the cervix for a period >2 hours in a woman who had normal cervical dilatation after entering the active phase of labor. This is applicable irrespective of a primigravida or a multigravida
  (2) Arrest of descent is when there is no descent of the presenting part for a period of >1 hour irrespective of primigravida or multigravida).

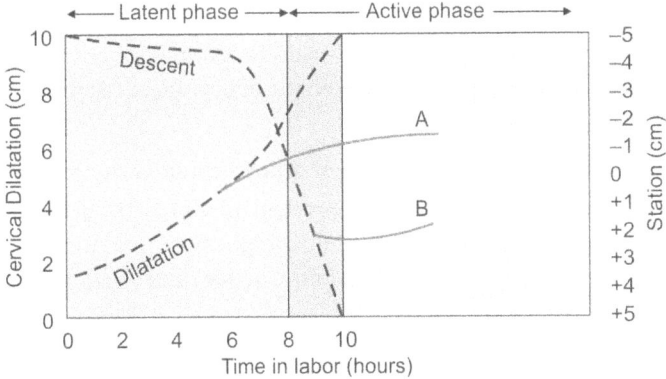

**Fig. 4.32:** Arrest disorders in the active phase of labor. (A): Secondary arrest of dilatation; (B) Arrest of descent. Normal dilatation and descent curves are shown with dotted lines.

*Q. What is meant by dystocia (difficult labor)? Mention the causes.*

**Ans. Dystocia (difficult labor)** is manifested by abnormally slow labor progress in relation to cervical dilation and descent of the presenting part.

**Causes of dystocia are:**

(1) **Fault in power:** Abnormal uterine contractions
(2) **Fault in the passage:** Contracted pelvis, pelvic tumor
(3) **Fault in the passage:** Malposition and malpresentation (face), fetal anomalies.

*Q. What are the different types of dysfunctional labor?*

**Ans.** (a) **Primary dysfunctional labor:** When the dysfunctional labor pattern starts following a normal latent phase. This is the commonest abnormal labor pattern. Augmentation of labor is done to correct it.

(b) **Secondary dysfunctional or arrest of labor:** When the active phase of labor commences normally, but stops or slows down significantly before the full dilation of the cervix. When this type of labor pattern seen in a multigravida, the risk of rupture uterus is high.

*Q. What are the etiology and management of the protracted active phase of labor?*

**Ans.** It may be due to inadequate uterine contractions. In such a situation, oxytocin augmentation of labor is successful. Otherwise, if it is due to cephalopelvic disproportion (CPD), cesarean delivery should be done.

*Q. What are the etiology and management of arrest disorder of labor?*

**Ans.** In the active phase, management depends on its etiology. Oxytocin augmentation is successful when it is due to inadequate uterine contractions. Cesarean section is indicated when it is due to fetal malpresentations, malpositions, cephalopelvic disproportion or asynclitism.

**Q. What is prolonged active phase of labor?**

**Ans.** When the rate of cervical dilation is slow (<0.5 cm/h) over 4 hours observation period after the woman has entered the active phase (4 cm cervical dilation) of labor.

**Q. What is secondary arrest cervical dilatation in active phase of labor?**

**Ans.** When a woman who had normal cervical dilation in the active phase of labor (>4 cm cervical dilatation) and she developed complete cessation of cervical dilatation for a period of 2 hours in the active phase of labor.

**Q. What is prolonged second stage of labor?**

**Ans.** When the duration of second of labor is more than 2 hours in a primi and more than one hour in a multi, it is called prolonged second stage of labor. However when the women is under regional anesthesia, the normal duration is extended to 3 hours in a primi and 2 hours in a multi.

**Q. What is prolonged latent phase of labor?**

**Ans.** Latent phase in said to be prolonged (abnormal) when it exceeds 20 hours in a primi or 14 hours in a multi. The average duration of latent phase in primi is 8.6 hours and that of a multi is 5.3 hours.

**Q. How do you manage a case with prolonged latent phase?**

**Ans.** Expectant management is usually done. Rest and analgesics are helpful. Most woman start normal cervical dilation when the active phase begins.

## OBSTRUCTED LABOR

**Q. What is obstructed labor?**

**Ans.** When there is arrest in the descent of the presenting part (for a period of ≥1 hour) due to some mechanical obstruction, in spite of good uterine contractions.

**Q. What are the common causes of obstructed labor?**

**Ans.** (a) Contracted pelvis and cephalopelvic disproportion.
(b) Abnormal presentations or positions, like transverse lie, brow presentation, occiput posterior position.
(c) Fetal malformations—hydrocephalus.

**Q. What are the effects of obstructed labor on the mother?**

**Ans.** (A) **Immediate complications:**
  (a) Dehydration
  (b) Metabolic ketoacidosis
  (c) Genital tract sepsis
  (d) Rupture of the uterus
  (e) Postpartum hemorrhage
  (f) Maternal death.

(B) **Late complications:**
  (a) *Genital tract fistula:*
    - Vesicovaginal
    - Rectovaginal.

**Q. What are the effects on the fetus?**

Ans. (a) Asphyxia
  (b) Acidosis
  (c) Intracranial hemorrhage
  (d) Infection
  (e) Increased perinatal morbidity and mortality
  (f) Fetal death.

**Q. Outline the management issues in a case with obstructed labor.**

Ans. (1) **Prevention:** Partographic management of labor and timely intervention can prevent it.

(2) **Actual management:**

Resuscitation of the patient:
  (a) Correction of dehydration, IV infusion of crystalloids (Ringer's solution).
  (b) Correction of electrolyte imbalance.
  (c) Control of sepsis (antibiotic therapy): Parenteral route (IV).
  (d) Blood sample to send for grouping and cross-matching.

(3) **Obstetric management:**
  (a) Cesarean delivery when the fetal condition is good.
  (b) When vaginal delivery is possible: Patient may be delivered by forceps or craniotomy (destructive operation) in a case with dead fetus.
  (c) Symphysiotomy as an alternative may be done.

CHAPTER 5

# Active Management of Labor

**Chapter Objectives**

**Knowledge and understanding of:**
- Labor monitoring and fetal surveillance
- Assessment of labor progress: Normal and abnormal
- Data interpretation
- Clinical judgment and management issues

❖ Labor Monitoring—Partography                                       217

❖ Intrapartum Electronic Fetal Monitoring—Cardiotocography            229

# LABOR MONITORING-PARTOGRAPHY

## THE SIMPLIFIED PARTOGRAPH (GOVERNMENT OF INDIA)

Government of India (GOI) is committed to meet the Sustainable Development Goals (SDG) (See p. 344) of less than 70 maternal deaths per 100,000 live births by the year 2030. National Population Policy (NPP) with its wings of National Health Mission (NHM) and Reproductive and Child Health (RCH-II) program ensures universal coverage of all births with skilled attendance both in the institution and at the community level. This also ensures emergency obstetric and neonatal care services for women and newborn.

With this initiative, **partographic recording** (Fig. 5.1) of the progress of labor has been introduced. Skilled attendance at birth (p. 349) and partographic labor recording facilitates timely referral and safe delivery.

Evidence-based practices have demonstrated that presence of skilled birth attendants (SBAs) can effectively reduce maternal mortality. SBAs are appointed to work at the outreach centers, subcenters (SCs), primary health centers (PHCs) and first referral units (FRUs).

Skilled birth attendants are trained to diagnose women in labor. They are skilled to differentiate true labor pain from false labor pains. They have the knowledge and skill to manage the different phases of labor (latent and active), stages of labor, monitoring of uterine contractions, cervical dilatation, FHR and maternal vitals at frequent intervals.

**Plotting of partograph:** It is started when the cervical dilatation is 4 cm or more when the active labor starts.
- The first recording is plotted on the alert line.
- The rest of the procedures are similar to that of WHO (See p. 220).
- Next plotting is done after 4 hours following another vaginal examination.
- When the labor plotting remains on the left of the alert line progress is considered satisfactory.
- When the alert line is crossed (the labor plotting moves on the right of the alert line), labor is considered abnormal (labor is prolonged or obstructed).
- In this case, woman needs to be referred urgently to the FRU. The partograph should also be sent along with the woman.
  - Crossing the action line (labor plotting on the right of the action line) indicates need for intervention. Therefore, by the time the action line is crossed, the woman should reach the FRU for necessary intervention.
  - The difference between the alert line and the action line is 4 hours.
  - So SBA is alerted once alert line is crossed. SBA should refer the woman soon and should not wait till the action line is crossed.
  - Other procedures (recording of uterine contractions, maternal vitals, FHR, liquor) are same as that of WHO (See p. 220).

**The transformational change** in relation to the care during delivery (intrapartum and immediate postpartum care) as introduced by NHM 2017 has been discussed in Chapter 9 (See p. 349).

**Q. What is active management of labor?**

Ans. It is the management of labor with active involvement of the consultant obstetrician. It has many components of which partography for assessment of labor progress and cardiotocography for fetal monitoring are important. AMOL has many advantages (see below).

**Q. What is a partograph?**

Ans. It is a composite graphical record of key data (cervical dilatation, descent of fetal head and FHR) against duration of labor in hours.

**Q. How a cervicograph is plotted?**

Ans. In cervicograph (Philpot and Castle-1972), the **alert line** starts at 4 cm (WHO) of cervical dilatation and ends at 10 cm (at the rate of 1 cm per hour). The **action line** is drawn 4 hours (WHO) to the right and parallel to the alert line.

**Q. What is the plotting of a cervicograph in a normal labor?**

Ans. In a normal labor, the cervical dilatation (cervicograph) lies either on the alert line or to the left of it (Zone-1).

**Q. What is the importance of alert and action lines?**

Ans. When the cervicograph crosses the alert line (Zone-2), it is abnormal. Patient needs to be critically assessed.

When it crosses the action line (Zone-3), patient should be reassessed by a senior person. Decision is to be made either for delivery (cesarean section) or augmentation depending upon the abnormality detected.

**Q. What are the advantages of partographic management of labor?**

Ans. (a) Early detection of dysfunctional labor
(b) Reduction in the complications of labor dysfunction
(c) Reduction in duration of labor (12 hours)
(d) Early detection of fetal hypoxia
(e) Reduction in the incidence of cesarean section
(f) Less need of analgesia
(g) Maternal anxiety is less due to support of the caregiver
(h) While working in the peripheral center, timely transfer of the mother could be done, once the diagnosis of dysfunctional labor is made.

## Q. What are the names associated with graphic analysis of labor (partograph)?

**Ans.** (a) Friedman Emanuel, 1954: Cervical dilatation and descent of fetal head.
(b) Philpott and Castle, 1972: Cervical graph with alert and action lines.
(c) Studd and Duignant, 1972: Nomogram, to assess mean cervical dilatation.

## Q. What are the components of a partograph?

**Ans.** (a) **Patient information:** Name, age, gravida, parity, hospital number, time of admission, time of rupture of membranes.
(b) **Fetal heart rate:** Recorded every half an hour.
(c) **Status of membranes and color of liquor:**
   O : Membrane absent
   I : Membranes intact
   R : Membranes ruptured
   C : Membranes ruptured—liquor clear
   M : Liquor—meconium stained
   B : Liquor—blood stained.
(d) **Cervical dilatation** expressed in cm. Alert and action lines are drawn (Fig. 5.1).
(e) **Descent of fetal head:** Assessed by abdominal examination (p. 185, Figs. 4.18A and B) or by vaginal examination in relation to station.
(f) **Hours** is the time elapsed since the onset of active phase of labor. **Time** is the actual time of examination (Fig. 5.1).
(g) **Uterine contractions:** Number of contractions in 10 minute time period and their duration in seconds. They are shaded accordingly (Fig. 5.1).
(h) **Drugs and fluids:** To record oxytocin—in mIU/minute. Oxytocin drop rate is to be escalated (doubled) at an interval of 30 minutes till adequate contractions are obtained. Drugs are recorded when given.
(i) **Pulse and blood pressure:** Pulse—to record every 30 minutes and is marked with a dot (•), BP is measured in every 4 hours and is marked with arrows (b).
(j) **Temperature:** To record every 2 hours.
(k) **Urine:** To record for volume, protein and acetone when passed (usually 2-3 hours).

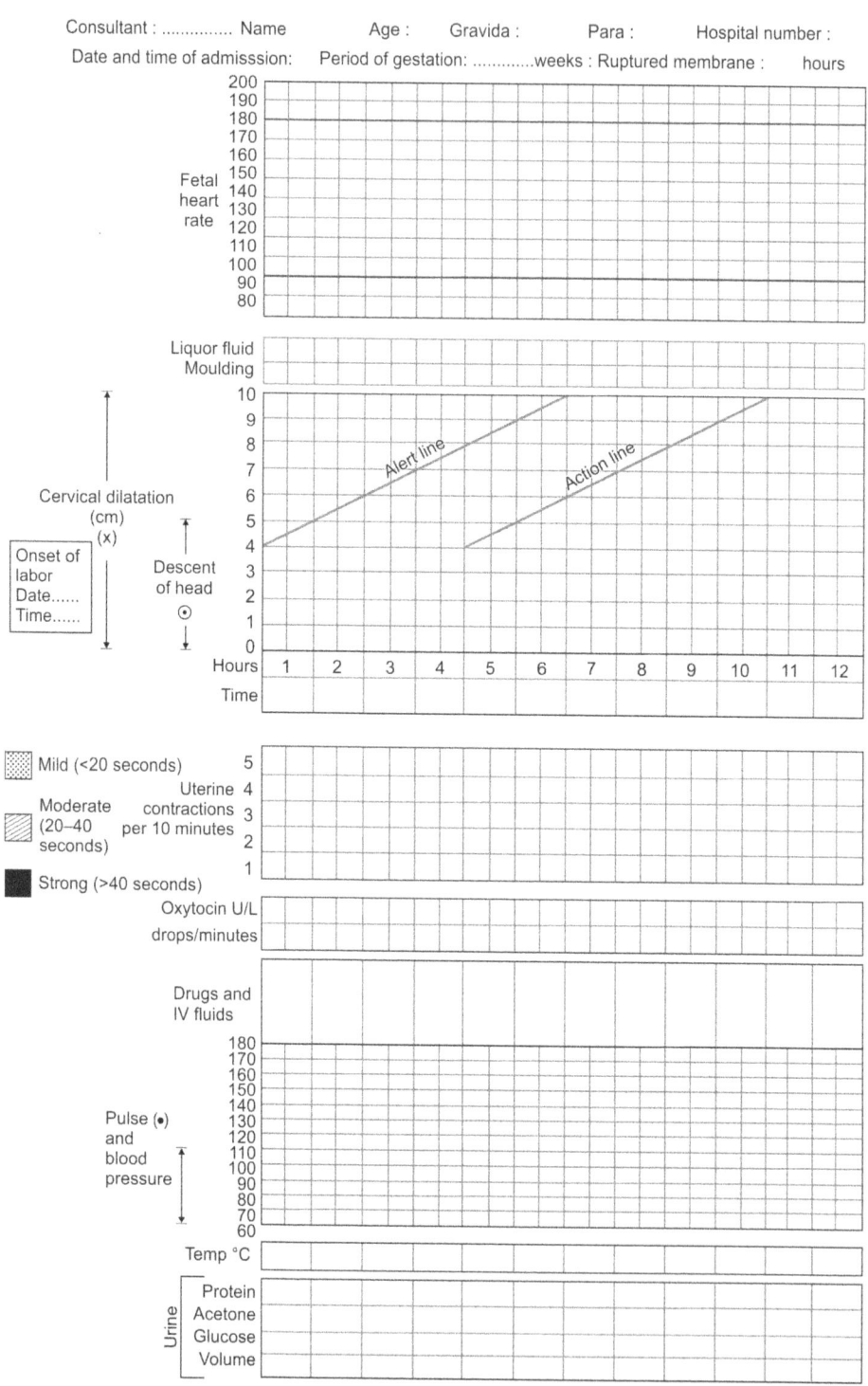

**Fig. 5.1:** Partograph 1 : WHO Partograph (modified).

## INDUCTION OF LABOR

Induction of labor (IOL) means the initiation of labor with uterine contractions by methods (medical, surgical, mechanical or combined) for the purpose of vaginal delivery. It is done after the period of fetal viability (28 weeks).

**Q. What are the common indications of IOL?**

Ans. (a) Pre-eclampsia
 (b) Eclampsia
 (c) Postmaturity
 (d) IUFD
 (e) Antepartum hemorrhage
 (f) Diabetes mellitus.

**Q. What are the contraindications of IOL?**

Ans. (a) Cephalopelvic disproportion
 (b) Malpresentation (transverse lie)
 (c) Placenta previa
 (d) Previous cesarean delivery.

**Q. What are the methods of IOL?**

Ans. (a) **Medical:** Oxytocin, prostaglandins ($PGE_2$, $PGE_1$)
 (b) **Surgical:** Stripping of the membranes, artificial rupture of membranes
 (c) **Mechanical:** Foley's catheter
 (d) **Combined methods:** Medical followed by surgical or surgical followed by medical methods.

Augmentation of labor means acceleration of labor process when it is already initiated. It is commonly done in cases with uterine inertia, or following induction of labor or in the active management of labor.

## Oxytocin Infusion Dose Calculation

Start oxytocin 1 unit in 500 mL Ringer lactate at the rate of 15 drops/min [(dose = 2 milliunits (mU)/min)] [15 drops = 1 mL; oxytocin is stored in refrigerator] [1 unit = 1000 milliunits (mU)]

After 30 minutes, to increase drip rate to 30 drops/min—(4 mU/min)

Dose of oxytocin need to be adjusted when high concentration oxytocin is to be given and volume of fluid is to be low (see table below). Infusion pump may be used alternatively.

| Amount of oxytocin (Unit in 500 mL) | Drop rate (per min) | Oxytocin infusion rate in milliunits/min (mU/min) |
|---|---|---|
| 1 unit | 15 drops | 2 |
| 1 unit | 30 drops | 4 |
| 2 unit | 30 drops | 8 |
| 4 unit | 30 drops | 16 |

**Q. What are the different parameters for observation following oxytocin infusion?**

**Ans.** (1) Rate of flow (concentration: mU/min)
(2) Uterine contractions
(3) Uterine relaxations
(4) FHR monitoring
(5) Assessment of progress of labor.

**Q. What are the indications for stopping the oxytocin infusion?**

**Ans.** (1) Onset of abnormal uterine contractions (uterine tachysystole)
(2) Evidences of fetal distress
(3) Maternal distress (maternal hypotension).

**Q. What are the different routes of oxytocin administration?**

**Ans.** (1) Controlled IV infusion is commonly used for induction or augmentation of labor.
(2) IV or IM: 5-10 units after birth of the baby (active management of third stage of labor).
(3) IM as syntometrine (See p. 326)
(4) Buccal tablets or nasal spray—limited use on trial basis.

**Q. How the quality of care should be maintained during induction of labor?**

**Ans.** (National Health Mission—2017):
(a) Respectful maternity care should be maintained. It always ensures positive outcomes.
(b) Induction or augmentation of labor should be done only with sound clinical indication.
(c) Privacy of the woman (providing separate labor room/cubicle) should be maintained.
(d) A birth companion of her choice should be allowed during the course of induction/labor.

## PARTOGRAPH FOR NORMAL LABOR

### Case Summary

*Mrs KN, 23 years old, G-2, P-1, L-1 (P1+0+0+1) was admitted at 6 am on 13-10-2010 with labor pain following a term pregnancy. Her first pregnancy ended in spontaneous vaginal delivery. She had spontaneous rupture of membranes 1 hour prior to her admission. On examination, she was normotensive, uterine contractions were mild to moderate (2-3 per 10 minutes) and FHS was 130 bpm and regular. Pelvic examination revealed: Cervix 60% effaced; os : 2 cm, membranes absent and liquor—clear. Her partograph is shown in the **Figure 5.2: Partograph 2**.*

**Q. What was the cervical dilatation at 8 am?**

**Ans.** Cervix became 4 cm dilated.

## Chapter 5 • Active Management of Labor

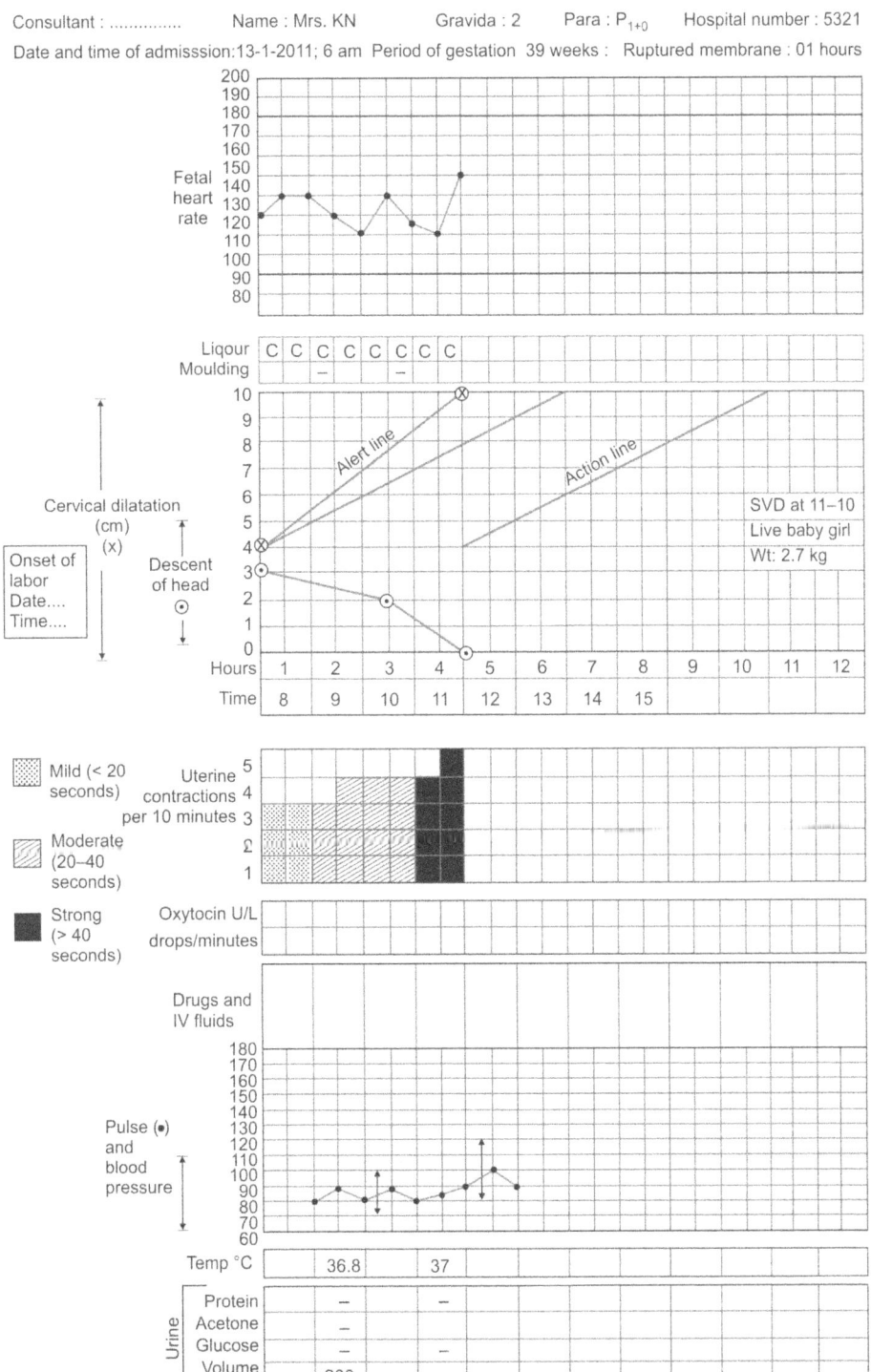

**Fig. 5.2:** Partograph 2.

**Q. How long she took to enter into the active phase of labor?**

**Ans.** During admission at 6 am, she was 2 cm dilated and by 8 am she became 4 cm. It is by 2 hours since admission that she entered the active phase of labor.

**Q. What should be the normal rate of cervical dilatation for her?**

**Ans.** As she is P1+0+0+1, her cervical dilatation should ideally be 1.5 cm/h.

**Q. At what time she became fully dilated?**

**Ans.** At 12.00 hours (6 hours since admission) she became fully dilated.

**Q. What was the duration of the active phase of labor?**

**Ans.** 4 hours.

**Q. How were the uterine contractions during the course of labor?**

**Ans.** During the first hour, contractions were mild each lasting <20 seconds.

For the next 2 hours, the frequency of uterine contractions were 3–4/10 minutes and each lasted about 20–40 seconds.

In the last 1 hour, contractions were really strong. Number of contractions increased to 4–5 and each lasted for ≥40 seconds.

**Q. How was the fetal heart rate during the course of labor?**

**Ans.** During the entire course of labor, the FHR varied from 120–150 bpm. There was no bradycardia or tachycardia or any irregularity.

**Q. How was the blood pressure of the woman during the course of labor?**

**Ans.** BP remained between 110/70 mm Hg and 120/80 mm Hg.

**Q. Did Mrs KN require any augmentation of labor?**

**Ans.** No. She progressed normally. There was no need of augmentation for her.

**Q. What was the level of fetal head when she was admitted?**

**Ans.** Head was 3/5th palpable above the brim (Crichton's method). Head was not engaged at the time of admission.

## PARTOGRAPH FOR ABNORMAL LABOR

### Case Summary

*Mrs CL, 31 years old, G5P3, A1, L3 (P3+0+1+3) was admitted in labor following a term pregnancy. Her partograph is shown in **Figure 5.3: Partograph 3**.*

**Q. Discuss the partographic observation of Mrs CL during admission at 8 am.**

**Ans.** Mrs CL had :
(1) Cervical dilatation : 4 cm
(2) Fetal head : 3/5th palpable above the brim (not engaged)
(3) Uterine contraction : Mild, each lasting for <20 seconds

(4) FHR : Between 130 and 140 bpm, regular
(5) Liquor : Clear
(6) Blood pressure : 130/80 mm Hg.

Mrs CL was in active phase of labor.

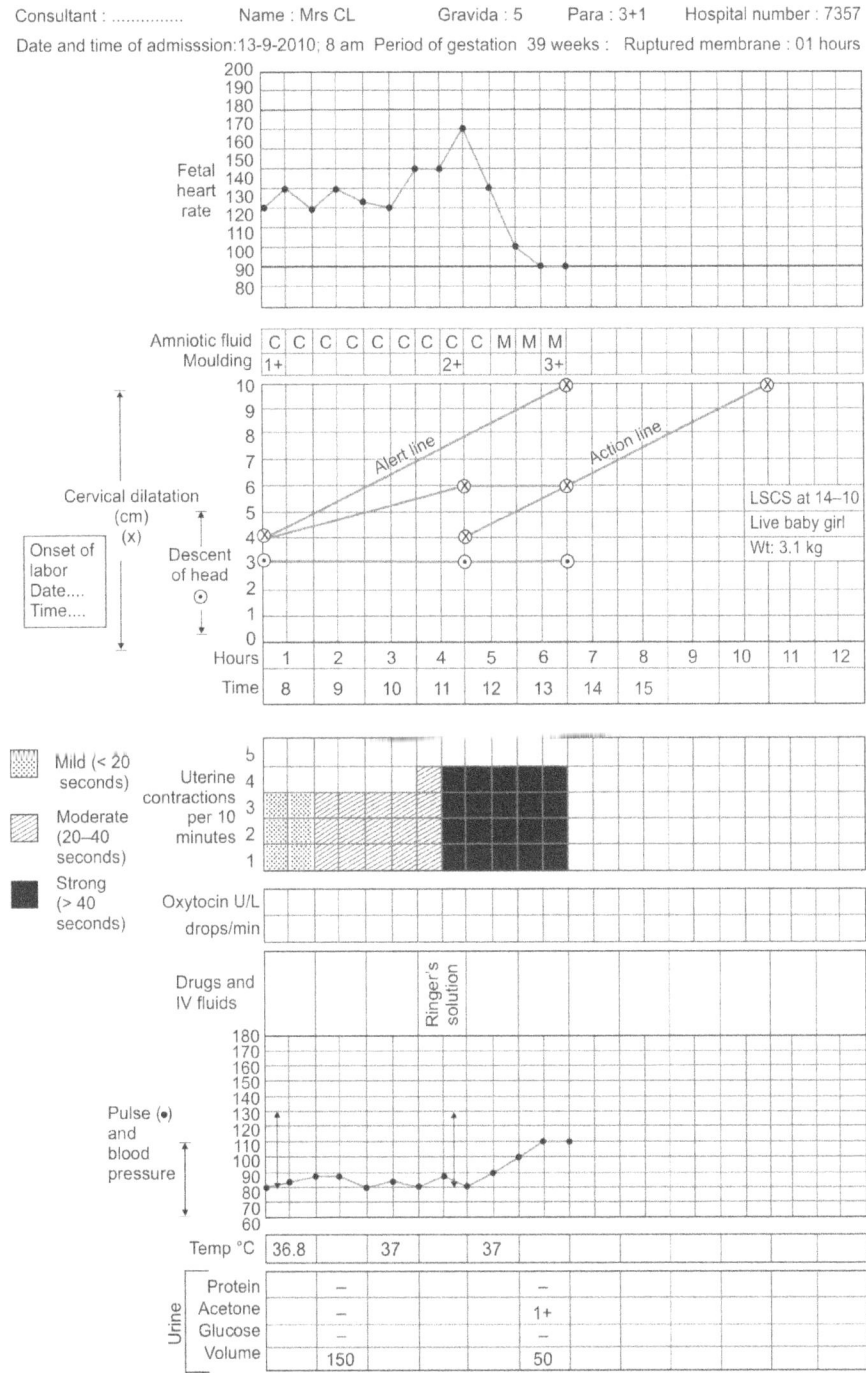

Fig. 5.3: Partograph 3.

**Q. Discuss her labor progress observed after 4 hours of labor (12.00 hours).**

**Ans.** (1) Cervical dilatation : 6 cm dilated. But it has crossed the alert line.
(2) Fetal head : 3/5th brim, no descent of head since admission.
(3) Uterine contractions : 3/4 in 10 minutes time, each lasting for >40 seconds.
(4) FHR : >160 bpm (tachycardia) but coming down steeply upto 100 bpm (bradycardia) by the next hour.
(5) Liquor : Clear.
(6) Moulding : 2+.

**Comments:** Cervical dilatation increased by 2 cm over a period of 4 hours. For Mrs CL, it was much less (normally 1.5/h). Cervicograph is on the right side of the alert line. There is no change in the descent of the presenting part in spite of the fact that uterine contractions were adequate. Presence of tachycardia and bradycardia with moulding indicate adverse fetal response in relation to the progress of labor.

*Ringer's solution was started to maintain her hydration and normal metabolic status.*

**Q. Discuss the partograph as recorded during the course of Mrs CL's labor at 14.00 (2 pm).**

**Ans.** (1) Cervical dilatation : 6 cm. It has touched the action line
(2) Fetal head : 3/5th above the brim. No descent at all.
(3) Uterine contraction : 3-4 in 10 minutes time each lasting ≥40 seconds.
(4) FHR : Significant bradycardia <110 bpm.
(5) Liquor : Meconium stained.
(6) Moulding : 3+.

**Comments:** Mrs CL had no further dilatation of the cervix since the last observation at 12 pm (2 hours) and there is no descent of the presenting part. Fetal bradycardia, moulding of the head, meconium-stained liquor were observed. Partographic analysis of labor revealed arrest of dilatation and descent in the active phase of labor despite adequate uterine contractions. This indicates labor is obstructed. Owing to this observation along with presence of fetal distress, labor was terminated. Cesarean delivery was performed at 2–10 pm.

**Q. How can you evaluate critically that partograph can reduce the problems of prolonged and obstructed labor?**

**Ans.** See SAQ p. 243.

## Case Summary

*Mrs Bani Kumari, a 26-year-old primigravida was admitted in labor following a term pregnancy. Her partograph is shown in* **Figure 5.4: Partograph 4.**

**Q. Discuss the partographic observation of Mrs Bani at 10 am (Fig. 5.4 partograph 4).**

**Ans.**
- Cervix was 4 cm dilated
- Uterine contractions were 2 in 10 minutes and each lasted less than 20 seconds

## Chapter 5 • Active Management of Labor

### Identification data

**Name:** Mrs. Bani Pillai  **W/o:** Ramaraju  **Age:** 26 years  **Parity:** Primigravida  **Reg No.:** 23780

**Date and time of admission**
11th march 2011, 10 am

**Date and time of ROM:**
11th march 2011, 10 am

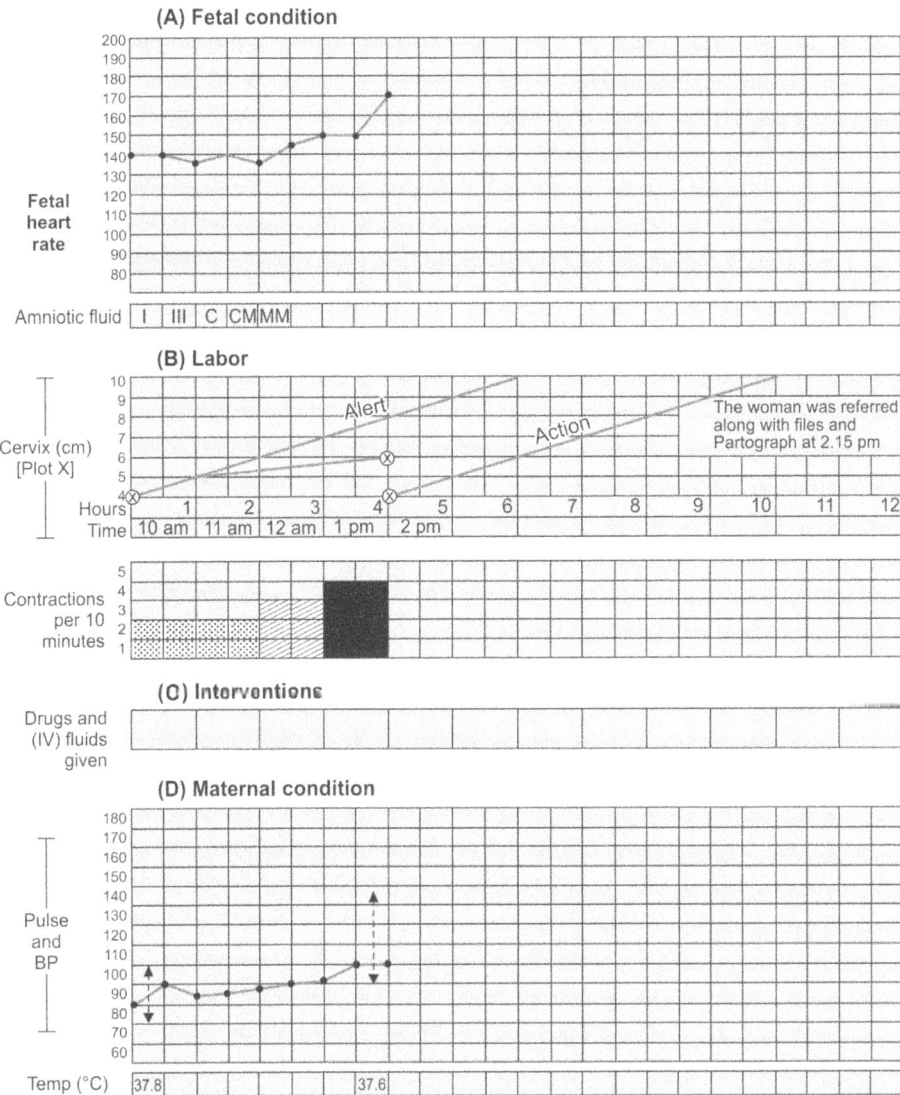

**Fig. 5.4:** Partograph 4.

- FHR was 140/min
- Blood pressure was 100/70 mm Hg
- Temperature was 37°C
- Pulse was 80/min.

**Q. Discuss her partographic observation at 2 pm.**

**Ans.**
- Cervix was 6 cm dilated
- Liquor was meconium-stained
- Uterine contractions were 4 in 10 minutes and each lasted for 45 seconds
- FHR was 170/min
- Maternal pulse was 100/min, temperature was 37.6°C and blood pressure was 140/90 mm Hg.

**Q. Why she was referred?**

**Ans.** Labor was monitored by an ANM at a peripheral center. Labor plotting had moved on the right of the alert line. Labor is prolonged, liquor was meconium-stained, FHR was 170/min. BP was 140/90 mm Hg. She needed intervention. Therefore, she was referred to the nearby FRU where she reached by 30 minutes.

## INTRAPARTUM ELECTRONIC FETAL MONITORING—CARDIOTOCOGRAPHY

**Q. What do you understand by intrapartum fetal monitoring?**

**Ans.** It simply means to watch the fetal behavior during the course of labor.

**Q. Is there any additional stress to the fetus even during the course of a normal labor?**

**Ans.** Yes. During the course of labor, there are certain changes that put the fetus under stress even in a normal labor. There are:
 (a) During uterine contractions, there is curtailing of uteroplacental circulation—so the fetus may develop hypoxia.
 (b) Head compression during labor may affect the vital centers of the fetal brain.
 However, in a compromised fetus and/or in an abnormal labor, fetal distress may appear more frequently compared to a normal labor.

**Q. What are the different methods of intrapartum fetal monitoring?**

**Ans.** (1) Clinical, (2) Biophysical and (3) Biochemical.

**Q. What are the advantages of CTG over clinical monitoring?**

**Ans.** (i) Early detection of fetal hypoxia
 (ii) Improvement of intrapartum fetal death
 (iii) Improvement of perinatal mortality
 (iv) Important document for medicolegal purpose.

**Q. What are the drawbacks of CTG?**

**Ans.** (i) Instruments are expensive
 (ii) Trained personnel are needed to interpret a trace
 (iii) Due to false prediction cesarean delivery rate may go high.

**Q. What is a nonstress test (NST)?**

**Ans.** It is an antenatal observation. It is the association of FHR acceleration with fetal movements. When present, it indicates a healthy fetus. This is reliable screening test.

**Q. What are the causes of fetal tachycardia (FHR >160 bpm)?**

**Ans.** See Table 5.1.

**Q. What are the causes of fetal bradycardia (FHR <100 bpm)?**

**Ans.** See Table 5.1.

| Table 5.1: Causes of fetal bradycardia. | |
| --- | --- |
| Causes of fetal tachycardia (FHR >160 bpm) | Causes of fetal bradycardia (FHR <110 bpm) |
| (a) Drugs to mother : (i) Beta-sympathomimetic agents used to inhibit preterm labor (isoxsuprine, ritodrine), (ii) vagolytic : Atropine<br>(b) Infection — both maternal and fetal<br>(c) Anemia — both maternal and fetal<br>(d) Fetal hypoxia | (a) Fetal hypoxia and acidosis<br>(b) Fetal sepsis and anomalies<br>(c) Use of local anesthetic drugs and epidural analgesia<br>(d) Drugs to mother, e.g. pethidine, antihypertensives (methyldopa, propranolol) and $MgSO_4$<br>(e) Fetal heart conduction defect (SLE) |

**Q. Mention the criteria of a reassuring (reactive) trace?**

**Ans.**
- Baseline FHR between 100 and 160 bpm
- Baseline variability >5 bpm
- Two accelerations in 20 minutes observation
- No deceleration or may be an early deceleration.

**Q. When a CTG trace pattern is called abnormal?**

**Ans.** Abnormal trace pattern (pathological) includes:
- **Baseline FHR:** <100 bpm or >180 bpm.
- **Baseline variability:** <5 bpm for >90 minutes or sinusoidal pattern.
- **Acceleration:** None in 40 minutes observation.
- **Deceleration:** Late deceleration >30 minutes or single prolonged deceleration >3 minutes or atypical variable decelerations.
- **Sinusoidal pattern**.

**Q. What are the reasons for decreased baseline variability?**

**Ans.**
(1) Fetal sleep
(2) Infection
(3) Maternal medications (pethidine, propranolol, $MgSO_4$)
(4) Fetal hypoxia
(5) Fetal heart conduction defect (SLE).

**Q. What are the indications of continuous electronic monitoring of the fetus?**

**Ans.** When the risks of intrapartum fetal hypoxia is high, continuous electronic fetal monitoring is suggested.
**The conditions are:**
(1) Intrauterine growth restriction (IUGR)
(2) Meconium-stained liquor
(3) Maternal hypertension/diabetes
(4) Previous cesarean delivery
(5) Malposition (OP) or presentation (breech).

## INTERPRETATION OF A CARDIOTOCOGRAPH

**Q. What is baseline FHR?**

Ans. It is the mean level of FHR between the peaks and depressions. It is expressed as beats per minute (bpm).

**Q. What is the baseline variability?**

Ans. It is the oscillation of baseline FHR excluding the accelerations and decelerations. A baseline variability of 10–25 bpm is a sign of fetal well-being.

**Q. What is an acceleration?**

Ans. Acceleration is the increase in FHR by 15 bpm or more lasting for at least 15 seconds.

**Q. What does an acceleration signify?**

Ans. Acceleration denotes a healthy fetus. However, the significance of absence of acceleration is uncertain.

**Q. What is a deceleration?**

Ans. It is the decrease in FHR below the baseline by 15 bpm or more and lasting for ≥15 seconds.

**Q. What are the different types of decelerations? What is the significance of each type?**

Ans. (A) *Early deceleration:* It is due to head compression (Type I dips).
(B) *Late deceleration:* Indicates uteroplacental insufficiency and fetal hypoxia (Type II dips).
(C) *Variable deceleration:* It may be due to cord compression.

**Q. What is a reassuring (reactive) CTG?**

Ans. Presence of ≥2 acceleration of ≥15 bpm above the baseline and lasting for ≥15 seconds, in a 20 minutes observation is a reassuring pattern.

**Q. What features in a CTG are suggestive of a healthy fetus?**

Ans. Presence of accelerations and a normal baseline variability (10–25 bpm) denote a healthy fetus.

## Case Summary

*Mrs SL 26 years old school teacher, presents in her first pregnancy at 36 completed weeks of gestation with diminished fetal movements. She was normotensive and without any obstetric and medical complications of pregnancy. Cardiotocograph was done (Fig. 5.5) and is shown in Figure 5.6, Cardiotocograph-1.*

**Q. What is the baseline FHR for Mrs SL?**

Ans. 150 beats/minute (bpm).

**Q. What is the baseline variability?**

Ans. 10–20 bpm.

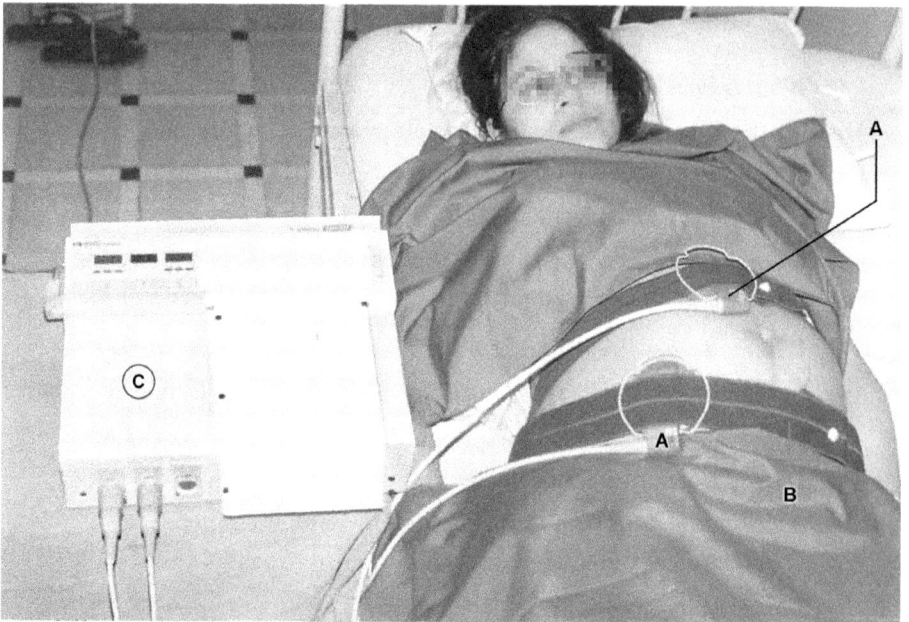

**Fig. 5.5:** Cardiotocography is in progress using abdominal transducers.
A : Abdominal transducers (external monitoring)
B : Abdominal belt to keep transducers in position
C : CTG machine; FHR tracing is being recorded

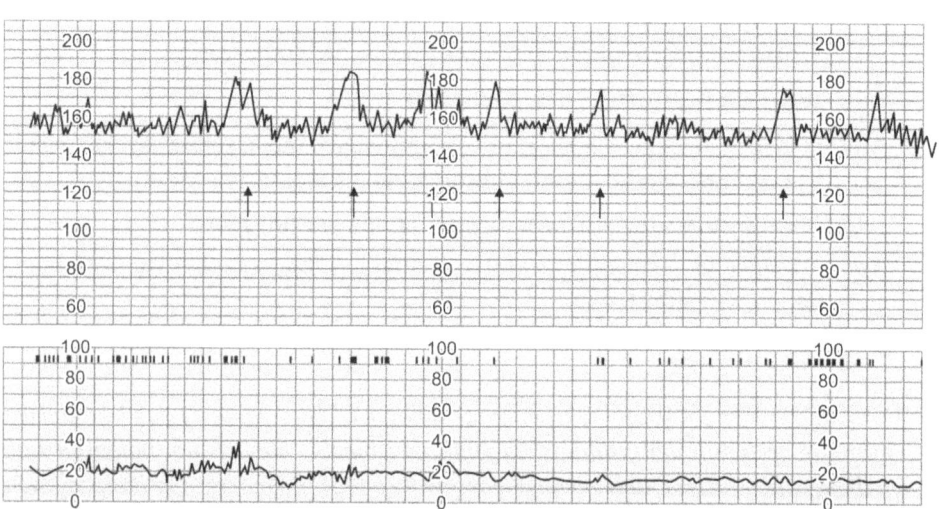

**Fig. 5.6:** Cardiotocograph–1: CTG trace of Mrs SL fetal movements (black blocks) with cardiac accelerations are seen.

**Q. Is there any sinusoidal pattern?**
**Ans.** Nil

**Q. How many acceleration are there in the trace?**
**Ans.** Six within the period of 20 minutes.

**Q. Is there any deceleration?**
**Ans.** Nil.

**Q. What about the nonstress test?**
**Ans.** Fetal movements are evidenced by black blocks in the graph. Simultaneous with the fetal movements, there is acceleration of FHR.

**Q. How do you categorize this CTG trace?**
**Ans.** All the four features are normal (reassuring). It is a normal trace indicating a healthy fetus.

**Q. What about the tocograph in the trace?**
**Ans.** Tocograph showed absence of uterine contractions.

## Case Summary

*Mrs ZC, 26 years old housewife, P0+0+0+0 was admitted at 35.4 weeks of gestation because she was epileptic and the baby was small for gestation. A 30 minutes cardiotocography (CTG) trace was done when she complained of diminished fetal movements. The CTG trace is shown in the Figure 5.7, Cardiotocograph-2.*

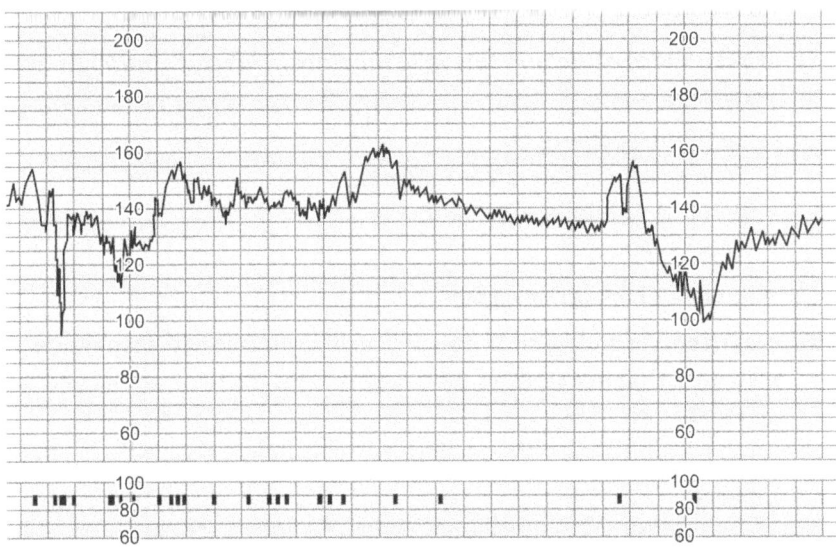

**Fig. 5.7:** Cardiotocograph–2: Abnormal nonstress test showing repeated decelerations 40 bpm and lasting >3 minutes.

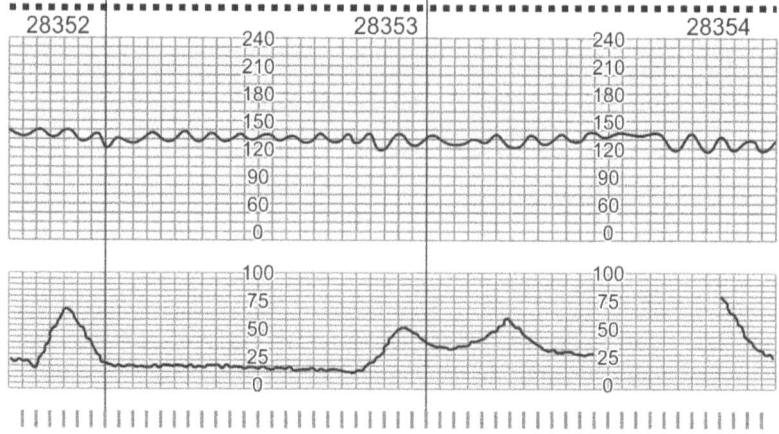

**Fig. 5.8:** Cardiotocograph–3: Sinusoidal pattern showing reduced baseline variability.

***Q. What abnormalities are shown in the trace?***

**Ans.** Baseline fetal heart rate was 140 bpm with unprovoked repeated decelerations (20-40 bpm) lasting for more than 3 minutes.

***Q. What would be the next plan of management?***

**Ans.** Patient should be admitted for continuous monitoring and for biophysical scoring. Further CTG showed in the trace as below (Fig. 5.8: Cardiotocograph-3)

***Q. What abnormalities are shown in the trace? This trace pattern remained persistent.***

**Ans.**
- Sinusoidal pattern
- Fetal baseline heart rate is 135 bpm
- Baseline variability is ≤5 bpm
- Acceleration : Nil.

***Q. What would be your advice?***

**Ans.** This trace is pathological. Fetus needs to be evaluated with biophysical profile including Doppler study of umbilical vessels, ductus venosus and middle cerebral artery.

***Q. Both the parameters revealed the fetus is hypoxic. What would be your advice?***

**Ans.**
- To organize delivery.
- On examination, cervix was found unfavorable. She was delivered by LSCS. The baby weighed 1.2 kg.

CHAPTER 6

# Obstetrics Short Questions

## Chapter Objectives

**Short questions:**
- Model answers are provided to develop the art of writing in a concise way with important and updated information.
- Discussion need to be focused.

❖ Obstetrics Short Questions with Answers 236

## Q. 1 Magnesium sulfate is the drug of choice in the management of eclampsia—Discuss.

**Ans.** Eclampsia is the leading cause of maternal death in India. Magnesium sulfate is used in severe pre-eclampsia **to prevent seizures (prophylactic use)**. It is used in eclampsia **to control seizures as well as to prevent its recurrence**.

Other drugs occasionally used in the management of eclampsia are Lytic cocktail (Menon's regimen), Diazepam therapy (Lean's regimen) and Phenytoin therapy. These drugs have got no prophylactic value.

Moreover, compared to these drugs magnesium sulfate has got the superiority in the following areas:

(a) It is given either by IM (pritchard) or by IV regimen (zuspan)—it is relatively simple to administer.
(b) In majority of cases—clinical monitoring is sufficient enough to continue the drug. Clinical monitoring parameters are:
   (i) Presence of knee jerks
   (ii) Urine output is >30 mL/hour
   (iii) Respiratory rate is 12/minute. Rarely serum magnesium level estimation is needed. (Normal therapeutic level is 4–7 mEq/L).
(c) Compared to other drugs it **prevents seizures more effectively** and **prevent its recurrence**.
(d) It acts by reducing motor end plate sensitivity to acetylcholine and it blocks neuronal calcium influx. It induces **dilatation of cerebral and uterine vessels** which is distinctly beneficial. Moreover **it does not alter maternal sensorium**. This is a major advantage over other drugs.
(e) It has excellent results with significantly **reduced maternal mortality (3%) and morbidity**.
(f) Compared to other drugs, it has **no detrimental effect on the fetus or the neonate**. This is a major advantage over the other drugs.
(g) **Side effects** (muscular paresis, respiratory failure) **are rare** once drug dose is monitored clinically and carefully. However, 10% calcium gluconate, 10 mL IV slowly is an effective antidote.
(h) Compared to other drugs, perinatal mortality is also very low with $MgSO_4$. The **other drugs have got significant fetal and neonatal depression effect**.

Considering all these benefits over the other drugs, magnesium sulfate is considered the drug of choice in eclampsia.

[(For further details: See p. 333-336 (Drugs in Obstetrics)].

## Q. 2 Active management of third stage of labor should be done in all cases—discuss.

**Ans.** The third stage is the most crucial stage of labor. Unless managed properly it can lead to the following complications like:
  (i) Postpartum hemorrhage
  (ii) Shock
  (iii) Uterine inversion
  (iv) Retention of placenta
  (v) Pulmonary embolism
  (vi) Maternal death.

Previous uneventful first and second stage may become abnormal in the third stage and may lead to maternal death. To prevent such complications active management of third stage of labor (AMTSL) is helpful.

**Procedure of active management of third stage:** Injection oxytocin 10 units IV (slowly)/IM or injection methergin 0.2 mg IV (slowly) is given to the mother within 1 minute following birth of the baby. Injection oxytocin is preferred as it has less side effects compared to methergin (nausea, vomiting and rise in BP).

The **principles** of active management of third stage of labor are:
  (a) To stimulate powerful uterine contractions following birth of the baby by giving **parenteral (IM/IV) oxytocin.**
  (b) To facilitate the **early separation of placenta.**
  (c) To excite **uterine contractions (massaging the uterus)** to expedite the delivery of the placenta by controlled cord traction.
  (d) To **prevent** postpartum hemorrhage.

The significant **advantages** of active management of third stage of labor are:
  (a) Third stage blood loss is reduced approximately to one-fifth
  (b) Duration of third stage is reduced to its half.

However, timing of injection is important. Active management therefore needs more trained nursing personnel in the labor ward to give the injection in time.

Besides the normal cases, this management is certainly valuable in cases that are likely to develop postpartum hemorrhage (anemia, hydramnios, twins, grand multiparity, previous history of postpartum hemorrhage (PPH) and delivery under anesthesia).

There are **few contraindications** of this management especially for methergin. These cases are women with heart disease, severe pre-eclampsia and in cases with twins until the 2nd baby is born.

However, injection oxytocin is safe in such cases compared to methergin. Considering all the benefits, active management should be done in almost all cases in the third stage of labor.

## Q. 3 Maternal mortality is mostly avoidable—Discuss.

**Ans.** Maternal mortality ratio (MMR) in India is high (130/100,000 live births—SRS 2014-2016). In India, lifetime risk of dying for a woman during pregnancy is 0.3% compared to one in 49,000 in developed countries.

The **direct causes** (Fig. 6.1) of maternal deaths are due to hemorrhage (27%), infection (11%), hypertension during pregnancy (14%), unsafe abortion (8%), and obstructed labor (9%).

The important **indirect causes** (28%) of deaths are anemia, viral hepatitis and heart disease (p. 340).

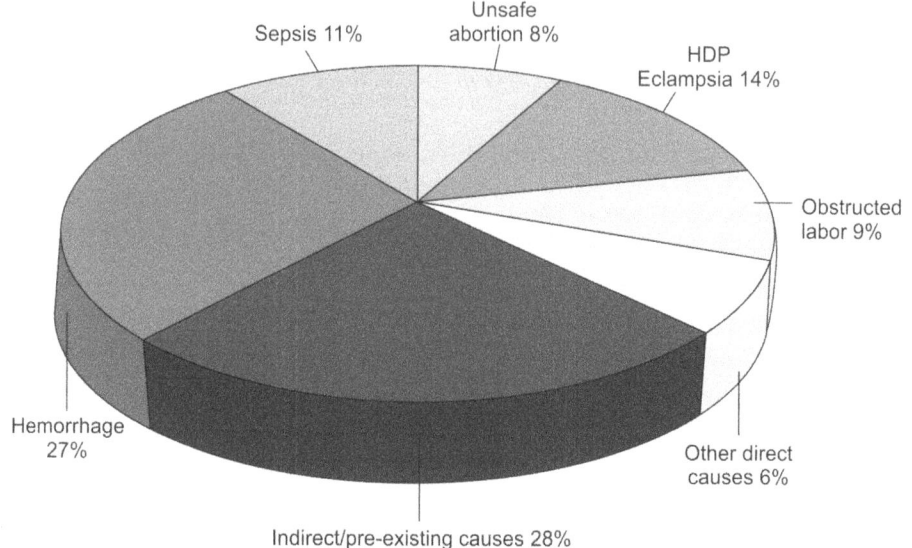

**Fig. 6.1:** Important causes of maternal deaths (WHO, 2014-2016).

The **factors associated** with high maternal mortality are advanced women's age, high parity and unintended pregnancy.

The **important social factors** associated are:
(a) Illiteracy
(b) Ignorance
(c) Unregulated fertility
(d) Poor socioeconomic condition
(e) Underutilization of existing healthcare services
(f) Lack of communication and referral facilities.

The **important steps** to reduce maternal mortality are:
(a) Utilization of basic antenatal, intranatal and postnatal care with quality.
(b) Presence of skilled birth attendant to prevent complications of labor and delivery.
(c) Availability of emergency obstetric care, safe abortion services and easy access to family planning services.

(d) Improvement of legislative and policy action to remove social inequalities on grounds of gender.
(e) To ensure accountability to improve quality of care and equity.

Moreover there are certain proven interventions to reduce maternal deaths. They are

(a) **Hemorrhage** [antepartum hemorrhage (APH), PPH, abortion, ectopic pregnancy]: Proven interventions are to correct anemia, skilled attendant at birth, prevention and treatment of hemorrhage, use of oxytocics in time, to replace the blood loss by transfusion when indicated.
(b) **Infection** (labor and puerperium): Clean delivery practices, skilled birth attendant, use of antibiotics—when infection is evident.
(c) **Hypertension** (pre-eclampsia, eclampsia): Early detection, antiseizure prophylaxis ($MgSO_4$) and appropriate referral.
(d) **Unsafe abortion**: Safe abortion services, use of antibiotics.
(e) **Obstructed labor**: Use of partograph, early diagnosis, and timely intervention or referral.
(f) **Anemia prevention:** Routine supplementation of iron and folic acid during pregnancy.
(g) **Treatment** against hookworm, malaria and hospital admission when needed.
(h) **Medical disorders in pregnancy** (diabetes, jaundice, chickenpox)—appropriate intervention or referral for optimum care.

Combining all the above factors (health, social and policy actions) and by proper interventions against the major causes, maternal mortality can be reduced significantly in India.

## Q. 4 Prenatal counseling is a must—Discuss.

**Ans.** Prenatal counseling means **evaluation and then counseling a woman about pregnancy, its course and the likely outcome well before the time of actual conception**.

The objective of prenatal counseling is that woman should enter the pregnancy in an optimal state of health which would be safe both to herself and fetus. Otherwise many adverse factors begin to exert their effects by the time woman is seen in the antenatal clinic.

Generally women are first seen in the antenatal clinic at around 14 weeks of gestation. By the time they are seen, organogenesis is completed.

Preconceptional phase evaluation **helps to identify the high-risk factor**. At the same time, it helps to organize care to reduce or to eliminate risk factor so that pregnancy outcome is improved.

*Few examples of such benefits are:*

(a) **Folic acid supplementation (4 mg a day)** starting 4 weeks before conception and continued up to 12 weeks of pregnancy. This can reduce the incidence of **neural tube defects**.
(b) Women with **medical complications (hypertension and diabetes) in pregnancy**, need education and treatment before conception. This is done to minimize complication like IUGR (hypertension).
(c) Control of diabetes mellitus before pregnancy is important. This is to reduce the risk of fetal malformations, macrosomia and intrauterine fetal death (IUFD).
(d) Many drugs used during the nonpregnant state should be avoided during pregnancy because of fetal hazards. **Warfarin, valproate are replaced with other drugs like heparin and levetiracetam respectively for the safety of the fetus.**

This can only be done once the woman is seen and counseled before pregnancy (prenatal counseling). Therefore prenatal counseling is a must to improve the pregnancy outcome.

## Q. 5 External cephalic version has got a place in the management of breech presentation—Discuss.

**Ans.** External cephalic version (ECV) is a **maneuver done externally to change the fetal presentation** and to bring the fetal head to the lower pole of uterus. The success rate of version is about 60–70%. Version is usually done from 37 weeks onwards up to early labor.

**Successful version has the following benefits:**
(a) Reduction in the incidence of breech presentation at term.
(b) Reduction in the incidence of vaginal breech delivery.
(c) Reduction in the incidence of associated complications.

However, it is true that not all cases of breech presentation are fit to be considered for ECV.

**Contraindications of ECV**
(a) Antepartum hemorrhage
(b) Uterine malformation
(c) Oligohydramnios
(d) Multiple pregnancy
(e) Contracted pelvis
(f) Previous cesarean delivery, etc.

Moreover **ECV has got some complications** of its own. Complications are:
(a) Fetal distress
(b) Placental abruption
(c) Premature rupture of membranes
(d) Rupture of uterus
(e) Amniotic fluid embolism
(f) Fetal death, etc.

These may necessitate immediate delivery.

Considering all the benefits and the risks, it appears that **each case should be selected carefully excluding the contraindications.**

**Each case needs proper evaluation before and after the maneuver.**
(1) Cardiotocography should be done before and after the procedure to assess fetal well-being.
(2) Tocolytics may be used.
(3) Epidural analgesia has also been used.
(4) Anti-D immunoglobulin should be given to a Rh-ve woman after the procedure.
(5) ECV is done at or beyond 36 weeks and in the labor ward.
(6) Facilities for cesarean delivery must be present, in case any complications develop during ECV procedure.

Therefore it appears on critical evaluation that external cephalic version has got a place in the management of breech presentation in a well-selected case.

### Q. 6 Twin pregnancy is a high-risk one—Discuss.

**Ans. High-risk pregnancy** is defined as one which is complicated with factor(s) that adversely affects the pregnancy outcome—maternal or perinatal or both. Considering this, twin pregnancy outcome is affected adversely by many factors. The adverse outcome affects the health of the fetus, neonate or mother.

| Complications of twin pregnancy that affects the maternal health are |
|---|
| (a) Nausea |
| (b) Vomiting |
| (c) Anemia |
| (d) PIH and pre-eclampsia |
| (e) Polyhydramnios/oligohydramnios |
| (f) Preterm labor |
| (g) Malpresentation |
| (h) Antepartum hemorrhage |
| (i) Mechanical distress (dyspnea, palpitation) |
| (j) Prolonged labor |
| (k) Operative interference |
| (l) Postpartum homorrhage |

| The fetal hazards are |
|---|
| (a) Miscarriage |
| (b) Vanishing twin |
| (c) Fetus papyraceus |
| (d) Preterm birth |
| (e) Fetal anomalies |
| (f) Discordant growth |
| (g) Intrauterine death of one fetus |
| (h) Twin transfusion syndrome |
| (i) Cord prolapse |
| (j) Locked twins and increased |
| (k) Perinatal mortality. |

**Complications are more in monochorionic twins.** Perinatal mortality is markedly increased due to prematurity. Considering all these complications affecting the mother, fetus and neonate, twin pregnancy is considered as a "high-risk pregnancy".

The importance of defining the high-risk situation is to anticipate the complications. Simultaneously, we have to adopt the preventive measures to avoid or to minimize the complications. Early diagnosis with ultrasonography is important to make the management plan. Chorionicity can be diagnosed around 12 to 13 weeks of pregnancy. Anemia can be prevented by antenatal supplementation of increased amount of iron and folic acid. This can meet up the increased demand and thereby can prevent complications due to anemia. Preterm labor is common in twins. Prophylactic use of corticosteroids (Inj Betamethosone/dexamethasone) should be given to prevent respiratory distress syndrome of the newborn.

Similarly postpartum hemorrhage is a major threat to the mother. This is commonly due to atonicity of the uterus as it is hugely enlarged during pregnancy. So twin pregnancy needs careful antenatal care and intrapartum care to prevent all these complications. Such a woman should be delivered in a hospital equipped with neonatal intensive care unit (NICU).

### Q. 7 Introduction of partograph has reduced the incidence of prolonged labor and cesarean delivery—Discuss.

**Ans.** Partograph is a **composite graphical record** of cervical dilatation, descent of fetal head, FHR and well-being of both fetus and mother. All these are depicted in a single sheet of paper against the duration of labor in hours. The components of a partograph are designed to assess the progress of labor and the well-being of the mother and fetus.

In **cervicograph** (Philpott and Castle, 1972), the **alert line** starts at 4 cm of cervical dilatation (WHO—4 cm) and ends at 10 cm dilatation (at the rate of 1 cm/hour).

The **action line** is drawn 4 hours (WHO—4 hours) to the right and parallel to the alert line.

**In a normal labor, the cervicograph (cervical dilatation) should be either on the alert line or to the left of it.** Labor is said to be **abnormal** when cervicograph crosses the alert line and falls on **zone 2**. Here the case needs careful reassessment. Intervention is required (ARM, oxytocin or delivery), when it crosses the action line and falls on **zone 3**.

**Partograph has got many advantages.** The main advantage is that it can detect deviation from normal course of labor early.

In a partograph (WHO), the labor process is divided into two phases:

(i) **Latent phase** that ends when the cervix is 4 cm dilated
(ii) **Active phase** starts from cervical dilatation of 4 cm and ends at 10 cm dilatation.
WHO Partograph is plotted from the active phase of labor. In the active phase, cervix should dilate at least 1 cm/hour. First stage of labor is considered **prolonged** when the rate of cervical dilatation is <1 cm/hour in primigravida and <1.5 cm/hour in multigravida.

Similarly if the rate of descent of the fetal head is <1 cm/hour in a primigravida and <2 cm/hour in a multigravida it is called **prolonged**.

**Secondary arrest** can be diagnosed when the active phase of labor commences normally but stops or slows down significantly for 2 hours or more prior to full dilatation of the cervix.

**Obstructed labor** can be diagnosed when the progressive descent of the presenting part is arrested in spite of good uterine contraction. This is often associated with maternal features of dehydration, exhaustion and sepsis. Fetal distress often is there. **Partograph can detect both prolonged labor or obstructed labor early before any adverse effect on the mother or the fetus sets in.** Partograph abnormality suggests either early referral to an equipped center or an early intervention. In majority of cases, intervention is in the form of ARM with or without oxytocin. When intervention is done timely, majority of cases result in successful vaginal delivery. So introduction of partograph has reduced the incidence of prolonged labor and cesarean delivery.

## Q. 8 Exclusive breastfeeding should be encouraged.

**Ans. Exclusive breastfeeding means giving nothing orally other than colostrum and breast milk.** Breastfeeding has got **several advantages,** whereas **artificial feeding has got several disadvantages**. Considering the benefits of exclusive breastfeeding, all babies regardless of the type of delivery should be given **early and exclusive breastfeeding** up to 6 months of age.

| Benefits of early and exclusive breastfeeding |
|---|
| (a) Breast milk has got the **ideal composition** of a food for the newborn (fat, protein and carbohydrate) with low osmotic load. |
| (b) **Protection against** infection and deficiency states: <br>   (i) • **Lactoferrin**, lysozyme, interferon <br>      • **Long chain Ω-3 fatty acids** prevent infection <br>   (ii) **Vit D** protects against rickets <br>   (iii) **Passive immunity** (IgA, sIgA, IgG): Prevents infection from gastrointestinal (GI) tract. |
| (c) **Breast milk is readily available**, more convenient, no cost, no preparation, better for neurodevelopment. |
| (d) **Natural contraception** |
| (e) **Additional advantages**: Laxative action, no risk of allergy, psychological—mother-child bonding, helps uterine involution, reduces the risk of rickets and scurvy. |

| Short- and long-term risks of artificial feeding |
|---|
| (a) Infection—diarrhea |
| (b) Sudden infant death syndrome |
| (c) Chronic diseases |
| (d) Childhood obesity |
| (e) Adult obesity |
| (f) Atopic dermatitis |
| (g) Reduced intelligence quotient |
| (h) Type II diabetes mellitus |
| (i) Hypertension |

**Considering all the benefits of breast milk and the long-term as well as short-term risks of artificial feeding exclusive breastfeeding should be encouraged.**

**Maternal benefits of breastfeeding are:**
(a) Psychological attachment (mother baby bonding)
(b) Enhances involution of the uterus
(c) Protection against breast cancer
(d) Protection against ovarian cancer
(e) Protection against unplanned pregnancy. This is due to lactalional menorrhea (LAM) effect. (Dutta, Obs 9/e, p. 521)
(f) Lowers the risk of cardiovascular disease.

## Q. 9 Iron should be given to all antenatal mothers—Discuss.

**Ans. Iron deficiency anemia** is the common type of anemia in pregnancy especially in the tropical countries. In a healthy individual, daily intake of dietary iron is about 15 mg. Daily loss is about 1.5 mg. Daily absorption of iron from duodenum is about 1.5 mg. With an absorption rate of 10%, the normal daily intake can meet up the daily normal loss of iron. But considering the socioeconomic status, several factors interferes with the normal amount of daily iron intake and absorption.

(a) Presence of phosphate, phytate in the food containing mainly carbohydrate, **impairs the absorption of iron** on the other hand, vitamin C, orange juice increase the absorption of iron.

(b) Intestinal infestation with hookworm, amebiasis and conditions like diarrhea, hypochlorhydria **reduces iron absorption**.

(c) During pregnancy, there are several reasons for poor iron absorption. These conditions are:
   (i) Inadequate intake of diet due to nausea, vomiting in pregnancy
   (ii) Presence of chronic infections like asymptomatic bacteria and tuberculosis.

(d) Conditions in pregnancy where **iron loss is more**:
   (i) Loss through sweat and/or repeated pregnancies at short intervals
   (ii) Pre-existing anemia due to excessive blood loss during menstruation
   (iii) Bleeding in pregnancy (APH, piles)
   (iv) Chronic infections—urinary tract and malaria. Many women enter pregnancy with a pre-existent anemic state.

(e) Sometimes, the **demand of iron in pregnancy is increased**. Conditions are:
   (i) Multiple pregnancy
   (ii) Pregnancies that are too frequent (<2 years of last delivery)
   (iii) Teenage pregnancy.

During pregnancy, **fetus is generally not affected** due to placental transfer of iron from the mother. As a result **mother suffers from iron deficiency**. Total amount of iron needed during pregnancy is about 1,000 mg. The amount of iron absorbed from the diet and that mobilized from the store are inadequate to meet this demand of pregnancy. Therefore, most women develop iron deficiency anemia. This results in depletion of the maternal reserve iron. The woman who has got sufficient reserve iron and is on a balanced diet is unlikely to develop anemia during pregnancy. But due to increased demand of iron during pregnancy, her reserve iron is utilized. Therefore, she runs the risk of developing anemia during puerperium unless the extra demand of iron is met with.

Therefore, considering all the factors supplementation of iron should be given to all antenatal women. Depending upon the severity of anemia and the duration of pregnancy, iron may be given orally, or parenterally (IM or IV infusion). Women with severe anemia in pregnancy and who are intolerant to oral iron may be given iron preparation by IV route (Dutta, Obs 9/e, p. 250).

### Q. 10 Once cesarean delivery is not always cesarean delivery—Discuss.

**Ans.** Long back (1916), Edward Cragin said, "once a cesarean section, always a cesarean section". This was said to reduce the complications of pregnancy with prior cesarean delivery mainly the rupture of uterus. Currently, the scenario has changed because of many developments in obstetric management.

Women with prior cesarean delivery is a 'high-risk' one. She needs regular antenatal check-up, timely admission in hospital and delivery under supervision. However, woman needs individualization as regard the decision for subsequent mode of **delivery**. This may be vaginal birth after cesarean—trial of labor (VBAC-TOL) or repeat cesarean delivery. There are **several factors to be considered before making such a decision**. These are:

(i) Indications of primary cesarean section (CS)—recurrent or nonrecurrent
(ii) Type of primary CS (lower segment or classical)
(iii) Number of previous CS
(iv) Estimated weight of the baby
(v) Adequacy of the pelvis
(vi) Presence of any associated obstetric complications in the present pregnancy.

**Women for VBAC-TOL:**
(i) Previous lower segment CS with transverse scar
(ii) Nonrecurrent indication
(iii) Previous one or two lower segment cesarean delivery
(iv) Adequate pelvis for the fetus
(v) Without any other obstetric complications (placenta previa)
(vi) Where continued labor monitoring is possible
(vii) Availability of other resources like anesthetist, blood transfusion and emergency CS facilities round the clock are there.

**Women should be counseled and informed consent should be taken**. Many women (60–70%) deliver successfully vaginally after previous CS once all the above mentioned selection criteria are fulfilled.

**Benefits of successful VBAC are:** Avoidance of operative delivery, anesthesia, less hospital stay. Morbidity is less both to the mother and neonate.

**Successful VBAC is commonly observed in women who have:**
(i) Previous vaginal delivery
(ii) Where primary CS was done due to nonrecurrent indication (breech presentation, fetal distress)
(iii) Women who start their labor spontaneously
(iv) Where primary cesarean section was done during labor rather than electively.

**Advantages of successful VBAC are** reduced incidence of postpartum morbidity, infection, blood transfusion and hospital stay.

Therefore, all women with prior delivery by cesarean section need not necessarily **be delivered by cesarean section during the next pregnancy**. She could be delivered successfully by VBAC-TOL provided she is selected carefully with all the criteria as discussed above. She needs to be monitored carefully during labor.

## Q. 11 Evaluate critically the role of ultrasound scan examination in modern obstetric practice.

**Ans.** Ultrasound scan examination is considered an asset in modern obstetric practice. The information obtained by USG scan **in the first trimester** especially using transvaginal scan is immense. Diagnosis of pregnancy is made with ultrasound appearance of gestational sac, yolk sac, and fetal pole. Furthermore fetal, viability, location (intrauterine or extrauterine), number, gestational age are the invaluable information obtained by USG. Ultrasound parameters (nuchal thickness, nasal bone) are used to detect fetal anomaly also.

In the first trimester of pregnancy, commonly the transvaginal ultrasound is used.

**The second trimester scan** has the major importance of **fetal anomaly detection**. However, these soft markers need for confirmation with some other invasive procedure which again needs the help of sonography. Commonly used sonographic markers of chromosomal anomalies are choroid plexus cyst, short femur, cleft lip/palate, low set ears, nuchal translucency, renal anomalies and cardiac defects.

**Fetal biometry** is done for gestational age determination in the second trimester. Commonly used parameters are biparietal diameter (BPD), head circumference (HC), abdominal circumference (AC) and femur length (FL). The variation is 10–14 days.

Estimated fetal weight could be determined also with all the parameters.

**Obstetric intervention:** Ultrasonography can be used as an adjunct to many interventions in obstetrics like amniocentesis, CVS or cordocentesis and intrauterine fetal transfusion.

**Doppler ultrasound** is of value in assessing fetal well-being with fetal blood flow study in the umbilical artery, middle cerebral artery. Doppler USG is helpful for assessing a fetus complicated with IUGR, Rhesus alloimmunization, placenta previa, and management of twin pregnancy (determination of chorionicity).

**USG for coexistent pathology:** Ultrasound scan can detect any coexistent pathology (ovarian cysts) during pregnancy.

**USG is valuable in postpartum period** to detect any retained bits of placenta or the diagnosis of deep vein thrombosis. Unfortunately, it has the limitations and that it suffers from the misuse. Ultrasound examination during pregnancy may cause anxiety to the woman due to its exposure to the fetus.

Considering the benefits of use in obstetric practice, ultrasonography is of immense value provided it is used rationally.

## Q. 12 Prophylactic forceps delivery has got a place—Discuss.

**Ans.** Forceps delivery is done to expedite the process of delivery during the second stage of labor. Provided the criteria are fulfilled prior to forceps operation and the operator is an experienced one, it is beneficial both for the mother as well as the baby.

Indications of forceps operation may be:
 (i) Maternal (inadequate expulsive efforts)
 (ii) Fetal (fetal distress)
 (iii) Others (prolonged second stage of labor).

**Prophylactic forceps** are the applications of forceps in the second stage of labor to deliver the fetus when some complications either to the fetus or the mother are being anticipated. Therefore, it is done to cut short the second stage of labor. It is done before any maternal and/or fetal complication actually develops.

Commonly, it is a low forceps delivery.

The common indications of prophylactic forceps are:
 (i) Eclampsia
 (ii) Heart disease
 (iii) Severe pre-eclampsia
 (iv) Prior cesarean delivery
 (v) Patients under epidural analgesia.

The benefits of prophylactic use of forceps are:

**In eclampsia:** Repeated convulsions and its associated complications: Cerebrovascular complications, cardiac failure, pulmonary edema can be reduced.

In **heart disease:** Risks of cardiac failure can be reduced.

**In severe pre-eclampsia:** Risk of eclampsia can be reduced

**In prior cesarean delivery:** Risk of scar rupture can be reduced.

**In women under epidural analgesia:** Risk of prolonged second stage and the associated risks of fetal distress can be reduced.

Therefore, prophylactic forceps delivery is beneficial both for the mother and the baby in some selected cases. However, prophylactic forceps should not be applied until the criteria of low forceps are fulfilled. The operator must be an experienced one.

### Q. 13 Prophylactic oxytocin is better than ergometrine in management of postpartum hemorrhage—Discuss.

**Ans.** Ergometrine is a powerful oxytocic. It excites powerful myometrial contraction which lasts for 3 hours. It is very effective when used as a prophylaxis against postpartum hemorrhage in the active management of third stage of labor. However in spite of its beneficial effects, it is not completely free from risks and side effects.

**There are certain risks of its use:**
(a) It causes nausea and vomiting. These side effects are more common.
(b) It should not be given to any woman who is suffering from **organic cardiac disease**. It causes rapid squeezing of blood from uteroplacental circulation into the systemic circulation. There is overloading of the right heart and the risk of heart failure.
(c) When given in a woman with **severe pre-eclampsia and eclampsia**, there is further sudden rise of blood pressure due to its vasoconstrictor effect. This may precipitate further convulsions or other complications (cerebral hemorrhage).
(d) In a woman with suspected **multiple pregnancy**, if given after the delivery of the first baby, the second baby suffers from hypoxia. This is due to tetanic contraction of the myometrium.
(e) It should not be given to a **Rh-negative woman**, as the risks of fetomaternal hemorrhage is more.

Besides the above mentioned contraindications, methergin has also got few other side effects.

**The Important side effects are:**
Rise in blood pressure, bronchospasm, poor lactation and even myocardial infarction.

On the other hand, **oxytocin** is also an effective uterotonic drug. It acts physiologically over the uterine musculature. It maintains the law of polarity. Oxytocin works faster than ergometrine. Oxytocin is much safer than ergometrine. It is very effective and has got less side effects and complications. Therefore, oxytocin is a better substitute in such cases.

## Q. 14 All pregnant women should undergo hemoglobin estimation during antenatal booking—Discuss.

**Ans. Hemoglobin estimation**

Estimation of hemoglobin and testing of ABO and Rh grouping are recommended as a routine to all pregnant woman throughout the world. These two tests are essential for all pregnant women for the following reasons:

During pregnancy, any woman with hemoglobin level, <11 g/dL is considered anemic (WHO). Moreover any woman with hemoglobin level—9 g/dL needs investigation to find out the cause of anemia and treatment.

**Anemia** is a common problem in many countries throughout the world during pregnancy. Anemia is a major (20%) cause of maternal death in India. It is entirely a preventable death. Benefits of estimating hemoglobin during pregnancy are many. Antenatal check-up gives us an opportunity for screening anemia during pregnancy early. Once detected the woman is thoroughly investigated to find out the cause of anemia. This is helpful to treat anemia specifically. Once diagnosed and appropriately treated, many complications of anemia in pregnancy, labor and puerperium can be prevented.

**Complications of anemia** like cardiac failure, pre-eclampsia, infection, postpartum hemorrhage or shock could be avoided. Thus, maternal mortality can be reduced significantly.

**Deficiency anemia**, mainly the iron deficiency anemia is common in India. Depending upon the severity of iron deficiency treatment could be started by giving adequate diet and oral or parenteral iron or even blood transfusion. Women who are intolerant to or noncompliant with oral iron are treated with parenteral IV iron preparation (iron sucrose). This will help to build up her hemoglobin early before the woman goes into labor. Blood transfusion may be given in few cases depending upon the duration of pregnancy and levels of hemoglobin.

Thorough investigations can diagnose few **cases of the hemoglobinopathies** which are again not uncommon in India. Special management can be initiated so that maternal and perinatal deaths are avoided in such cases also. Thus estimation of hemoglobin is of immense value for all pregnant woman during antenatal booking.

### Q. 15 All pregnant women should have ABO, Rh grouping in pregnancy—Discuss.

**Ans. ABO and Rh grouping:** In the modern society, knowledge of ABO and Rh grouping is essential to all individual not to speak of a pregnant woman. Accident and emergency never come with prior intimation. Prior knowledge of ABO and Rh saves much time in an emergency situation. This is in terms of either receiving blood transfusion or donating blood.

Pregnancy complication like ectopic pregnancy, antepartum hemorrhage, postpartum hemorrhage are often faced as emergency and are managed with urgent transfusion with appropriate group, type and cross-matching. Obstetric hemorrhage is a major cause of maternal death in India. Prior knowledge of ABO, Rh saves much valuable and golden moments to save a life.

This knowledge also helps in prearranging donors or blood in a case when there is scarcity of blood availability or in cases with uncommon ABO-Rh grouping (Rh-negative woman).

Women who are found Rh-negative are further investigated (indirect Coombs' test, amniocentesis, cordocentesis) to assess the severity of fetal affection during pregnancy and also for treatment. This helps to improve perinatal outcome in a rhesus negative woman.

The knowledge of ABO-Rh grouping of the woman is also helpful in the diagnosis of jaundice and certain hemolytic disease of the newborn (Mother: O and fetus A or B).

Therefore, the testing ABO-Rh grouping is of utmost importance to all pregnant woman in the antenatal clinic.

## Q. 16 Emergency obstetric care is one of the effective strategies for preventing maternal deaths in India—Discuss.

**Ans.** Emergency obstetric care (EmOC) is the care provided emergently (urgently) to a pregnant woman during the time of emergency arising out of any obstetric complication.

In India lead causes of maternal deaths are:

(a) **Obstetric hemorrhage** due to PPH, APH and hemorrhage related to abortion, ectopic pregnancy and molar pregnancy.
(b) **Hypertensive disorders in pregnancy:** Pre-eclampsia, eclampsia and HELLP syndrome.
(c) **Sepsis:** Puerperal sepsis and septic abortion.
(d) **Obstructed labor** and **rupture uterus.**
(e) **Medical disorders in pregnancy:** Anemia and jaundice (viral hepatitis).

These complications often arise as an emergency and without any warning. **In India, three delays are the important causes of maternal deaths.**

**Three delays are:**

(a) **Delay** in detecting the problem and deciding to seek care
(b) **Delay** to reach the healthcare facility
(c) **Delay** in receiving the care at the center.

These delays prevent women with obstetric complications to access and receive treatment in time. Most of these women are admitted with a grave condition. Unless they are provided with an appropriate intervention urgently, most of them would die. Interventions may be different for an individual case.

For example, blood volume replacement (crystalloids, colloids, blood transfusion) and use of oxytocics in a case with atonic PPH are the essential emergency obstetric care.

Case of eclampsia and severe pre-eclampsia are often seen as an emergency in the peripheral centers. Injection magnesium sulfate need to be given as an emergency to arrest the convulsions and also prophylactically.

Time is an important factor for these women to avail the EmOC. Once emergency care is provided, rest of the care could be organized with referral and time. It is now well known that nonavailability of EmOC is the root cause of maternal mortality. However, it is important to remember that not only the EmOC must be timely available but it should be a quality care. Only then it would be effective to prevent maternal deaths.

Therefore, EmOC is one of the effective strategies in preventing maternal deaths in India.

### Q. 17 Only antenatal care cannot prevent all maternal deaths— Discuss.

**Ans.** Antenatal care (ANC) is the periodic, regular and systematic supervision of a woman during pregnancy. ANC is mainly focussed to screen the high-risk cases and to improve maternal health through education, counseling and care.

In India, lead causes of maternal deaths are:
(i) Hemorrhage
(ii) Hypertensive disorders
(iii) Sepsis
(iv) Obstructed labor and rupture uterus
(v) Medical disorders in pregnancy like anemia, jaundice.

Antenatal care is an important part of the total care during pregnancy, labor and puerperium. However, ANC cannot prevent all obstetric complications that arise suddenly and without any warning during pregnancy, labor and puerperium.

Delay in treatment or no treatment may end in maternal deaths due to complications arising at any of the stage of pregnancy, labor or puerperium. Therefore, emergency obstetric care (EmOC) is an essential service to save mothers from death.

It has been known that majority (75%) of maternal deaths occur during intrapartum or immediate postpartum period and the rest (25%) occur in antenatal period. This highlights the importance of the time of labor.

Therefore, good antenatal care alone cannot reduce maternal mortality entirely. Only a good ANC cannot ensure an uneventful intrapartum and postnatal periods. This is because many complications during labor and immediate puerperium are grave and may arise suddenly and unpredictably. Risk screening approach in ANC has many limitations. Interventions made during ANC may not have a major impact in reducing MMR. Management done during ANC are not the same to manage the complications of labor and puerperium. Risk screening in ANC may not identify all women at risk of deaths. Every pregnancy is at risk till she passes the course of labor and purperium uneventfully. Therefore, only ANC cannot prevent all maternal deaths.

## Q. 18 Oxytocin should be used judiciously in the management of—Discuss.

**Ans. Oxytocin** is a nonapeptide released from the posterior pituitary. Synthetic oxytocin is currently used in obstetrics as a powerful uterotonic drug. Common indications of use are: 1. **Therapeutic** (mainly) and 2. **diagnostic** (not commonly used).

(1) **Therapeutic use** may be in (A) pregnancy, (B) labor, and (C) puerperium.
- (a) **Pregnancy**: Early pregnancy—to induce abortion, to stop bleeding in cases following evacuation of uterus (incomplete abortion).
- (b) **Late pregnancy:** To induce labor.
- (c) **Labor:** Augmentation labor (therapeutic), **active management of third stage of labor (Preventive use against PPH).**
- (c) **Puerperium:** To control postpartum hemorrhage.

(2) **Diagnostic use:** Use of oxytocin is very much beneficial. But it must be used judiciously otherwise complications occurs that may endanger the mother, baby or the both. **Oxytocin stress test is not commonly done.**

One must be careful to exclude the **contraindication of its use** in late pregnancy and labor like:
- (a) Grand multipara
- (b) Contracted pelvis
- (c) History of prior cesarean delivery
- (d) Malpresentation
- (e) Presence of fetal distress
- (f) Obstructed labor.

Moreover when oxytocin is being used in infusion, it has to be monitored very carefully. Otherwise many complications may occur.

**The important complications are:**
- (a) **Uterine hyperstimulation**—leading to fetal distress
- (b) **Uterine rupture**—leading to maternal and fetal death
- (c) **Fetal distress**—due to fetal hypoxia
- (d) **Others**—water intoxication and hypotension.

For all these reasons, use of oxytocin must be judicious to get the benefits otherwise complications may occur.

## Q. 19 Active management of third stage of labor should be done as a routine—Discuss.

**Ans.** The principles of third stage labor management are:

(a) To ensure strict vigilance

(b) To follow the guidelines strictly in practice.

The **purpose** is to prevent complications, mainly the postpartum hemorrhage (PPH). **PPH is the lead cause of maternal deaths in India.**

**Active management is preferred** over expectant management.

**Advantages are:**

(a) Active management of third stage of labor (AMTSL) stimulates powerful uterine contractions when given within 1 minute of delivery of the baby. It is given by injection IM (WHO) soon following birth of the baby.

(b) There is early separation of placenta.

(c) Third stage blood loss is reduced to one-fifth.

(d) There is shortening of the duration of third stage to about 5-7 minutes (to half) instead of the average of 15 minutes.

**Procedures**

Injection oxytocin 10 IU intramuscular (IM) (preferred) or methergin 0.2 mg IM is given to the mother within 1 minute of delivery of the baby (WHO).

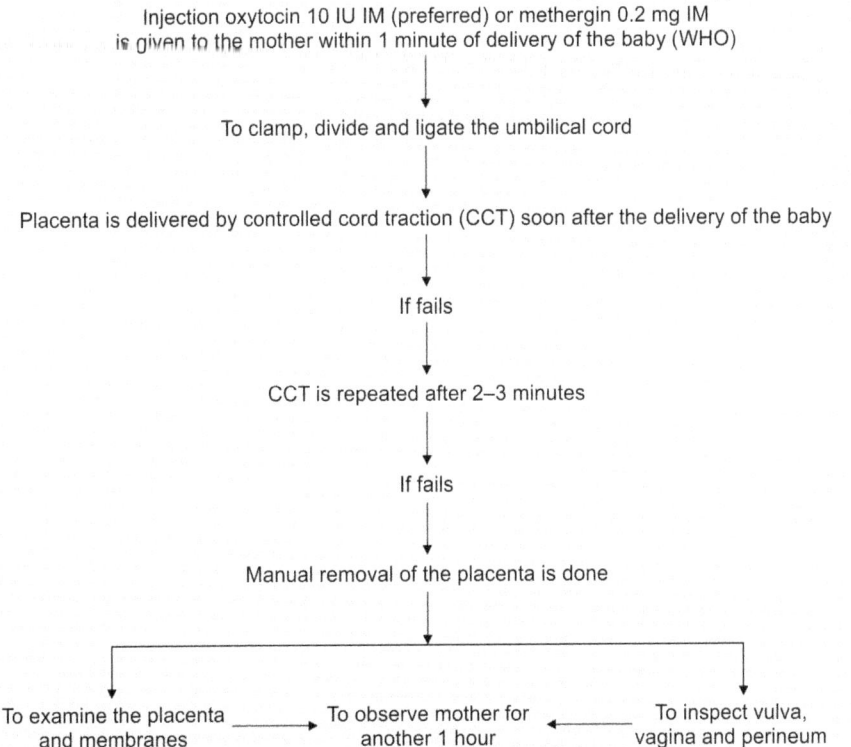

**SPACE FOR NOTES**

# CHAPTER 7

# Operative Obstetrics

**Chapter Objectives**
**To demonstrate knowledge and understanding of:**
- Surgical anatomy of abdomen and the pelvic organs
- Outlines of common surgical procedures
- Case selection (indications of surgery)
- Principles of the surgical procedure
- Principles of homeostasis and hemostasis
- Postoperative care
- Surgical complications and management
- Follow-up procedures

- ❖ Dilatation and Evacuation (D and E)     258
- ❖ Suction Evacuation     259
- ❖ Manual Vacuum Aspiration (MVA)     260
- ❖ Episiotomy     261
- ❖ Forceps Delivery     263
- ❖ Ventouse Delivery     268
- ❖ Cesarean Section     269
- ❖ Destructive Operations     277

## DILATATION AND EVACUATION (D AND E)

**Indications:**
(i) Incomplete abortion
(ii) Inevitable abortion
(iii) MTP (6-8 weeks)
(iv) Evacuation of hydatidiform mole.

**Principal steps:** The preliminary steps are:

(A) Antiseptic cleaning with savlon/povidone-iodine solution
(B) Perineum is draped with sterile towels.

   (i) Sim's posterior vaginal speculum is introduced, anterior lip of the cervix is grasped by an Allis tissue forceps. The uterine sound is avoided as it may cause perforation or bleeding.

   (ii) The cervix is dilated using the metal dilator (Hegar's or Hawkin Ambler's) (Figs. 7.1A and B) up to the desired extent.

   (iii) The products are removed by the ovum forceps. The uterine cavity is curetted gently by a blunt curette. Injection methergin (0.2 mg) is given IV.

   (iv) The speculum and the Allis forceps are removed. The uterus is massaged bimanually. The vagina and perineum are cleaned and a sterile vulval pad is placed.

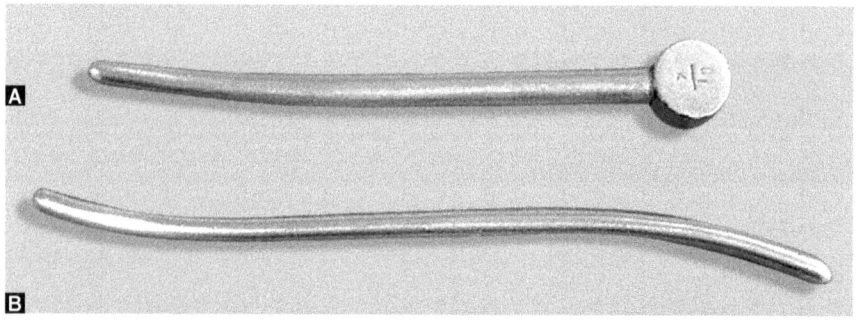

**Figs. 7.1A and B:** Cervical dilators: (A) Hawkin-Ambler, (B) Das/Hegar's dilator.

**Complications of D and E operation**

*Immediate:*
(i) Hemorrhage
(ii) Injury (cervix)
(iii) Uterine perforation
(iv) Infection (sepsis)
(v) Shock.

*Remote*:
 (i) Pelvic inflammation
 (ii) Infertility
 (iii) Cervical incompetence
 (iv) Uterine synechiae.

> **Q. How do you manage a case of uterine perforation diagnosed during D and E?**
>
> **Ans.** (A) Small perforation with a sound or with a small size dilator—usually conservative management is done. Patient is kept admitted, and the vital parameters, bleeding P/V are monitored.
> (B) When the perforation is a big one patient may need laparotomy or laparoscopy to manage the perforation.

## SUCTION EVACUATION

**Indications:**
 (i) Medical termination of pregnancy (first trimester)
 (ii) Incomplete abortion
 (iii) Inevitable abortion (first trimester)
 (iv) Hydatidiform mole.

**Important steps:**
(1) Initial steps up to dilatation of the cervix are the same as discussed in D and E operation.
(2) The suction cannula (Fig. 7.2) is filled to the suction apparatus. The cannula size is generally the same to the weeks of pregnancy to be terminated (e.g. size 7 is for 7 weeks of pregnancy). The cannula is introduced into the uterus.
(3) The pressure (negative) of the suction machine is raised to 400–600 mm Hg. The cannula is moved up and down and also rotated within the uterine cavity to get the curette like effect. **The end point of suction is denoted by:**
  (i) No more material is being sucked out
  (ii) Gripping of the cannula by the uterus
  (iii) Grating sensation
  (iv) Appearance of bubbles in the cannula.

**Fig. 7.2:** Plastic suction cannula (Karman's type).

(4) The vacuum is broken and the cannula is withdrawn. The uterine cavity is gently curetted by a blunt flushing curette.
(5) The vagina and vulva are cleaned and a vulval pad is placed.

**Q. What are the complications of suction and evacuation?**

Ans. Complications are similar to D and E (see above). However, the risk of uterine perforation is less.

**Q. What are the signs of completion of the procedure?**

Ans.
- No more products of conception is seen to come out
- Air bubbles are seen to come out
- Uterus contracts around the cannula (gripping effect)
- Gritty sensation is felt.

**Q. How the cannulas are sterilized?**

Ans. The cannulas are sterilized with ethylene oxide and remain sterile as long as the package is intact.

## MANUAL VACUUM ASPIRATION (MVA)

**Q. How to charge the aspirator?**

Ans. (1) To check the instruments (Figs. 7.3 and 7.4):
  (a) The valve, cap, liner all are in place
  (b) The plunger is pushed all the way inside the cylinder
  (c) Collar stop in place.
(2) Push the valve buttons downwards and forwards until they lock.
(3) Pull the plunger back until the arms snap outward and catch on the cylinder base. The aspirator is now charged.

**Q. Outline the procedure of MVA.**

(Initial steps are the same as that of suction evacuation)

Ans. (a) The appropriate size cannula is inserted and the cannula tip should go beyond the internal OS and to remain inside the uterine cavity.
(b) The cannula is attached to the charged aspirator.

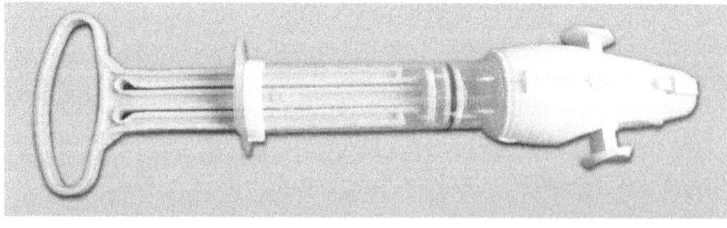

**Fig. 7.3:** Manual vacuum aspiration (MVA) syringe.

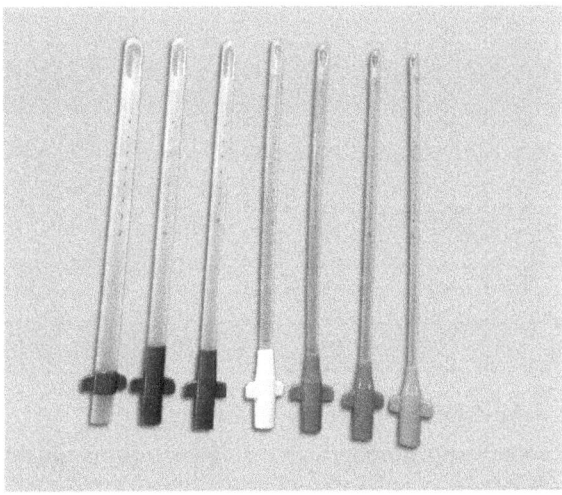

Fig. 7.4: Manual vacuum aspiration (MVA) cannula.

(c) Buttons are released to create vacuum.
(d) Products of conception are evacuated by rotating the cannula 180° in each direction and also with in and out motion.
(e) When finished, the buttons are depressed and the instruments are withdrawn. If the procedure needs to be repeated, the aspirator is emptied, recharged and may be used again or a second aspirator may be used.

**Q. What are the signs of completion of the procedure?**
**Ans.** Same as that of suction evacuation.

**Q. How the cannulas are sterilized?**
**Ans.** The cannulas (Fig. 7.4) are sterilized with ethylene oxide and remain sterile as long as the package is intact.

## EPISIOTOMY

**Q. What are the common indications of episiotomy?**
**Ans.** (i) Rigid perineum
 (ii) Malpresentation and malposition: Breech delivery, face to pubis delivery, shoulder dystocia
 (iii) Operative vaginal delivery: Forceps, ventouse
 (iv) Previous perineal surgery: Pelvic floor repair.

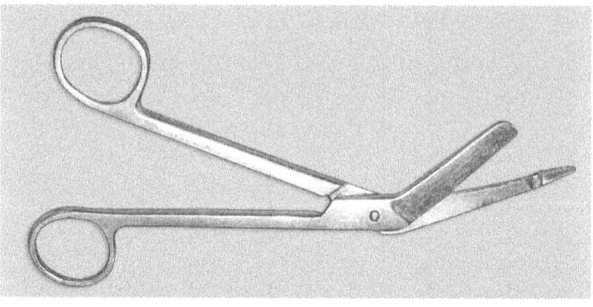

Fig. 7.5: Episiotomy scissors.

**Q. What are the different types of episiotomy?**

**Ans.** Figure 7.5 shows episiotomy scissors. Episiotomy could be made as:
  (i) Mediolateral
  (ii) Median
  (iii) Lateral
  (iv) J-shaped.

However, commonly mediolateral episiotomy is done. Mediolateral episiotomy is safe and it can be extended if necessary. However, blood loss may be little bit more.

**Q. What are the structures cut in episiotomy?**

**Ans.** (i) Posterior vaginal wall
  (ii) Superficial and deep transverse perineal muscles including bulbospongiosus and levator ani
  (iii) Fascia covering those muscles
  (iv) Transverse perineal branches of pudendal vessels and nerves
  (v) Subcutaneous tissue and skin.

**Q. What are the important steps in the repair of episiotomy?**

**Ans.** Repair of episiotomy is done in three layers.
  (1) Vaginal mucosa and submucosal tissues
  (2) Perineal muscles
  (3) Skin and subcutaneous tissues.

Suture material commonly used is No "0" chromic catgut for all the layers, interrupted sutures are used. In that case patient could be discharged after 24–48 hours.

**Q. Mention some of the important complications of episiotomy.**

**Ans.** (A) Immediate, (B) Remote.
  (A) **Immediate:**
    (i) Extension of the incision to involve rectum. This is more common in median episiotomy.
    (ii) Vulval hematoma
    (iii) Infection and wound dehiscence
  (B) **Remote:**
    (i) Dyspareunia
    (ii) Painful scar.

## FORCEPS DELIVERY

**Q. What are the different varieties of obstetric forceps?**

**Ans.** Varieties are:
(a) Long curved obstetric forceps with or without axis traction (Das's variety) device (Fig. 7.6).
(b) Short curved (Wrigley's) forceps
(c) Kielland's (rotational) forceps.

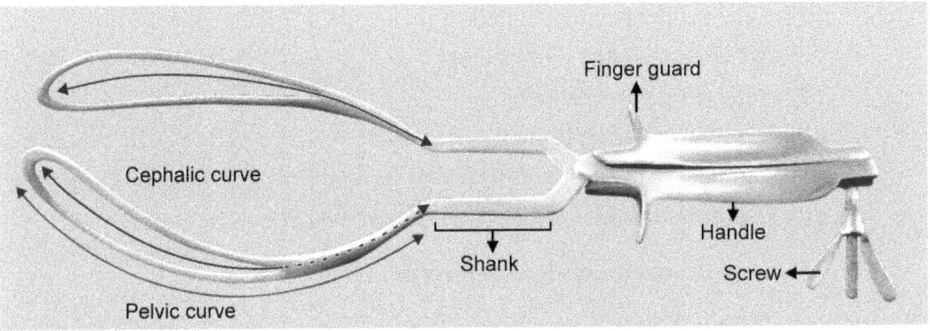

**Fig. 7.6:** Long curved obstetric forceps.

**Q. What are the different parts of a long curved obstetric forceps?**

**Ans.** p. 301.

**Q. What are the different types of forceps delivery?**

**Ans.** Types of forceps delivery are:
(a) Outlet forceps (commonly done)
(b) Low forceps
(c) Mid forceps, and
(d) High forceps (abandoned).

**Q. What are the different functions of the obstetric forceps?**

**Ans.** p. 301.

**Q. What are the indications of forceps delivery?**

**Ans.** Indications are grouped into (A) Maternal, (B) Fetal, and (C) Others.
(A) **Maternal:**
  (i) Maternal distress
  (ii) Cardiac disease
  (iii) Severe pre-eclampsia.

(B) **Fetal:**
  (i) Fetal distress
  (ii) Aftercoming head of vaginal breech delivery.
(C) **Others:** Prolonged second state of labor.

**Q. What are the conditions that should be fulfilled prior to application of forceps?**

**Ans.** The important ones are:
(a) Fetal head must be engaged
(b) Cervix must be fully dilated
(c) Membranes must be ruptured
(d) Pelvis must be adequate
(e) Bladder must be emptied
(f) Fetal head position, rotation and station must be correctly known
(g) Patient's consent (verbal or written) to be taken.

**Q. What are the complications of forceps delivery?**

**Ans.** Complications are:
(A) Maternal and (B) Fetal

(A) **Maternal**
  (i) Injury—vaginal laceration and cervical injury
  (ii) Postpartum hemorrhage
  (iii) Infection

(B) **Fetal**
  (i) Cephalhematoma
  (ii) Intracranial hemorrhage
  (iii) Injury to face.

**Q. What is prophylactic forceps?**

**Ans.** *See* p. 302.

**Q. What is trial of forceps?**

**Ans.** *See* p. 302.

**Q. What is failed forceps?**

**Ans.** *See* p. 302.

Chapter 7 • Operative Obstetrics

## PROCEDURE OF LOW FORCEPS DELIVERY

### Case Summary

Mrs AS, 34 years old lady, was seen in labor in her first pregnancy. It was a term pregnancy that had spontaneous onset of labor. She progressed into the second stage of labor uneventfully. After one and half hour of second stage of labor fetal bradycardia was observed. It remained persistent for another 10 minutes. She was reassessed. Pelvic examination fulfilled the criteria for low forceps delivery. She was prepared for low forceps delivery.

### LOW FORCEPS DELIVERY (Figs. 7.7 to 7.14)

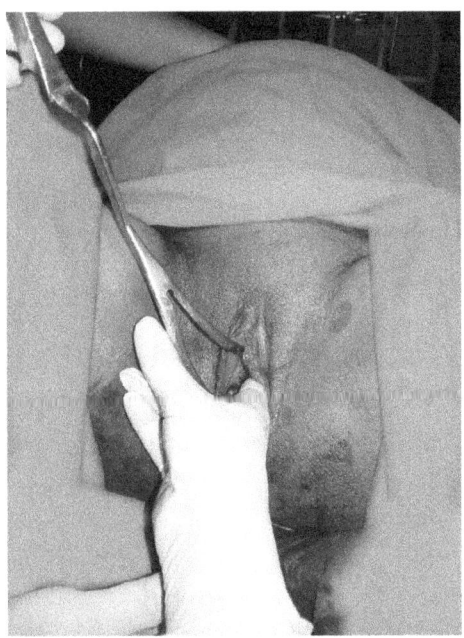

Fig. 7.7: Left blade of the forceps is introduced first. The left handle is hold by the three fingers (index, middle and the thumb) of the left hand. Thumb pressure is used to introduce the blade under guidance of the fingers of the right hand.

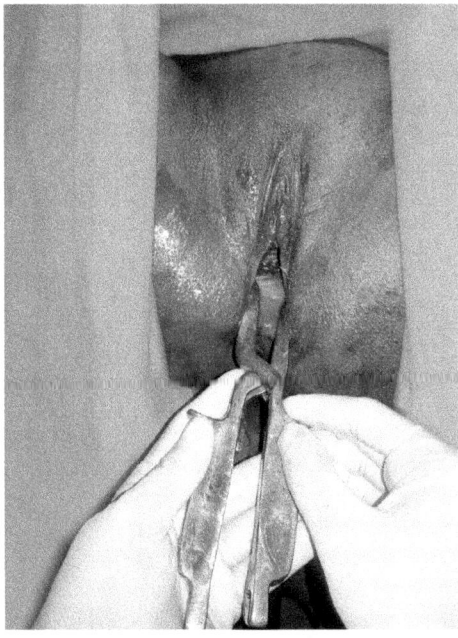

Fig. 7.8: Locking of the blades. Blades are locked easily when applied correctly (bimalar, biparietal placement).

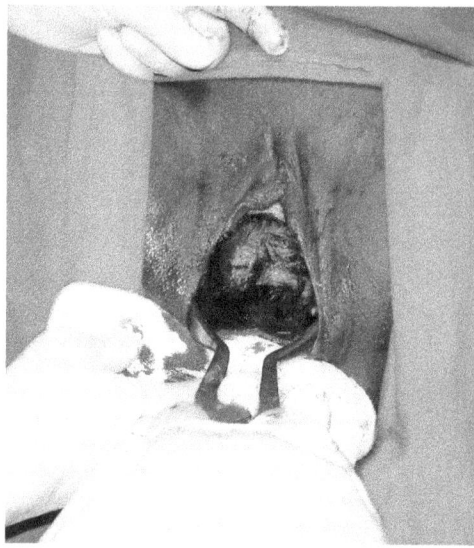

**Fig. 7.9:** Direction of pull: First—downwards and backwards until the head is in perineum → Straight and horizontal (seen) towards the operator.

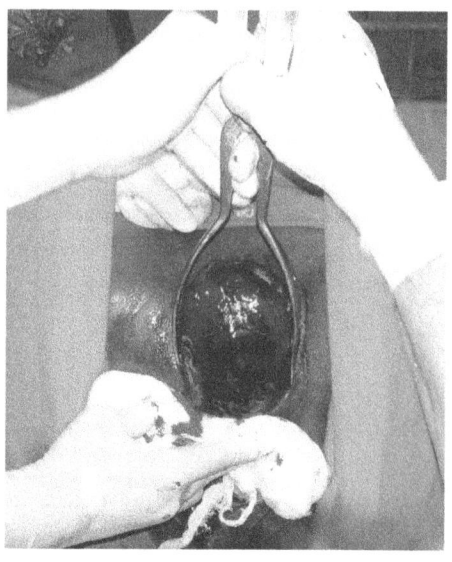

**Fig. 7.10:** Pull is now changed and directed upwards and forwards towards the mother's abdomen. The head is delivered slowly by extension.

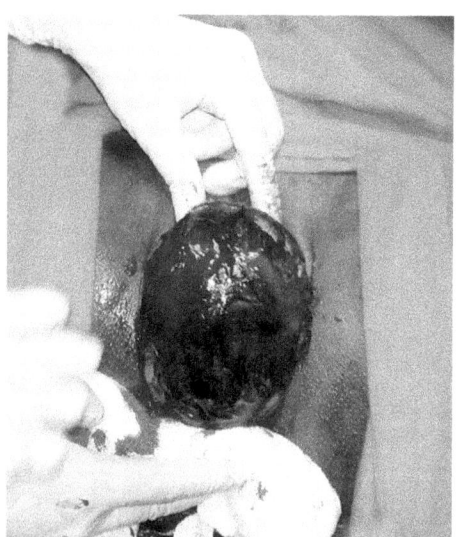

**Fig. 7.11:** The blades are removed. Head is delivered slowly. Ritgen's maneuver is seen.

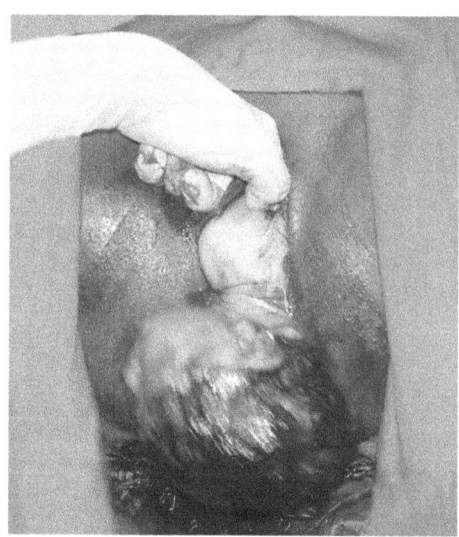

**Fig. 7.12:** Delivery of the shoulder. Note that the bisacromial diameter lies in the anteroposterior diameter of the outlet of the pelvis. Also note that the anterior shoulder is being released slowly from under the symphysis pubis.

Chapter 7 • Operative Obstetrics

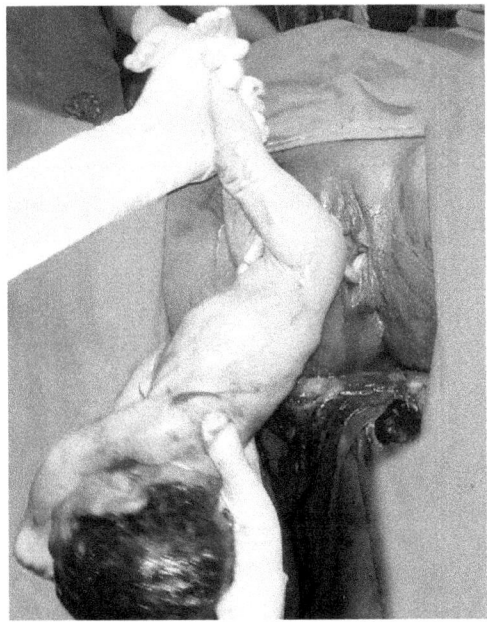

**Fig. 7.13:** Delivery of the trunk and that of the baby was done completely.

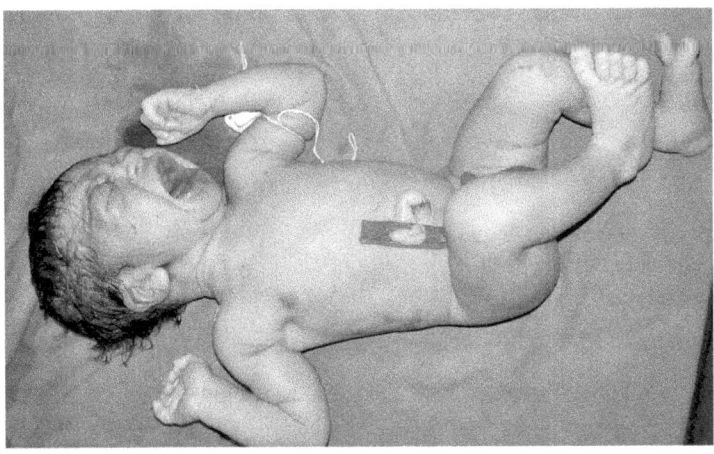

**Fig. 7.14:** Immediate care of the newborn was done. Cord clamping and Apgar rating was done (Apgar score: 8 and 10).

## VENTOUSE DELIVERY

**Q. How ventouse works?**

**Ans.** Ventouse is an instrumental device (Fig. 7.15) used to assist delivery by creating a vacuum between the cup and fetal scalp.

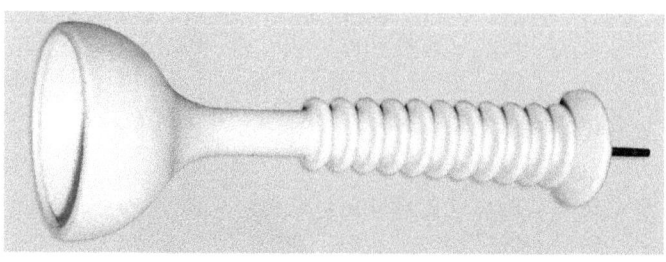

**Fig. 7.15:** Ventouse cup—Silastic.

**Q. What are the indications of ventouse delivery?**

**Ans.** Indications are the same as that of forceps delivery. Common indications are:
  (a) Maternal exhaustion
  (b) Fetal distress
  (c) Prolonged second stage of labor.

**Q. What conditions should be fulfilled before application of ventouse?**

**Ans.** Criteria to be fulfilled are the same as that of forceps. This is according to the guidelines (ACOG 2000).

**Q. What is the flexion point?**

**Ans.** It is an imaginary site located midsagittally on the fetal head about 6 cm behind the center of the anterior fontanelle or 2 cm in front of the posterior fontanelle.

Traction force centered over this site by either ventouse or forceps, promotes flexion and brings the smallest cranial diameter to the pelvis.

**Q. What are the contraindications of ventouse delivery?**

**Ans.** Important contraindications are:
  (a) Any presentation other than vertex
  (b) Preterm fetus <34 weeks.

**Q. What are the advantages of ventouse over forceps?**

**Ans.** Important advantages of ventouse over the forceps are:
  (a) It can be used in unrotated head (occiput posterior position) as it helps autorotation.
  (b) It does not occupy any space like the forceps.
  (c) Perineal and pelvic floor injuries are less.
  (d) Easier to learn and apply.

**Q. What are the advantages of forceps over ventouse?**

**Ans.** Advantages of forceps over ventouse are:
  (a) Forceps can quickly deliver the baby as in a case of fetal distress.
  (b) Higher rate of successful delivery compared to ventouse (ventouse has higher failure rates).
  (c) Forceps are used effectively where moderate force is required.
  (d) It can be used for any gestational age fetus.

**Q. What are the complications of ventouse delivery?**

**Ans.** Important complications of ventouse delivery are:
  (A) Neonatal:
      (a) Scalp abrasion
      (b) Cephalhematoma (less)
      (c) Retinal hemorrhage.
  (B) Maternal: Injuries are less compared to forceps.

## CESAREAN SECTION

**Q. Mention some of the common indications of cesarean section.**

**Ans.** Common indications are:
  (1) Failed induction of labor
  (2) Cephalopelvic disproportion
  (3) Previous cesarean delivery
  (4) Fetal distress
  (5) Antepartum hemorrhage
  (6) Malpresentation (Breech).

**Q. Mention the important steps in lower segment cesarean section.**

**Ans.**
  (a) Preoperative preparation
  (b) Anesthesia—general or spinal or epidural
  (c) Antiseptic painting (povidone iodine 7.5%) and draping.
  (d) Skin incision—suprapubic transverse (commonly used).
  (e) Opening up of the peritoneal cavity—Doyen's retractor is introduced.
  (f) Peritoneal incision → lower segment transverse incision → uterine muscle incision → lower segment transverse.
  (g) Delivery of the head—the membranes are ruptured → Doyen's retractor is removed. The hand is insinuated and the palm is placed below the head. The head is delivered by the hand → suctioning of the baby's mouth is done.
  (h) Delivery of the trunk of the baby is done slowly. The cord is clamped and cut in between two clamps. The baby is handed over to the pediatrician/nurse. Doyen's retractor is reintroduced.
  (i) To wait for spontaneous separation of placenta
  (j) Delivery of the placenta and membranes slowly and completely.

(k) Repair of the uterine wound. The margins of the uterine wounds are picked up by Allis tissue (Green Armytage) forceps (Total 4; one on each corner of the incision and one each on upper and lower margin).

**Q. What are the complications of cesarean section?**

**Ans.** The complications are mainly maternal. These may be:

(A) **Intraoperative:**
- Extension of uterine incision
- Injury to bladder, ureter
- Hemorrhage
- Fetal/neonatal: Inadvertent injury, scalpel cut.

Complications due to anesthesia:
(a) Regional—hypotension, total spinal
(b) General—aspiration (Mendelson's) syndrome, atelectasis

(B) **Postoperative:**
- Immediate: Postpartum hemorrhage (PPH), shock, infections (wound)
- Remote: Incisional hernia, scar rupture in future pregnancy.

## OPERATIVE PROCEDURE OF LOWER SEGMENT CESAREAN SECTION

### LOWER SEGMENT CESAREAN SECTION (FIGS. 7.16 TO 7.27)

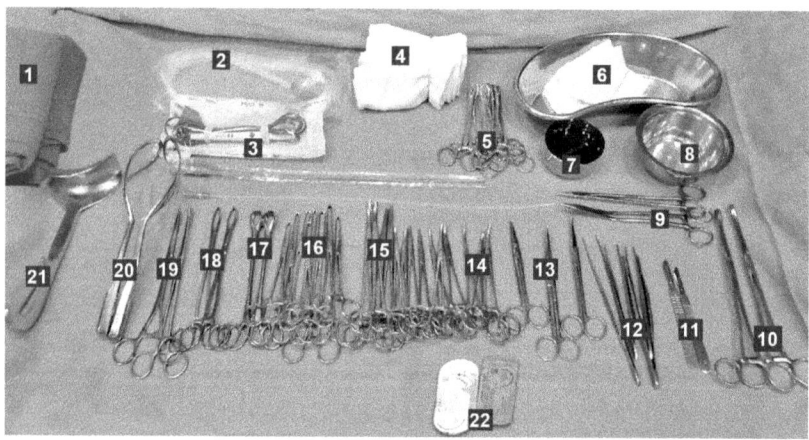

**Fig. 7.16:** Operation trolley with all the instruments for cesarean section. 1. Towels for drapping, 2. Suction tube (with cannula), 3. Electrodiathermy set, 4. Mops (large swabs), 5. Towel clips, 6. Kidney dish, gauze pieces, 7. Bowl with povidone iodine, 8. Empty bowl, 9. Needle holders (curved and straight variety), 10. Sponge holding forceps, 11. Knives, 12. Dissecting forceps (toothed and non-toothed), 13. Scissors (3), 14. Artery forceps (short variety), 15. Kocher's forceps, 16. Allis tissue forceps, 17. Lanes tissue forceps, 18. Little Wood's forceps, 19. Green Armytage forceps, 20. Obstetric forceps, 21. Doyen's retractor, 22. Suture packets.

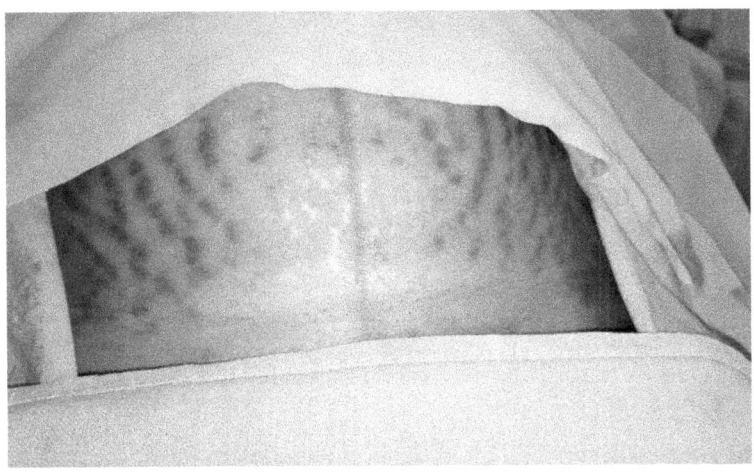

**Fig. 7.17:** Abdomen is painted with povidone iodine solution and is draped with sterile towels. Only the area of operation is exposed.

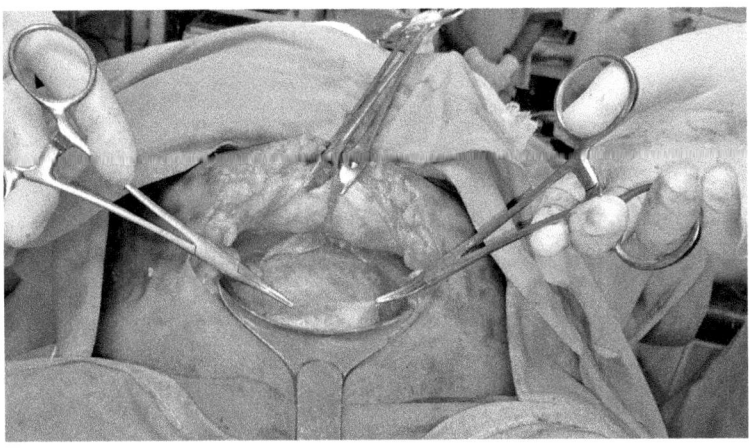

**Fig. 7.18:** Abdomen is opened by modified Pfannenstiel incision. Loose peritoneum of the uterovesical pouch is being stretched out and shown. It is incised transversely.

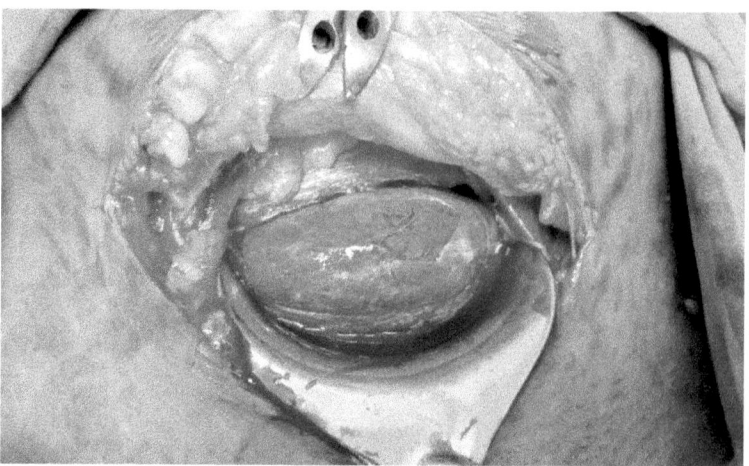

**Fig. 7.19:** Uterine muscle incision (low transverse) has been made in this lower segment of the uterus (LSCS). The amniotic membrane is seen to bulge out with the pressure of amniotic fluid. This amniotic membrane needs to be ruptured to deliver the baby. Doyen's retractor is seen in place.

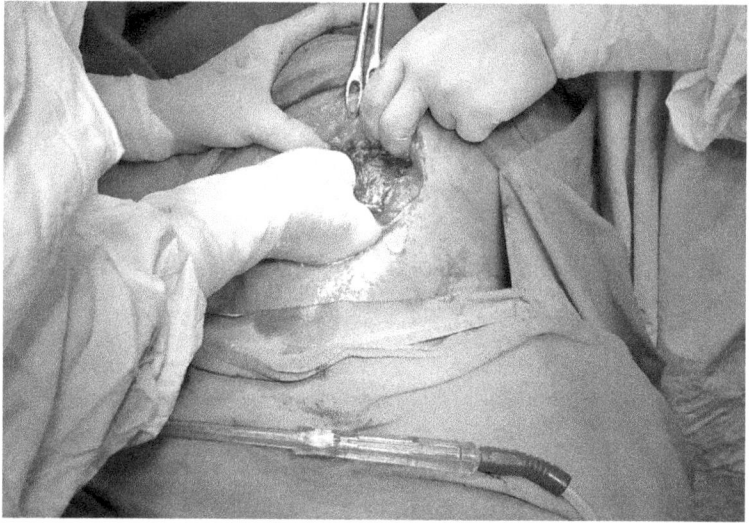

**Fig. 7.20:** Delivery of the head.

The amniotic fluid is sucked out following rupture of the membranes. Doyen's retractor is removed. The head is delivered slowly with the fingers of the right hand, insinuated between the head and the lower uterine flap. Assistant applies some pressure on the fundus at this time.

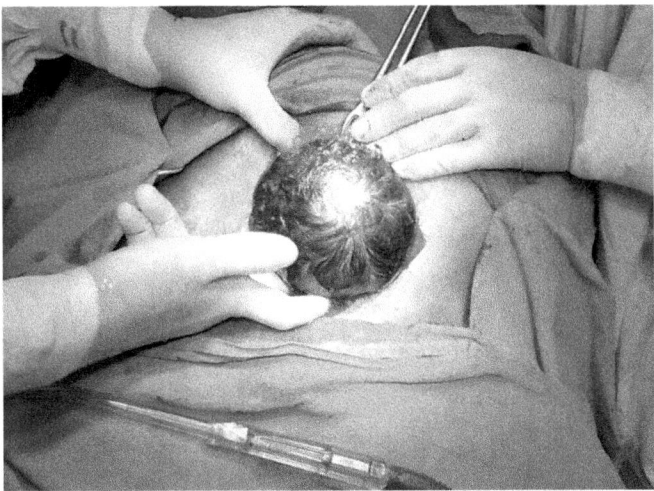

**Fig. 7.21:** Delivery of the baby is on progress. It is to be done slowly. The head is delivered by elevation and flexion using the fingers to act as a fulcrum. Note that Doyen's retractor has been taken out.

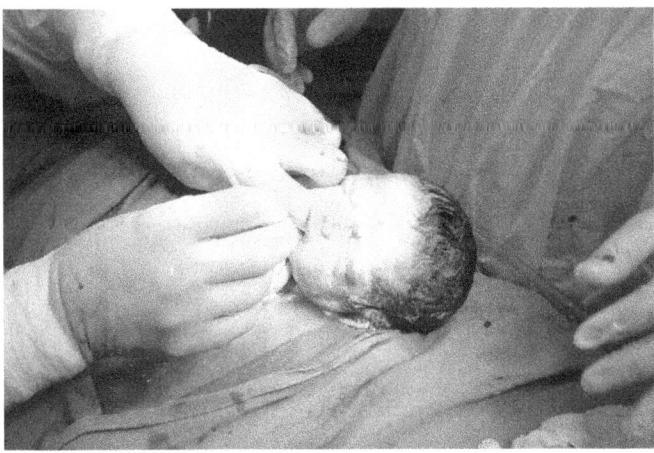

**Fig. 7.22:** Delivery of the head in cesarean section. Suctioning of the mouth, pharynx, are being done gently before delivery of the trunk.

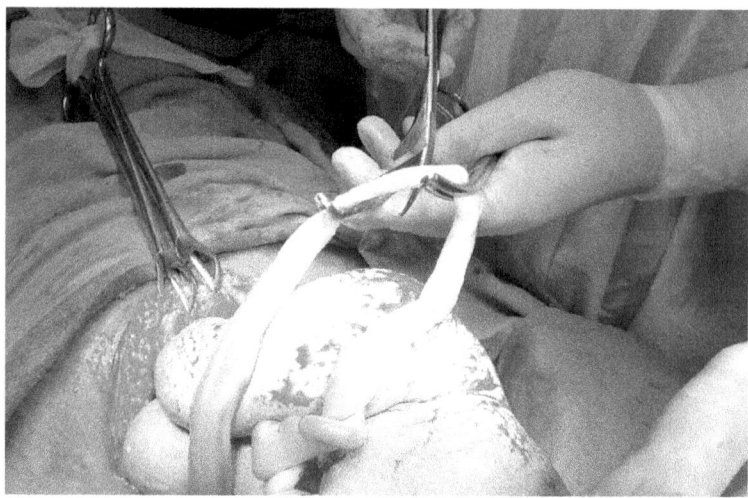

**Fig. 7.23:** Baby is delivered slowly. The cord is clamped and cut in between (See details of steps in the CD incorporated). Baby is handed over to the neonatologist for immediate care of the newborn.

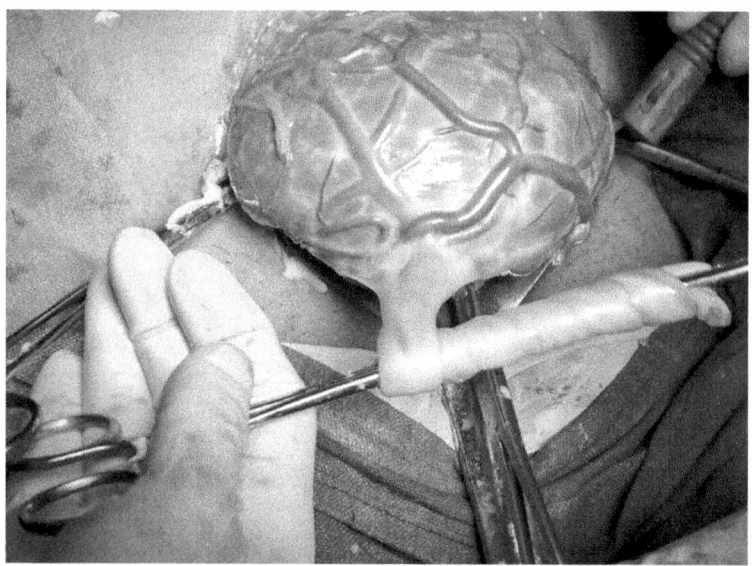

**Fig. 7.24:** Delivery of the placenta and membranes: Placenta is allowed to separate spontaneously. Placenta is delivered by traction on the cord (right hand). Simultaneously the uterus is pushed upwards using the left hand. Note the abdominal retractor (Doyen's) is reintroduced.

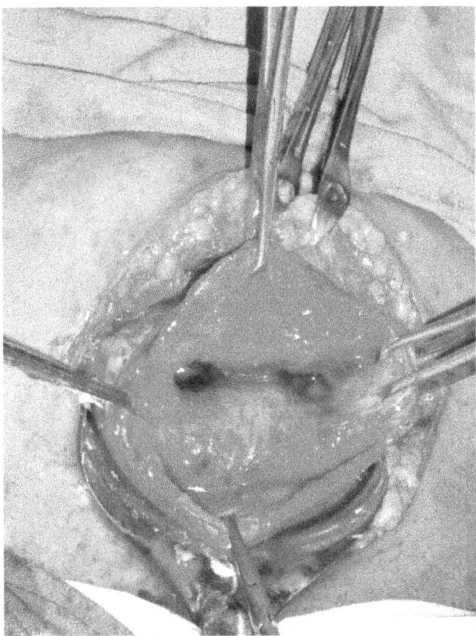

**Fig. 7.25:** The uterine wound is seen following delivery. Usually four Allis's tissue forceps (Green Armytage forceps) are used to hold the incision margins, two (one each) on the angles of incision. Another two (one each) on the upper and lower uterine flap.

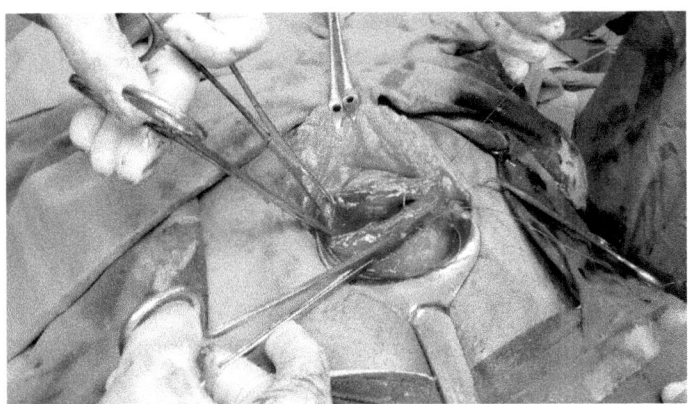

**Fig. 7.26:** Suturing of the uterine wound. It is done in two or three layers. It may be done keeping the uterus in the abdominal cavity or delivering it out (eventration). Suture material is no. '0' chromic catgut or Vicryl-0 with round bodied needle. A continuous running suture taking deeper muscles is made. A similar suture is placed taking the superficial muscles overlapping the first layer. Nonclosure of the visceral peritoneum is preferred.

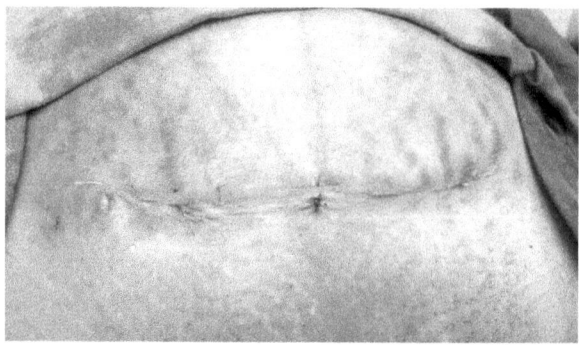

**Fig. 7.27:** Closure of the abdomen.
The mops are removed and the number verified. Peritoneal toileting is done. Doyen's retractor is removed. The abdomen is closed in layers. The vagina is cleaned of blood and blood clots. A sterile vulval pad is placed.

**Q. What measures are taken to overcome the difficulties during the delivery of the head during cesarean delivery?**

**Ans.** Difficulties are faced in cases following prolonged labor. The fetal head is often tightly wedged deep in the pelvis. The commonly practiced methods in such a situation are:

(a) The hand is insinuated between the lower uterine flap and fetal head. The palm is placed below the head. The head is hooked out by elevation and flexion using the hand as a fulcrum. The assistant exerts the fundal pressure only when the head comes out through the incision line.

(b) **Push method:** An assistant is asked to push the head with an upward pressure by a hand in the vagina. This method is often successful to dislodge the head from the point of impaction. Once this is done the surgeon hooks out the head as the method described above. The risks involved in this method are: Extension of uterine incisions, increased hemorrhage and rarely fetal skull fracture.

(c) **Pull method:** The fetal legs are grasped and the fetus is delivered slowly first, buttocks, then the trunk and finally the head. Sometimes, the lower segment transverse incision may need to be extended to make it as J-, U- or inverted T-shaped to create more space.

(d) **Patwardhan's technique:** Shoulders are delivered first one after the other through the incision. The back is placed anteriorly to make the occiput anterior. The fetal trunk is delivered in a flexed manner by pulling down the legs through incision opening. The head is delivered as in breech extraction. The risks of this method are: Extension of the incision margins, increased blood loss and fetal trauma.

**Q. What are the difficulties in delivery of floating head during cesarean delivery?**

**Ans.** (a) The lower segment transverse incision is made and the membranes are ruptured. The liquor is allowed to drain: The head gradually settles down to the lower segment. The hand is insinuated between the lower uterine flap and head. The palm is placed below the head. The head is lifted out by elevation and flexion using the hand as a fulcrum. The assistant exerts fundal pressure only when the head comes out through the incision line.
(b) Delivery by forceps (Wrigley's forceps) (Fig. 7.28): Forceps blade(s) single blade (as vectis) or both the blades can be used to deliver the head.
(c) Ventouse may also be used as an alternative.

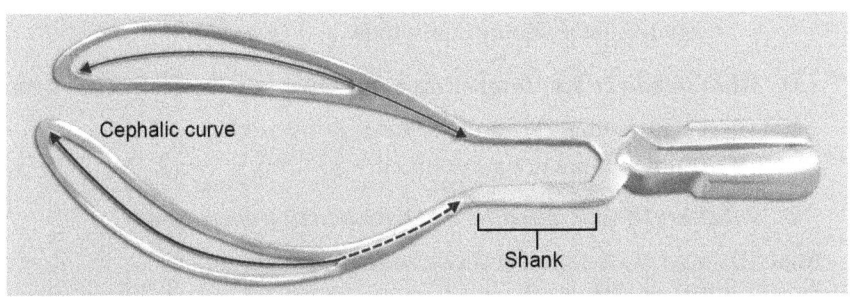

**Fig. 7.28:** Short-curved obstetric forceps (Wrigley's forceps).

## DESTRUCTIVE OPERATIONS

**Q. Name some of the destructive operations.**

**Ans.** Figure 7.29 shows Oldham's perforator. Some of the destructive operations are:
  (i) Craniotomy
  (ii) Evisceration
  (iii) Decapitation
  (iv) Cleidotomy.

**Q. What are the indications of craniotomy?**

**Ans.** (i) Fetus with hydrocephalic head either living or dead.
(ii) Obstructed labor with a dead fetus in cephalic presentation.

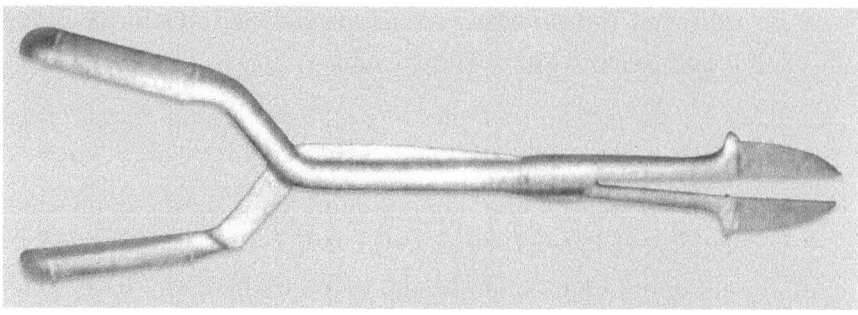

**Fig. 7.29:** Perforator (Oldham's).

**Q. What are the contraindications of craniotomy?**

**Ans.** (i) Severely contracted pelvis where the fetus cannot be delivered even if the head contents are evacuated

(ii) Rupture of uterus—laparotomy should be done. Rupture uterus must be excluded before doing craniotomy.

**Q. What should be the postoperative care following any destructive operation?**

(i) A self-retaining (Foley's) catheter is inserted for 3–5 days.

(ii) Antibiotics are to be continued.

**Q. What are the complications of a destructive operation?**

**Ans.** (i) Injury to the uterus, cervix, vagina

(ii) Rupture of uterus

(iii) Postpartum hemorrhage—atonic and/or traumatic

(iv) Shock

(v) Injury to the adjacent organs: Vesicovaginal or rectovaginal fistula

(vi) Puerperal sepsis

(vii) Subinvolution

(viii) Prolonged ill health.

# CHAPTER 8

# Practical Obstetrics

- ❖ Obstetric Instruments — 280
- ❖ Specimens — 312
- ❖ Imaging Studies — 316
  - ➤ Ultrasonogram — 316
  - ➤ Magnetic Resonance Imaging (MRI) — 323
- ❖ Drugs in Obstetrics — 324
  - ➤ Oxytocics — 324
  - ➤ Antihypertensives — 331
  - ➤ Anticoagulants — 333
  - ➤ Anticonvulsants — 333
  - ➤ Tocolytic Drugs — 336

# OBSTETRIC INSTRUMENTS

**Chapter Objectives**

**Basic knowledge and understanding of:**
- Identification of the instrument
- Uses
- Related surgical procedures with its use (obstetric)
- Complications out of its use (as applicable)

## CLINICAL THERMOMETER (FIG. 8.1)

Celsius temperature scale (°C) is SI derived unit and is known as celsius after the name of the scientist who introduced it. *Conversion of fahrenheit to celsius*—subtract 32, multiply by 5 and then divide by 9. *Conversion of Celsius to Fahrenheit*—multiply by 9, divide by 5 and then add 32.

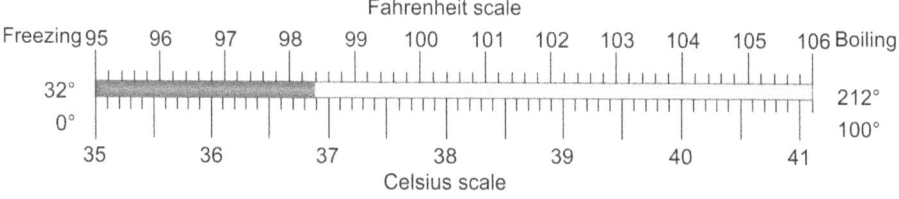

**Fig. 8.1:** Clinical thermometer.

## DIPSTICKS (URO-DIP REAGENT STRIPS) FOR URINALYSIS (FIG. 8.2)

**Principle:** Reagent strips are used for rapid determination of the following in urine:

- Urobilinogen
- Glucose
- Bilirubin
- Ketones
- Specific gravity
- Blood
- PH
- Protein
- Nitrite
- Leukocytes
- Ascorbic acid

**Specimen collection:** Urine is collected in a clean dry container that allows all the test field of the strip to be completely immersed. Use of fresh morning specimen is commonly used.

**Test procedure:**
(1) Dip the strip into urine up to the test required, for no more than 2 seconds.

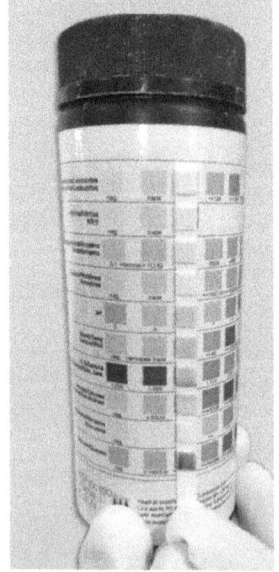

**Fig. 8.2:** Dipsticks (Uro-dip reagent strips) for urinalysis.

(2) Turn the strip on its side and tap on a piece of tissue paper to remove any excess of urine.
(3) To compare the colors of reagent pads within a minute with the color chart on the vial under good light keeping the strip horizontal to prevent any possible mixing of chemicals between the adjacent pads.

**Results:** Each color block gives a range of values. Positive result for nitrites suggests infection.

## RUBBER CATHETER (FIG. 8.3)

**Description:** It is made of rubber. It has different sizes. Slit openings are (usually two) there close to the tip one on either side for drainage of bladder.

**Sterilization:** Boiling.

**Uses:** It is used to empty the bladder in cases with retention of urine during—

(a) **Pregnancy** [retroverted gravid uterus];
(b) **Labor:**
   (i) When the woman fails to pass urine by herself
   (ii) Before and after any operative interventions (Forceps delivery, *See* p. 263, Destructive operations, *See* p. 277);
(c) **Postpartum**
   (i) During management of postpartum hemorrhage *See* p. 107, retained placenta;
(d) **Other uses**
   (i) As a tourniquet
   (ii) To administer $O_2$ when nasal catheter is not available
   (iii) As a mucus sucker—when it is attached to a mechanical or electric sucker.

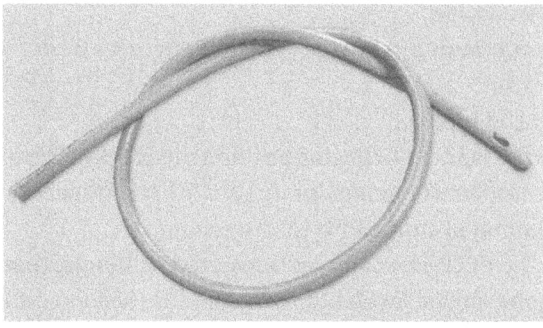

Fig. 8.3: Simple rubber catheter.

*Self-assessment:*

   Q. *What is the length of female urethra?*
   **Ans.** It is 4 cm.

**Q. What are the causes of retention of urine during pregnancy, labor and puerperium?**

**Ans.** Common causes are:
(a) Retroverted gravid uterus
(b) During labor (due to pain and spasm)
(c) During management of PPH
(d) Following operative delivery (forceps).

**Q. Why a metal catheter is not used in obstetrics?**

**Ans.** To avoid trauma to the soft and vascular urethra.

## FOLEY'S SELF-RETAINING CATHETER (FIG. 8.4)

**Description:** It is made of silicon rubber. The catheter tip has two slit openings one on either side for drainage of urine. The other end goes to the urinary bag for collection of urine. The catheter has two channels within. One channel for drainage of urine and the other channel is used to push some water through it. Water inflates the catheter bulb that makes the catheter self-retaining. The bulb capacity is written on the catheter. The catheters are of different sizes. The commonly used sizes in female are 14F, 16F or 18F.

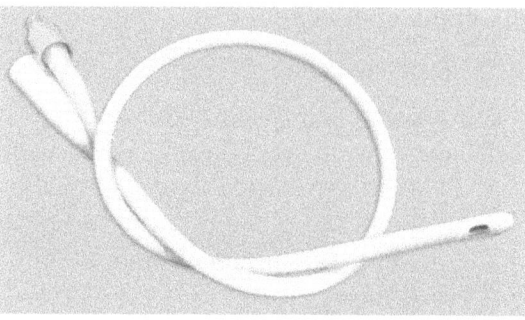

Fig. 8.4: Foley's catheter.

**Sterilization:** It is available in a sterile package following sterilization with ethylene oxide (ETO). It is disposable.

**Uses:** It is used for continuous drainage of bladder in cases with:
(i) Eclampsia (p. 75),
(ii) Retroverted gravid uterus,
(iii) To give rest to the bladder following any destructive operation
(iv) In a case with suspected bladder injury (p. 278). It is usually kept for 7–10 days,
(v) In the management of atonic PPH (p. 108), and
(vi) To control atonic PPH. The catheter is inserted within the uterine cavity and the catheter balloon is inflated with normal saline. The balloon provides a tamponade (p. 109) to the uterine surface. The catheter drains the blood from the uterine cavity if there is any.

*Self-assessment:*

**Q. What are the indications of continuous bladder drainage?**

**Ans.** (a) Eclampsia
(b) In the management of PPH
(c) Retroverted gravid uterus
(d) In the management of obstetrics shock (see above).

**Q. What are the causes of PPH?**

**Ans.** Common causes are expressed as: 4 Ts
 (1) **Tone** (atonicity—enlarged uterus)
 (2) **Trauma** (genital tract injuries—vagina, cervix)
 (3) **Tissues** (retained tissues, bits of placenta)
 (4) **Thrombin** (coagulopathy—DIC).

**Q. What are the causes of atonic PPH?**

**Ans.** When the uterus is hugely enlarged:
 (a) Multiple pregnancy
 (b) Polyhydramnios
 (c) Big baby, others—prolonged labor, grand multipara, uterine fibroid, anemia, APH.

## SIMS' DOUBLE-BLADED POSTERIOR VAGINAL SPECULUM (FIG. 8.5)

**Description:** This double-bladed speculum has a groove in the handle (located in between the blades). This groove is in continuity at either end with the concave inner surface of each blade. The purpose of the groove is to allow drainage of blood, urine (in case of VVF), or secretions to collect such body fluid samples for tests.

The blades are of unequal breadth to facilitate introduction into the vagina depending upon the space available (narrow blade in nulliparous and the wider blade in parous women).

**Sterilization:** Boiling or autoclaving.

**Uses:** It is used in obstetrics
 (i) To inspect the cervix and vagina to detect any injury following delivery
 (ii) To clean the vagina following delivery
 (iii) To inspect the cervix and vagina to exclude any local cause for bleeding in APH (Cusco's speculum preferred)
 (iv) During D and E operation (p. 258).

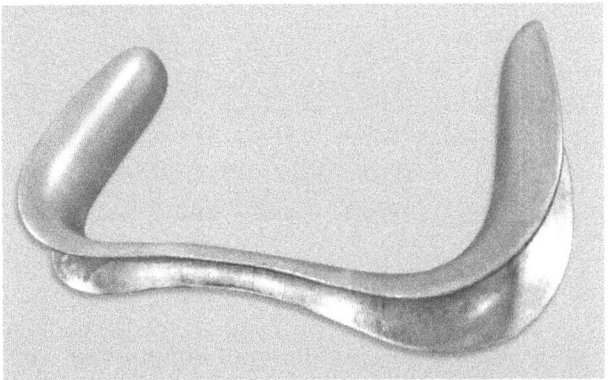

**Fig. 8.5:** Sims' double-bladed posterior vaginal speculum.

*Self-assessment:*

**Q. What are the common sites of traumatic PPH?**

**Ans.** Trauma to the genital tract are the common causes. Injury to the cervix, vaginal vault, lacerated injury to the vagina, perineal injury, rarely rupture of uterus.

**Q. How do you diagnose traumatic PPH?**

**Ans.** Usually uterus remains contracted. A through clinical and speculum examination is needed. A good light source is needed for examination. Repair of injuries are done under anesthesia. Catgut sutures are commonly used.

**Q. What are the indications of D + E?**

**Ans.** See p. 258.

**Q. What are the local (extra-placental) causes of APH?**

**Ans.** See p. 100.

**Q. What is Sims' position and what is Sims' triad?**

**Ans.** See p. 405.

## CUSCO'S BIVALVE, METALLIC, SELF-RETAINING, ADJUSTABLE, VAGINAL SPECULUM (FIG. 8.6)

**Description:** It has two blades joined by screws that allow the blades to open and close around a transverse axis. The blades are concave inside. The handle is designed to open and close the blades and to adjust the space with the blades with a separate rod and screw system. This also makes the blades self-retaining during examination. This speculum does not need any assistant to hold it.

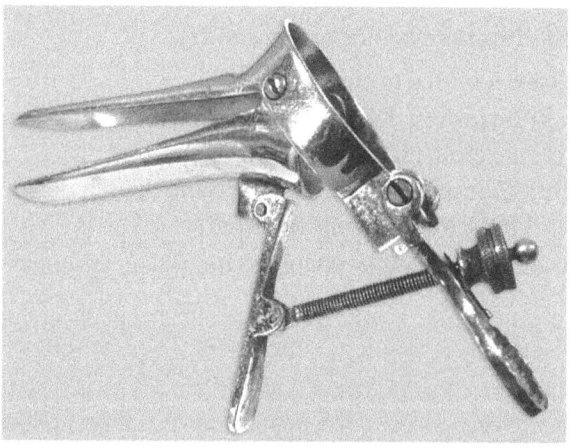

Fig. 8.6: Cusco's bivalve self-retaining vaginal speculum.

**Sterilization:** Boiling or autoclaving.

**Uses:**
(i) To visualize the cervix and vaginal fornices for any local cause (polyp and ectopy) of APH
(ii) To inspect the cervix and to prepare cervical smear for cytology screening
(iii) To detect leakage of liquor from the cervical os in a case of suspected PROM.

## MULTIPLE TOOTHED VULSELLUM (FIG. 8.7)

**Description:** It is a long metallic instrument having the handle at one end with a catch. The other end has teeth (3–4) which bite the tissue when grasped to have a fixed grip. The instrument has a smooth curvature which allows good vision of the tip while working at a depth.

**Sterilization:** Boiling or autoclaving.

**Uses:** It is used to catch hold the anterior lip of the cervix in D + E operation, suction evacuation (p. 259). As it produces trauma to the soft and vascular cervix, Allis tissue forceps is used instead.

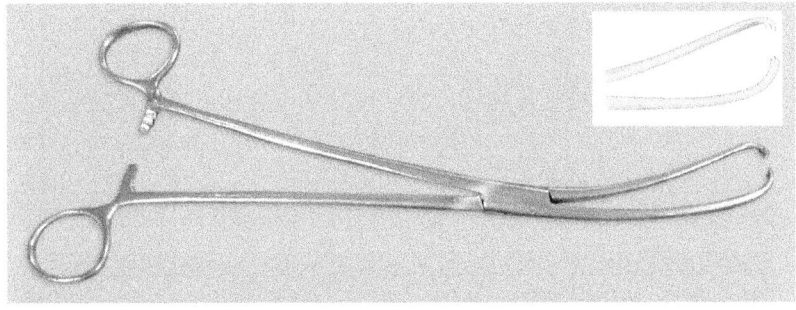

**Fig. 8.7:** Multiple toothed vulsellum.

## ALLIS TISSUE FORCEPS (FIG. 8.8)

**Description:** It is a metallic instrument having two ends. One end is the handle with the provision of ratchet and catch. The other end has the arrangement of multiple teeth (4–6). The blades allow some space within locked position so that the tissue hold is not crushed. This forceps may be of different sizes.

**Uses:**
 (i) To catch hold of the anterior lip of the cervix in D + E operation
 (ii) To hold the apex of the episiotomy wound during repair
 (iii) To catch hold of the margins of the peritoneum, rectus sheath, vaginal mucosa during repair
 (iv) To catch hold of the torn ends of the sphincter ani externus prior to suture in repair of complete perineal tear
 (v) To catch hold the margins and angles of the uterine flaps in lower segment cesarean section (LSCS) after the delivery of the baby as an alternative to Green Armytage hemostatic clamp.

**Self-assessment:**

 *Q. What is episiotomy?*

 **Ans.** It is a surgically planned and deliberate incision over the perineum and the posterior vaginal wall to increase the space during the second stage of labor.

**Q. What are the obstetric causes of perineal tear?**
Ans. *See* p. 410-411.

**Q. What are the different degrees of perineal tear?**
Ans. *See* p. 410-411.

**Q. When and how a recent perineal tear is repaired?**
Ans. *See* p. 410-411.

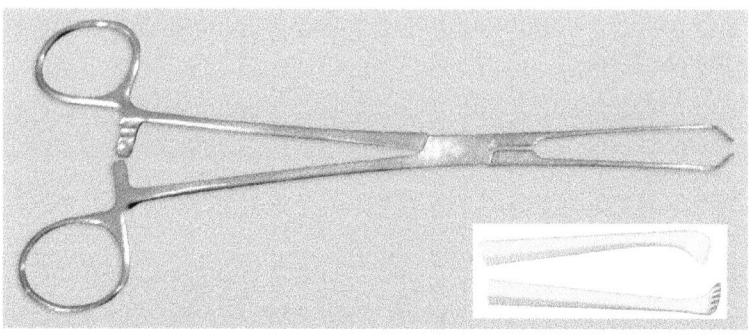

Fig. 8.8: Allis tissue forceps.

## LITTLE WOOD'S FORCEPS (FIG. 8.9)

**Description:** It is a metallic instrument used to hold tissues. The design is similar to that of Allis tissue forceps except that the blades are curved with concavity inwards. Uses are similar to that of Allis tissue forceps.

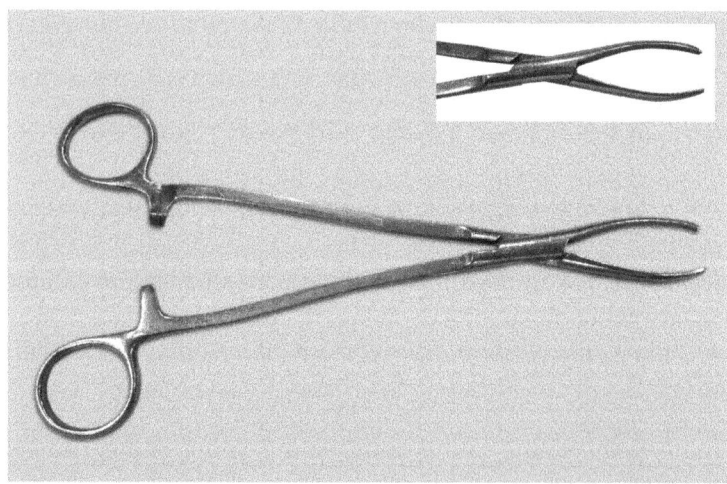

Fig. 8.9: Little wood's forceps.

# LONG STRAIGHT HEMOSTATIC FORCEPS (FIG. 8.10)

**Description:** It is a long metallic instrument. It has a handle at one end provided with a ratchet and catch. The blades, on the other side, are having transverse serrations on the inner surface. Spencer wells variety either straight or curved are commonly used.

**Use:** This is not commonly used in obstetrics. It can be used to clamp the pedicle while removing the uterus (hysterectomy) as in rupture uterus. The umbilical cord may be clamped as an alternative to Kocher's forceps.

*Self-assessment:*

    Q. What are the causes of rupture uterus?

Ans. See p. 313.

    Q. How to suspect scar dehiscence?

Ans. See p. 43.

    Q. How a case of rupture uterus is managed?

Ans. See p. 313-314.

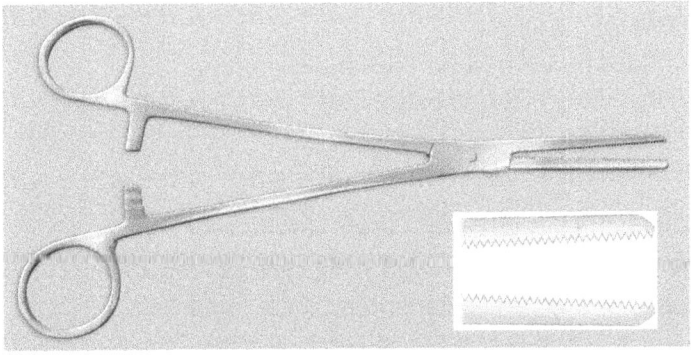

Fig. 8.10: Long straight hemostatic forceps.

# KOCHER'S HEMOSTATIC FORCEPS (FIG. 8.11)

**Description:** It is a long metallic instrument having handle (ratchet and catch) at one end and the tissue holding blades are on the other end. This instrument has a tooth at the tip of one blade and a corresponding groove on the other blade. This names the instrument is used to hold tissues (umbilical cord) firmly when locked and the risk of slipping is negligible.

**Sterilization:** Boiling or autoclaving.

**Uses:**

(i) To clamp the umbilical cord/for better grip and effective crushing effect to occlude the vessels

(ii) In low rupture of the membranes as surgical induction of labor or augmentation of labor.

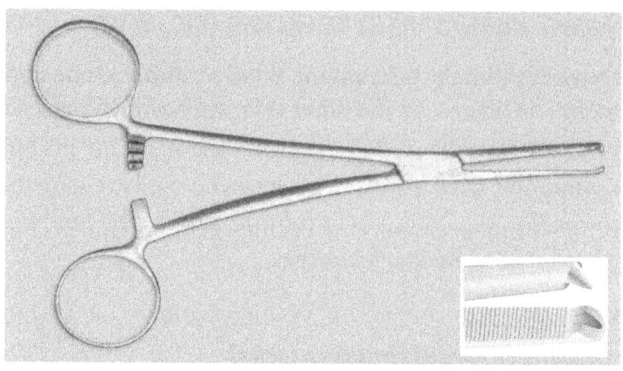

**Fig. 8.11:** Kocher's hemostatic forceps.

*Self-assessment:*

**Q. Describe the structures of umbilical cord.**

**Ans.** The important structures are:
(a) Covering epithelium
(b) Wharton's jelly
(c) Blood vessels—two arteries and one vein
(d) Remnants of the umbilical cord—yolk sac, vitelline duct
(e) Allantois
(f) Obliterated extraembryonic coelom.

**Q. What is the significance of single umbilical artery?**

**Ans.** It is frequently associated with congenital malformations of the fetus. Renal, genital anomalies and the trisomy 18 are common.

**Q. What are the indications of induction of labor?**

**Ans.** See p. 221.

**Q. What are the indications of surgical induction of labor?**

**Ans.** Common surgical indications are: Pre-eclampsia, eclampsia, abruptio placenta, chronic hydramnios, and along with (following) medical induction.

**Q. What are the dangers of induction of labor (medical and surgical)?**

**Ans. Surgical induction:** Cord prolapse, amnionitis, accidental injury to the placenta, bleeding
**Medical:** Related to individual method.
**PGs:** Uterine hyperstimulation, tachysystole, fetal distress, meconium-stained liquor, infection.
**Oxytocin:** Hyperstimulation, fetal distress, uterine rupture.

**Q. What is the preinduction cervical scoring system?**

**Ans. Bishop's** preinduction cervical scoring system is used. Total score is 13. **Favorable** score is 6–13. **Unfavorable** score is 0–5.
5 parameters are studied
**Cervix:** Dilatation, effacement, consistency and position.
**Head:** Station.

**Q. What immediate attention we should pay following ARM?**

**Ans.** The followings are important: To check the—
(a) Color of liquor
(b) Status of the cervix
(c) Station of the head
(d) Cord prolapse if any
(e) FHR pattern thereafter
(f) Sterile vulval pad is placed.

# LONG STRAIGHT SCISSORS (FIG. 8.12)

**Uses:** It is commonly used:
(i) To cut the umbilical cord,
(ii) To make episiotomy,
(iii) To cut suture materials as in cesarean section.

*Self-assessment:*

**Q. When should the umbilical cord be clamped and cut?**
**Ans.** *See* p. 188.

**Q. What are the indications of early cord clamping and cutting?**
**Ans.** *See* p. 188.

**Q. At what distance from the umbilicus the cord is clamped and cut?**
**Ans.** *See* p. 188.

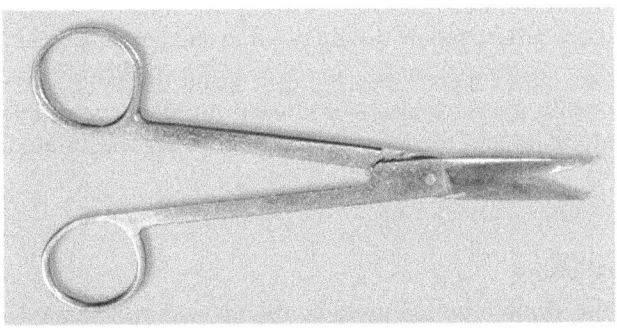

**Fig. 8.12:** Long straight scissors.

## UTERINE SOUND (FIG. 8.13)

It is an olive pointed, graduated, malleable, metallic uterine sound.

**Uses:**
(i) To know the position (ante-or retroversion) of the uterus and the length of the uterocervical canal prior to dilatation of the cervix in D + E operation,
(ii) To sound the uterine cavity to detect any foreign body (IUCD),
(iii) It acts as a first dilator of the cervical canal.

*Self-assessment:*

Q. What are the instruments required for D + E or suction evacuation?

**Ans.** See p. 258, 259.

Q. What are the important steps of S + E or D + E?

**Ans.** See p. 258-260.

Q. What are the complications of S + E or D + E operation?

**Ans.** See p 258-260.

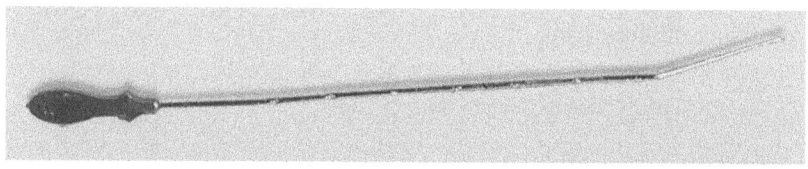

Fig. 8.13: Uterine sound.

## CERVICAL DILATORS (FIGS. 8.14A AND B): HAWKIN-AMBLER (FIG. 8.14A) AND DAS OR HEGAR'S DILATORS (FIG. 8.14B)

**Hawkin-Ambler**

**Description:** It is a single-ended metallic cervical dilator. The disc shaped end is the handle and the other pointed side is the dilating end. It has a smooth curvature with the tip directing upwards to follow the anteversion and anteflexion of the uterus.

It has got 16 sizes, the smallest one being 3/6 and the largest one being 18/21. The number is arbitrary in the scale of Hawkin-Ambler. The smaller one denotes measurement at the tip and the larger one measures the maximum diameter at the base in mm.

**Sterilization:** Boiling or autoclaving.

**Das or Hegar's dilators**

**Description:** This double-ended metallic dilator with a S-shaped curvature. The minimum size is 1/2 and the maximum size is 11/12. The number represents the diameter in mm. Both the sides are used with the lower number first.

**Use:** It is used in dilatation of the cervical canal prior to evacuation operation. Das/Hegar's dilators both are functionally the same.

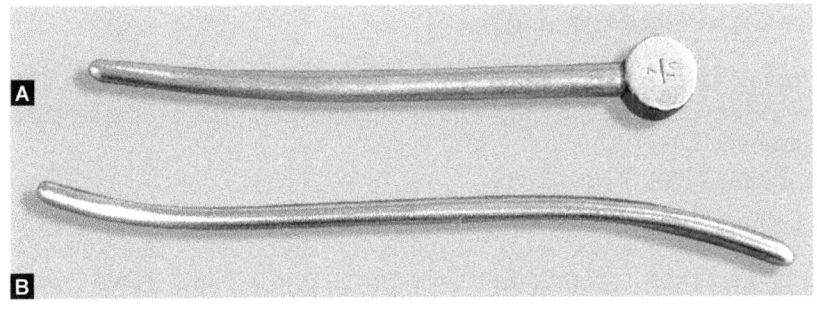

**Figs. 8.14A and B:** Cervical dilators: (A) Hawkin-Ambler; (B) Das/Hegar's dilator.

**Degree of dilatation required:**
 (i) Incomplete abortion—sufficient to introduce the index finger (usually 16/19),
 (ii) In suction evacuation—one size smaller than the size of the suction cannula,
(iii) In MTP by D + E—sufficient dilatation to introduce ovum forceps (usually 9/12).

*Self-assessment:*
    *Q. How to know the end point of suction procedure?*
  Ans. *See* p. 259.

    *Q. What is the management protocol when there is uterine perforation?*
  Ans. *See* p. 259.

    *Q. What are the indications of laparotomy following perforation?*
  Ans. Laparoscopy is helpful to assess the situation. Laparotomy is indicated in the following situations:
    (1) Lateral uterine wall injury with intraperitoneal hemorrhage or broad ligament hematoma
    (2) Suspected injury to bowel and/or omentum
    (3) Deterioration of vital signs during the period of observation
    (4) Perforation prior to complete evacuation.

## FLUSHING CURETTE (FIG. 8.15)

**Description:** It is a long metallic instrument with a channel inside. The stout end is used as the handle and the other end is spoon-shaped and fenestrated. This end is used as the blunt curette. The channel present inside the curette was designed to flush the endometrial cavity with antiseptic solution. Currently flushing system is not used. It is a blunt curette used in the operation of D + E. Previously, it was used to flush the uterine cavity with lukewarm antiseptic solution passing through the communicating channel.

*Self-assessment:*

Questions are similar as in Figs. 8.13 and 8.14.

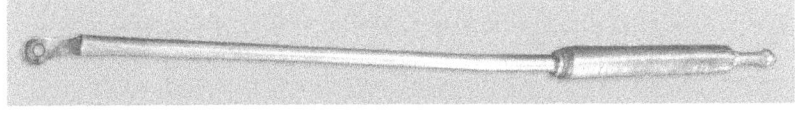

**Fig. 8.15:** Flushing curette.

## DOYEN'S RETRACTOR (FIG. 8.16)

**Description:** It is long metallic instrument. It has a stout handle at one end. The other end has a wide retracting blade (fan-shaped and curved). It needs an assistant to hold the instrument.

**Sterilization:** Boiling or autoclaving.

**Uses:** It is used to retract the abdominal wall as well as the bladder for proper exposure of lower uterine segment during LSCS. It is to be introduced after opening the abdomen; to be temporarily taken off while the baby is delivered, to be reintroduced after delivery of the baby and finally to be removed after toileting the peritoneal cavity.

*Self-assessment:*

**Q. List the types of CS.**

**Ans.** (a) Lower segment cesarean section (commonly done)
(b) Classical or upper segment cesarean section (rarely done).

**Q. What are the different types of uterine incisions for cesarean section?**

**Ans.** (a) Lower segment (LS) transverse incision (common)
(b) LS vertical
(c) LS 'J'-shaped
(d) Inverted 'T'-shaped incision
(e) Upper segment vertical incision.

**Q. What are the common indications of LSCS?**

**Ans.** *See* p. 269.

**Q. Describe the principal steps of LSCS.**

**Ans.** *See* p. 269-270.

**Q. Discuss the merits and demerits of LSCS over classical CS.**

**Ans.** *See* Dutta Obs 9/e, p. 552 Table 37.4.

**Q. What are the complications of CS?**

**Ans.** *See* p. 270.

**Q. What measures should be taken to reduce the rate of cesarean delivery?**

**Ans.** Important measures are:
(a) Partographic monitoring of labor
(b) Active management of labor
(c) Practice of ECV in selected cases with breech presentation
(d) Assisted vaginal breech delivery in selected cases
(e) Practice of VBAC in a selected case.

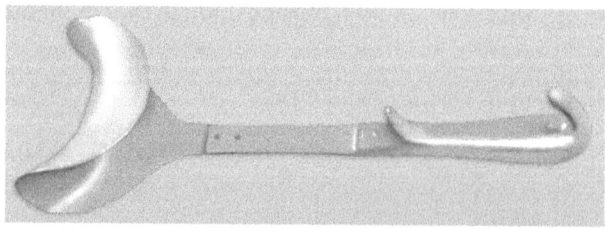

Fig. 8.16: Doyen's retractor.

## SPONGE HOLDING FORCEPS (FIG. 8.17)

**Description:** It is a long metallic (steel) instrument. It has two ends:
(1) One end is the handle with ratchet and catch.
(2) The other end is ring-shaped with transverse serration inside for better grip.

**Sterilization:** Boiling or autoclaving.

**Uses:**
(i) Toileting the vulva, vagina and perineum prior to and following delivery
(ii) Antiseptic painting of the abdominal wall prior to cesarean section
(iii) To catch hold the membranes if it threatens to tear during delivery of the placenta
(iv) To catch hold the cervix (2 pairs are needed) for inspection in suspected cervical tear
(v) to catch hold the cervix during encirclage operation.

*Self-assessment:*

Q. *What antiseptic solutions are commonly used to clean the vulva and vagina prior to and following delivery?*

Ans. *See* p. 258.

Q. *How the antiseptic painting of the abdominal wall is done before CS and what antiseptic solution is commonly used?*

Ans. *See* p. 271.

Q. *What happens if bits of placental tissue or membranes are left behind?*

Ans. (a) Postpartum hemorrhage
(b) Infection
(c) Pain
(d) Anemia
(e) Subinvolution of uterus.

Q. *How a cervical tear is repaired?*

Ans. Repair is done under general anesthesia with good light. The apex of the tear is identified. Two sponge holding forceps are used to hold the lips of the cervix. Vertical mattress sutures are placed using vicryl.

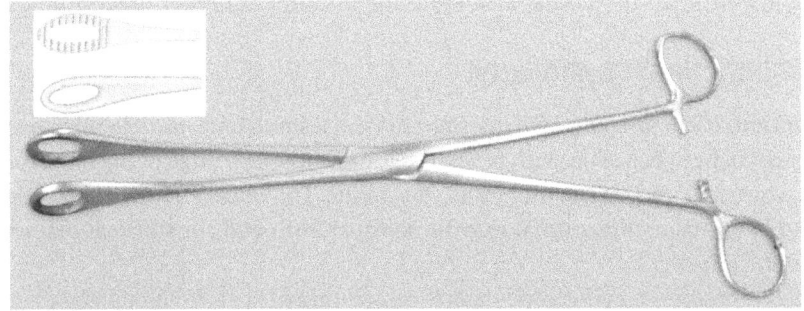

**Fig. 8.17:** Sponge holding forceps.

## OVUM FORCEPS (FIG. 8.18)

**Description:** It is a long metallic (steel) instrument with two ends and a shaft. The handle has no catch. For this reason risk of crushing any tissue, if it is grasped inadvertently is less. The fenestrated end has no serrations inside. This way ovum forceps differs from a sponge holding forceps.

**Sterilization:** Autoclaving or boiling.

It has got no catch and the blades are slightly bent and fenestrated. Absence of catch minimizes uterine injury, if accidentally caught. It prevents crushing of the conceptus. It is to be introduced with the blades closed, to open up inside the uterine cavity, to grasp the products and to take out the instrument with a slight rotatory movement. The rotatory movements not only facilitate detachment of the products from the uterine wall but also minimize the injury of the uterine wall, if accidentally grasped.

*Self-assessment:*

Q. *How to differentiate it from a sponge holding forceps?*

Ans. See above.

Q. *How the absence of catch made it advantageous?*

Ans. See above.

Q. *What are the indications of its use?*

Ans. It is used to evacuate the uterus. It is introduced inside the uterine cavity with blades closed. The blades are opened inside the uterine cavity to grasp the products of conception which are then taken out.

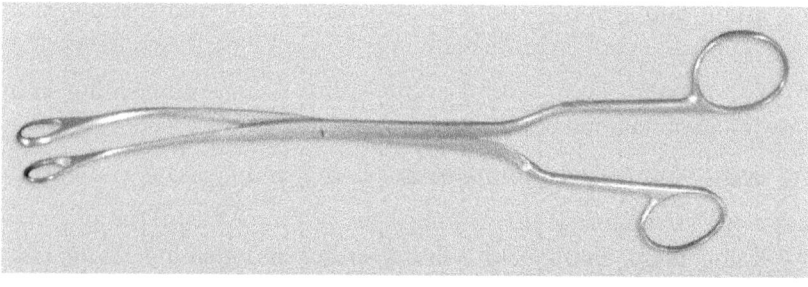

Fig. 8.18: Ovum forceps.

## UTERINE CURETTE (FIG. 8.19)

**Description:** It is a long metallic instrument with a small fenestrated end at each side and a shaft in between. The shaft is used as the handle. The edge of the fenestration is sharp at one end and on the other end, it is blunt. The blunt and the sharp edges are directed in opposite direction. It may be sharp at both ends or sharp at one end and blunt at the other.

**Uses:** Its common use in obstetrics is in the operation of D + C for incomplete abortion. In D + E operation, the curettage is done by blunt curette as the uterine wall is very soft. It can also be used in D + C operation 1 week following evacuation of hydatidiform mole.

**Sterilization:** Boiling or autoclaving.

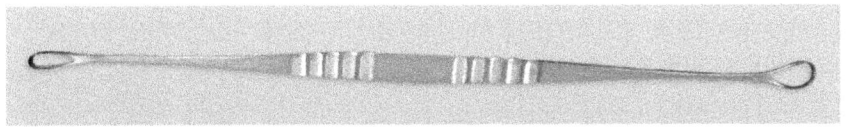

**Fig. 8.19:** Uterine curette.

*Self-assessment:*

**Q. What is the place of curettage following evacuation of hydatidiform mole?**

Ans. Gentle curettage may be done after 5–7 days. This helps to remove the necrotic decidua, tissues and the attached vesicles. It reduces the vaginal bleeding. The curetted materials are sent for histopathological examination.

**Q. What are the drawbacks of vigorous curettage?**

Ans. Risk of perforations of the uterus is high.

## UTERINE DRESSING FORCEPS (FIG. 8.20)

**Description:** It is a long metallic instrument with a handle with ratchet and catches at one end and the transversely serrated long blades at the other end. The instrument has a smooth S-shaped curve designed to accommodate the blades within the urine cavity.

The instrument is most often confused with laminaria tent introducing forceps. The blades are transversely serrated while in the latter, there is a groove on either blade.

**Sterilization:** Boiling or autoclaving.

**Uses:**
(i) To swab the uterine cavity following D + E with small gauze pieces
(ii) To dilate the cervix in lochiometra or pyometra.

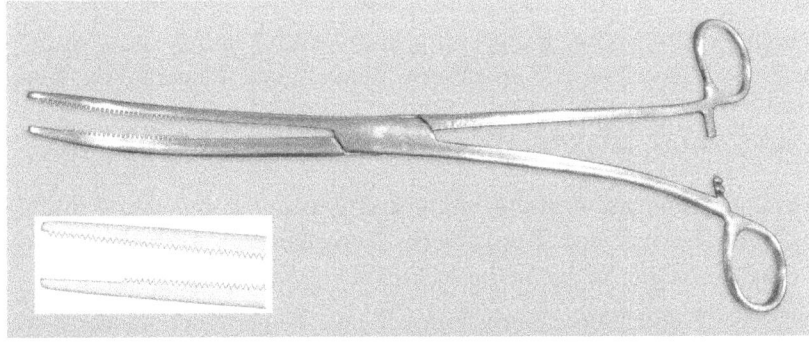

**Fig. 8.20:** Uterine dressing forceps.

## LAMINARIA TENT AND THE TENT INTRODUCING FORCEPS WITH LAMINARIA TENT (FIG. 8.21)

The instrument is almost similar to uterine dressing forceps. There is a groove on either blade to catch the laminaria tent.

**Laminaria tent:** It is dehydrated, compressed, Chinese seaweeds. It is sterilized by keeping it in absolute alcohol at least for 24 hours. Usually more than one tents are to be introduced to prevent dumbling of the ends. It produces slow dilatation of the cervical canal, as it swells up due to hygroscopic action.

**Isabgol tents (Isogel):** It is dried granules prepared from the husks of "certain mucilaginous tropical seeds".

*Self-assessment:*

   Q. *What are the other alternatives of tent used for slow dilatation of the cervix?*
   Ans. *See* above.

   Q. *What is postabortion care?*
   Ans. It includes:
      (a) Treatment of any complications to be done urgently
      (b) Family planning counseling and referral services
      (c) Linkage to other family planning services
      (d) Male partner is to be involved.

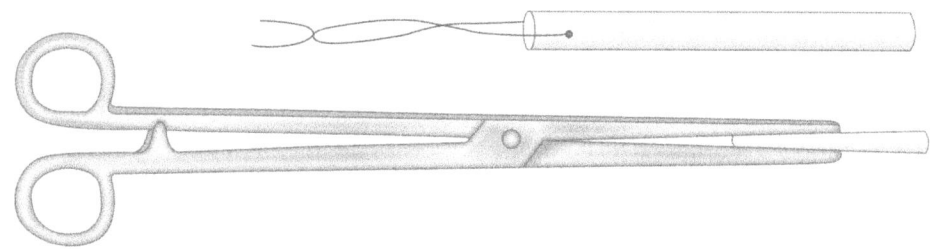

Fig. 8.21: Laminaria tent and the tent introducing forceps with laminaria tent.

## MANUAL VACUUM ASPIRATION SYRINGE (FIGS. 8.22 TO 8.24)

**Use:** Manual vacuum aspiration (MVA) is used for evacuation of the uterus (MTP) by creating a vacuum. It is used up to 12 weeks of pregnancy.

**Other uses:** Evacuation of the uterus in cases of:
  (i) Menstrual regulation
  (ii) Incomplete/missed abortion (up to 12 weeks)
  (iii) Molar pregnancy (up to 12 weeks)
  (iv) Anembryonic sac (p. 114)
  (v) Endometrial sampling/biopsy.

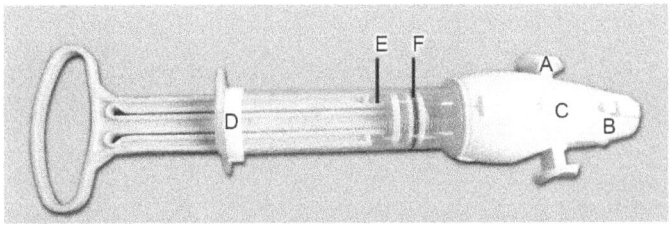

**Fig. 8.22:** MVA syringe (Ipas MVA plus).
A. Valve button
B. Cap
C. Hinged valve with valve liner within
D. Collar stop
E. Cylinder
F. Plunger O-ring

**Advantages of MVA:**
 (i) Simple
 (ii) Safe
 (iii) Can be done as an outpatient basis (without electricity)
 (iv) With local anesthesia
 (v) Effective (98%)
 (vi) Less traumatic
 (vii) Takes less time (10–15 minutes).

*Self-assessment:*

Q. *What are the methods of termination of pregnancy in the first trimester?*

Ans. The commonly used methods are:
 (A) **Medical:**
   (a) Mifepristone
   (b) Mifepristone and misoprostol (PGE1)
   (c) Others—methotrexate
 (B) **Surgical:**
   (a) Menstrual regulation
   (b) Manual vacuum aspiration (MVA/EVA)
   (c) Suction evacuation (S/E)
   (d) Dilatation and evacuation (D/E).

Q. *What are the complications of MVA?*

Ans. See p. 260.

Q. *How one can ensure that the procedure is completed?*

Ans. See p. 260.

Q. *What are the precautions that we should take?*

Ans. See p. 260.

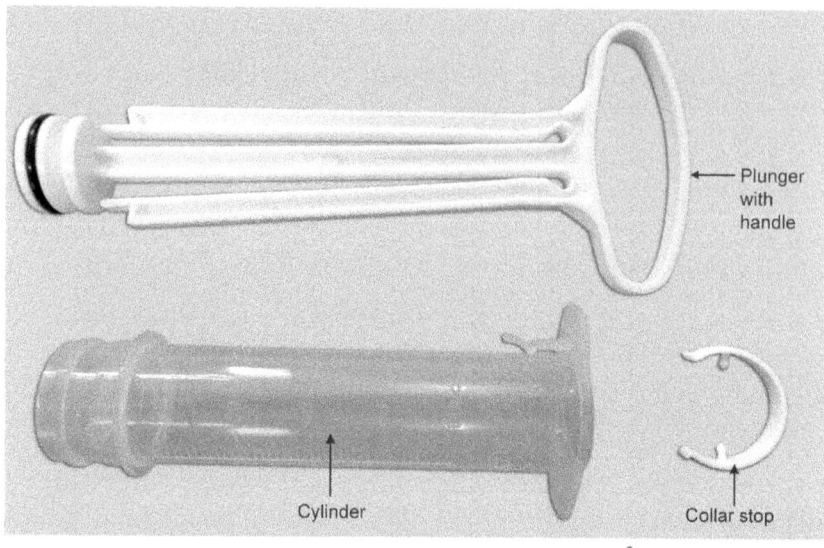

**Fig. 8.23:** Parts of MVA syringe.

**Parts of MVA syringe** (Fig. 8.23):
 (i) Cylinder
 (ii) Hinged valve (valve liner inside)
 (iii) Valve cap
 (iv) Valve button
 (v) Plunger with handle
 (vi) Collar stop
 (vii) Cannula— dimensions and sizes are similar to Karman's (*see* Fig. 8.25). The winged adaptor is fixed at the base (Fig. 8.24).

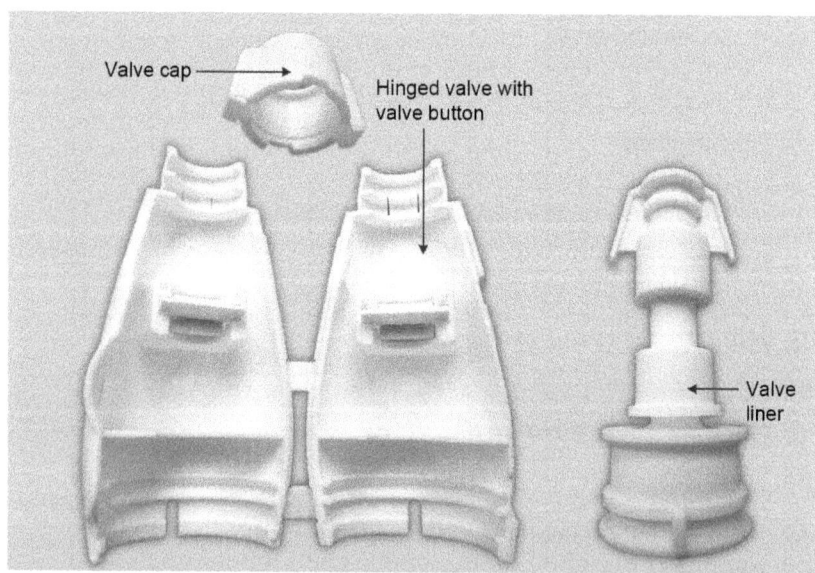

**Fig. 8.24:** Valve cup and valve liner.

## PLASTIC SUCTION CANNULA (KARMAN'S TYPE) (FIG. 8.25)

It is of different sizes and the approximate size required for a particular case equals to the weeks of pregnancy to be terminated. The plastic cannula has got advantages over the metallic one—as it causes less damage to the uterine wall and the product sucked out is visible. **The vacuum must be broken before its withdrawal.** It is of different sizes (4, 5, 6, 7, 8, 9, 10, and 12 mm). It is used for S + E and MVA.

*Self-assessment:*

    Q. *How is the size of the cannula determined?*

Ans. *See* p. 259.

    Q. *During S + E procedure, how is the cannula to be moved?*

Ans. *See* p. 259.

    Q. *How much suction pressure is generally used?*

Ans. *See* p. 259.

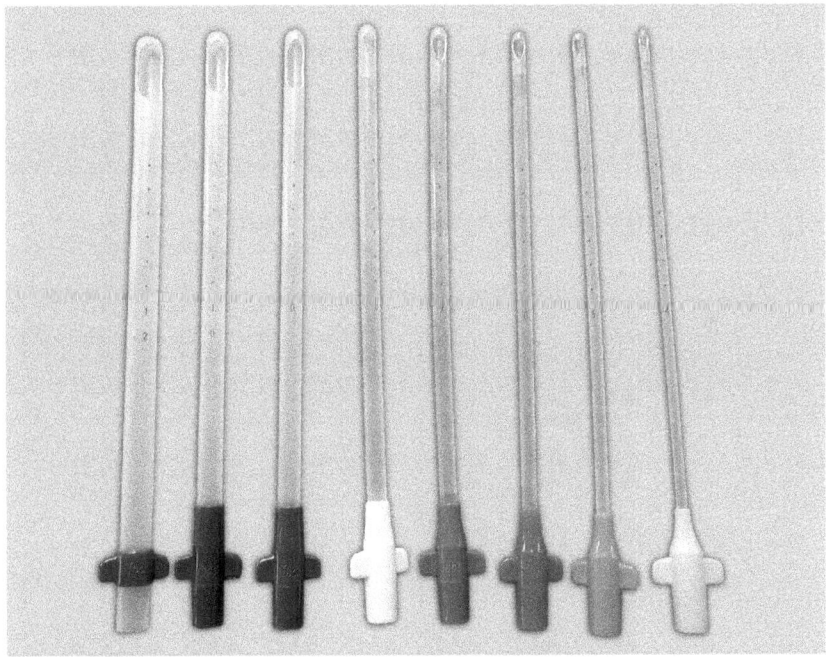

Fig. 8.25: MVA—cannulas of different sizes; the winged adaptor.

## OPERATION TROLLEY FOR SUCTION AND EVACUATION (FIG. 8.26)

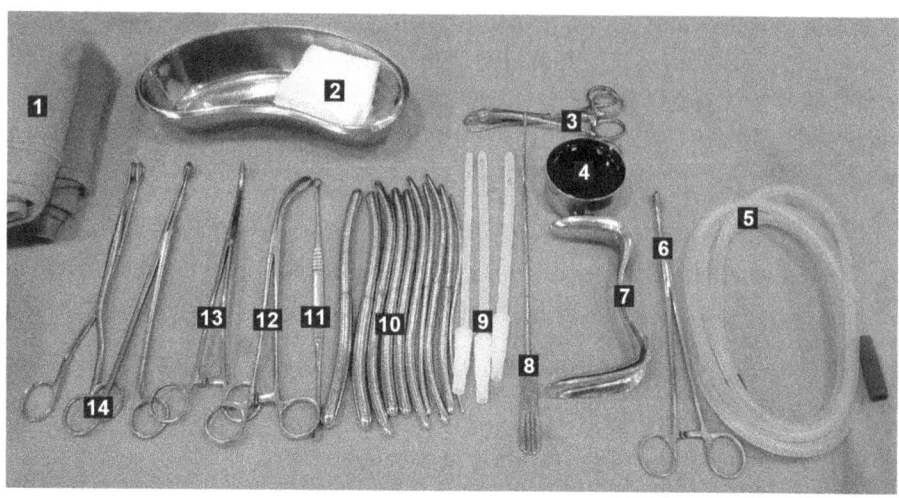

**Fig. 8.26:** Operation trolley for suction and evacuation.
1. Towels for drapings, 2. Kidney dish with sterile gauze pieces, 3. Towel clip, 4. Bowl with povidone iodine, 5. Suction tube, 6. Sponge holding forceps, 7. Sim's posterior vaginal speculum, 8. Uterine sound, 9. Suction cannulas (3), 10. Cervical dilators (Hegar's), 11. Uterine curette (sharp and blunt), 12. Multiple toothed vulsellum, 13. Uterine dressing forceps, 14. Ovum forceps (2)

## LONG CURVED OBSTETRIC FORCEPS (FIG. 8.27)

It is commonly used in low forceps operation.

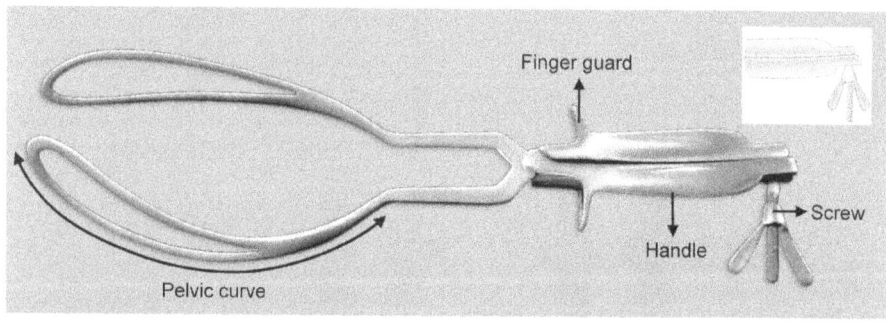

**Fig. 8.27:** Long curved obstetric forceps.

*Self-assessment:*

**Q. What are the different types of obstetric forceps?**

**Ans.** (1) Long curved obstetric forceps with or without axis traction during (Fig. 8.27).
(2) Short curved forceps (*see* Fig. 8.28).
(3) Kielland's forceps (*see* Fig. 8.29).

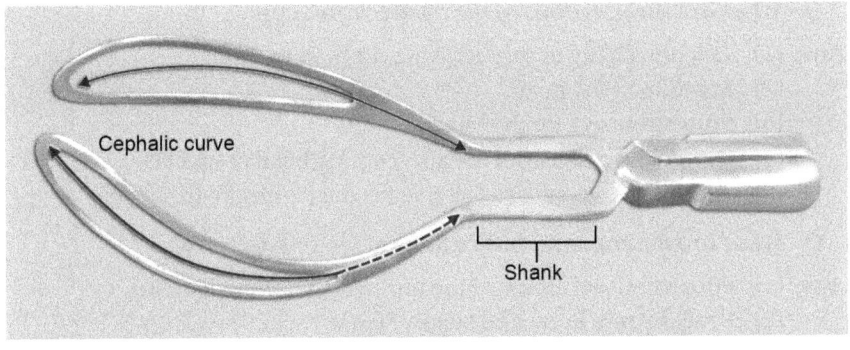

**Fig. 8.28:** Short-curved obstetric forceps (Wrigley's forceps).

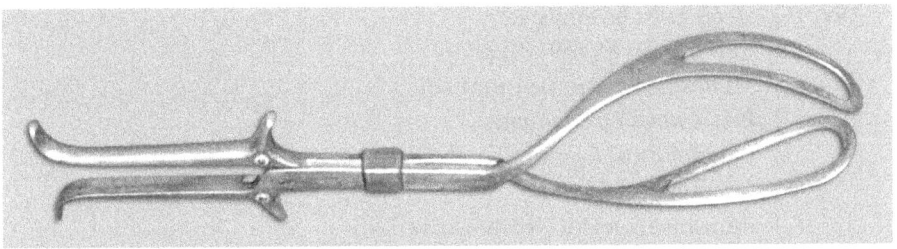

**Fig. 8.29:** Kielland's forceps.

***Q. What are the different parts and the curvatures?***

**Ans.** (1) **Parts of forceps:**
  (a) Blades—two (right and left)
  (b) Shank
  (c) Lock
  (d) Handle
(2) **Curvatures:**
  (a) Pelvic curve—curve on the edge
  (b) Cephalic curve—curve on the flat surface.

***Q. How do you identify the blades?***

**Ans.** (1) The tip of blade should point upwards
(2) Cephalic curve is to be directed inwards
(3) Pelvic curve is to be directed forwards.

***Q. What are the different types of forceps application?***

**Ans.** (1) **Outlet forceps:** Fetal skull; at pelvic floor, sagittal suture is in antero-posterior diameter of the pelvis
(2) **Low forceps:** Station is at +2 or more
(3) **Mid forceps:** Head is engaged but station is above +2 cm
(4) **High forceps (abandoned):** Head is not engaged.

**Q. What are the functions of the obstetric forceps?**

**Ans.** (1) Traction (20 kg in primigravida, 13 kg in multi)
(2) Rotation of the head
(3) Protective cage for the head
(4) Controlled delivery of the aftercoming head of breech
(5) One blade may be used as a vectis during cesarean section.

**Q. What are the common indications of forceps delivery?**

**Ans.** (1) Poor expulsive efforts of the mother (maternal distress)
(2) Fetal distress in second stage of labor
(3) Prolonged second stage of labor
(4) To cut start the second stage of labor.

**Q. Conditions to be fulfilled before applications of forceps.**

**Ans.** (1) Head must be engaged
(2) Cervix must be fully dilated
(3) Membranes must be ruptured
(4) Pelvis must be adequate
(5) Bladder must be emptied
(6) Adequate analgesia
(7) Informed consent (written or verbal).

**Q. What are the steps of forceps application?**

**Ans.** (1) Identification of the blades
(2) Introduction of left blade first
(3) Introduction of right blades
(4) Locking of the blades
(5) Traction
(6) Delivery of the head of the baby
(7) Removal of the blades
(8) Delivery of the baby.

**Q. What is the direction of pull during delivery?**

**Ans. Direction:**
(a) **Outlet forceps delivery:** Straight horizontal then upwards and forwards.
(b) **Low forceps delivery:** Downwards and backwards → the straight pull → finally upwards and forwards.

**Q. What are the difficulties in forceps delivery?**

**Ans.** Difficulties may be:
(A) During application of the blades due to:
  (a) Incompletely dilated cervix or
  (b) Unrotated head or
  (c) Non-engaged head.
(B) During locking of blades due to: Unrotated head
(C) During traction due to: Undiagnosed occiput posterior.

**Q. What is prophylactic forceps?**

**Ans.** When forceps are applied to shorten the second stage of labor in anticipation to some complications either to mother or to fetus.
Indications are:
(i) Eclampsia,
(ii) Fetal growth restriction (FGR).

**Q. What is trial forceps?**

**Ans.** It is a tentative attempt of forceps delivery in a case with suspected midpelvic contraction with a preamble declaration that the procedure may be abandoned, if moderate force fails to overcome the resistance and to deliver the baby. In that case baby is delivered by immediate cesarean section. The trial of forceps delivery is conducted in an operation theater keeping everything ready for cesarean section so that no time is wasted to deliver the baby. It has the advantage of reducing many unnecessary cesarean sections.

**Q. What is failed forceps?**

**Ans.** When there is failure of forceps delivery in spite of deliberate attempt to deliver the baby. Common reasons are:
(a) Incompletely dilated cervix
(b) Cephalopelvic disproportion
(c) Unrotated head.

## SHORT CURVED OBSTETRIC FORCEPS (WRIGLEY'S FORCEPS) (FIG. 8.28)

It can only be used as outlet forceps for extraction of the head.

*Self assessment:*

**Q. How do you differentiate short curved forceps from long curved forceps?**

**Ans.** The short curve forceps is also known as Wrigley's forceps. The points of differentiation are:
(a) Lighter
(b) Short in total length
(c) Reduction in the lengths of:
   (i) Shank
   (ii) Handle
(d) It has a marked cephalic curve but less pelvic curve.

**Q. Define outlet forceps.**

**Ans.** *See* p. 301.

**Q. What is the direction of pull?**

**Ans.** *See* p. 266.

## KIELLAND'S FORCEPS (FIG. 8.29)

It is usually used as rotation forceps in deep transverse arrest of occipitoposterior position of the head or in unrotated vertex or face presentation.

*Self-assessment:*

**Q. How do you identify the blades?**

**Ans.** See p. 301.

**Q. Discuss its special advantages over the long-curved forceps.**

**Ans.** Advantages over long curved forceps are:
(i) This can be used in unrotated
(ii) Facilitates grasping the head with correction of asynclitism.

**Q. What are the methods of application?**

**Ans.** Methods of application are:
(a) Wandering method (superior blade first). It is commonly done.
(b) Direct method
(c) Classical method.

**Q. What are the hazards of its use?**

**Ans.** Complications are:
(A) Fetal: Facial injury—bruising or laceration, skull fracture, intracranial hemorrhage.
(B) Maternal: Perineal injury—sulcus tear, vaginal laceration.

## FORCEPS' AXIS TRACTION DEVICES (FIG. 8.30)

It includes axis traction rods (right and left) and handle. The rods are assembled in the blades of long-curved obstetric forceps prior to introduction and lastly the handle is attached to the rods. The devices are required where much forces are necessary for traction as in midforceps operation. These are less commonly used now.

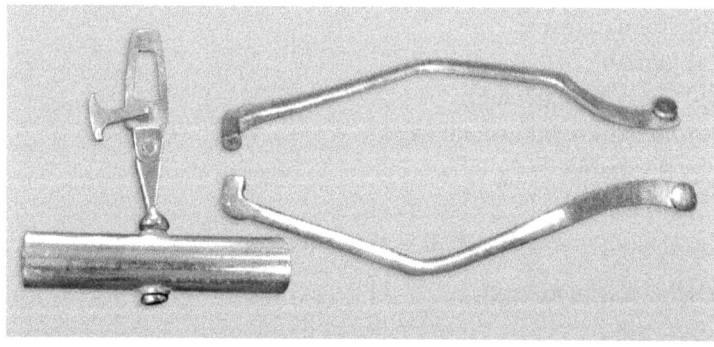

**Fig. 8.30:** Forceps' axis traction devices.

***Advantages:*** Axis traction devices are used in midcavity delivery and in cases following manual rotation of the head. It provides traction in the correct axis of the pelvic curve. Less force is needed to deliver the head.

*Self-assessment:*

**Q. What is understood by operative vaginal delivery?**

**Ans.** The different operations that are done to assist the process of vaginal delivery. The commonly performed procedures are:
(a) Forceps
(b) Ventouse
(c) Destructive operations (craniotomy).

## EPISIOTOMY SCISSORS (FIG. 8.31)

It is bent on edge. The blade with blunt tip goes inside the vagina. This is designed to avoid trauma to the baby while making the perineotomy (incision).

*Self-assessment:*

**Q. What are the common indications of episiotomy?**

**Ans.** See p. 261.

**Q. Should episiotomy be made in all cases?**

**Ans.** Episiotomy is recommended in selected cases only. It should not be done as a routine in all cases.

**Q. Discuss the types of episiotomy.**

**Ans.** See p. 262.

**Q. What structures are cut during episiotomy?**

**Ans.** See p. 262.

**Q. What are the complications of episiotomy?**

**Ans.** See p. 262.

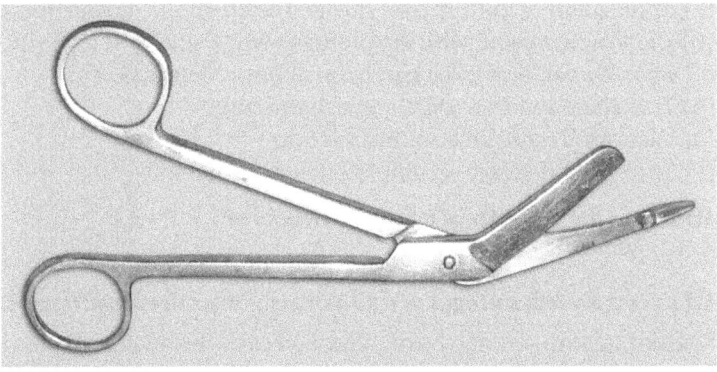

Fig. 8.31: Episiotomy scissors.

# VENTOUSE CUP WITH TRACTION DEVICE (FIGS. 8.32A AND B)

Ventous cup is used during delivery to a baby using vacuum extractor. The cup is attached to the baby's head by suction. Since the scalp is sucked into the cup during delivery, it produces a temporary swelling on the infant's head known as 'chignon' which disappears within few hours. The cup has got various sizes (*See* p. 241 Figs. 8.32A to C).

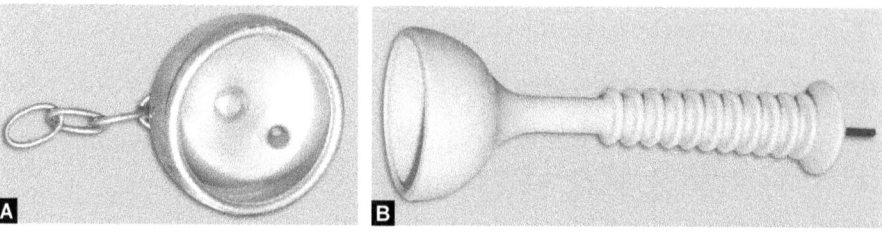

**Figs. 8.32A and B:** Ventouse cup: (A) Metal; (B) Silastic.

*Self-assessment:*

**Q. What are the indications of its use?**
**Ans.** *See* p. 268.

**Q. List its advantages over forceps.**
**Ans.** *See* p. 268.

**Q. What are the conditions to be fulfilled for its application?**
**Ans.** The conditions are the same as in forceps delivery (ACOG 2000).

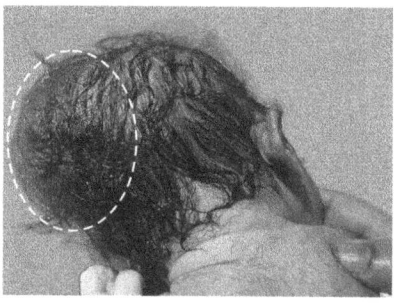

**Fig. 8.32C:** Chignon.

**Q. Describe the methods of its use.**
**Ans.** Methods are:
(a) Application of the cup over the fetal scalp on the flexion point.
(b) Vacuum is created with the pump slowly.
(c) Effective vacuum is 0.8 kg/cm² in about 10 minutes.
(d) Traction is made at right angle to the cup.
(e) Vacuum is reduced once head is born.
(f) The rest of delivery is completed in a normal way.

**Q. What are the hazards of ventouse delivery?**
**Ans.** *See* p. 269.

**Q. What are the advantages of a silastic cup over the metallic one?**
**Ans.** Silastic cups are soft, can be molded, and cause less trauma. It can be applied over the scalp easily.

**Q. What is flexion point?**
**Ans.** *See* p. 268.

**Q. What is chignon?**
**Ans.** It is an artificial caput succedaneum, as the scalp is sucked into the cup during the process of delivery. Chignon usually disappears within few hours (*See* Fig. 8.32C).

## GREEN ARMYTAGE HEMOSTATIC FORCEPS (FIG. 8.33)

**Description:** It is a long metallic instrument. Handle is at one end with ratchet and catch. The other end is the tissue holding broad end. This end has got transverse serrations.

**Uses:** This forceps is used in lower segment cesarean section. Total four forceps are ordinarily required—one for each angle and one for each flap. Its functions are hemostasis and to catch hold of the margins so that they are not missed during suture. It cannot be used in classical cesarean section. Alternative to this Allis tissue forceps may be used.

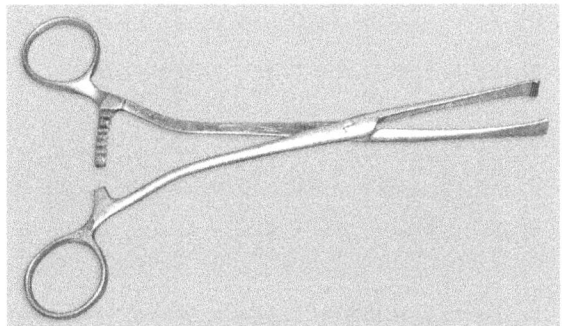

**Fig. 8.33:** Green armytage hemostatic forceps.

*Self-assessment:*

*Q. What are the factors responsible for rise in CS rate?*

Ans. Common factors are:
(a) Rise in primary cesarean delivery
(b) Rise in induction of labor and failed induction rates
(c) Decline in vaginal breech delivery
(d) Decline in operative vaginal delivery
(e) Fear of litigation
(f) CS on maternal request.

*Q. What are the methods of suturing the uterine wound?*

Ans. See p. 275.

*Q. List the criteria for VBAC.*

Ans. See p. 45.

*Q. What are the intraoperative complications of CS?*

Ans. See p. 270.

*Q. What is the significance of the name Green armytage?*

Ans. See p. 691.

## MUCUS SUCKER (FIGS. 8.34A AND B)

**(A) Disposable, (B) Metal**—it is used to suck out the mucus from the naso-oropharynx following delivery of the head of the baby. To be of value, the mucus should be sucked prior to the attempt of respiration, otherwise the tracheobronchial tree may be occluded leading to inadequate pulmonary aeration and development of asphyxia neonatorum. The metal sucker requires a **sterile simple rubber catheter** to be fitted at one end and a sterile piece of gauze to the other end. Currently electric or the disposable sucker is being used.

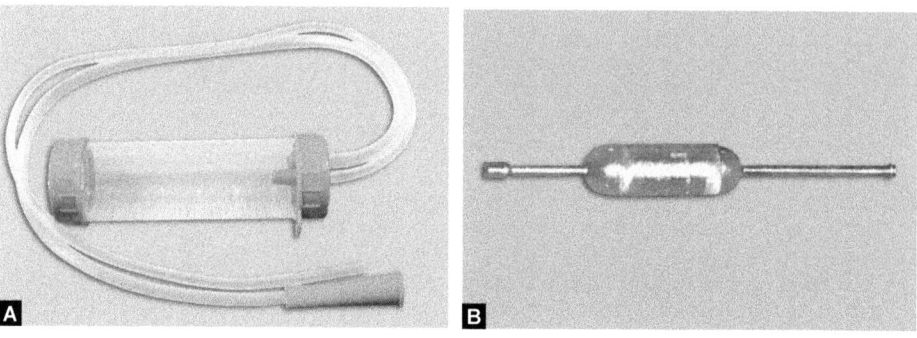

**Figs. 8.34A and B:** (A) Mucus sucker—disposable; (B) Mucus sucker—metal.

*Self-assessment:*

**Q. Discuss immediate care of the newborn.**

**Ans.** See p. 188.

**Q. Discuss the management of the cord round the neck.**

**Ans.** Immediately following delivery of the head, the neck is palpated to exclude any cord loop. When it is present and if it is found loose, it is slipped over the head and the baby is delivered. When it is tightly applied, it is cut in between two Kocher's forceps placed 2.5 cm apart.

**Q. What are the causes of asphyxia neonatorum?**

**Ans.** Common causes are:
(a) **Maternal conditions:** Anemia, eclampsia, cardiovascular disorders
(b) **Placental insufficiency:** Abruptio placenta, cord compression
(c) **Maternal medications:** Pethidine, morphine
(d) **Labor problems:** Dysfunctional labor, prolonged labor, obstructed labor
(e) **Birth trauma:** Forceps/ventouse delivery, breech delivery
(f) **Postnatal factors:** Postnatal hypothermia, sepsis.

**Q. How Apgar scoring is done?**

**Ans.** See p. 188.

**Q. How do you manage an asphyxiated neonate?**

**Ans.** See Obst. Text 9th Ed. p. 440-441.

# CORD CLAMP (DISPOSABLE) (FIG. 8.35)

It is made of plastic and is supplied in a sterile pack. The serrated surface and the lock make its grip firm. It occludes the umbilical vessels effectively. The cord clamp is to be kept in place until it falls off together with the detached stump of umbilical cord.

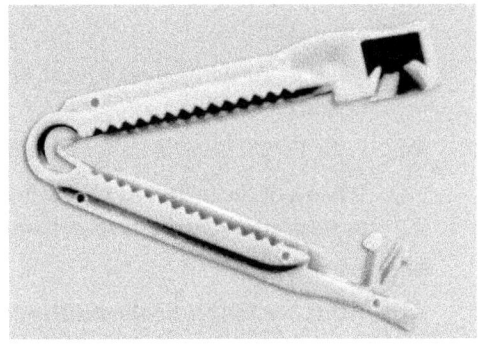

Fig. 8.35: Cord clamp (disposable).

*Self-assessment:*

Q. *What is the purpose of the cord clamp that is applied on the maternal end?*

Ans. *See* p. 188.

Q. *What are the different abnormalities of cord attachment?*

Ans. Common abnormalities are:
  (a) Attached at the margin of placenta—Battledore placenta
  (b) Attached to the membranes—Velamentous placenta.

Q. *What is the significance when the cord is unduly long or short?*

Ans. **Short cord:**
  (a) Malpresentation
  (b) Fetal distress in labor
  (c) Failure in ECV
  (d) Placental abruption
  **Long cord:**
  (a) Cord prolapse
  (b) True knot formation
  (c) Cord entanglement.

# PINARD'S STETHOSCOPE (FIG. 8.36)

**Uses:** It should be held firmly at right angle to the point on the abdominal wall. The ear must be firmly closed to the aural end. **It should not be touched by hand while listening.**

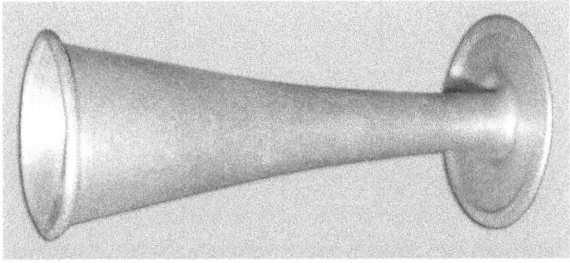

Fig. 8.36: Pinard's stethoscope.

*Self-assessment:*

**Q. Earliest at what weeks, FHS could be detected with a stethoscope?**
Ans. See p. 322.

**Q. Earliest at what weeks fetal heart beat could be visible on ultrasound examination?**
Ans. With TVS, it is visible after completed 5 weeks of gestation.

**Q. What are the different sites where maximum intensity of FHS is obtained in relation to fetal presentation and position?**
Ans. See p. 22.

**Q. What are the clinical conditions where FHS may not be audible?**
Ans. Maternal obesity, hydramnios, occiput posterior position.

## PERFORATOR (OLDHAM'S) (FIG. 8.37)

The instrument is required in craniotomy to perforate the skull bone for decompression of the fetal head.

*Self-assessment:*

**Q. What are the indications of craniotomy?**
Ans. See p. 227.

**Q. What are the contraindications of craniotomy?**
Ans. See p. 278.

**Q. What are the conditions to be fulfilled prior to craniotomy?**
Ans. (a) Cervix must be fully dilated
(b) Baby must be dead (hydrocephalus being excluded).

**Q. What specific postoperative care is essential in such a case?**
Ans. See p. 278.

**Q. Describe important steps of the operation.**
Ans. See p. 278.

**Q. What procedure should be done after delivery of the placenta?**
Ans. See p. 278.

**Q. What are the complications of destructive operations?**
Ans. See p. 278.

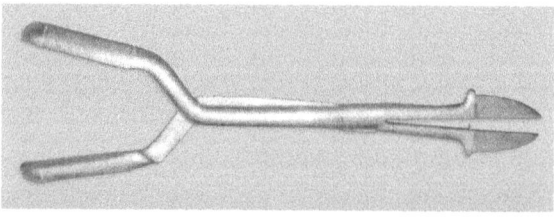

**Fig. 8.37:** Perforator (Oldham's).

## GIANT VULSELLUM (FIG. 8.38)

It is used in destructive operation especially in evisceration to have a good grip of the fetal parts for giving traction.

*Self-assessment:*

Q. *What is meant by neglected shoulder presentation?*
Ans. It is meant to direct all the serious complications that may arise out of shoulder presentation when a woman is in labor and is left uncared.

Q. *Mention the postoperative care following any destructive operation.*
Ans. *See* p 278.

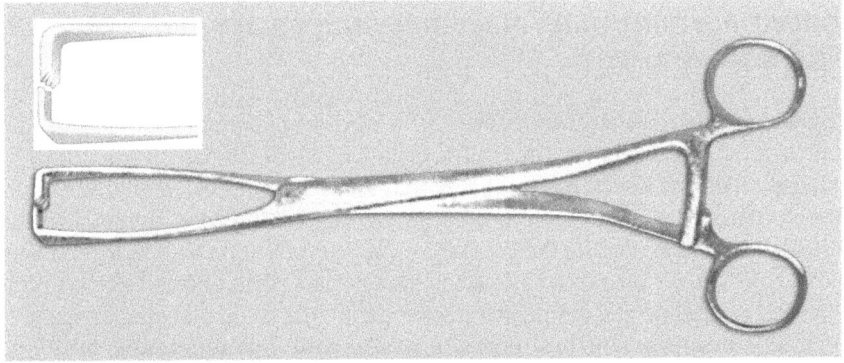

Fig. 8.38: Giant vulsellum.

## PROCESSING OF INSTRUMENTS

**A. Disinfection** is done by any one of the methods: Immersing instruments in (i) boiling water for 20 minutes, (ii) 2% glutaraldehyde (cidex) solution for 20 minutes or, (iii) 0.5% chlorine solution for 20 minutes (0.5% of chlorine solution is made by adding 3 teaspoons (15 g) of bleaching powder in 1 liter of water).

**B. Cleaning:** Instruments are disassembled and washed on all surfaces in running (*preferably warm*) water. The cannulas should be flushed repeatedly.

**C. Sterilization:** Either by (i) autoclaving at 121°C (250°F) under pressure of 15 lbs/in$^2$ (106 kPa) for 30 minutes or, (ii) immersing in 2% glutaraldehyde (cidex) solution for 10 hours. All metallic instruments are sterilized by autoclaving or boiling. Rubber goods (catheters) are sterilized by boiling.

## SPECIMENS

### Chapter Objectives
**Good knowledge and understanding of:**
- Macroscopic description of the organ(s) with associated pathology
- Surgical procedures done in relation to such pathology
- Obstetric (maternal and fetal) complications related to this pathology
- Expected histopathology
- Management options
- Follow-up management

### NORMAL PLACENTA AND PLACENTA SUCCENTURIATA (FIGS. 8.39A AND B)

Photographs showing maternal surface of a normal placenta (Fig. 8.39A) and the fetal surface of a placenta succenturiata. (Fig. 8.39B). Maternal surface looks rough and shaggy. It shows 15–20 convex polygonal areas as lobes or cotyledons bounded by fissures. Membranes are seen at the margin. Fig. 8.39B shows the fetal surface of a placenta succenturiata. The fetal surface looks smooth and shiny as it is covered by amnion layer. The umbilical cord is attached at/or near the center. There is one small lobe (size of a cotyledon) situated at a distance from the main placental margin. It has vascular communication (arrow mark). It is a placenta with a succenturiate lobe.

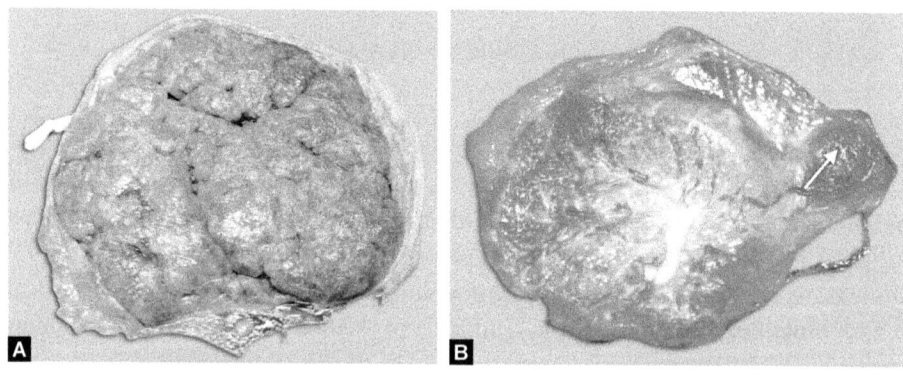

**Figs. 8.39A and B:** (A) Normal placenta (maternal surface); (B) Placenta succenturiata (fetal surface). Vascular communication is seen (arrow showing).

*Self-assessment:*

    **Q. What are the surfaces of a normal placenta and how they could be identified?**

  **Ans.** *See* above.

**Q. What is the weight of a normal placenta?**

**Ans.** Normal placenta weighs around 500 g.

**Q. What is the normal attachment of a placenta?**

**Ans.** Placenta is implanted to the upper part of the body of the uterus, close to the fundus. It may be on the anterior or posterior wall of the uterus.

**Q. What is the clinical significance of placenta succenturiata?**

**Ans.** Increased risk of abortion, antepartum hemorrhage.

**Q. What other abnormalities of placenta are commonly seen?**

**Ans.** Battledore placenta (cord inserted at the margin of placenta).

## RUPTURE UTERUS (FIG. 8.40)

It is a specimen of gravid uterus showing ragged, irregular, blackish necrosed margin along the lateral wall of the uterus. Cervix is not seen. It is a specimen of rupture uterus. Subtotal hysterectomy with conservation of ovaries had been done.

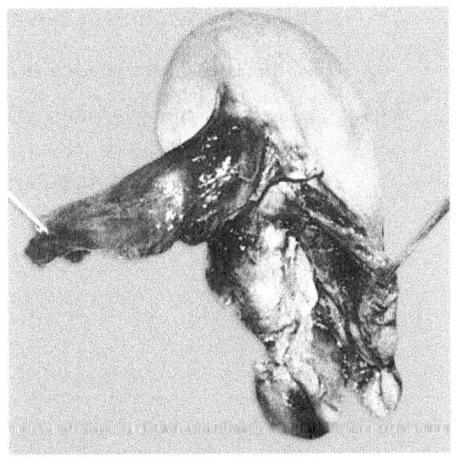

Fig. 8.40: Rupture uterus.

*Self-assessment:*

**Q. What are the common causes of rupture uterus?**

**Ans.** (a) Obstructed labor
(b) Injudicious oxytocin use in labor
(c) Rupture of uterine scar (CS).

**Q. What are the common types of rupture uterus?**

**Ans.** Types are:
(a) **Spontaneous rupture:**
 (i) Grand multipara
 (ii) Obstructive: Obstructed labor
(b) **Scar rupture:** Scarred uterus—CS or myomectomy and
(c) **Iatrogenic rupture:** Injudicious oxytocin use in labor, ECV, internal version.

**Q. Differentiation of uterine scar dehiscence from scar rupture?**

**Ans.** *See* p. 42-43.

**Q. How the diagnosis of rupture uterus (spontaneous as well as scar) is made?**

**Ans.** *See* p. 42-44.

**Q. How do you manage a case of rupture uterus?**

**Ans.** Resuscitation and laparotomy. Resuscitation includes: IV infusion of crystalloids (normal saline) and blood transfusion. Resuscitation and laparotomy are done simultaneously. Laparotomy and hysterectomy (commonly subtotal hysterectomy) are done. Repair of uterus may be done in selected cases with scar rupture. Repair and bilateral tubal ligation may also be done.

## UNRUPTURED TUBAL ECTOPIC PREGNANCY (FIGS. 8.41A AND B)

It is a photograph (endoscopic panoramic view) of an unruptured tubal ectopic pregnancy. Ectopic pregnancy is seen at the region of ampulla of the tube (right).

*Self-assessment:*

Q. *How a case of acute (ruptured) tubal ectopic pregnancy is diagnosed?*

Ans. **Symptoms:** Amenorrhea, acute abdominal pain, vaginal bleeding,
**Signs:** Pallor, features of hypotension, shock, positive pregnancy test.

Q. *How a case of unruptured tubal ectopic pregnancy is diagnosed?*

Ans. (i) Estimation of serum β-hCG (positive in low concentration ≥1500 IU/L)
(ii) On TVS: Adnexal mass, empty uterine cavity
(iii) Laparoscopy (confirmaton of diagnosis, Fig. 8.41B).

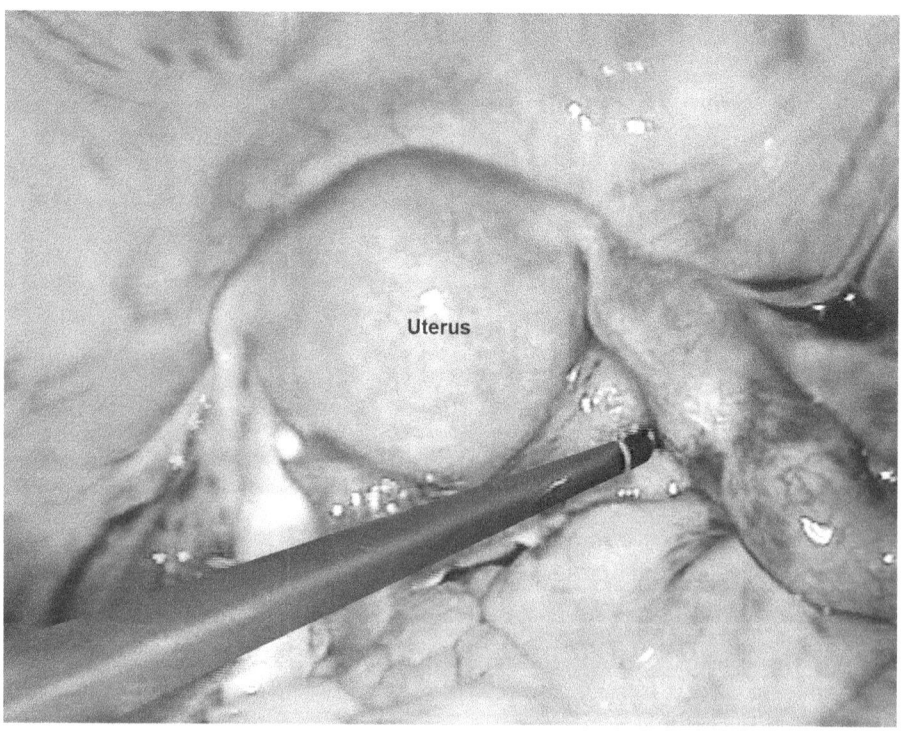

Fig. 8.41A: Unruptured tubal ectopic pregnancy (laparoscopic view).

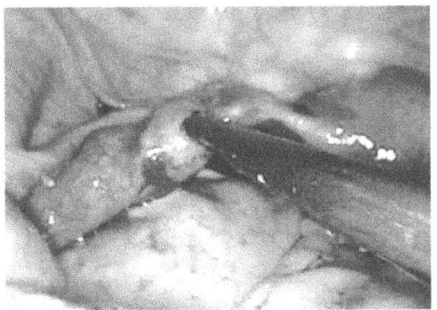

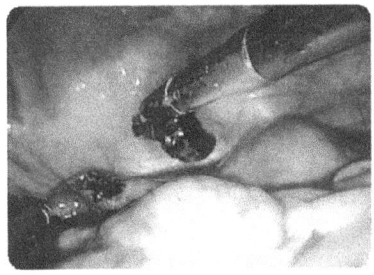
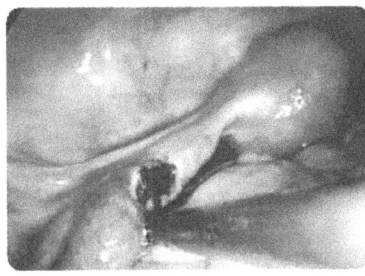

**Fig. 8.41B:** Unruptured tubal ectopic pregnancy. Salpingostomy is being done laparoscopically.

***Q. How do you manage a case of acute tubal ectopic pregnancy?***

**Ans.** Resuscitation and laparotomy. Blood transfusion is often needed.

***Q. How do you manage a case of an unruptured tubal pregnancy?***

**Ans.** Management of an unruptured tubal ectopic pregnancy depends on several factors like:
   (a) Serum β-hCG levels
   (b) Gestational sac size
   (c) Patient's hemodynamic stability
   (d) Presence of fetal cardiac motion.

**Management options are:**
(1) Expectant—observation
   Indications are:
      (i) β-hCG is <1500 IU/L
      (ii) Gestational sac is 4 cm.
      (iii) No visible fetal heart beat on TVS
      (iv) On TVS, no evidence of gastational. Sac rupture or bleeding P/V
      (v) Patient is hemodynamically stable.
(2) Medical (methotrexate-IM). Generally, it is given IM 50 mg/m² as a single dose.
(3) Surgical—laparoscopically or laparotomy: Salpingostomy or salpingectomy
(4) Follow-up is done till β-hCG becomes negative.
Rh-negative woman should be given anti-D immunoglobulin IM.

# IMAGING STUDIES

> **Chapter Objectives**
> **Imaging studies**
> Basic knowledge and understanding of:
> - Ultrasonogram and magnetic resonance images for:
>   – Rational use
>   – Assessment of fetal well-being and maternal health
>   – Interpretation of results
>     - Adverse effects (if any)
>   – To screen/diagnose maternal and fetal complications

## ULTRASONOGRAM

### Gestational Sac (Fig. 8.42)

*Q. What is seen in the ultrasonogram?*

Ans. A well-defined gestational sac (GS) within the uterine cavity is seen. The sac is located eccentrically within the uterine cavity.

*Q. What is the usual location of the GS within the uterine cavity?*

Ans. GS is normally located eccentrically within the uterine cavity. This is an important observation to differentiate it from a pseudosac.

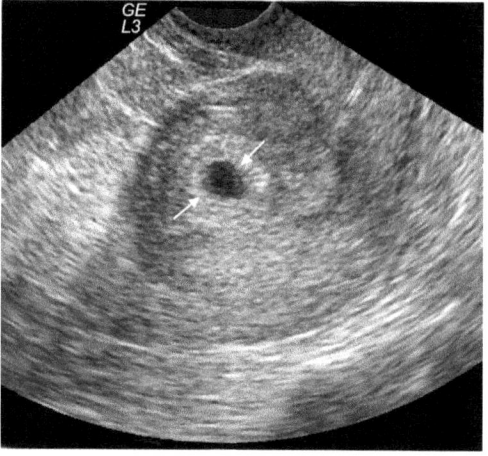

Fig. 8.42: Gestational sac.

*Q. How ultrasonographically can we differentiate a normal gestation sac from a pseudosac?*

Ans. Normal gestation sac is eccentric in position within the endometrium of fundus or body of the uterus. Pseudogestational sac is irregular in outline and usually located centrally in the uterus. The pseudosac remains empty and has no double decidual sign.

*Q. What is double decidual sign?*

**Ans.** Double decidual (Fig. 8.43) sign of gestational sac is due to the interface between the decidua and chorion. It appears as two distinct layers of the wall of the gestation sac.

*Q. At what early weeks of gestation the GS could be seen?*

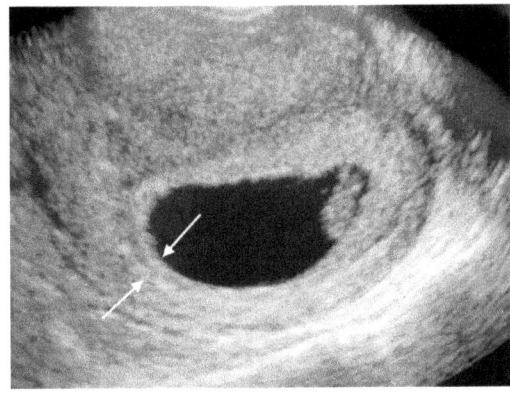

**Fig. 8.43:** Double decidual sign.

**Ans.** Gestation sac could be seen as early as 4.5–5 weeks period with the use of transvaginal ultrasonography.

*Q. How is the shape of the gestation sac?*

**Ans.** Normal gestation sac appears round in early weeks and gradually it becomes oval in shape.

*Q. What is the significance of the diagnosis of gestation sac?*

**Ans.** (a) Presence of an intrauterine gestational sac is a reliable evidence of intrauterine pregnancy.
(b) Presence of gestation sac outside the uterine cavity suggests ectopic pregnancy.
(c) Fetal gestational age could be estimated measuring the *mean sac diameter* (M3D)
(d) Abnormal size of the GS is an indication of abnormal outcome.

## Yolk Sac (Fig. 8.44)

*Q. When does yolk sac appear?*

**Ans.** Yolk sac (YS) is the first structure seen normally within the GS. Yolk sac is seen normally with transabdominal sonography (TAS) when the mean GS diameter is 10–15 mm. With the use of transvaginal sonography (TVS), yolk sac is seen with the mean sac diameter of 8 mm (5.5 weeks)

*Q. What are the significance(s) of the detection of yolk sac?*

**Ans.** (a) Presence of yolk sac is diagnostic of intrauterine pregnancy
(b) Presence of yolk sac differentiates an early intrauterine GS from a pseudo sac
(c) Number of yolk sacs and the number of amniotic sacs are the same.

*Q. What are the functions of the yolk sac?*

**Ans.** (a) It plays an important role in embryonic development by transfer of nutrients
(b) Fetal angiogenesis starts in the wall of the yolk sac
(c) Fetal hematopoiesis occurs in the yolk sac
(d) Primitive gut is formed from the dorsal wall of the yolk sac.

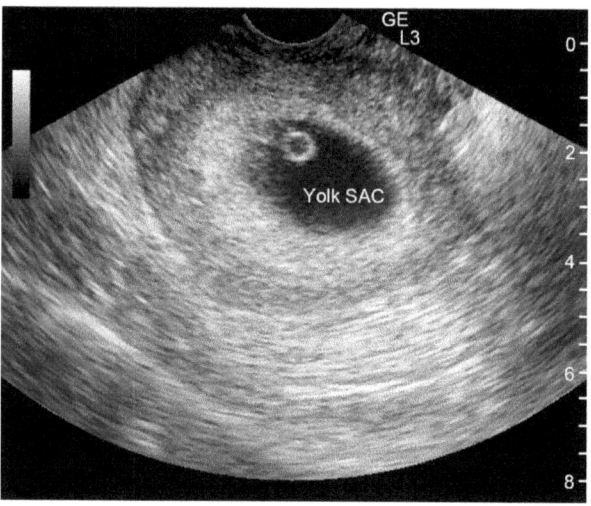

**Fig. 8.44:** Ultrasound showing yolk sac.

## Crown Rump Length (Fig. 8.45)

**Q.** *At what time of gestation the embryo appears?*

**Ans.** Embryo first appears adjacent to the yolk sac at 6 week of gestation.

**Q.** *How the CRL is measured?*

**Ans.** Crown rump length (CRL) is measured with caliper placed from the top of the head to the end of bottom (excluding the limbs).

**Q.** *What is the importance of CRL measurement?*

**Ans.** (a) Measurement of CRL in the first trimester can predict the fetal gestational age more accurately (± 5-7 days).
(b) Screening of aneuploidy is best done by late first trimester ultrasonography.

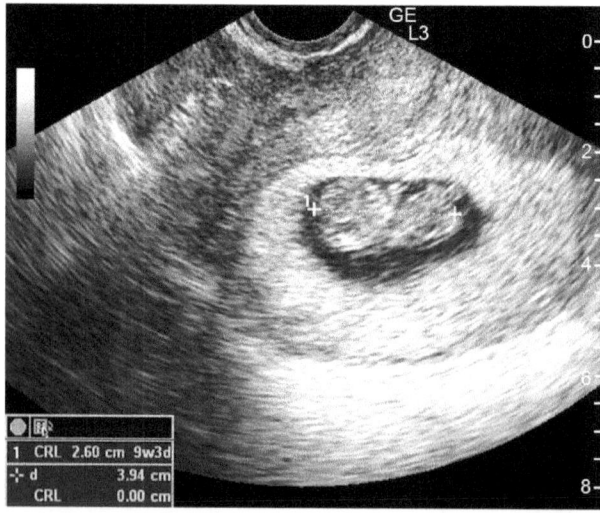

**Fig. 8.45:** Ultrasound showing crown rump length.

## Embryonic Cardiac Activity

**Q. What period of gestation embryonic heart begins to beat?**

Ans. Tubular embryonic heart begins to beat at 36-37th day of gestational age.

**Q. What is the rate of embryonic heart?**

Ans. Normal embryonic cardiac activity is >100 beats per minute.

**Q. What is the significance of detection of embryonic cardiac activity?**

Ans. Presence of cardiac activity indicates a viable embryo. Absence of embryonic cardiac activity is the most important factor to predict poor pregnancy outcome.

## Fetal Cardiac Activity

**Q. What is the normal fetal heart rate?**

Ans. Normal fetal heart rate varies between 100 and 160 beats per minute.

**Q. How early diagnosis of intrauterine fetal death (IUFD) could be made using sonography?**

Ans. Sonography can make the diagnosis of IUFD earliest. The evidences of IUFD are:
(a) Absence of fetal cardiac motion
(b) Absence of all other fetal movements during a careful observation period with sonography.
(c) Careful observation of absent fetal cardiac activity with real time sonography is a strong presumptive evidence of fetal death.

## Biparietal Diameter and Head Circumference (FIG. 8.46)

It is an ultrasonogram showing the fetal head. In this view, biparietal diameter (BPD) and head circumference (HC) had been measured as a part of fetal biometry (Fig. 8.46).

*Self-assessment:*

**Q. What is the importance of BPD measurement?**

Ans. BPD is most accurate for assessment of fetal gestational age from 14-24 weeks (variation ± 8 days).

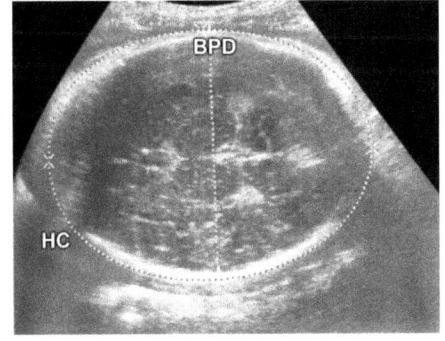

Fig. 8.46: BPD and HC.

**Q. How BPD is measured?**

Ans. It is measured from outer edge of proximal skull to the inner edge of the distal skull. It is measured at the level of thalami and cavum septum pellucidum.

**Q. What is the importance of HC?**

**Ans.** Head-shaped dolichocephaly (flattened) or (brachycephaly) rounded is known. HC is more reliable than BPD.

**Q. What other fetal parameters are measured to determine fetal gestational age?**

**Ans.** Femur length (FL) and abdominal circumference (AC). AC is measured at the level of fetal stomach and umbilical vein.

## Ultrasonogram Showing Two Fetal Heads in Twin Pregnancy (Fig. 8.47)

*Self assessment:*

**Q. How the diagnosis of twin pregnancy can be made clinically?**

**Ans.** See p. 87.

**Q. What other information can be obtained from sonography besides the confirmation of diagnosis?**

**Ans.** See p. 87.

**Q. What are the complications (maternal and fetal) of twin pregnancy?**

**Ans.** See p. 87.

**Q. Outline the management of twin pregnancy in labor.**

**Ans.** See p. 88.

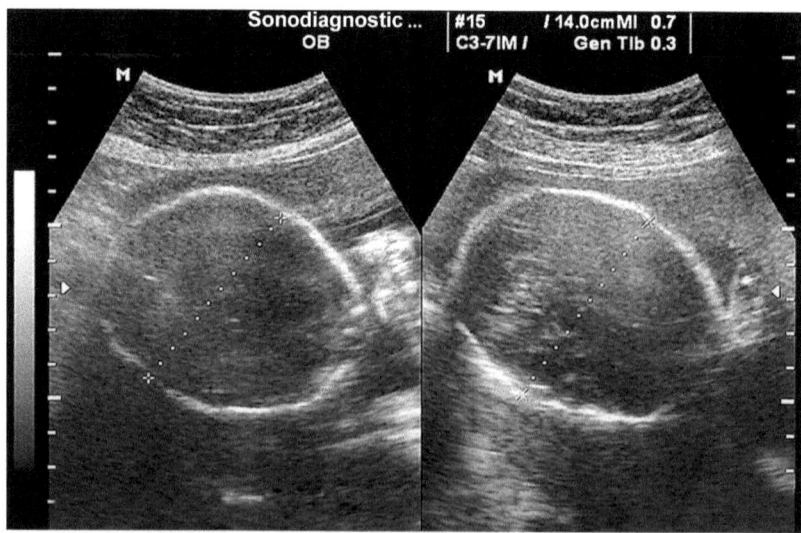

**Fig. 8.47:** Ultrasonogram showing two fetal heads in twin pregnancy.

## Ultrasonogram: Placenta Previa (Fig. 8.48)

It is an ultrasonogram showing placenta previa where the placenta is seen implanted over the anterior wall of the lower segment approaching the internal os.

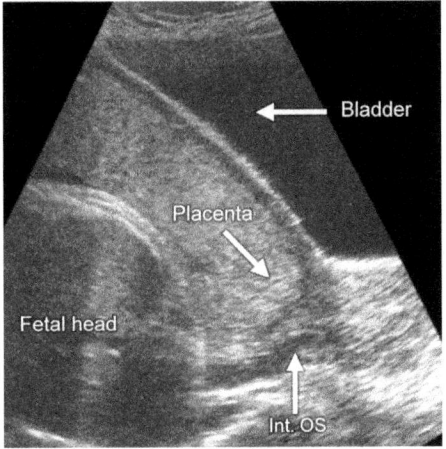

Fig. 8.48: Ultrasonogram: Showing placenta previa.

*Self-assessments:*

Q. *What are the common causes of antepartum hemorrhage?*

Ans. *See* p. 100.

Q. *What are the types of placenta previa?*

Ans. *See* p. 101.

Q. *How do you differentiate a case of placenta previa from abruptio placenta?*

Ans. *See* p. 103.

Q. *What are the complications of placenta previa?*

Ans. *See* p. 101.

Q. *How do you manage a case of placenta praevia?*

Ans. *See* p. 102.

## Ultrasonogram: Hydatidiform Mole (Figs. 8.49A and B)

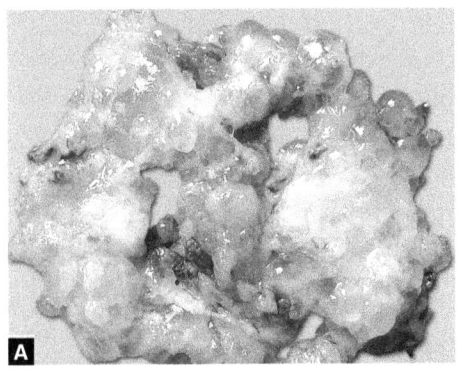
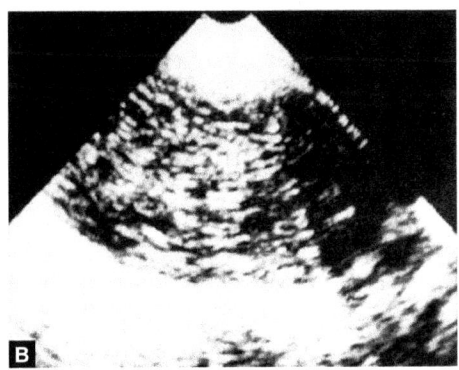

Figs. 8.49A and B: (A) Showing grape-like vesicles of varying sizes. These are the tissues of molar pregnancy; (B) An ultrasonogram showing snowstorm appearance of a molar pregnancy.

*Self-assessment:*

Q. *How a case of molar pregnancy commonly presents?*

Ans. *See* p. 423-424.

**Q. What are the complications of a molar pregnancy?**

Ans. Hemorrhage, shock, pre-eclampsia, sepsis, acute pulmonary insufficiency and rarely coagulation failure. The late complications are development of persistent trophoblastic neoplasia and choriocarcinoma.

**Q. How do you manage a case of hydatidiform mole?**

Ans. Principles of management are—(a) Supportive therapy (blood transfusion), (b) Suction evacuation of the uterus and (c) Follow-up (p. 424-426).

## Doppler (Ultrasound) Fetal Monitor—(A) Device and (B) in use (Figs. 8.50A and B)

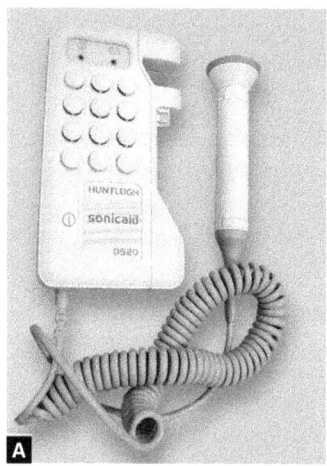
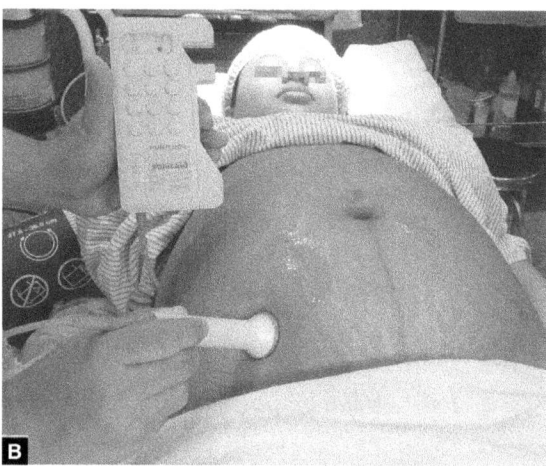

**Figs. 8.50A and B:** Doppler (ultrasound) fetal monitor is being used.

*Self-assessment:*

**Q. Earliest at what weeks the FHS could be detected with a doppler.**

Ans. Using Doppler ultrasound fetal cardiac motion could be detected as early as 7th week of pregnancy. FHS is heard using a hand held Doppler at around 10th week of pregnancy.

**Q. What are the other alternatives when FHS is not audible with a stethoscope?**

Ans. (a) Hand held Doppler, (b) CTG, (c) Ultrasound for cardiac motion.

**Q. What are the advantages of EFM over the clinical?**

Ans. See p. 229.

**Q. What are the causes of fetal bradycardia?**

Ans. See p. 230.

**Q. What are the characteristics of an abnormal CTG?**

Ans. See p. 230.

**Q. What other tests could be done when a CTG is abnormal?**

Ans. See p. 234.

## MAGNETIC RESONANCE IMAGING (MRI)

Magnetic resonance imaging (Fig. 8.51) is useful to obtain high soft tissue contrast and for acquisition of images in different planes. MRI could be used for assessment of: **A. Fetal:** Anatomy survey, fetal biometry and also as a complement to sonography. **B. Maternal:** Cerebral vascular flow study, evaluation of placenta previa and accreta.

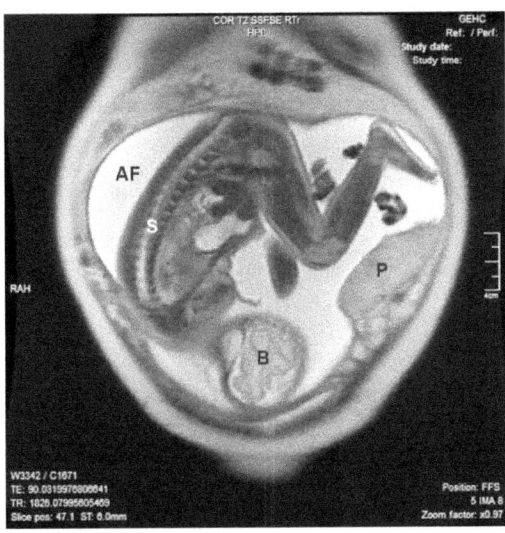

Fig. 8.51: A sagital balanced M R image of a fetus at 31 weeks of gestation (AF = amniotic fluid; S = spine; P = placenta; B = brain).

**Q. Is MRI safe in pregnancy?**

**Ans.** MRI has got no ionizing radiation effect. MRI studies during pregnancy are found safe to the fetus and mother.

**Q. Is there any complications of MRI?**

**Ans.** MRI needs a higher level of cooperation from the patient. The patient is placed on a table that goes into a space surrounded by the magnet. Claustrophobia has been observed in about 5% of patients. Movement of the fetus during MR sequence may distort the images.

**Q. What are the contraindications of MR imaging ?**

**Ans.** Common contraindications are :
(a) Cardiac pacemaker
(b) Ocular metallic foreign body
(c) Cochlear prosthesis
(d) Magnetic dental implants.

# DRUGS IN OBSTETRICS

**Chapter Objectives**

**Good knowledge and understanding with the effects on mother and fetus:**
- Rational therapy in relation to period of gestation (safety issues)
- Drug dose, route of administration and duration
- Response evaluation
- Adverse effects

## OXYTOCICS

Oxytocics or ecbolics are the drugs that stimulate myometrial contractions. Drugs belonging to this group are (Fig. 8.52):
- Oxytocin
- Methylergometrine (methergin)
- Prostaglandins: $PGE_1$, $PGE_2$, $PGF_{2\alpha}$
- Carbetocin.

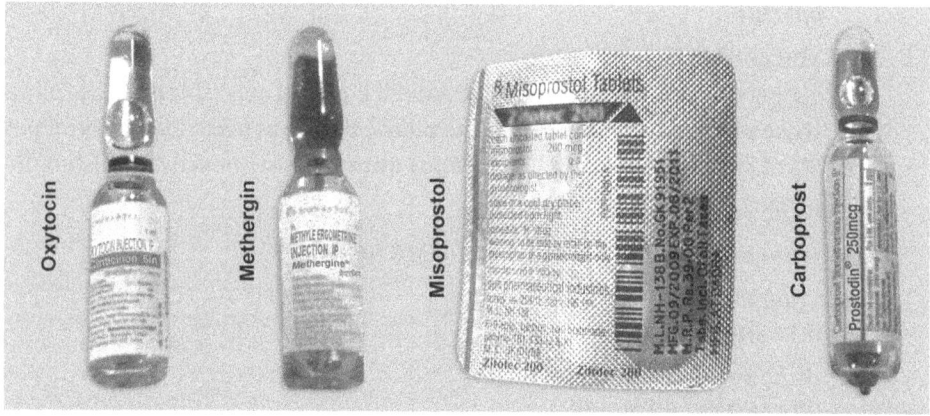

Fig. 8.52: Oxytocics: Oxytocin, methergin, misoprostol ($PGE_1$); carboprost ($PGF_2\alpha$), prostin ($PGE_2$).

## Oxytocin

Oxytocin is a nonapeptide. It stimulates myometrial contractions during pregnancy, labor and puerperium.

Storage: Injection—refrigerate 2°–8°C. Stable for 3 months at room temperature 15°–25°C.

Synthetic oxytocin—syntocinon is commonly used. (One ampule containing 5 IU/mL).

**Mode of administration:** IV—slow, IV infusion, and IM

**Onset of action:** IV—almost immediate, IM: 3-5 minutes.

**Duration of action:** IV—20 minutes to 1 hour. IM: 2-3 hours.

**Indications of use:**

**Pregnancy:**
(a) Early:
- To accelerate abortion process (inevitable and missed)
- To expedite to expulsion of molar pregnancy
- To control bleeding following evacuation of the products of conception from the uterus.

(b) Late: To induce labor.
(c) Labor: Active management of third stage of labor.
(d) Postpartum: To control (prophylactic) PPH.

> **Q. What are the side effects and dangers of oxytocin use?**
>
> **Ans. Maternal:** Arrhythmia, headache, nausea, vomiting, uterine hyperstimulation, uterine rupture and water intoxication.
> **Fetal:** Fetal distress, hypoxia and fetal death.
> **Rare side effects are:** Hyponatremia, DIC, anaphylactoid reactions (shock).
> **Contraindications:** Grand multipara, contracted pelvis, malpresentation, fetal distress and obstructed labor.
>
> **Q. What are the precautions of use?**
>
> **Ans.** Monitoring of fetomaternal conditions are important. Water intoxication due to large infusion volumes and electrolyte imbalance are to be avoided. Variable speed infusion pump is preferred.
>
> **Q. What is carbetocin? What are its contraindications and side effects?**
>
> **Ans. Carbetocin:** It is a longer acting oxytocin derivative.
> **Indications:** Prevention of PPH due to uterine atony following cesarean delivery.
> **Dose:** It is given by slow IV injection. 100 µg in 1 mL is for 1 dose. It is given over 1 minute.
> **Contraindications:** Pre-eclampsia, elampsia and epilepsy.
> **Side effects:** Chills, chest pain, hot flush, tachycardia, tremor, and hypotension. It is avoided in cases with hepatic and renal impairment.

## Methergin (Methylergometrine)

It is a semisynthetic ergot alkaloid that acts directly on the myometrium. Methergin stimulates powerful (tetanic) uterine contractions. (1 ampoule = 0.2 mg/mL).

**Routes of administration:** IM, IV and per oral

**Onset of action:** IV—40 to 60 seconds; IM—6-7 minutes; oral—10 minutes

**Duration of action:** 3 hours.

**Indications of use:**
(a) In the active management of third stage of labor.
(b) To control atonic postpartum hemorrhage.

(c) To control hemorrhage following evacuation operation in cases with incomplete/missed abortion or molar pregnancy.

**Hazards:**
(a) Nausea and vomiting
(b) Arrhythmias, bradycardia, chest pain, vasoconstriction, pulmonary edema, and hypertension.
(c) Rise in blood pressure, myocardial infarction and bronchospasm.

**Contraindications of use:**
(1) In twin pregnancy until the second baby is delivered
(2) Organic heart disease—may cause heart failure
(3) Severe preeclampsia
(4) Eclampsia
(5) Rh-negative mother
(6) Sepsis
(7) Vascular disease, severe cardiac disease
(8) Labor in the process of:
   (i) Induction
   (ii) First and second stage.

**Q. What are the side effects of methylergometrine?**

Ans.
- Nausea
- Tinitus
- Vasoconstriction
- Vomiting
- Palpitation
- Myocardial infarction
- Headache
- Transient hypertension

**Q. What are the reasons that prophylactic ergometrine should not be given to all cases?**

Ans. *See* SAQ, p. 249.

**Q. What is syntometrine and what are the benefits of its use?**

Ans. Injection syntometrine is a combination of ergometrine 0.5 mg and oxytocin 5 IU/mL.

**Indications and dose:**
(a) In the active management of third stage of labor.
(b) Management of PPH due to uterine atony
(c) Hemorrhage following incomplete abortion

**Dose:** 1 mL. IM for one dose.

**Dose:** It is given by IM injection. It has the benefits of using the two drugs. Onset of action is quick due to oxytocin and the duration of action is longer due to ergometrine. It is can be used in the active management of third stage of labor.

**Q. How to monitor a woman in labor with oxytocin infusion for augmentation of labor?**

Ans. The important parameters of observation are: Partographic monitoring of labor is to be done:
(1) To record the rate of flow of oxytocin infusion (mIU/min).

(2) Uterine contractions per 10 minutes.
   **Uterine contractions:**
   (a) Number of contractions,
   (b) Duration of contractions (in seconds),
   (c) Intensity of contraction,
   (d) Period of relaxation.
(3) FHR monitoring by auscultation every 30 minutes or by continuous EFM
(4) Assessment of the progress of labor.
   (a) Dilation of the cervix,
   (b) Descent of the presenting part,
   (c) Station,
   (d) Position of the presenting part,
   (e) Color of the liquor.
(5) Any side effects or hazards of oxytocin use (*see* below).

# PROSTAGLANDINS (PGE$_1$, PGE$_2$, PGF$_{2\alpha}$)

**Use in obstetrics:**
(1) Induction of abortion: PGE$_1$, PGE$_2$
(2) Induction of labor: PGE$_1$, PGE$_2$
(3) Cervical ripening: PGE$_2$, PGE$_1$
(4) Management of atonic PPH: PGE$_1$, PGF$_{2\alpha}$ (See p. 108).

**Q. What are prostaglandins? What are the commonly used prostaglandins in obstetrics?**

**Ans.** Prostaglandins are the derivatives of prostanoic acid. Of the many varieties PGE$_2$, PGF$_2\alpha$, PGE$_1$, PGI$_2$ are commonly used in clinical obstetric practice.

**Q. What are the common indications for the use of prostaglandins in obstetrics?**

**Ans.** Common indications of use in obstetrics are:

| A. Early pregnancy | B. Late pregnancy |
|---|---|
| • Medical termination of pregnancy | • Ripening the cervix prior to induction of labor |
| • Induction of abortion (missed miscarriage) | • Induction of labor |
| • Termination of molar pregnancy | • Augmentation (acceleration) of labor |
| • Medical management of tubal ectopic pregnancy | • Management of atonic postpartum hemorrhage especially in a case unresponsive to oxytocin or ergometrine |

**Q. What PGs are commonly used obstetrics?**

**Ans.** Of the many varieties: PGE$_2$, PGF$_2\alpha$ and PGE$_1$ are commonly used in obstetrics.

**Q. What are the adverse effects with the use of prostaglandins?**

**Ans.** (a) Hypersensitivity to the compound
(b) Uterine scar rupture ($PGE_1$)
(c) Deterioration of organ functions in the presence of active cardiac, pulmonary, renal or hepatic disease
(d) Hypotension ($PGE_2$)
(e) Bronchospasm ($PGF_2\alpha$)

**Q. What are the different preparations of prostaglndins available for clinical use?**

**Ans.** $PGF_2\alpha$: Used by parenteral route
**Methyl analogue of $PGF_2\alpha$ (carboprost,** containing 250 µg/mL).

**Q. What is the dose schedule for $PGF_2\alpha$?**

**Ans. Dose:** Carboprost ($PGF_2\alpha$) is given by deep intramuscular injection, 250 µg. It is repeated if required at intervals every 15 to 90 minutes. Total 8 doses (2 mg) maximum could be given.
Medicinal form available: Injection Carboprost trometamol 250 µg. deep IM.

**Q. What are the side effects of $PGF_2\alpha$?**

**Ans.** Side effects of $PGF_2\alpha$ (Carboprost tromethamine):
- Nausea
- Vomiting
- Diarrhea
- Hyperthermia
- Bronchospasm
- Pain at the injection site
- Flushing
- Cardiovascular collapse
- Headache
- Pulmonary edema.

**Obstetric Complications**
(a) Cervical tears (bucket handle), lacerations
(b) Hyperstimulation of the uterus
(c) Meconium stained liquor
(d) Fetal distress, low Apgar scores
(e) Rupture of uterus.

**Q. What are the contraindication for the use of $PGF_2\alpha$?**

**Ans.** (a) Untreated pelvic infection
(b) Cardiac, renal, pulmonary, hepatic disease
(c) Bronchial asthma
(d) Scarred uterus.

## Prostaglandin $E_2$ (Prostin $E_2$)

Prostaglandin $E_2$ is widely used. It has got less side effects also.

**Q. What are the different preparations available for prostaglandin $E_2$?**

**Ans.** (a) **Vaginal tablet:** It contains 3 mg of dinoprostone (Prostin $E_2$). It is inserted in the prosterior fornix followed by 3 mg after 6–8 hours (maximum 6 mg).

(b) **Vaginal pessary (Propess):** It is available with a retrieval device so that it could be taken out if needed. The pessary releases dinoprostone approximately 5 mg over 12 hours. It is removed when cervical ripening is adequate. It is to be removed 30 minutes before, if oxytocin is to be used. Dose not to be repeated.

(c) **Dinoprostone gel (Prostin $E_2$ gel):** 500 µg is inserted into the cervical canal below the level of internal OS. It can also be inserted as $PGE_2$ gel, 1 mg high up in the posterior fornix for induction of labor. It may be repeated after 6 hours, if needed.

Prostin $E_2$ vaginal gel and vaginal tablets are not bioequivalent.

**Cautions of use:** History of asthma, glaucoma, scarred uterus, cardiac, hepatic or renal impairment.

**Contraindications:** Unexplained vaginal bleeding during pregnancy, scarred uterus, grand multipara, multiple pregnancy, placenta previa, untreated pelvic infection, CPD, ruptured membranes, active cardiac and pulmonary disease.

**Side effects**
- Nausea
- Vomiting
- Diarrhea
- Uterine hypertonus
- Amniotic fluid embolism
- Fetal distress
- Bronchospasm
- Uterine rupture
- Shivering
- Pyrexia (temporary)
- Abruptio placenta
- Cardiac arrest
- DIC

## Prostaglandin $E_1$ (misoprostol)

Misoprostol is the methyl ester of $PGE_1$. Primarily, it has been used for peptic ulcer disease.

Q. *What are the indications of use of $PGE_1$?*

Ans. Indications of use during:

(A) **Early pregnancy**
(1) Medical termination of pregnancy: (a) First trimester, (b) Second trimester.
(2) Incomplete abortion
(3) Missed abortion.

(b) **Late pregnancy (Off level: Unlicensed use)**
(1) Ripening of cervix
(2) Induction of labor.

(c) **Labor**
(1) Augmentation of labor
(2) Active management of third stage of labor
(3) Management of severe postpartum hemorrhage unresponsive to oxytocin and ergometrine.

(d) **Routes of administration**
Misoprostol can be used with all the following routes:
(a) Oral
(b) Sublingual
(c) Buccal

(d) Vaginal
(e) Rectal.

Medicinal forms: Misoprostol tablets: 25 µg, 50 µg, 100 µg or 400 µg per tablet is available.

**Q. What is the dose schedule of misoprostol?**

**Ans.** Dose schedule varies depending upon the indication of use and also the route:

(a) For MTP in the first trimester, it is given 400 µg to 800 µg vaginally (preferably) or orally.
(b) MTP in the second trimester: 400 µg to 800 µg given vaginally (high bioavailability).
(c) For abortion process—200 µg to 400 µg vaginally
(d) For ripening of the cervix induction of labor: 25 µg to 50 µg vaginally or orally at interval of 3-6 hours.
(e) For management of third stage of labor (AMTSL): 600 µg tablets is given orally or rectally. It is convenient for women with home delivery. It can be given by a community health worker.
(f) For atomic PPH, it is given rectally 600 µg to 1,000 µg.

**Q. What are the side effects its use?**

**Ans.** Common side effects are: Nausea, vomiting diarrhea, chills, shivering, hyperthermia.

**Worse side effects are:**
(a) Uterine hyperstimulation (tachysystole)
(b) Fetal heart rate abnormally
(c) Meconium passage in the liquor
(d) Rupture uterus (rare).

**Q. What are the contraindications for the use of misoprostol?**

**Ans.** (a) Prior history of cesarean delivery
(b) Any other scar in the uterus (myomectomy).

**Q. How to make the selection of an appropriate oxytocic in obstetrics?**

**Ans.** All the oxytocics have got their place in obstetrics:

(1) To **control hemorrhage** following delivery: Atomic PPH or abortion.
   (a) **Methylergometrine** is a life-saving drug.
   (b) In a **refractory case of atomic PPH: $PGF_2\alpha$** (IM/Intramyometrial).
   (c) **$PGE_1$ (misoprostol)** 1,000 mg (rectal) is effective especially for home delivery to prevent PPH.
(2) **Induction of labor:**
   (a) With favorable preinduction cervical (Bishop) score: Either oxytocin or prostaglandin ($PGE_2$ gel/$PGE_1$ tablet).
   (b) Cervical score unfavorable especially in cases with IUFD, early weeks of gestation: Prostaglandins ($PGE_2$, $PGE_1$) have got distinct advantages over oxytocin. Misoprostol has certain advantages over $PGE_2$.

(3) **Augmentation or acceleration of labor**: Oxytocin is commonly used.
(4) **Induction of abortion**: Prostaglandins (misoprostol-PGE$_1$) is superior over oxytocin. However, oxytocin may supplement the effects of PGs in the process.
(5) **In the active management of third stage of labor (AMTSL):**
   (a) Oxytocin 10 IU IM is recommended (WHO), immediately following the delivery of the baby. Side effects are less.
   (b) Methylergometrine is an alternative in a selective case (when oxytocin is not available). It has more side effects.
   (c) Prostaglandin E$_1$ (misoprostol) 600 µg orally or rectally could be given in a case with home delivery.
   (d) Injection syntometrine (injection ergometrine 0.5 mg and oxytocin 5 units/mL) could be given IM following delivery of the baby.

**Q. What are the advantages of misoprostol on the other oxytocics?**

**Ans.** Misoprostol PGE$_1$ has the following superiority over the others:
(a) It is cheap
(b) Stable at room temperature (no refrigeration needed)
(c) It has long shelf-life
(d) Ease of administration: Oral, sublingual, rectal, vaginal (see above)
(e) No need of any injection
(f) Less side effects (less bronchospasm)
(g) Failure of induction is less
(h) Induction delivery interval is short
(i) Patient many remain ambulatory following its use
(j) More effective than oxytocin and dinoprostone for induction of labor.

# ANTIHYPERTENSIVES

## Labetalol

It is used as an antihypertensive in pregnancy. It works as a combined α and β adrenergic receptor blocking agent. It has mild α and predominant β-adrenergic receptor blocking actions. Labetalol blocks the β adrenoreceptors in the heart and in addition, it has an arteriolar vasodilating action. It lowers the peripheral vascular resistance.

It is also used parenterally for the control of hypertensive crises in pregnancy.

**Dose:**
- Orally 100 mg TID; may be increased maximum up to 2.4 g daily.
- IV injection (hypertensive crisis): 20–40 mg IV over at least 1 minute. It may be repeated at every 10–15 minutes, until the desired effect is observed, maximum up to 200 mg.

**Side effects:** Postural hypotension, tremors, headache, bronchospasm, congestive cardiac failure. *Efficacy and safety* with short-term use appear equal to methyldopa.

**Contraindications and precautions:** Asthma, cardiac failure, hepatic disorders and bradycardia. Labetalol may block the signs of acute hypoglycemia.

## Methyldopa

It works as a central and peripheral antiadrenergic drug. Once in the brain, it is converted into α-methylnorepinephrine by the enzyme dopa decarboxylase. α-methylnorepinephrine lowers arterial blood pressure through activation of $\alpha_2$-adrenergic receptors and also by lowered sympathetic outflow. It is effective and is proved to be safe both for the mother and fetus.

**Dose:** It is given orally 250 mg, 2–3 times daily. Dose may be increased to a maximum 3 g daily in divided doses.

**Side effects:** Maternal: dry mouth, postural hypotension, sedation, bradycardia, headache, depression, hepatitis, hemolytic anemia, mild psychosis, constipation, sleep disturbances, hallucinations.

**Fetal:** Intestinal ileus, bradycardia. Breastfeeding should be avoided as it is present in breast milk.

**Contraindications and precaution:** Hepatic disorders, psychic patients, congestive cardiac failure and postpartum depression.

## Nifedipine (calcium cannel blocker)

It causes direct arteriolar vasodilatation.

**Dose:** 5 to 10 mg three times a day, maximum may be 60 mg/day.

**Side effects:** Flushing, hypotension, tachycardia, headache, palpitation and inhibition of labor.

**Caution:** Simultaneous use of $MgSO_4$ due to synergistic effect.

## Hydralazine

It works by peripheral vasodilatation as it relaxes the arterial smooth muscle. It is used as an adjunct to other agent like methyldopa or β blockers. It increases the cardiac output and renal blood flow. It is prescribed for cases with moderate-to-severe hypertension (adjunct therapy) and in cases with hypertensive crisis in pregnancy.

**Dose:** Orally—25 mg twice daily, may be increased maximum up to 100 mg a day.

**Intravascular (IV):** 5–10 mg diluted with 10 mL normal saline may be repeated after 20–30 minutes maximum up to 20 mg.

**Side effects:**

**Maternal:** Rashes, tachycardia, palpitation, hypotension, flushing, arrhythmia, lupus like syndrome (following long-term therapy), thrombocytopenia.

**Fetal:** Reasonably safe.

**Neonatal:** Thrombocytopenia.

**Contraindications and precautions:** Severe tachycardia, systemic lupus erythematosus, high output failure, hepatic and renal impairment, breastfeeding (harmful effects are not known but the infant need to be monitored for the risk of neonatal thrombocytopenia to monitor infant).

## ANTICOAGULANTS

### Heparin

It inhibits the action of thrombin. It enhances the action of antithrombin III, and increases factor Xa inhibitor.

It is used for the initial treatment of deep vein thrombosis (DVT) and pulmonary embolism (PE).

**As prophylaxis,** it is used in high-risk patients, patients undergoing surgical procedures (cesarean section, hysterectomy).

**Dose:** Loading dose of 5,000–10,000 units followed by continuous IV infusion of 15–25 units/kg/h (with monitoring).

**Pregnancy:** 5,000–10,000 units SC every 12 hours (with monitoring).

### Low Molecular Weight Heparin

Low molecular weight heparin (LMWHs) (Enoxaparin) are effective and safe as unfractionated heparin. They have longer duration of action. They are used with single daily SC injection. Prophylactic regimen of LMWH does not need monitoring.

Dalteparin sodium (Fragmin): Daily SC injection, 200 units/kg body weight maximum up to 18,000 units or enoxaparin sodium-SC injection: 40 mg twice daily based on early pregnancy body weight (up to 50 kg).

**Side effects: Maternal**—hemorrhage, thrombocytopenia, hyperkalemia, osteoporosis (prolonged use) and alopecia.

**Fetal:** Does not cross the placenta, and these drugs are not teratogenic

**Contraindications and precautions:** Hemorrhagic disorders, thrombocytopenia, peptic ulcer, severe hypertension, recent cerebral hemorrhage, hepatic and renal impairment.

**Antidote:** Protamine sulfate.

## ANTICONVULSANTS

Commonly used anticonvulsants are: Magnesium sulfate ($MgSO_4$), diazepam and phenytoin.

### Magnesium sulfate ($MgSO_4$, $7H_2O$)

**Magnesium sulfate:** It is the drug of choice in the management of eclampsia (See SAQ, p. 236). It is a membrane stabilizer and neuroprotector. It is given IV or IM. Monitoring of drug dose is simple.

Magnesium sulfate is continued for 24 hours after the last seizure or delivery whichever is later. Therapeutic level of serum Mg is 4–7 mEq/L. Antidote to $MgSO_4$ toxicity is—injection calcium gluconate 10 mL (10%) to be given slow IV.

**Pharmacology:** Magnesium (Mg) is essential mineral present mostly in the intracellular compartment. It decreases release of acetylcholine at the neuromuscular junction and also reduces the sensitivity of motor end plate to acetylcholine. Magnesium has got its, depressant effects on CNS and respiratory system. These effects are antagonized by calcium. Magnesium causes vasodilation. When used in pregnancy, magnesium reduces uterine vascular resistance and increases the uteroplacental blood flow. This is beneficial to the mother as it reduces the systemic arterial pressure. It is also beneficial to the fetus to increase the fetoplacental blood circulation.

### Uses of $MgSO_4, 7H_2O$:
(a) **Prevention and control of seizures in obstetrics**—eclampsia, severe pre-eclampsia (prophylactic use).
(b) **Tocolysis** (preterm labor).
(c) **Neuroprotector:** It is given to mother to prevent neonatal cerebral palsy in cases with preterm labor (<34 weeks) and birth.

**Dose schedule:** Eclampsia, preeclampsia, tocolysis.
(a) **Intramuscular dose schedule:**
  - $MgSO_4$ 4 g 20% solution IV slowly (1 g/minute)
  - $MgSO_4$, 10 g 50% solution; 5 g deep IM in the upper and outer quadrant of each buttock.
  - $MgSO_4$ 5 g 50% solution deep IM every 4 hours on alternate buttock.
  - In case of recurrence of fits: $MgSO_4$ 2 g IV 20% solution slowly (at the rate of 1 g/min).
(b) **Intravenous dose schedule:**
  - 4 g diluted in 100 mL of normal saline given over 15–20 minutes
  - 1–2 g/h in 100 mL of normal saline. Controlled infusion device (infusion pump) is preferred.
  - Monitor for magnesium toxicity.
(c) **Tocolysis:** Dose schedule the same as that in eclampsia.
(d) **Neuroprotection:** Dose schedule is the same as used in the management of eclampsia.
(e) **Arrhythmias, hypomagnesemia:**
  - IV—10 mg/kg (20% solution) of $MgSO_4$ over 15–20 minutes then IV infusion 1 g/h. Controlled infusion device (infusion pump) is preferred.
  - IM—10 mg/kg every 6 hours four doses.

*Plasma levels of $MgSO_4$:*
  - Normal plasma level: 1.5–2.2 mEq/L
  - Therapeutic plasma level: 4–6 mEq/L
  - Magnesium is eliminated via the kidneys.
  Supplied as injection 10% (0.8 mEq/100 mg/mL), 50% (4 mEq/500 mg/mL).

**Pharmacokinetics:**

| | |
|---|---|
| Onset of action: | IV: Immediate |
| | IM: Within an hour |
| Peak effect: | IV: Few minutes |
| | IM: 1–3 hours |

Duration of action: IV: 30 minutes
IM: 3–4 hours.

**Drug interaction:**
(a) It potentiates the effects of both depolarizing and nondepolarizing group of muscle relaxants.
(b) Potentiates the CNS depressant effects of sedatives, narcotics, volatile anesthetics.

**Monitoring parameters of $MgSO_4$:**
- Respiratory rate: 16/min
- Urine output: 30 mL/h
- Presence of deep tendon reflexes (Patellar reflex)
- Serum level of magnesium should be <10 mEq/L.

**Toxicity of magnesium:**
(a) Respiratory depression
(b) Neuromuscular paralysis
(c) Renal suppression.

**Precautions of use and management of magnesium toxicity:**
- Life-threatening hypermagnesemia:
  - Calcium gluconate 1 g IV (10 mL—10%)
  - Fluid loading and forced diuresis.
- Periodic measuring of plasma magnesium level in selected cases besides clinical monitoring (*see* above). Knee jerk reflex to be tested before each dose of magnesium sulfate. Repeat dose should be withheld when knee jerks are absent.
- Magnesium is contraindicated in patients with—a) heart block and b) myasthenia gravis.

**Side effects/toxicity of magnesium sulfate**
- Cardiovascular:
  - Hypotension
  - Heart block
  - Circulatory collapse.
- CNS: Depressed reflexes; flaccid paralysis
- Pulmonary: Respiratory paralysis
- Metabolic hypocalcemia
- Others: Flushing, sweating.

> **Q. Magnesium toxicity resulting in maternal death is rare.**
> **Ans.** $MgSO_4$ is the drug of choice to treat and prevent subsequent convulsion in eclampsia. Recurrence of fits following $MgSO_4$ therapy is only 10%.
> In these cases, bolus of 2 g of magnesium sulfate can be given IV over 3–5 minutes.
> Magnesium toxicity should be considered in those women who do not regain consciousness. Compared to the other drugs (diazepam, phenytoin

and lytic cocktail) MgSO$_4$ was associated with significantly lower rate of recurrent seizures (9.4% versus 23.1%) and lower rate of maternal deaths (3% versus 4.8%).

**Q. How to adjust the dose and the percentage concentration of MgSO$_4$?**

**Ans.** 1 ampoule of injection MgSO$_4$ 50% contains 1 g of MgSO$_4$ in 2 mL. For IV injection concentration of MgSO$_4$ should not exceed 20%. To make it 20%, 1 part of magnesium sulfate injection 50%, need to be diluted with at least 1.5 parts of water for injection.

4 g magnesium sulphate is in 8 mL.

To make it 20% another 1.5 parts of water for injection is to be added,
e.g.: {8 mL + (8×1.5 = 12 mL) = 20 mL}.

It is convenient to use a 20 mL syringe and to draw initially the 4 ampoule of MgSO$_4$ (8 mL) and the rest is filled up by water injection to make it 20% in 20 mL. For IM injections 50% concentration does not need any change.

## TOCOLYTIC DRUGS

Tocolytics are drugs that inhibit uterine contractions. Tocolytics are commonly used in the management of preterm labor. The commonly used drugs are—calcium channel blockers (nifedipine), magnesium sulfate, betamimetics (ritodrine) or oxytocin antagonists (atosiban).

## Betamimetics

Ritodrine is given as IV infusion. Isoxsuprine (duvadilan) can be given orally or as IV infusion. Drugs are effective for short-term benefit.

**Side effects:** Headache, palpitation, tachycardia and pulmonary edema, hyperglycemia, hypokalemia.

## Calcium Channel antagonists (Nifedipine, Nicardipine)

**Nifedipine:** These drugs interfere with the inward displacement of calcium ions through the cell membranes. These drugs influence the myocardial cells and the cells of the vascular smooth muscle. Nifedipine relaxes the vascular smooth muscles and dilates the coronary and peripheral arteries. It is used for the management of hypertension, hypertensive crises as well as for tocolysis.

**Dose: Oral**—10–20 mg every 4–6 hours.

**Side effects:** Headache, flushing, tachycardia, palpitation, nausea, fall in blood pressure, visual disturbances.

**Contraindication and precautions:** Aortic stenosis, ischemic chest pain, hypotension, poor cardiac reserve, diabetes mellitus, arrhythmias, hyperthyroidism.

**SPACE FOR NOTES**

CHAPTER 9

# Maternal Health: India and Global Scenario

**Chapter Objectives**

**To demonstrate knowlege and of understanding of:**
- MMR and targets to reduce maternal deaths
- SDGs, MDGs and their targets
- NHM, RCH-II and JSSK guidelines on maternal and newborn care

- ❖ Maternal Mortality Ratio (MMR), Maternal Mortality Rate and Lifetime Risk     339
- ❖ Sustainable Development Goals (SDG 3)     344
- ❖ Millennium Development Goals (MDG 4 and 5) and Sustainable Development Goals (SDGS)     345
- ❖ National Health Mission (NHM) and Reproductive and Child Health-II (RCH−II)     348
- ❖ Janani Shishu Suraksha Karyakram (JSSK) a Government of India (GOI) Scheme     350
- ❖ Maternal Health Beyond 2030     357

## MATERNAL MORTALITY RATIO, MATERNAL MORTALITY RATE AND LIFETIME RISK

### Levels of Maternal Mortality Ratio by Regions

| Region | MMR per 100,000 live births | Maternal mortality rate | Lifetime risk | % to total maternal deaths |
|---|---|---|---|---|
| India | 130 | 8.8 | 0.3% | 100.0 |
| EAG and Assam | 188 | 16 | 0.67% | 52.5 |
| South (subtotal) | 77 | 4.7 | 0.2% | 21.5 |
| Other (subtotal) | 93 | 5.4 | 0.2% | 26 |

**EAG and Assam, southern subtotal, other subtotal, and India:** 2014–2016
(EAG: Empowered Action Group States and Assam)

### Levels of Maternal Mortality Ratio, 1997–2016

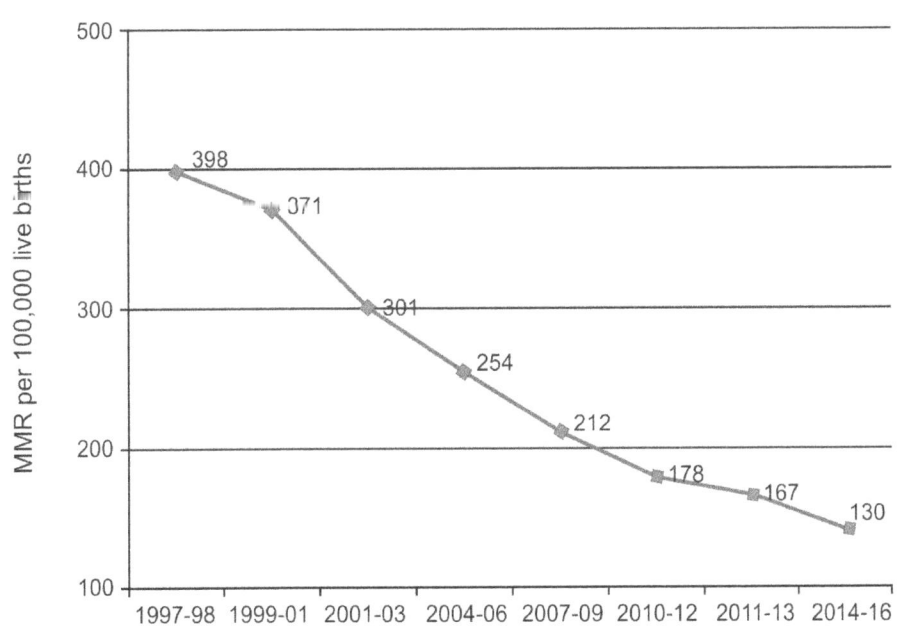

(RGI: Register General of India, SRS: Sample Registration System)

## Percentage of Total Maternal Deaths in India, 2014–2016

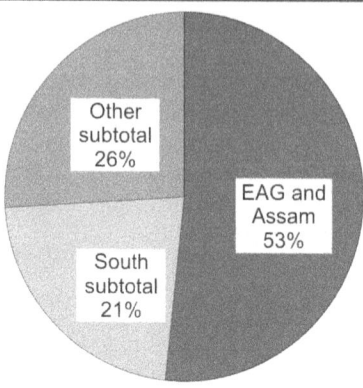

Maternal mortality and neonatal death matter of great concern worldwide. Maternal death is a strong indicator of the quality of healthcare delivery system for any country.

## Statewise Maternal Mortality Ratio in India (SRS 2014–2016)

| India 130/100,000 Live births | | | | | |
|---|---|---|---|---|---|
| States in India that have reached the MDG target and the states that are in close proximity to MDG are as below: | | | | | |
| Kerala | Maharashtra | Tamil Nadu | Andhra Pradesh | Telengana | Gujarat |
| 46 | 61 | 66 | 74 | 81 | 91 |
| West Bengal | Punjab | Madhya pradesh | Odisha | Uttar pradesh | Assam |
| 101 | 122 | 173 | 180 | 201 | 237 |

## Global Estimates of the Causes of Maternal Deaths (WHO: 2014—2016)

| Causes | Percentage (%) |
|---|---|
| • Hemorrhage | 27% |
| • Hypertension | 14% |
| • Sepsis | 11% |
| • Unsafe abortion | 8% |
| • Embolism | 3% |
| • Obstructed labor | 9% |
| • Other direct | 6% |
| • Indirect causes | 28% |

**NB:** Hemorrhage and hypertension account for more than half (53%) of all maternal deaths

## Global Causes of Deaths Among Children Ages 0–59 Months (WHO)

| Neonatal (41%) | | Postneonatal (59%) | |
|---|---|---|---|
| Causes | Percentage (%) | Causes | Percentage (%) |
| • Preterm | 12 | • Pneumonia | 14 |
| • Birth asphyxia | 9 | • Infections | 9 |
| • Sepsis | 6 | • Non-communicable diseases | 4 |
| • Pneumonia | 4 | | |
| • Congenital | 3 | • Meningitis | 2 |
| • Tetanus | 1 | • Pertussis | 2 |
| • Diarrhea | 1 | • AIDS | 2 |
| • Other neonatal | 5 | • Malaria | 8 |
| | | • Injury | 3 |
| | | • Measles | 1 |
| | | • Diarrhea | 14 |

**Magnitude of the problem:** Globally, there is an estimated 3,03,000 maternal deaths in 2015. The MMR is 216 per 1,00,000 live births for 183 countries. Lifetime risk is 1 in 180. Developing region accounted for approximately 99% (3,02,000) of the estimated total maternal deaths in 2015. Sub-Saharan Africa accounted alone for approximately 66% (2,01,000) followed by Southern Asia (66,000).

*For every one woman that dies, another 20 women suffer some serious and/or life-long disability (morbidity).*

**Maternal health in India:** Currently maternal mortality in India is 130 per 100,000 live births (SRS: 2014-2016). India is committed to meet the MDG 5 target of less than 100 deaths per 100,000 live births by the year 2015.

In India, approximately 22% of birth takes place at home and of these about 5.7% of births are attended by a skilled person. Presence of an SBA at every birth, along with availability of an effective referral system, can reduce maternal morbidity and mortality to a considerable extent.

Evidence-based practices have demonstrated that presence of skilled birth attendant (SBA) can effectively reduce maternal mortality.

**Government of India pointed out three types of delays** that results in an increase in maternal mortality and morbidity.

**Delay – I:** **Delay in recognizing the problem and deciding to seek care** (Lack of birth preparedness).

**Delay – II:** **Delay in reaching the health facility** (due to nonavailability of transport, referral facility, lack of complication readiness).

**Delay – III:** **Delay in receiving treatment** at the center (due to unequipped health facility, lack of trained personnel, medicines, blood, etc. lack of facility readiness).

### Goals and Targets to Reduce Maternal Deaths in India

| Organization | Year | Target of MMR reduction | Target year set |
|---|---|---|---|
| 1. National Population Policy (NPP) | 2000 | MMR <100 per 100,000 LB | 2010 |
| 2. National Health Policy (NHP) | 2002 | MMR <100 per 100,000 LB | 2010 |
| 3. National Rural Health Mission (NRHM) | 2005 | MMR <100 per 100,000 LB | 2012 |
| 4. 8th MDG 4 and 5 | 1990 | IMR <30 per 1,000 LB | 2015 |
| | | MMR reduction by 75% | |
| | | IMR reduction by 66% | |
| 5. Sustainable Developmental Goals | 2015 | MMR reduction $\leq$70 per 100,000 LB | 2030 |
| | | NMR $\leq$12 per 1,000 LB | |

**Q. How do you define a maternal death and what is maternal mortality ratio?**

**Ans.** Maternal death is defined as the death of a woman while pregnant or within 42 days of termination of pregnancy, irrespective of the duration and site of pregnancy, from any cause related to or aggravated by pregnancy or its management but not due to accidental or incidental causes.

**Maternal mortality ratio** is expressed in terms of maternal death per 100,000 live births. In India, MMR is 130 per 100,000 live births. In the developed world, it is below 12 per 100,000 live births. Globally, it is 216/100,000 LB.

**Maternal mortality rate** is defined as the number of maternal deaths to women in the ages 15–49 per 100,000 women in that age group.

**Lifetime risk** is defined as the probability that one woman of reproductive age (15–49 years) will die due to complications of pregnancy, childbirth or puerperium, assuming that chance of death is uniformly distributed across the entire reproductive span. In india, it is 0.3%.

## Maternal Near Miss

**Q. What do you understand by the term maternal near miss (MNM) or severe acute maternal morbidity (SAMM)?**

**Ans.** MNM or SAMM is understood in simpler term in this way.

Pregnancy labor/delivery, puerperium
⇩
Complications
⇩
Maternal morbidity due to the complications of pregnancy, labor or puerperium
⇩
Severe morbidity
⇩
Severe life-threatening morbidity
⇩
Management

| **Maternal near miss** | **Maternal death** |
| --- | --- |
| (the woman survived) | (the woman died) |

**Q. How do you define maternal near miss or SAMM?**

**Ans.** A woman who nearly died but survived a complication that occurred during pregnancy, childbirth or within 42 days of termination of pregnancy.

**Q. What is understood by maternal near miss?**

**Ans.** **Maternal near miss** is defined as a woman who nearly died but survived a complication that occurred during pregnancy, childbirth or within 42 days of termination of pregnancy (WHO). Any life-threatening complication of pregnancy that results in an organ dysfunction is identified as maternal near miss. The classification of causes are the same as that of maternal deaths. Maternal near miss is also an important indicator for assessment of the quality of care provided to a pregnant woman for that country.

**Q. What are the common life-threatening conditions in pregnancy, labor and puerperium?**

**Ans.** (a) Hemorrhage (APH, PPH, ectopic pregnancy and abortion)
(b) Hypertensive disorders in pregnancy (pre-eclampsia and eclampsia)
(c) Sepsis (puerperal, postabortal)
(d) Other systemic disorders: Renal failure, pulmonary edema, disseminated intravascular coagulopathy (DIC).

## SUSTAINABLE DEVELOPMENT GOALS (SDG 3)

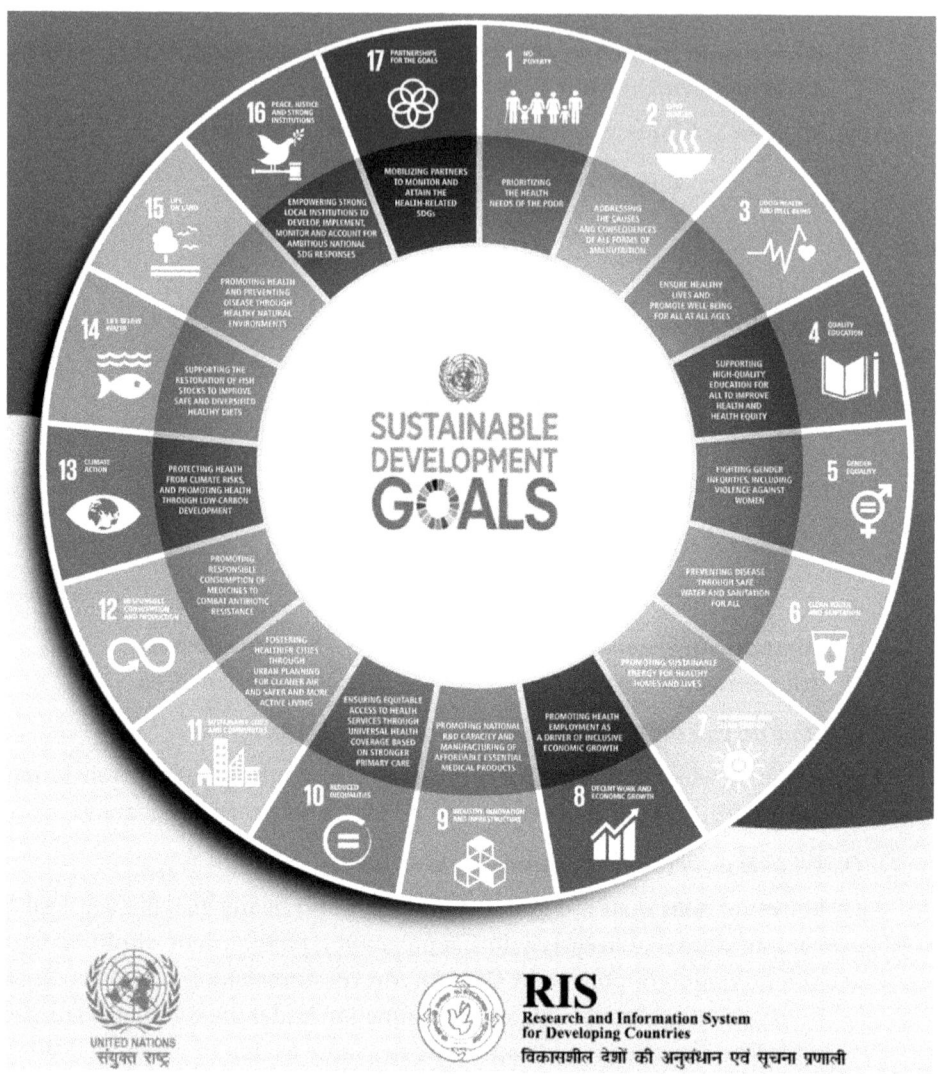

| SDG Health-related Targets ||
|---|---|
| **SDG 3 targets** | **Other linked targets** |
| 3.1 By 2030, reduce the global maternal martality ratio to less than 70 per 100,000 live births | 2.1 By 2030, end hunger and ensure access by all people in particular the poor and people in vulnerable situations, including infants to safe nutritious and sufficient food all year round |
| 3.2 By 2030, end preventable deaths of newborns and children under 5 years of age with all countries aiming to reduce neonatal mortality to at least as low as 12 per 1,000 live births and under 5 mortality to at least as low as 25 per 1,000 live births | 2.2 By 2030, end all forms of malnutrition, including achieving, by 2025, the internationally agreed targets on stunting and wasting in children under 5 years of age, and address the nutritional needs of adolescent girls, pregnant, lactating women and older persons |

## Chapter 9 • Maternal Health: India and Global Scenario

| | |
|---|---|
| 3.3 By 2030, end the epidemics of AIDS, tuberculosis malaria and neglected tropical disease and combat hepatitis, water-borne disease and other communicable diseases | 5.6 Ensure universal access to sexual and reproductive health and reproductive rights as agreed in accordance with the program of action of the International Conference on Population and Development and the Beijing Platform for Action and the outcome documents of their review conferences |

**Q. What is the sustainable development goals (SDGs)?**

**Ans.** SDGs, initiated by WHO, UNICEF, UNFPA, WORLD BANK Group, and UNPD estimates make global targets for ending preventable maternal mortality (EPMM). By 2030, every country should reduce its maternal mortality ratio by at least two-thirds from the 2010 baseline and no country should have an MMR higher than 140 deaths per 100,000 live births (twice the global targets). (WHO-2015).

**Q. How SDG is going to work to meet the challenges?**

**Ans.** MDGs 5 in 2000, initiated an unprecedented and ongoing global conversation about how maternal mortality should be measured. It also stressed the need of good data collection. At the same time it designed what strategies could be employed to save lives. Hundreds and thousands of women are still dying during childbirth and/or from pregnancy-related complications each year, 80% of which is preventable. SDG is a call to action across all regions of the globe both the developed and developing, to end preventable maternal mortality on a global level by 2030.

### SDGs Time-bound Targets

| Goal No. | Goals | Indicators | Target by 2030 |
|---|---|---|---|
| 3.1 | Reduce maternal mortality | Maternal mortality ratio (MMR) | 70 per 100,000 live births or less |
| 3.2 | Reduce neonatal mortality | Neonatal mortality rate | 12/1000 live births or less |

## MILLENNIUM DEVELOPMENT GOALS (MDG 4 and 5) AND SUSTAINABLE DEVELOPMENT GOALS (SDGs)

**Q. What is understood by MDGs?**

**Ans.** These are global movements of academics, governments, international agencies, healthcare professional associations, donors and nongovernmental associations with the Lancet as key partners for effective interventions to improve maternal, newborn and child health. The interventions also include policies, financial flow and equity.

**Q. How to achieve the target of reducing maternal deaths keeping in mind the experience of MDGs?**

**Ans.** To achieve this global goal, it requires countries to reduce their MMR by at least 7.5% each year between 2016 and 2030. Based on this point estimates for average annual reduction, three countries with an MMR more than 100 nearly reached or exceeded this reduction rate between 2000 and 2015: Cambodia, Rwanda and Timor-Leste. The recent success of these countries in rapidly reducing maternal mortality proved that this goal is possible to achieve.

**Q. What are the strategies designed by WHO for the success in reducing maternal mortality?**

**Ans.** WHO recently published five strategies towards ending preventable maternal mortality (EPMM). (Examples with country's names are given that have made significant reductions in maternal mortality).

**Q. What are the five strategies and the names of the countries that they have achieved the targets?**

**Ans. The five strategies for achieving the targets are:**
  (1) Addressing inequities in access to and quality of sexual, reproductive, maternal and newborn health care (Ethiopia, Vietnam).
  (2) Ensuring universal health coverage for comprehensive sexual, reproductive, maternal and newborn health care (Rwanda, Bangladesh).
  (3) Addressing all causes of maternal mortality, reproductive and maternal morbidities, and related disabilities (Nepal, Maldives).
  (4) Strengthening health systems to respond to the needs and priorities of women and girls (Indonesia, Cambodia).
  (5) Ensuring accountability to improve quality of care and equity (Mangolia, India).

*Names of the countries that have made significant reductions in maternal mortality are mentioned within the parenthesis.*

**Q. How the strategies are to be implemented?**

**Ans.** Strategic framework and program implementation are to be done with:
  (1) Empowering women, girls and communities
  (2) Protecting and supporting the mother–baby dyad care
  (3) Ensuring country ownership, leadership and supportive legal, technical and financial frameworks
  (4) Applying a human rights framework to ensure that high-quality reproductive, maternal and newborn health care is available, accessible and acceptable to all who need it (WHO-2015).

**Q. What other areas we need to improve upon to achieve this target?**

**Ans.** WHO stresses on the need for good quality data collection. Each country need civil registration and vital statistics (CRVS) systems. Under reporting need to be avoided. Actual number and the cause of deaths can help to make correct strategies to reduce maternal deaths.

**Q. What are the different tools for improving data collection?**

**Ans.** The tools for improving data collection are:
(1) **Confidential enquiry into maternal deaths (CEMD) with established Central registration and vital statistics (CRVS)** can reduce under reporting of maternal deaths due to misclassification. It has been proved very effectively in England and Wales since 1952.
(2) **Maternal death surveillance and response (MDSR):** It helps continuous monitoring of maternal deaths. It identifies the trends, the causes of maternal deaths, and is effective in reducing the deaths. MDSR is recently established in Cameroon, Democratic Republic of Congo, India and few other countries.
(3) **Digital Innovations:** Mobile devices, (mHealth tools) can help registration of pregnancies, notifications of births and deaths. This can link information directly to the district and national level health management and vital statistical systems.

**Q. What is the outcome of MDG 5 and how we should look into it?**

**Ans.** Among the 95 countries, 9 countries with an estimated MMR reduction of 75% or more have achieved MDG 5. These 9 countries have been placed in the **first category**. The **second category**, that are making progress are the 39 countries with an estimated MMR reduction of 50% or more. The **third category**, countries making insufficient progress, comprises 21 countries with an estimated MMR reduction of 25% or more, and at the **fourth and final category** includes 26 countries that have made no progress; they have an estimated MMR reduction of less than 25%.

**Q. What is the current situation in India?**

**Ans.** The states in India that have reached MDG target in 2007-2009 are Kerala, Tamil Nadu, Maharashtra, Gujrat and Andhra Pradesh, Telangana. The sates that are in close proximity to MDG target are West Bengal, Karnataka, Punjab and Haryana.

# NATIONAL HEALTH MISSION (NHM) AND REPRODUCTIVE AND CHILD HEALTH-II (RCH–II)

## The Key Maternal Health Strategies in NHM and RCH – II

- Providing essential obstetric care, quality antenatal care (ANC) and postnatal care (PNC).
- Providing skilled attendance at every birth
- Promoting institutional delivery
- Maintaining strict asepsis
- Providing kangaroo mother care
- Operationalizing emergency obstetric care
- Strengthening referral system
- Safe abortion services
- Services to deal reproductive tract infections (RTI) and sexually transmitted infections (STIs).

## Procedures and Drugs Permitted for use by Skilled Birth Attendants (ANMS, LHVS and SNS)

| Sl. no. | | Condition |
|---|---|---|
| 1. | Labor management | • Partograph plotting for every labor<br>• Safe delivery and care to newborn |
| 2. | Active management of third stage of labor (AMTSL) | • Use of uterotonic drugs (oxytocin/tablet misoprostol)<br>• Controlled cord traction<br>• Uterine massage |
| 3. | Prevention of PPH | • AMTSL<br>• Use of oxytocin 10 IU IM or giving misoprostol 600 µg (for home deliveries) |
| 4. | Management of PPH | • Giving injection oxytocin 10 IU IM<br>• Administering 20 IU oxytocin in 500 mL Ringer lactate, IV at 60 drops per minute<br>• Referring to FRU |
| 5. | Management of eclampsia | • Giving one dose of Injection $MgSO_4$ (10 mL) of 5 g, deep IM in each buttock<br>• Referring to RFU |
| 6. | Vaginal or perineal tears | • Identifying tears<br>• Managing first degree tears by use of pad and pressure |
| 7. | Management of puerperal infections/PROM/ secondary PPH | Giving first dose of the following antibiotics and referring:<br>• Injection gentamicin 80 mg IM<br>• Capsule ampicillin 1 g PO<br>• Tablet metronidazole 400 mg PO |
| 8. | Incomplete abortion with bleeding | Digital removal of retrained products of conception |
| 9. | Cases with preterm labor (<34 weeks) | • Corticosteroid therapy (Injection: deep IM<br>• Betamethasone or Dexamethasone) with schedule dose (See p. 193). This is to prevent respiratory distress syndrome of the the newborn. |

**Q. Who is a skilled birth attendant?**

**Ans. Skilled birth attendant (SBA)** is defined as an accredited health professional (doctor, midwife or nurse) who has been educated and trained to achieve proficiency in the skills, needed to manage normal (uncomplicated) pregnancies, childbirth and the immediate postnatal period and in the identification, management and referral of complications in women and newborns. Besides doctors, SBAs include auxiliary nurse midwives (ANMs), lady health visitors (LHVs) and staff nurse (SNs). SBAs are trained and made competent to take certain life-saving measures.

**Q. What is the action plan for NHM?**

**Ans.** National Health Mission (NHM) action plan is to:
  (a) Strengthen all primary health centers (PHCs), community health centers (CHCs) and first referral units (FRUs).
  (b) Provide basic and comprehensive emergency obstetric care (EmOC) and essential newborn care (see below).
  (c) Janani Shishu Suraksha Karyakram (JSSK) under the umbrella of NHM is to implement the interventions in all the states and union territories (UTs) with a special focus on **low-performing states (LPS)** that they have low institutional deliveries (Uttar Pradesh, Uttarakhand, Bihar, Jharkhand, Madhya Pradesh, Chattisgarh, Assam, Rajasthan, Odisha, Jammu and Kashmir). The remaining states have been named as **high performing states**.

## National Health Mission Guidelines for Maternal and Newborn Care (2017)

**Q. What is the transformational change in relation to the care during delivery (intrapartum and immediate postpartum care) as introduced by NHM 2017?**

**Ans.** According to National Health Mission (NHM)—2017, it is the respectful maternity care that should be practised. It ensures positive outcomes for both the mothers and newborns. It also supports cognitive development of the babies later in life.

**Q. What all we understand by respectful maternity care?**

**Ans.** This is an essential and comprehensive care. It includes respect for women's autonomy, dignity, privacy, feelings, choices, freedom from ill treatment and coercion and consideration for personal preferences including option for companionship during the maternity care.

**Q. How we should practice respectful maternity care while managing a woman in labor?**

**Ans.** It includes:
  (a) As a healthcare professional, we should provide privacy to the pregnant woman during the intrapartum period. She should be provided a separate labor room or a private cubicle.

(b) Presence of a birth companion of her choice during the course of her labor.
(c) Freedom to choose a comfortable position during birthing (squatting, standing. etc.)
(d) Use of labor beds instead of tables
(e) To place the baby on mother's abdomen following birth.
(f) Initiation of breastfeeding within one hour of birth.
(g) We should adhere to the clinical protocols for the management of labor.

**Q. What are the practices that we should not do in the respectful management care?**

**Ans.** (a) Any verbal or physical abuse of pregnant woman.
(b) Induction or augmentation of labor without sound clinical indications.
(c) Insisting on conventional lithotomy position for the delivery.
(d) Immediate clamping or cutting of the umbilical cord.
(e) Separating the baby from the mother for routine care and procedures.
(f) Out of pocket expenditures (OOPE) on drugs, diagnostics, including the demand by the staff for gratuitous payment by the families for celebrations of the baby's birth.

**Q. What are the objectives of providing such transformed RMC care?**

**Ans.** (a) To reduce maternal and newborn mortality and morbidity due to complications of pregnancy, labor, delivery and puerperium.
(b) To improve quality of care during labor, delivery and immediate postpartum period. It also ensures timely referral, and two-way follow-up system effectively.
(c) To enhance satisfaction of the beneficiaries visiting the health facilities.

## JANANI SHISHU SURAKSHA KARYAKRAM (JSSK)
### A GOVERNMENT OF INDIA (GOI) SCHEME

JSSK is an intervention for safe motherhood under the NHM. The main objective is to reduce maternal and neonatal mortality to promote institutional delivery. The scheme was launched in 12th April, 2005. This scheme is being implemented at all the states and UTs, with a special focus on **low-performing states (LPS)**. Under the JSY, accredited social health activist (ASHA) works as an effective link between the government and poor pregnant women in the village.

- JSSK focuses especially on poor pregnant women for states that have low institutional delivery (LPS).
- Each women (beneficiary) registered under the scheme, should have a JSY card along with MCH card.
- Each pregnant woman is eligible for cash assistance (in Rupees) for institutional delivery as mentioned here:

| Category | Rural area | | Total | Urban area | | Total |
|---|---|---|---|---|---|---|
| | Mother's package | ASHA's package | | Mother's package | ASHA's package | |
| LPS | 1,400 | 600 | 2,000 | 1,000 | 400 | 1,400 |
| HPS | 700 | 600 | 1,300 | 600 | 400 | 1,000 |

**Eligibility for cash assistance:**

**LPS:** All pregnant women delivering in government institutions or accredited private institutions.

**HPS:** Pregnant women below the poverty line.

**LPS and HPS:** All SC/ST women delivering in a government institutions or accredited private institutions.

## Key Areas in Antenatal Care [Government of India (GOI)]

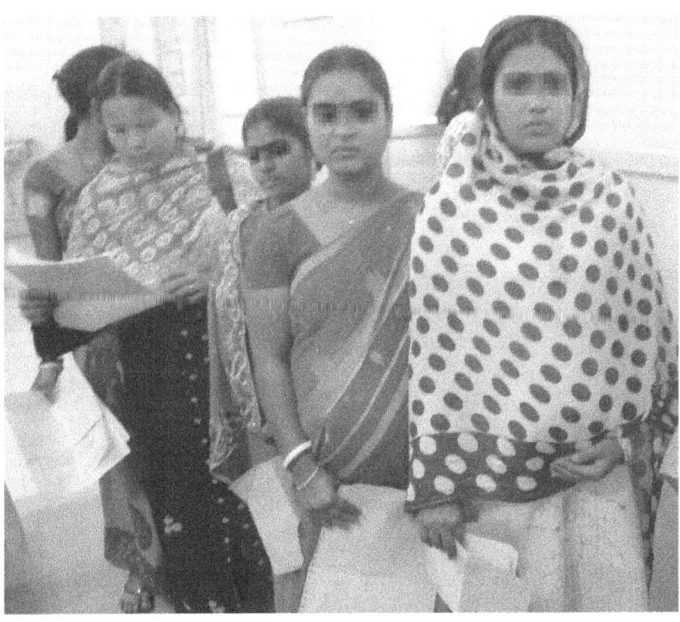

Fig. 9.1: Antenatal checkup.

**Care during pregnancy:**
- Detection of pregnancy by Nischay Pregnancy Test Kit.
- Register every pregnancy within 12 weeks.
- Ensure four antenatal visits to monitor the progress of pregnancy (Fig. 9.1).
- 2nd visit: 14–26 weeks., 3rd visit: 28–34 weeks., 4th visit: 36 weeks—to the expected date of delivery.
- Give every pregnant woman: Tetanus Toxoid (TT) injections and
- Iron folic acid (IFA) supplementation.

***IFA supplementation:*** She should take one IFA tablet daily during pregnancy and in the puerperium up to 6 months.
- Tablet calcium with vitamin D3 is also given throughout pregnancy and lactation.
- Record blood pressure and weight at every visit.

***Investigations:***
- To test blood for hemoglobin, urine for sugar and protein at every visit
- To advise and encourage the woman to opt for institutional delivery.
- To maintain proper records for better case management and follow-up.
- Not to give a pregnant woman any medication during the first trimester unless medically indicated.
- To determine the blood group including the Rh factor.
- To conduct the venereal disease research laboratory (VDRL)/rapid plasma reagin (RPR) test to rule out syphilis.
- To test the woman for human immunodeficiency virus (HIV).
- To check the blood sugar.
- To carry out the hepatitis B surface antigen (HBsAg) test.
- All women in the reproductive age group should be advised to have folic acid for 2–3 months preconception and continue with it during the first 12 weeks of pregnancy. This remarkably reduces the incidence of neural tube defects in the fetus A daily dose of 400 µg folic acid taken orally is the recommended daily dose.
- Low iodine levels during pregnancy can cause cretinism which can lead to mental physical retardation of the baby. So regular consumption of iodized salts is advised as a prophylactic measures

**Q. What are the symptoms indicating complications in pregnancy?**

**Ans.** The symptoms indicating complications in pregnancy are:
- Fever
- Persistent vomiting
- Abdominal pain not relieved with rest
- Abnormal vaginal discharge/itching
- Palpitations, easy fatigability
- Breathlessness at rest/on mild exertion
- Generalized swelling of the body, puffiness of the face
- Severe headache and blurring of vision
- Vaginal bleeding
- Decreased or absent fetal movement
- Leaking of watery fluid per vaginum (PV).

## Micro-Birth Plan: The Components

### A. Planning and preparing for birth (birth preparedness)

*Counselling*

*Registration of the pregnant woman:*
- Informing the woman about the dates of antenatal visits, schedule for TT injections and EDD.
- Identifying the place of delivery and the person who would conduct the delivery.
- Identifying a referral facility and the mode of referral.
- Taking the necessary steps to arrange for transport for the beneficiary.
- Registration of pregnant woman and filling up of the Maternal and Child Protection Card and JSSK card/below poverty line (BPL) certificates/necessary proofs or certificates for the purpose of keeping a record.

*Maternal Request for Home Delivery and the Counseling*
- If in spite of all the efforts, the pregnant woman decides to go for a home delivery, she is informed that there are situations when complications arise and a home delivery may be risky and potentially life-threatening.

**Q. How to counsel a woman with the benefits of institutional delivery?**

**Ans.** Benefits of institutional delivery are:
- Labor monitoring, active management of complications, emergencies of mother and postpartum monitoring are possible.
- Skilled staff provides specific care and attention to newborn babies in order to prevent neonatal mortality.
- Disposable delivery kits (DDKs) are to be made ready when she decides for home delivery in spite of counseling.
- DDKs are to be supplied to those pregnant women in the community who insist on having a home delivery.
- To explain the '*six cleans*' to such women. These are: Clean surface, clean hands, clean cord cut, clean cord tie, clean umbilical stump and clean perineum. Counsel and help them to maintain the 'six cleans' during delivery at home.
- To keep a record of such women and continue counseling them during all their subsequent antenatal visits to opt for an institutional delivery.
- To keep things ready to attend to such women at their home during delivery.
- The pregnant woman, her family members or the ASHA should call the ANM to conduct the delivery at home.

**The requirements during and immediately after delivery at home:**
- Presence of an ANM for conducting the delivery.
- The Maternal and Child Protection Card (for complete information regarding the antenatal period).
- Clean towels/cloth for drying and wrapping the baby.

- Clean clothes that have been washed and sun-dried for the mother and the baby.
- Sanitary pads/clean cloth for the mother.
- Supplies like injection oxytocin, tablet misoprostol, cord clamps, sterile surgical knife with blade, pediatric size bag and mask and other emergency drugs.
- A dry and comfortably warm environment/room.
- Food and water for the woman and the support person.

Advice the woman to go to the health facility or inform the ASHA to contact the SBA, if the woman has any one of the following signs which indicate the start of labor:
- A bloody, sticky discharge from the vagina ('show').
- Painful uterine contractions increasing in duration, frequency and intensity with the passage of time.

**Q. What are the danger signs during pregnancy, labor and puerperium?**

Ans. (a) **Maternal**
- Malpresentation
- Multiple pregnancy
- Any bleeding PV during pregnancy and after delivery (a pad is soaked in less than 5 minutes).
- Severe headache with blurred vision
- Hemoglobin <7 g%
- Convulsions or loss of consciousness
- Decreased or absent fetal movements
- High BP (>140/90 mm Hg) with proteins in the urine, and severe headache with epigastric pain.

(b) **Labor**
- Active labor lasting longer than 12 hours in a primipara and more than 8 hours in a multipara.
- Premature rupture of membranes (PROM) before 37 weeks.

(c) **Puerperium**
- Abdominal pain, features of septicemia, thrombophlebitis, breast complications (acute mastitis, breast abscess)
- Temperature more than 38°C
- Foul smelling discharge before or after delivery/abortion
- Perineal tear (2nd, 3rd and 4th degree).

**Note:** If the medical officer/ANM is not able to decide, she should send the case to the FRU or a 24 hour PHC.

## B. Care after delivery

*Postpartum care for mother and essential newborn care*

**Mother:**
- Look out for symptoms and signs of PPH and puerperal sepsis during postpartum visits as they are the major causes of maternal mortality.
- Advise the mother on colostrum feeding and exclusive breastfeeding.
- Advise the couple on family planning.

**Q. Mention the essential points in newborn care.**

Ans.
- To keep the baby warm
- Ensure care of the umbilicus, skin and eyes
- Ensure good suckling while breastfeeding
- Screen the newborn for danger signs
- Advise the mother and family members on immunization.

**Q. What are the key messages on breastfeeding?**

Ans.
- Initiate breastfeeding especially colostrum feeding within an hour of birth
- Not to give any prelacteal feeds
- To ensure good attachment of the baby to the breast
- Exclusively breastfeed the baby for 6 months
- Breastfeed the baby whenever he/she demands milk
- To follow the practice of rooming in.

**Q. What are the indications (danger signs) to refer a baby to the medical officer at the FRU?**

Ans.
- Baby is not breastfeeding
- Baby looks sick (lethargic or irritable)
- Baby has fever or feels cold to touch
- Breathing is fast or difficult
- There is blood in the stools
- Baby looks yellow, pale or bluish
- Baby's body is arched forward
- Body movements of the body, limbs or face are irregular
- The umbilicus is red, swollen or draining pus
- The baby has not passed meconium within 24 hours of birth
- Baby suffers diarrhea.

*Detection of Complication During Postpartum Period:*

**Q. What is puerperal sepsis and what are the features of puerperal sepsis?**

Ans. **Puerperal sepsis**: Puerperal sepsis is infection of the genital tract following childbirth till 42 days after delivery or abortion. Any two or more of the following signs and symptoms present are:
- Fever (temperature >38°C or >100.4°F)
- Lower abdominal pain and tenderness
- Abnormal and foul-smelling lochia, may be blood-stained
- Burning micturition
- Uterus tender and subinvoluted
- Feeling of weakness
- Vaginal bleeding
- Breast complications: Acute mastitis, breast abscess.

**Q. Discuss the importance of institutional delivery.**

Ans. To advise and encourage the woman to opt for institutional delivery (discussed above).

**Q. Who is an accredited social health activist (ASHA)? What is her role in the community?**

**Ans.** ASHA is a female (preferably a daughter-in-law) accredited social health worker of 25–45 years age. She is to work in a village with population >1,000 under the NRHM scheme. She is trained over a period of 3–4 weeks for this work.
- She acts as a link person among the beneficiary at the village level with the ANMs, LHVs, doctors at the FRU (Government).
- She arranges escort to the pregnant woman, sick child and provide DOTs, ORS, IFA tablets for the needful.
- She works along with Anganwadi workers (AWWs) and TBAs to provide service under JSSYK.

## Methods of Postpartum Contraception

Depot Medroxy Progesterone Acetate (DMPA), Intrauterine Contraceptive Device (IUCD), Female Sterilization (FS), No Scalpel Vasectomy (NSV). Emergency Contraception Pill (ECP) are the different measures that are available a woman following childbirth. Decision for choice is made depending on whether she is breastfeeding or not.

| Methods of postpartum contraception | | | | |
|---|---|---|---|---|
| Contraceptive method | DMPA | IUCD | Female Sterilization (FS) | NSV (For husband) |
| Breastfeeding (fully or nearly full or partial) | | | | |
| <6 weeks postpartum | Yes | Postplacental insertion within 10 minutes of delivery | While in hospital, postpartum sterilization after 24 hours to 7 days of childbirth | Any time following counseling |
| >6 weeks to <6 months postpartum | Yes | Immediate postpartum <48 hours of childbirth | >6 weeks postpartum | Yes, with counseling |
| >6 weeks postpartum | Yes | Postpartum >6 weeks | > 6 weeks postpartum | Yes, with counseling |
| Not breastfeeding | | | | |
| <21 days | Yes | | After 24 hours to 7 days after childbirth or | Any time with counseling |
| | | <48 hours after childbirth OR >6 weeks post-partum | | |
| >21 days | Yes | | >6 weeks postpartum | |

DMPA: depot medroxyprogesterone acetate; IUCD: intrauterine contraceptive device; FS: female sterilisation; NSV: no scalpel vasectomy

**Q. What are the components of essential obstetric care and what includes comprehensive emergency obstetric care (EmOC)?**

**Ans.** The components of essential obstetric care and comprehensive EmOC are:

| Essential obstetric care | Comprehensive EmOC (at FRUs under NRHM scheme) |
|---|---|
| • Early registration of pregnancy (<12 weeks)<br>• Minimum 4 antenatal visits (1st visit: 12-14 weeks; 2nd visit: 14-26 weeks; 3rd visit: 28-34 weeks and 4th visit: 36-40 weeks)<br>• Identification of high-risk factors<br>• Delivery: Institutional or with SBA<br>• Provision of prompt referral<br>• Postnatal care<br>• Essential newborn care<br>• Early and exclusive breastfeeding<br>• Family planning counseling | • Vacuum extractions<br>• Anesthetic services<br>• Blood transfusion facilities<br>• Cesarean delivery<br>• Manual removal of placenta<br>• Suction evacuation (MVA)<br>• Safe abortion services<br>• Contraceptive services (IUCDs)<br>• Sterilization operations<br>• Referral and transport facilities |

## MATERNAL HEALTH BEYOND 2030

## NATIONAL HEALTH POLICY (GOI–2017)

The National Health Policy 2017, aims the attainment of highest possible level of health and wellbeing for all at all ages through preventive and promotive health care system. There would be universal access to good quality health care services for all without any financial hardship. This would be achieved through increasing access, improving quality, and lowering the cost of health care delivery.

The policy recognizes the pivotal importance of Sustainable Development Goals (SDGs).

*The key policy principles are:*

(i) **Professionalism, Integrity and Ethics:** NHP demands high professional standard. Integrity and ethics are to be maintained.

(ii) **Equity:** Inequity to be reduced. This is to reduce disparity on the ground of gender, poverty, caste, disability or other forms of social and geographical barriers.

(iii) **Affordability:** The costs of care should be made affordable for all.

(iv) **Universality:** Prevention of exclusions on social, economic or on any other grounds.

(v) **Patient Centered and Quality of Care**: Gender sensitive, effective, safe, and convenient healthcare services to be provided with dignity and confidentiality.

(vi) **Accountability:** Financial and performance accountability, transparency in decision making, and elimination of corruption in health care systems are essential. It is applicable both in public and private care.

(vii) **Inclusive Partnerships**: A multistakeholder approach is accepted. Partnerships with academic institutions, and health care industry should be developed.
(viii) **Pluralism:** Patients who choose and when appropriate, should have access to Ayush Care Providers.
(ix) **Decentralization:** Decentralization of decision making and community level participation in health planning processes to be promoted side by side.
(x) **Dynamism and Adaptiveness**: Healthcare needs to be constantly improved based on new knowledge and evidence. Learning from the communities, from national and international knowledge partners, are designed to improve quality of care.

# Drug Therapy, Obstetric Charts, Graphs and Illustrations

CHAPTER

10

**Chapter Objectives**

**To demonstrate knowledge and understanding of:**
- Different drugs in obstetrics, risk of teratogenicity, dose schedule and side effects
- Critical periods in embryonic development
- Ultrasonographic estimation of gestational age

❖ Drug Therapy In Pregnancy and Teratogenicity     360
❖ Obstetric Charts and Graphs     363
❖ Critical Periods in Embryonic Development     365

# DRUG THERAPY IN PREGNANCY AND TERATOGENICITY

## Food and Drug Administration Fetal Risk Categories

| Category | Definitions |
|---|---|
| A | Well-controlled studies in pregnant women have failed to demonstrate a fetal risk |
| B | **No evidence of risk in humans:** Well-controlled studies in pregnant women have not shown any increased risk of fetal malformation despite adverse findings in animals. The chance of fetal harm is remote but remains a possibility |
| C | **Risk cannot be ruled out:** Adequate, well-controlled human studies are lacking. Animal studies have shown a risk to the fetus or are lacking as well. Potential benefit may outweigh the risk |
| D | **Positive evidence of risk:** Studies in human have demonstrated fetal risk. Potential benefits from use of the drug (life-threatening situation) may outweight the potential risk |
| X | **Contraindicated in pregnancy:** Proven fetal risks clearly outweight any possible benefit.<br>**Drugs in this group are:** Alcohol, ACE inhibitors, lithium, methotrexate, valproic acid, mifepristone, danazol, isotretinoin, radioactive iodine and others |

**Teratogen information databases:**
Organization of Teratology Information Services (OTIS): https://www.fda.gov/ScienceResearch/SpecialTopics/WomensHealthResearch/ucm256789.htm.

## Medications Categorized as Category X

- Aminopterin
- ACE inhibitors
- Coumarin derivatives
- Cyclophosphamide
- Danazol
- Diethylstilbestrol
- Ethanol
- Etretinate
- Fluconazole
- Isotretinoin
- Leuprolide
- Lithium
- Methotrexate
- Mifepristone/Misoprostol
- Phenytoin
- Quinine
- Radioactive iodine
- Trastuzumab
- Trimethadione
- Valproic acid

*Food and Drug Administration: Drug bulletin. Fed Reg 1980;44:37434.*

## Teratogens Known to Cause Malformations

| Infections | Drugs and chemicals | Physical agents |
|---|---|---|
| **Viruses** <br> • Rubella <br> • Cytomegalovirus <br> • Parvovirus B19 <br> • Herpes <br> • Varicella <br><br> **Others** <br> • *Toxoplasma* <br> • *Treponema pallidum* | • Phenytoin <br> • Tetracyclines <br> • Valproic acid <br> • Alcohol <br> • Folate antagonist <br> • Androgen hormones <br> • Carbamazepine <br> • Vitamin A excess <br> • Coumadin anticoagulants | • Ionizing radiation <br> • Lead <br> • Mercury |

**Q.** *What is a teratogen?*

**Ans. Teratogens** are substances that can cause fetal abnormalities in relation to structures, functions, growth restriction and/or death. A teratogen may be a substance, an organism or a physical agent.

**Q.** *What are the important criteria to determine teratogenicity?*

**Ans.** (1) The drug/agent must cross the placenta. The amount of placental transfer and teratogenicity depends on the drug quantity, protein binding, lipid solubility, molecular size and electrical charge of the molecule. Genotype of the conceptus is also important.

(2) Drug exposure during the period of organogenesis, day 31 (heart, CNS) to day 71 (palate, ear) after the LMP, is most vulnerable. Embryonic period between second to eight week after conception is the critical period for the structural defects. Risks of structural malformations are high during this period. In the fetal period (>8 weeks), growth of the fetus is affected and development of certain organs (minor malformations) may be there.

(3) It is difficult to establish the correlation between the drug exposure and the birth defects. This may be related incidentally and not causally. Animal studies are often insufficient, so also the case reports. Case control studies suffer for recall bias. Cohort studies are prospective. It needs time and are also expensive. Clinical trials involve randomized control trial (RCT). RCT can evaluate the areas of prevention and treatment regimen. Clinical trials for NTD, occurrence, recurrence and prevention have been successful. Periconceptional folic acid supplementation is a routine therapy now.

**Q.** *Mention some of the known teratogens to cause birth defects.*

**Ans.** Known teratogens to cause congenital fetal malformations and birth defects are:

(1) **Genetic:** 15–20%
(2) **Chromosomal abnormalities** ♦ 5–10%
    **Aneuploidy**
    ♦ Down syndrome
    ♦ Edward syndrome
    ♦ Turner syndrome
(3) **Environmental causes:**
    (a) Maternal infections: 1–3%
    (b) Maternal abuse of illicit substances: 1–4%
    (c) Drugs, chemicals, radiation and hyperthermia: 1–2%.
(4) **Unknown:** 65%.

**Q. What are the different antiepileptic drugs associated with birth defects?**

**Ans.** It is not certain whether the risk of fetal malformations is secondary to the underlying seizure pathology (epilepsy) or due to the exposure of medications. As regard the drugs, available data are limited. This is especially with the newer anticonvulsants.

**Q. What should be the guideline for the use of antiepileptic drug in pre-pregnancy?**

**Ans.** (a) The drug must be effective for seizure control
(b) Monotherapy to be maintained if possible
(c) Drug has least teratogenic effect
(d) Lowest dose as possible to maintain.

The table showing fetal malformations with different antiepileptic drugs is given below:

### Different Antiepileptic Drugs and Fetal Malformations

| Drug | Estimated incidence (%) | Pregnancy category (US-FDA) |
| --- | --- | --- |
| Valproate | 10.7 | D |
| Carbamazepine | 4.7 | D |
| Phenytoin | 7.3 | D |
| Phenobarbital | 4.9 | D |
| Lamotrigine | 2.9 | C |
| Levetiracetam | — | C |
| Topiramate | — | C |
| Oxcarbazepine | — | C |

## OBSTETRIC CHARTS AND GRAPHS

### Fetal Growth Parameters and Charts (Figs. 10.1 and 10.2)

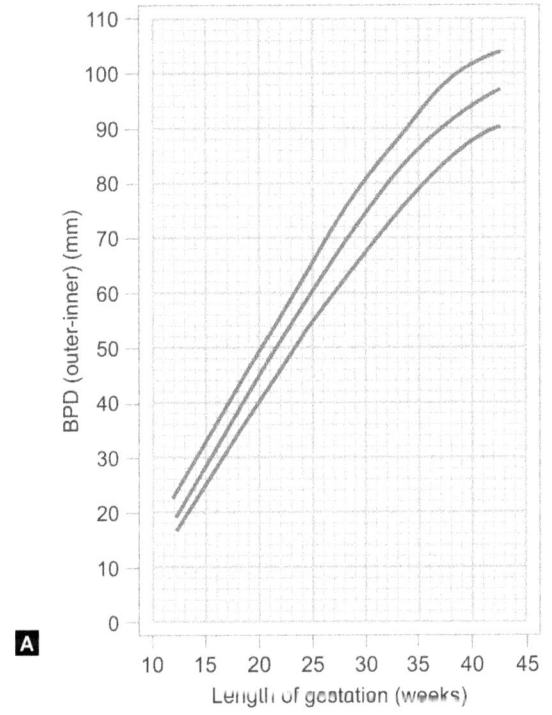

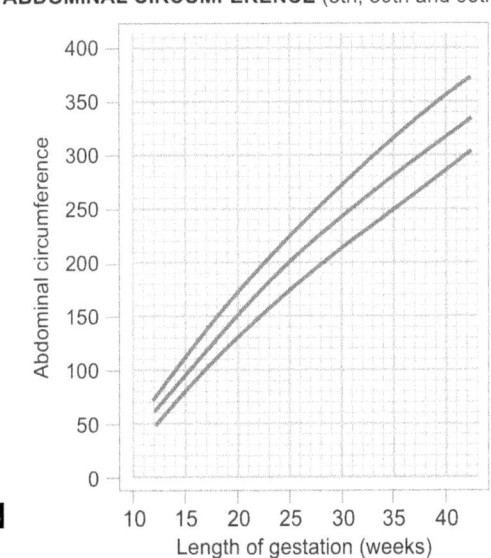

**Figs. 10.1A and B:** Ultrasonographic growth pattern of a normal fetus: (A) Biparietal diameter; (B) Abdominal circumference.

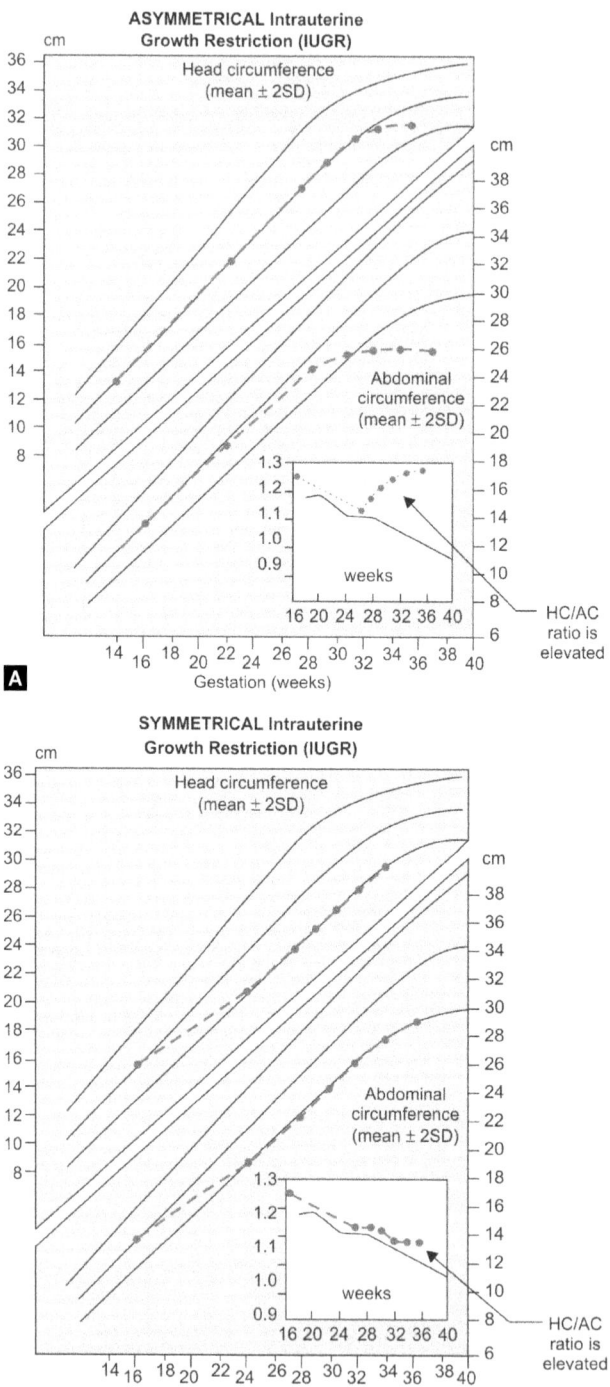

**Figs. 10.2A and B:** Ultrasonographic growth profile in a case of IUGR: (A) Ultrasonographic growth profile in a case of asymmetric IUGR shows, head circumference (HC) is maintained but abdominal circumference (AC) falls off around 30 weeks. The HC/AC ratio is elevated; (B) In symmetric IUGR, both the HC and AC are affected early. Therefore, HC/AC ratio remains normal.

## CRITICAL PERIODS IN EMBRYONIC DEVELOPMENT

| Postconception days | Important events in development |
|---|---|
| 1 | — |
| 5–7 | Implantation |
| 24–25 | Anterior neuropore closes |
| 26–27 | Posterior neuropore closes |
| 27–28 | Upper limb buds |
| 29–30 | Lower limb buds |
| 46–47 | Heart septations |
| 56–58 | Palate closes |
| 84 | Second trimester |

The classic teratogenic period is from day 31 after the LMP (28 day cycle) to 71 days

### First Trimester Ultrasonography Assessment Parameters
(a) Gestational sac
(b) Yolk sac
(c) Embryo and amnion
(d) Embryonic cardiac activity
(e) Umbilical cord.

### Estimation of Gestational Age
Determination is done with measurement parameters.
(a) Gestational sac: Mean sac diameter
(b) Crown-rump length (Fig. 10.3)
(c) Biparietal diameter (see Fig. 10.5).

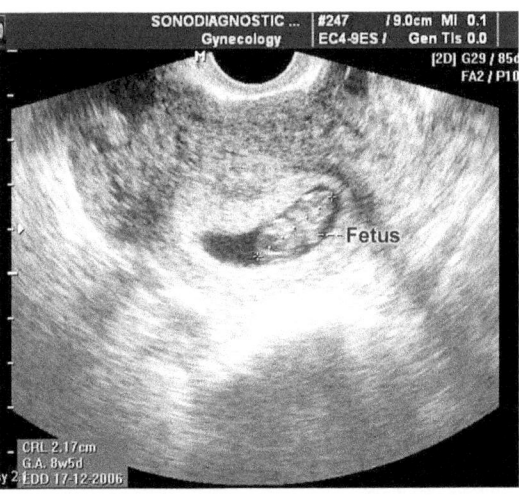

**Fig. 10.3:** Ultrasonogram showing crown-rump length (between the crosses) of a 8-0 week fetus. (*Courtesy:* Prof BN Chakravorty and Dr (Mrs) S Ghosh, IRM, Kolkata)

## Second Trimester Ultrasound for Fetal Anatomy Survey: Standard Sonogram

Organs surveyed are:
- **Head, neck, face**
- Midline falx, cerebellum, choroid plexus, lateral cerebral ventricles, cavum septum pellucidum, and upperlip
- **Chest:** Heart—four chamber view, outflow tracts
- **Abdomen:** Stomach, kidneys, bladder, umbilical cord insertion site into the abdomen, umbilical cord vessel number
- **Spine:** Cervical, thoracic, lumbar, and sacral
- **Extremities:** Arms, Legs—presence or absence
- **Gender:** As medically indicated.

## Obstetric Ultrasound

General survey parameters (ACR-2007):
- **Fetus:** Cardiac activity to document with M-mode
- **Presentation:** Cephalic, breech
- **Fetal number:** Single, twins (Fig. 10.4), triplets
- **Fetal:** Gestational age determination—measurements of—BPD (Fig. 10.5), HC (Fig. 10.6), abdominal circumference (AC) (Fig. 10.7), femur length (FL) (Fig. 10.8), amniotic fluid-volume.
- **Placenta:** Location
- **Fetal** growth profile
- **Fetal** weight.

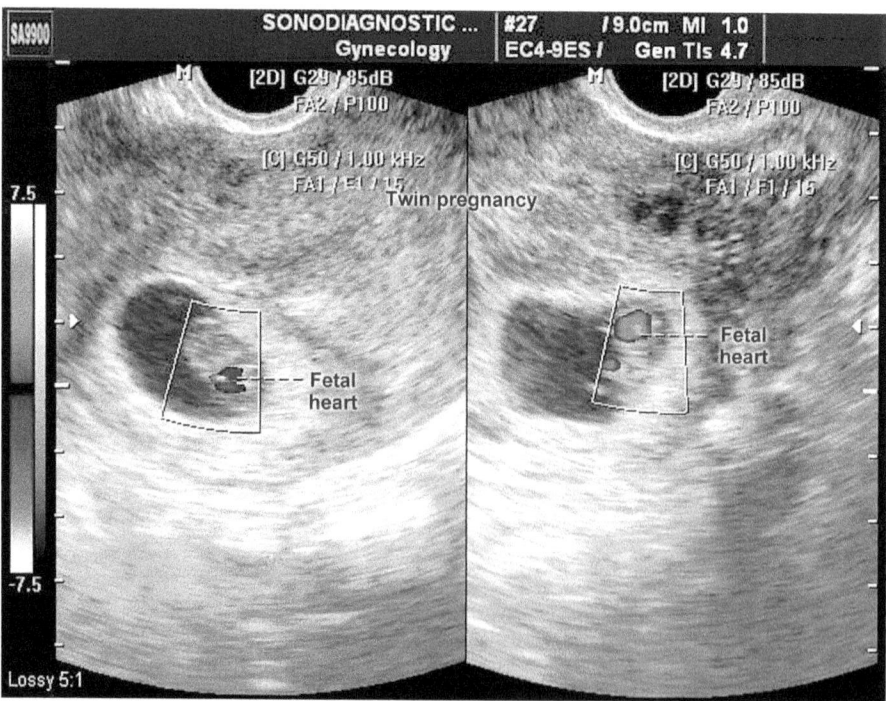

**Fig. 10.4:** Color Doppler scan (TVS) showing twin pregnancy with cardiac activity of both the fetuses

[*By courtesy:* Prof BN Chakravorty and Dr (Mrs) S Ghosh, IRM, Kolkata]

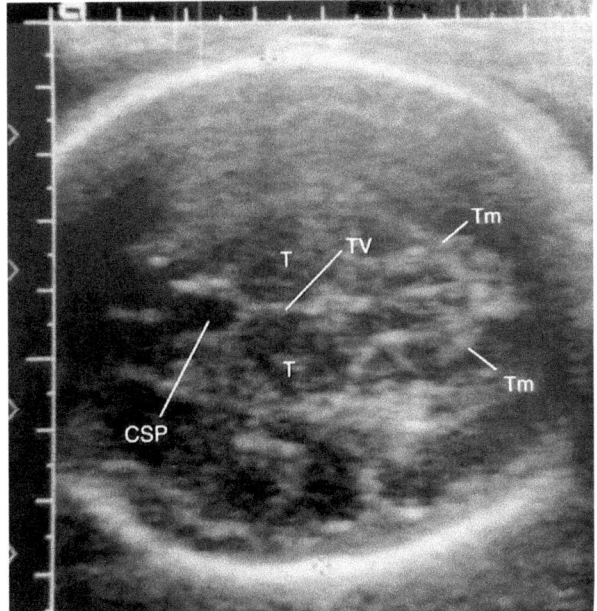

**Fig. 10.5:** Biparietal diameter (BPD) is measured at the level of thalami (T) and cavum septum pellucidum (CSP). Measurement is done from the outer edge of the skull to the opposite inner edge (parietal bone) and on a line perpendicular to the midline. Commonly the callipers are placed from the outer skull in the inner field to the inner skull in the far field. BPD is measured to assess: (i) fetal gestational age (most accurate between 12 and 18 weeks); (ii) fetal growth; and (iii) fetal weight. Head circumference is also measured by placing the dots (electronic callipers).

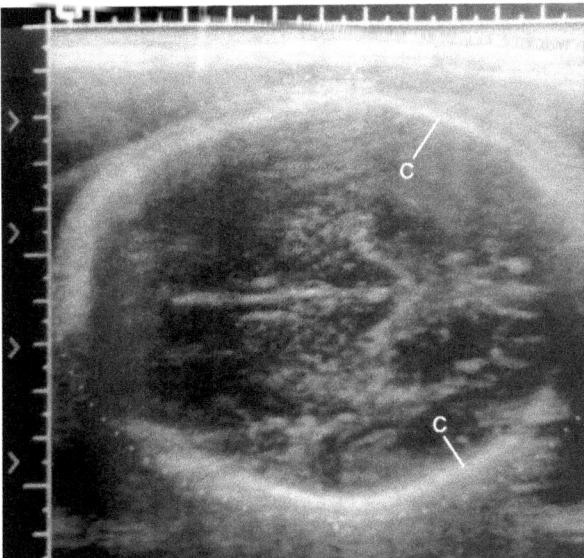

**Fig. 10.6:** Measurement of head circumference.

The transaxial plane of section is nearly the same as that of BPD. Callipers tracing dots are seen. Head circumference is measured around the outer side of the skull. Indications of measurement are the same as that of BPD. (C = cranium).

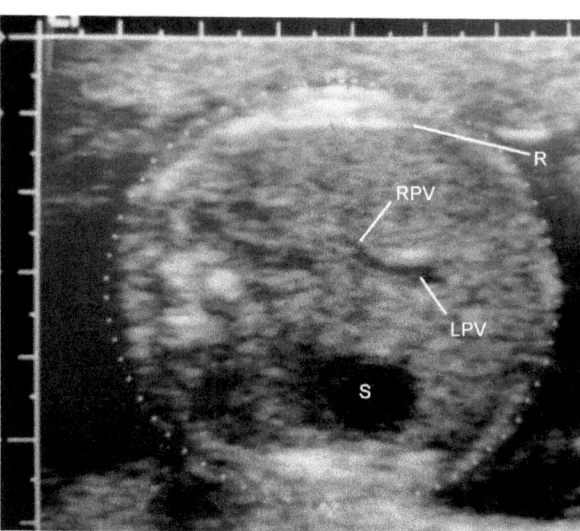

**Fig. 10.7:** Fetal abdominal circumference (AC) is measured at the level of umbilical vein (UV). Umbilical vein is seen within the substance of the liver. Dots have been placed to make this measurement. AC is measured to assess—(i) gestational age; (ii) intrauterine growth restriction (IUGR); (iii) macrosomia and (iv) fetal weight. Fetal stomach is demonstrated by S.
R = Rib; S = Stomach;
RPV = Right portal veins
LPV = Left portal veins
Abdominal circumference is measured with dots drawn around the outside of the skin.

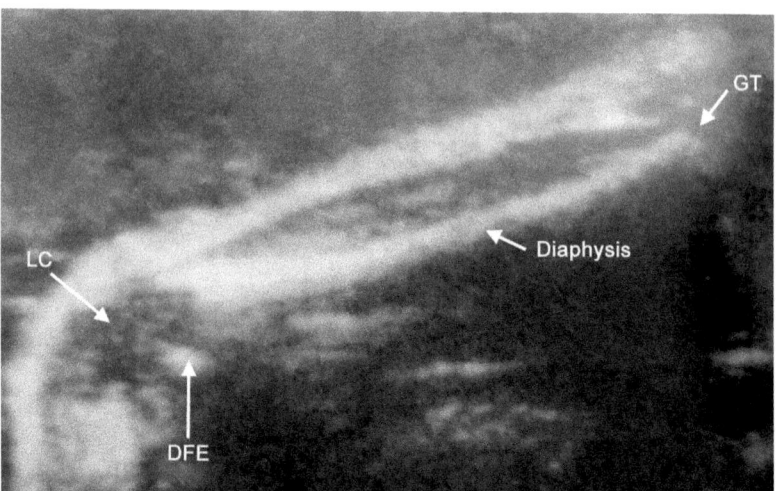

**Fig. 10.8:** Sonographic view of the fetal femur (femur length). measurement end points are between the two short arrows.
(GT = greater trochanter; LC = lateral condyle; DFE = distal femoral epiphysis).

## Fetal Structures Visualized by Ultrasonography (TVS) and Gestational Age

| Gestational age (weeks) | Structures visualized |
|---|---|
| 4 weeks and 3 days | Gestational sac |
| 5 weeks | Yolk sac |
| 6 weeks | Fetal pole, cardiac activity |
| 7 weeks | Upper limb buds, physiological midgut herniation |
| 8 weeks | Lower limb buds, stomach |
| 9 weeks | Spine, choroid plexus |

## Gestational Age Assignment by Ultrasonography

| Parameter | Gestational age (weeks) | Variability (days) |
|---|---|---|
| Crown-rump length (CRL) | 5–12 | ± 03 |
| Biparietal diameter (BPD) | 12–20 | ± 08 |
|  | 20–24 | ± 12 |
|  | >32 | ± 21 |
| Femur length (FL) | 12–20 | ± 07 |
|  | >36 | ± 16 |

**SPACE FOR NOTES**

# Gynecology

**SECTION 2**

- Gynecology Case Discussion — 373
- Special Topics — 433
- Gynecology Short Questions — 457
- Viva-Voce in Gynecology — 475
- Operative Gynecology — 496
- Practical Gynecology — 547
- Single Best Answer and Multiple Choice Questions — 650
- History in Obstetrics and Gynecology — 689

# CHAPTER 11

# Gynecology Case Discussion

## Chapter Objectives

**To demonstrate the knowledge and understanding of:**

- Benign gynecological diseases.
- Infections of the genital organs including Sexually transmitted disease (STIs).
- Functional anatomy of the perineum, other pelvic organs, colon, rectum and urinary bladder.
- Functional anatomy of the pelvic floor muscles, fascia and the ligaments.
- Neoplastic (both benign and malignant) gynecological conditions.
- To organize investigations and to interpret the results of investigations.
- Principles of medical/surgical management of gynecological problems and the follow up.

| | | | |
|---|---|---|---|
| ❖ | Case – 1 | Fibroid Uterus | 374 |
| ❖ | Case – 2 | Ovarian Tumor | 381 |
| ❖ | Case – 3 | Pelvic Organ Prolapse | 392 |
| ❖ | Case – 4 | Genitourinary Fistula | 403 |
| ❖ | Case – 5 | Ureteric Injury in Gynecology | 406 |
| ❖ | Case – 6 | Rectovaginal Fistula | 408 |
| ❖ | Case – 7 | Old Complete Perineal Tear | 410 |
| ❖ | Case – 8 | Pelvic Infections | 413 |
| ❖ | Case – 9 | Genital Tuberculosis | 416 |
| ❖ | Case – 10 | Abnormal Uterine Bleeding (AUB) | 418 |
| ❖ | Case – 11 | Hydatidiform Mole | 423 |
| ❖ | Case – 12 | Uterine Polyp | 428 |
| ❖ | Case – 13 | Infertility | 430 |

## OBJECTIVE STRUCTURED CLINICAL EXAMINATION (OSCE)

### CASE – 1 | FIBROID UTERUS

#### Case Summary

*Mrs DK, 45-year-old multiparous lady presents with the history of heavy, painful and irregular menstruation for the last 18 months. On examination, she was pale. Abdominal and pelvic examination revealed an irregularly enlarged firm mass arising from the uterus of about 14 weeks in size. The adnexae were unremarkable. Her recent cervical smear was normal.*

**Q. What is the provisional diagnosis?**

**Ans.** Fibroid uterus.

**Q. How can you confirm the diagnosis?**

**Ans.** Ultrasound scan (Fig. 11.1) or MRI (Fig. 11.2), less commonly needed.

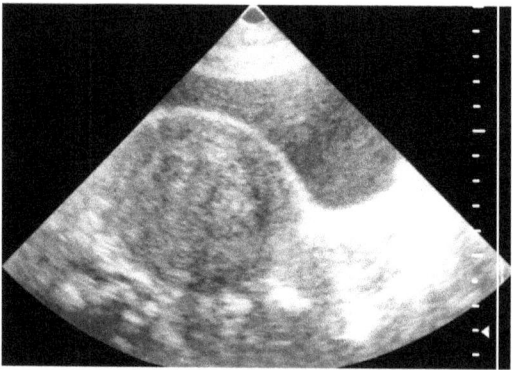

Fig. 11.1: Ultrasonography showing fibroid uterus.

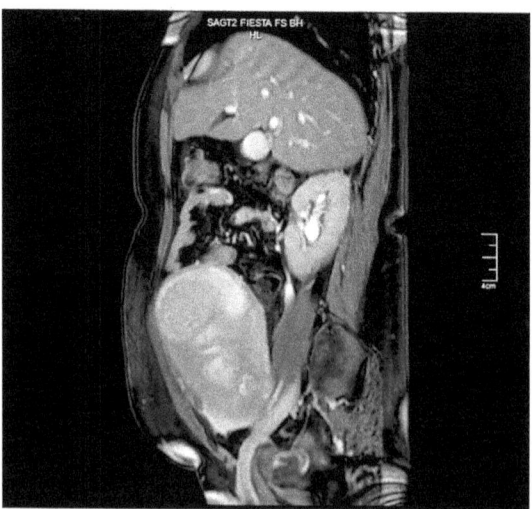

Fig. 11.2: MRI of a fairly large size fibroid (24 weeks of pregnancy size) arising from the body of the uterus.

**Chapter 11 • Gynecology Case Discussion** 375

***Q. What other symptoms and signs she may have presented with?***

**Ans.** *Symptoms due to anemia*: Tiredness, palpitation. Other symptoms like abdominal pain, pelvic pressure and symptoms due to degeneration.

***Q. What are the different types of uterine fibroid?***

**Ans.** According to the site of origin, fibroids may be:
   (A)  Body (corporeal)
   (B)  Cervical. Each type has been subdivided further (Fig. 11.3).

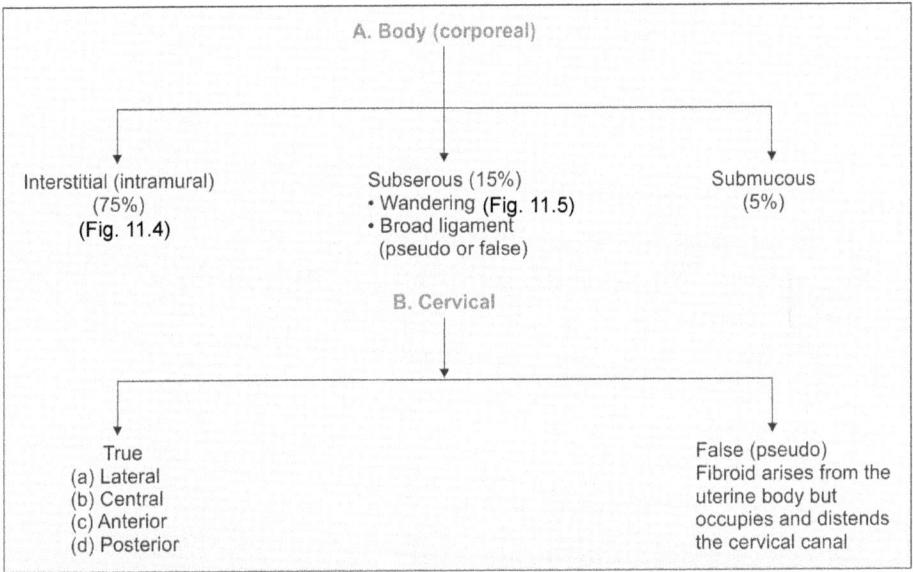

**Fig. 11.3:** Classification of fibroid.

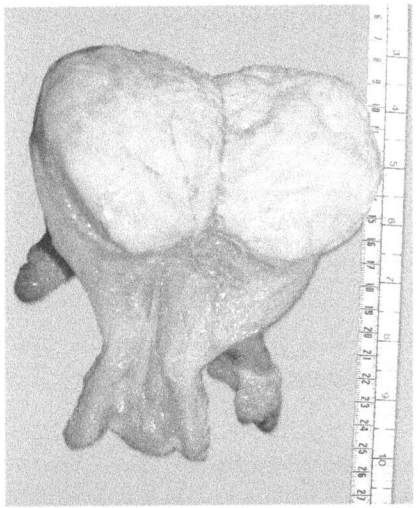

**Fig. 11.4:** Uterus is cut open to show the fibroid (interstitial).

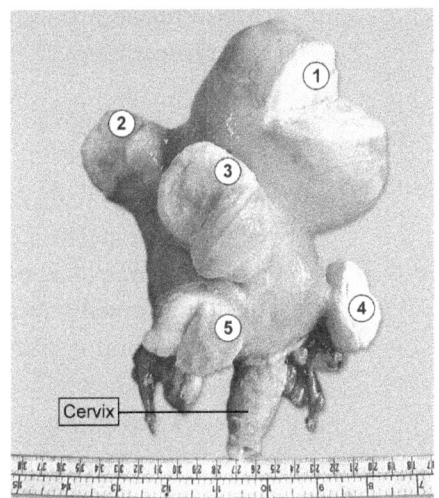

**Fig. 11.5:** Multiple subserous fibroid uterus. The fibroids are cut open to show the pseudocapsule and whorled appearance.
**Key:** 1, 2, 3, 4, 5: Cut section of fibroids.

**Q. What are the different secondary changes in fibroids?**

Ans. (a) Degenerations:
- (i) Hyaline (65%)
- (ii) Cystic (5–10%)
- (iii) Fatty
- (iv) Calcareous
- (v) Red (carneous degeneration)

(b) Atrophy

(c) Necrosis

(d) Infection

(e) Vascular changes

(f) Sarcomatous changes (0.1%).

**Q. What are the complications of fibroid?**

Ans. (a) Degeneration (mentioned before)

(b) Infection

(c) Torsion of a pedunculated fibroid

(d) Persistent menorrhagia → anemia

(e) Hemorrhage

(f) Polycythemia

(g) Sarcomatous change (0.1%).

**Q. What are the presenting symptoms?**

Ans. (a) Menstrual abnormalities:
- (i) Menorrhagia
- (ii) Metrorrhagia
- (iii) Dysmenorrhea

(b) Infertility

(c) Pain lower abdomen

(d) Lump abdomen

(e) Problems during pregnancy: Miscarriage, preterm labor, intrauterine growth restriction (IUGR).

(f) Pressure symptoms (more in cervical fibroid)
- Urinary symptoms: Dysuria, retention
- Bowel symptoms: Constipation
- Ureteric compression (rare): Hydroureter
- Others: Edema legs.

**Q. What are the causes of menorrhagia in fibroid uterus?**

Ans. (1) Increased endometrial surface area

(2) Interference with normal uterine contractility

(3) Increased vascularity, venous obstruction and congestion

(4) Endometrial hyperplasia due to hyperestrinism

(5) Pelvic congestion.

## Chapter 11 • Gynecology Case Discussion

**Q. What are the causes of infertility in fibroid uterus?**

**Ans. Uterine:** (i) Distortion and elongation of uterine cavity
 (ii) Congestion and dilatation of endometrial venous plexus → defective implantation
 (iii) Atrophy and necrosis of the endometrium over the submucous fibroid → defective nidation.
**Tubal:** (i) Cornual block due to cornual myoma
 (ii) Marked elongation of the tube over a big fibroid.
**Ovarian:** Anovulation
**Peritoneal:** Associated endometriosis.

**Q. What are the differential diagnosis of fibroid uterus?**

**Ans.** (1) *Pregnancy:* History of amenorrhea, symmetrical enlargement of uterus, urine for β-hCG, ultrasonography of lower abdomen.
(2) *Ovarian tumor:* Cystic, consistency, lower margin can be reached, moves side to side as well as from above downwards, notch is present between lump and uterus, movement of lump does not cause movement of cervix.
(3) *Chocolate cyst:* Fixed, tender mass, history of dysmenorrhea and dyspareunia.
(4) *Adenomyosis:* Age $\geq 40$ years, parous women, dysmenorrhea, smooth enlargement of uterus around 12 to 16 weeks.
(5) *Tubo-ovarian mass:* History of acute pelvic inflammation, pelvic pain and congestion, bilateral tender fixed mass with ill-defined margin.
(6) *Full bladder:* History of retention, on catheterization lump disappears.

**Q. What is the important observation during bimanual examination that can differentiate a fibroid uterus from an ovarian tumor?**

**Ans.** In a case of fibroid uterus:
 (i) The uterus is irregularly enlarged and the feel is firm to hard.
 (ii) Uterus is not felt separately from the mass and no groove is felt between the uterus and the mass.
 (iii) The cervix moves when the tumor is moved per abdomen and vice versa.

**Q. Give an outline of management of a case of fibroid uterus.**

**Ans. Management options depend on the following factors:**
 (a) Age
 (b) Presence of symptoms
 (c) Need of child bearing
 (d) Presence of any complications
**Management options available are:**
 (i) Conservative (observation)
 (ii) Medical
 (iii) Surgery for myomectomy (conservative) or hysterectomy. Surgery may be by laparotomy or by laparoscopy.

**Q. What is the place of medical management of fibroid uterus? What are the different agents used?**

**Ans.** Medical management may be done in few cases to improve the symptoms temporarily. Improvement of menorrhagia, anemia or pain could be there.

**Commonly used drugs:** Progestogens, danazol, antiprogestogens, GnRH analogs (agonists and antagonists).

**Other drugs:** COCs, DMPA, LNG-IUS, progesterone receptor modulators (ulipristal), anti-progesterone (mifepristone), GnRG receptor analogs (agonists, antagonists). Nonhormonal agents are: Tranexamic acid, aromatase inhibitors (letrozole, anastrozole).

**Q. What are the advantages and disadvantages of GnRH use?**

**Ans. Advantages:**
  (a) Reduces the size of myoma (60%)
  (b) Reduces the bleeding, improves anemia
  (c) Increases the possibility of laparoscopic procedure
  (d) Increases the possibility of vaginal hysterectomy.

**Disadvantages:**
  (a) Expensive
  (b) Menopausal symptoms
  (c) Hot flushes
  (d) Vaginal dryness
  (e) Loss in bone mineral density
  (f) Difficulties in surgery to get the correct plane of dissection
  (g) Risk of recurrence
  (h) Needs add back therapy to control the menopausal symptoms.

**Q. What are the indications of medical therapy?**

**Ans.** (a) Young woman desirous of child bearing

  (b) For improvement of anemia, control of bleeding, dysmenorrhea

  (c) To reduce the size of myoma before surgery.

**Q. What are the different types of surgery that can be done for fibroid uterus?**

**Ans.** (A) **Open surgery (Laparotomy)**
  (i) Myomectomy: Enucleation of fibroid (myoma) from the uterus and the uterus is preserved.
  (ii) Hysterectomy.

  (B) **Endoscopic surgery**
  (i) Laparoscopy:
  - Myomectomy
  - Myolysis (using laser)
  - Others: Laparoscopic myolysis using thermal or cryoprocedure.
  (ii) Hysteroscopy: Resection of a submucous myoma.
  (iii) Magnetic resonance-guided focussed ultrasound (MRgFUS) or MR high intensity focussed ultrasound (MR-HIFU).

  **The Exclusion criteria are:** Myoma >10 cm, uterus size >24 weeks, abdominal scars, other general contraindications of MRI.

  **Advantages are:** It is noninvasive, without any anesthesia, rapid recovery and return to work, and is well tolerated.

**Complications are:** Skin burns, venous thromboembolism, adjacent tissue injury.

(C) **Others:** Uterine artery embolization using polyvinyl alcohol microsphere. It is used for control of symptoms (to reduce the size of myoma and the uterus, also reduces menorrhagia, pain), when not controlled with other medical management.

**Side effects are:** Postembolization syndrome (25%), manifested with: malaise, nausea, pelvic pain, fever, leukocytosis, ovarian failure.
**Contraindications are:** Renal dysfunction, desire for pregnancy, large uterus, prior GnRH use, pelvic radiation, salpingectomy, pelvic infection, and drug allergy.

**Q. What is the treatment of choice for this patient (presented above)?**
**Ans.** Total abdominal hysterectomy with or without bilateral salpingo-oophorectomy (TAH and BSO). Oophorectomy should be done with her consent following counselling of risks and benefits.

**Q. What is the rationale behind the treatment (TAH and BSO)?**
**Ans.** This 45-year-old parous lady with a large fibroid was suffering from menorrhagia for a long time. Such a fibroid is unlikely to respond to medical therapy. Considering the risk of recurrence of myoma and the risk of recurrence of menorrhagia, myomectomy may not be a good option for this patient at this age.

**Q. Why are the normal ovaries removed during hysterectomy?**
**Ans. Benefits of oophorectomy are:**

(i) Protection against ovarian cancer (100%). Overall risk of ovarian carcinoma is less than 1% by the age of 70 years.

(ii) It reduces the risk of another laparotomy for chronic pelvic pain due to trapped ovarian syndrome (residual ovarian syndrome) or ovarian cyst formation, the overall risk of which is about 5–10%.

(iii) The conserved ovaries following hysterectomy loose their function soon due to interference with their blood supply during hysterectomy. There is early onset of menopause by 3–4 years. So the purpose of ovarian conservation is lost.

(iv) Moreover prophylactic oophorectomy protects against breast cancer (50%).

**Risks of prophylactic oophorectomy are:** Onset of premature (surgical) menopause and other health hazards (osteoporosis, ischemic heart disease). Psychological morbidities (irritability, mood swing, insomnia and depression) are also there. However, such a difficulty could be overcome by estrogen replacement therapy (ERT). Estrogen replacement therapy (ERT) is given in low doses (0.3 mg conjugated equine estrogen) and for short-term basis (5 years).

**Q. In a patient aged 30 years with a smaller fibroid, what other options she could have?**

Management options will depend upon few other factors apart from the age (*see* discussion above).

**Ans. Treatment options for the young woman with a smaller size fibroid.**
- Observation when there is no symptom.
- Medical therapy: Progestins, danazol, GnRH analogs. Ulipristal (progesterone receptor modulator), mifepristone (anti-progesterone), or LNG-IUD.
- Surgical: Myomectomy either by laparotomy, laparoscopy or by hysteroscopic resection (submucous variety).
- Embolization (embolotherapy) of uterine arteries.
- Desiccation (myolysis) of leiomyoma using laser has also been tried.
- Ultrasound or MRI guided therapy with 'High intensity focussed ultrasound' (HIFU).

## Chapter 11 • Gynecology Case Discussion

## CASE – 2 | OVARIAN TUMOR

### Case Summary

*Mrs PD, 20-year-old, newly married woman presents herself in the emergency with lower abdominal pain and heaviness. She was examined to have a cystic pelvic abdominal mass (Fig. 11.6). Sonography revealed a fairly large cystic mass arising from the pelvis. She was considered for emergency laparotomy. The findings are shown in the Figure 11.7. The uterus and the other ovary looked normal.*

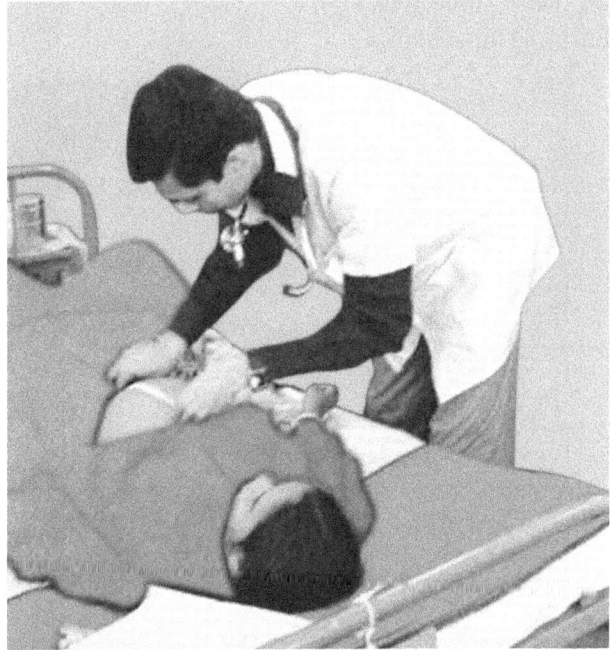

**Fig. 11.6:** Candidate performs clinical examination to measure the dimensions of a pelvic abdominal mass.

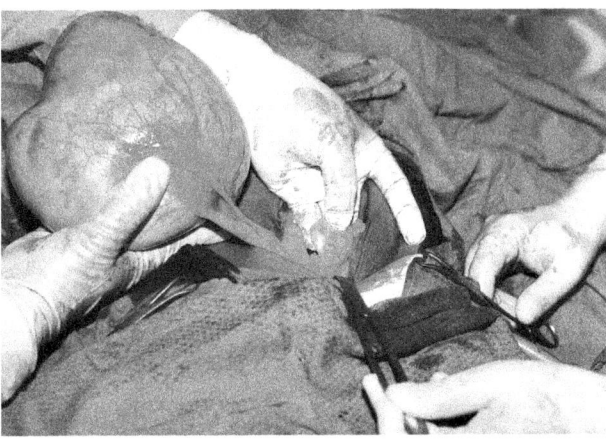

**Fig. 11.7:** Laparotomy showing ovarian tumor (right).

**Q. What is the diagnosis?**

**Ans.** Twisted ovarian cyst.

**Q. What are the differential diagnoses?**

**Ans.**
- Fibroid uterus
- Chocolate cyst
- Pregnancy
- Full bladder
- Mesenteric cyst (Fig. 11.8)
- Big hydrosalpinx (Fig. 11.9)
- Encysted tuberculosis.

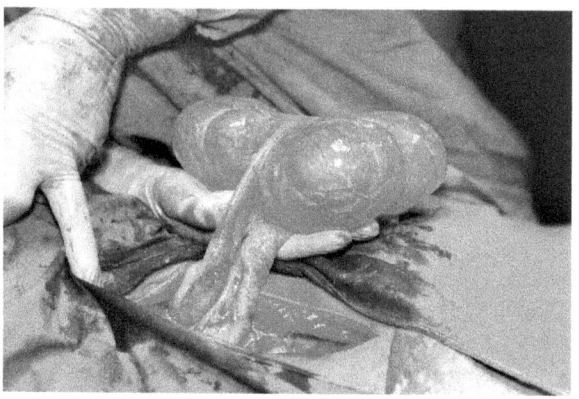

**Fig. 11.8:** Mesenteric cyst in a young woman who presented herself with the features of a twisted ovarian tumor.

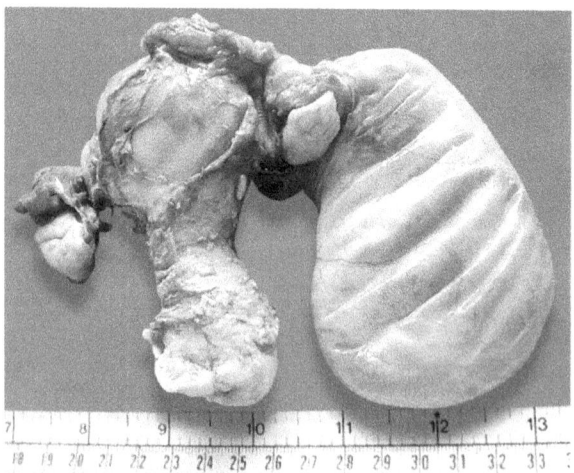

**Fig. 11.9:** Specimen of total hysterectomy with bilateral salpingo-oophorectomy showing a large hydrosalpinx (retort-shaped) of the left tube.

**Q. What investigations would have been done had she not been in acute pain?**

**Ans.** *Ultrasonography:* She had an ultrasonography done before coming to the hospital. USG revealed the picture as shown in Figure 11.10.

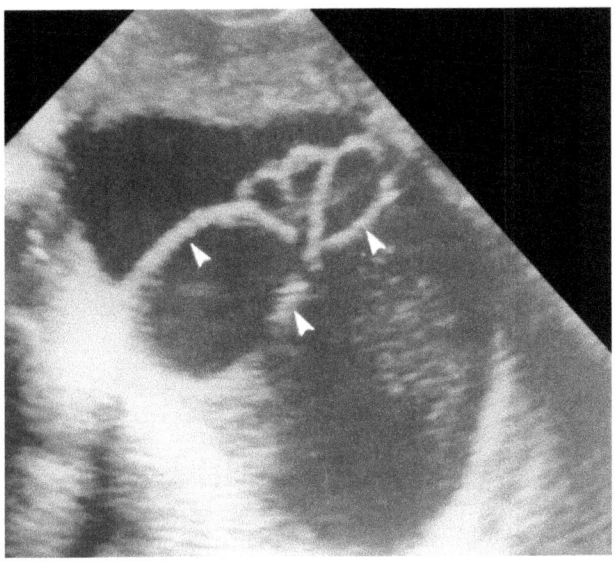

**Fig. 11.10:** Ultrasonographic view of ovarian tumor showing septations (arrow).

**Q. What surgical treatment should be appropriate for her?**

**Ans.** Ovarian cystectomy if ovarian tissue could be salvaged. Ovariotomy or oophorectomy—alternatively.

In either case, tissue should be sent for histological diagnosis.

**Q. What are the common ovarian tumors in this age group?**

**Ans. Germ cell tumors**—of which dermoid cyst is common.

Others are **epithelial cell tumors**—serous cystadenoma or mucinous cystadenoma.

**Q. What are the complications of benign ovarian tumor?**

**Ans.** (i) Torsion (Fig. 11.11)
(ii) Intracystic hemorrhage
(iii) Infection
(iv) Rupture
(v) Pseudomyxoma peritonei
(vi) Malignancy.

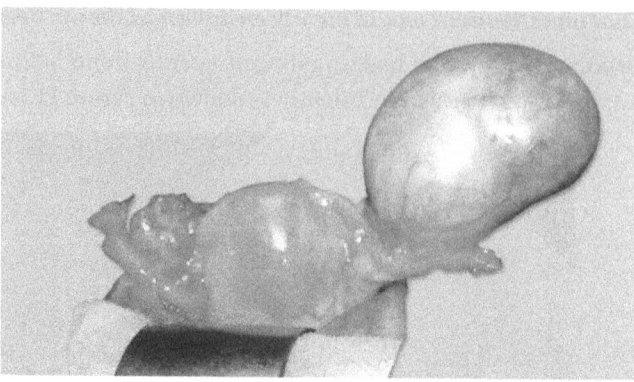

Fig. 11.11: Torsion of the left ovarian cyst.

**Q. What are non-neoplastic cysts of the ovary?**
Ans. (a) Follicular cysts
(b) Corpus luteum cyst
(c) Theca lutein and granulosa lutein cyst
(d) Polycystic ovarian syndrome (PCOS)
(e) Endometrial cyst (chocolate cyst).

**Q. What are the features of a functional cyst?**
Ans. (a) Usually <8 cm in diameter
(b) Regresses spontaneously
(c) Unilocular
(d) Usually contains clear fluid
(e) Usually without any complication.

**Q. Mention some of the common tumors of the ovary and their histogenesis?**
Ans. (A) **Epithelial tumor (70–80%)**
    (a) Serous cystadenoma
    (b) Mucinous cystadenoma
    (c) Endometrioid tumors.
(B) **Germ cell tumors of the ovary (15–20%)**
    (a) Dysgerminoma
    (b) Endodermal sinus cell tumor
    (c) Choriocarcinoma
    (d) Teratoma: (i) Immature and (ii) mature (dermoid).
(C) **Sex cord stromal tumors (3–5%)**
    (a) Granulosa cell tumor
    (b) Theca cell tumor
    (c) Sertoli cell tumor
    (d) Leydig cell tumor
    (e) Fibroma.
(D) **Others—unclassified.**
(E) **Secondary metastatic tumor (Krukenberg's tumor).**

**Q. How can you differentiate a benign ovarian tumor from a malignant one clinically during examination as well as during laparotomy (Fig. 11.12)?**

**Ans.** Features suggestive of malignancy for an ovarian tumor during **clinical examination** are:
(a) Tumor—bilateral (Fig. 11.12)
(b) Mobility—restricted or fixed
(c) Feel—solid/variegated
(d) Surface—irregular
(e) Ascites—present
(f) Nodules in POD—present.

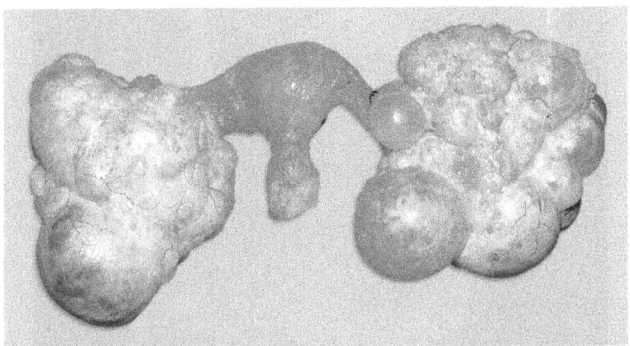

Fig. 11.12: Bilateral malignant ovarian tumor.

Features suggestive of malignancy of an ovarian tumor during **laparotomy** are:
(a) Ascites—present and often it is hemorrhagic
(b) Tumor on cut section; solid with hemorrhagic areas
(c) Peritoneal and/or omental metastatic deposits—present.

**Q. What is Meigs syndrome?**

**Ans.** Presence of ascites, right-sided hydrothorax (pleural effusion) in association with the presence of an ovarian tumor like fibroma, thecoma, Brenner or granulosa cell tumor is called Meigs syndrome.

**Q. On bimanual examination, how can you differentiate an ovarian tumor from a fibroid uterus?**

**Ans.** (a) The mass is felt separately from the uterus
(b) A groove is felt between the mass and the uterus
(c) On moving the mass per abdomen the cervix does not move
(d) The lower pole of the mass can be felt through the fornix.

**Q. What is pseudomyxoma peritonei?**

**Ans.** It is a condition of mucinous ascites usually secondary to mucinous tumors. It is often associated with mucinous cystadenoma of the ovary, mucocele of the appendix, gallbladder and also with intestinal malignancy.

**Q. What is the place of MRI in the management of an ovarian tumor?**

**Ans.** MRI is useful to make the diagnosis, to differentiate it from the uterus and to detect any solid areas and locularity (Fig. 11.13). It is especially useful in detecting a malignant tumor, enlargement of lymph nodes and to detect metastatic spread of the disease (omentum, diaphragm and pre-and para-aortic nodes).

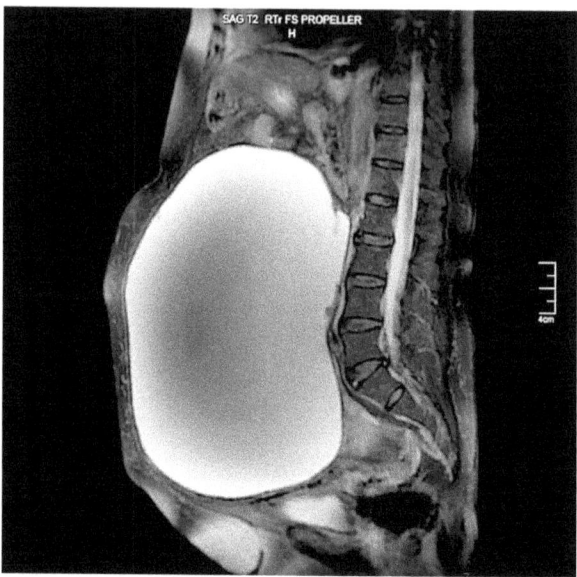

**Fig. 11.13:** MRI of a huge ovarian tumor occupying the whole abdomen.

**Q. What are the guidelines for surgery during laparotomy for such a case of ovarian tumor?**

**Ans.**
(i) A vertical incision is made
(ii) Peritoneal fluid if present is aspirated otherwise peritoneal washings with normal saline is collected and sent for cytology
(iii) The ovarian tumor is explored and nature (benign or malignant) is noted. (*see* discussion above)
(iv) Exploration is done for the other ovary, pelvic organs, omentum, liver, undersurface of the diaphragm and the periaortic group of lymph nodes for any metastatic deposits.

**Q. What are the different types of surgery that can be done in a case of benign ovarian tumor? What are the factors considered before such an operation?**

**Ans. The important factors considered are:**
(i) Age of the patient and her desire for future childbearing
(ii) Amount of healthy ovarian tissue available during surgery for preservation
(iii) Any high-risk factor for ovarian malignancy.

**Different types of surgery are:**

In a **young patient**: (i) Ovarian cystectomy or (ii) ovariotomy (salpingoo-ophorectomy).

In **parous women with age 40 years or above:** Total hysterectomy with bilateral salpingo-oophorectomy is done.

**Q. What is the common malignant tumor of the ovary?**

**Ans.** Malignant epithelial tumors are the most common (90%).

**Q. What is Krukenberg tumor of the ovary?**

**Ans.** It is a metastatic variety of malignant ovarian tumor.

**Q. What are the common primary sites for Krukenberg's tumor?**

**Ans.** Stomach, large bowel, breast and gallbladder.

**Q. What are the histological characteristics of a Krukenberg's tumor?**

**Ans.** *See* p. 615.

**Q. What is the importance of age in relation to ovarian tumor?**

**Ans.** Ovarian tumor can be observed at any age of a woman. Practically no age is immune to ovarian tumor (benign or malignant). However, nearly 60% of ovarian neoplasms found in the postmenopausal women are malignant.

Germ cell tumors of the ovary are commonly seen in the young and adolescent girls (14–20 years of age).

**Q. What are the common symptoms of ovarian tumors?**

**Ans.** (i) Majority are asymptomatic
(ii) Heaviness in lower abdomen
(iii) A gradually increasing abdominal mass
(iv) Pain in lower abdomen
(v) Respiratory distress (mechanical)
(vi) Usually no menstrual abnormality.

**Other symptoms** are more common when there are malignant changes.
- Dyspepsia, and flatulence
- Loss of appetite
- Appearance of abdominal pain and tenderness
- Rapid rate of tumor growth
- Loss of body weight.

**Q. Who are the high-risk women for developing ovarian malignancy?**

**Ans.** (a) Age of the woman, 40–60 years
(b) History of familial cancers (ovarian and breast)
(c) Postmenopausal palpable ovary.

**Q. What are the protective factors for ovarian malignancy?**
Ans. (a) Combined oral contraceptive pill use
  (b) Pregnancy
  (c) Breastfeeding
  (d) Aspirin.

**Q. What is the place of prophylactic oophorectomy while doing hysterectomy?**
Ans. See p. 379.

**Q. Name some hormone producing tumors of the ovary.**
Ans. Sex cord stromal tumor are known as 'functioning tumors' of the ovary as they produce hormones.
  (A) **Estrogen producing tumors**
    - Granulosa cell tumor
    - Theca cell tumor.
  (B) **Androgen producing tumors**
    - Sertoli cell tumor
    - Leydig cell tumor.

**Q. Which type of ovarian cyst undergoes torsion most often and why?**
Ans. Dermoid cyst because of moderate size, moderate weight (due to high fat content), free mobility and long pedicle.

**Q. What are the complications of benign ovarian tumor?**
Ans. Torsion, rupture, infection, impaction, intestinal obstruction, malignant change, pseudomyxoma peritonei, hemorrhage.

**Q. Management of an ovarian tumor?**
Ans. (A) **Investigations:**
  (i) Blood test: Complete hemogram
  (ii) Ultrasonography of pelvis
  (iii) X-ray—chest, abdomen
  (iv) Tumor markers CA-125 and HE4.

(B) **Management outline:**
  (i) **In women of reproductive age group:**
    - Asymptomatic simple cyst <5 cm do not require any treatment.
    - Cysts 5–8 cm require follow up.
    - Cyst >8 cm after menopause or before puberty or solid tumor at any age need to be evaluated by MRI/TVS and serum CA-125.
      Laparoscopic approach is considered to be gold standard for management of benign ovarian masses that are smaller in size.

      If the cyst is multilocular, bilateral and with echogenic nodules along with CA-125 raised, laparotomy and surgical removal is a must. In young women with bilateral benign ovarian cyst, cystectomy is preferable to oophorectomy.
  (ii) **Age more than 45 years:**
      Total abdominal hysterectomy with bilateral salpingo-oophorectomy is done.

**Q. What are the different modes of spread in a case of epithelial carcinoma of the ovary?**

**Ans.** (i) Transcoelomic
(ii) Direct
(iii) Lymphatics
(iv) Blood-borne.

**Q. What are the different modes of therapy in a case of malignant ovarian tumor?**

**Ans.** (i) Surgery (first choice)
(ii) Chemotherapy
(iii) Combination therapy
(iv) Radiotherapy.

**Q. What are the different types of surgery that can be done in the management of a case with malignant ovarian tumor?**

**Ans.** (a) Total hysterectomy with bilateral salpingo-oophorectomy, infracolic omentectomy and sampling of para-aortic lymph nodes
(b) Cytoreductive surgery (debulking procedure)
(c) Biopsy: USG/CT guided biopsy may be done in cases with advanced ovarian malignancy with comorbid conditions for consideration of neo-adjuvant chemotherapy.
(d) Unilateral salpingo-oophorectomy: This is rarely done in selected cases of younger age group of women to preserve fertility.

**Q. What are the common chemotherapeutic agents used in the management of epithelial ovarian cancer?**

**Ans.** (A) **Single agent**
(a) Platinum compounds: Carboplatin and cisplatin
(b) Taxane compounds: Paclitaxel and docetaxel
(c) Alkylating agents: Ifosfamide and cyclophosphamide.

(B) **Combination chemotherapy**
(a) Carboplatin and paclitaxel
(b) Cisplatin and paclitaxel
(c) CAP (cyclophosphamide, adriamycin and cisplatin).

**Q. Borderline ovarian tumors.**

**Ans.** These tumors are intermediate in position between benign and the malignant in terms of histology and prognosis.
(1) Nuclear atypia
(2) Stratification of the epithelium
(3) Microscopic papillary projections
(4) Cellular pleomorphism
(5) Mitotic activity.

They are characterized by atypical epithelial proliferation **without stromal invasion (differentiating features from ovarian carcinoma).**

**Treatment:**

Unilateral oophorectomy is optimum for the young women. When there is bilateral ovarian involvement or peritoneal spread, total hysterectomy with bilateral salpingo-oophorectomy with infracolic omentectomy is done.

**Q. What are the clinical features of malignant ovarian tumor?**

**Ans. Symptoms:**
- Abdominal distension
- Abdominal discomfort, pain
- Difficulty in eating and to move around
- Weight loss
- Urinary symptoms (urgency on frequently)
- Features of hormone production in hormone producing tumor.

**Signs:**
- Cachexia
- Solid, irregular, bilateral, fixed lump
- Ascites
- Nodules in POD.

**Q. What are the investigations you like to do in a case of suspected malignant ovarian tumor?**

**Ans.**
- **Ultrasonography**: Pelvis and whole abdomen
- **Chest X-ray**
- **Tumor markers**: Serum CA-125, LDH, α-fetoprotein, hCG
- **Contrast-enhanced computed tomography (CECT)** whole abdomen: It is helpful in detecting peritoneal deposits, metastasis of the omentum, pre- and para-aortic lymph node metastasis and for other metastatic survey (liver, diaphragm). It can be used in cases for detecting recurrence of ovarian carcinoma.
- **MRI**: It is used for surveying metastatic disease. Metastasis in pelvis, peritoneum, pre- and para-aortic lymph nodes, liver, omentum and distant sites (lung).
- **FNAC** (limited palace).
- **Positron emission tomography (PET):** It uses 18F-fluro-2-deoxy-glucose (FDG). This compound is absorbed by the cancer cells, later on it is detected by scanning. PET differentiates cancer tissues from normal tissues. PET when combined with CECT can detect small volume of metastatic disease. It is more sensitive than CT or MRI.

**Q. What is ROMA?**

**Ans.** It is the risk of ovarian malignancy algorithm. It consists of serum CA-125 and HE4 (human epididymal protein) values that are computed in an algorithm. This also includes menopausal status.

**Q. What is RMI?**

**Ans.** It is the risk of malignancy index. It combines three presurgical features:
**Levels of serum CA-125 level (CA-125)**
Menopausal status (M)
Ultrasound score (U)
RMI: U × M × CA125.
**Ultrasound score** = 1 point each for: multilocular cysts, solid areas, ascites, bilateral lesions, metastasis
M = Menopausal status (premenopausal = 1, post-menopausal = 3)
CA-125 = Serum CA-125 level in U/mL.
According to NICE guideline patient with an RMI—score >250 should be referred to a gynecologic oncology center for multidisciplinary team management.

**Q. What is treatment of epithelial ovarian cancer?**

**Ans. Early stage disease (1A, 1B, 1C)** surgical staging, total abdominal hysterectomy, bilateral salpingo-oophorectomy with total omentectomy and grading of the tumor are done. Chemotherapy is considered depending upon the grading of the tumor. Stage 1A grade 3 tumors and above: most patients are given chemotherapy.
**Advanced stage disease**—staging, cytoreductive surgery (hysterectomy, bilateral salpingo-oophorectomy, omentectomy and resection of peritoneal metastasis) followed by 6 cycles chemotherapy (carboplatin and paclitaxel).

**Q. What is neoadjuvant chemotherapy?**

**Ans.** It is done in advanced stages like stage III and IV of ovarian carcinoma. Initially, 3 cycles chemotherapy followed by surgery and again 3 cycle chemotherapy is given. It improves surgical resectibility of the tumor mass and the survival outcome.

**Q. What is second look operation?**

**Ans.** It is performed on a patient who has no clinical evidence of disease after a prescribed course of chemotherapy. It is done to determine the response to therapy.

**Q. Treatment of germ cell neoplasm.**

**Ans.** Surgery is required for diagnosis, staging and treatment. In contrast to epithelial ovarian carcinoma, most germ cell tumors can be safely treated with fertility preserving surgery rather than TAH+BSO. They are highly sensitive to chemotherapy (BEP—Bleomycin, Etoposide, and Cisplatin).

**Q. What are the reasons for poor outcome of ovarian cancers?**

**Ans.** (a) Late diagnosis
(b) No effective screening procedure available
(c) Limitations of cytoreductive surgery.

## CASE – 3 | PELVIC ORGAN PROLAPSE

### Case Summary

Mrs PL, 53-years old, multiparous lady presents with the problem of descent of her uterus. She has also some amount of backache and dragging feel in the vagina and walking difficulty. Examination revealed the findings (Fig. 11.14).

**Q. What is the diagnosis?**

**Ans.** Genital prolapse.

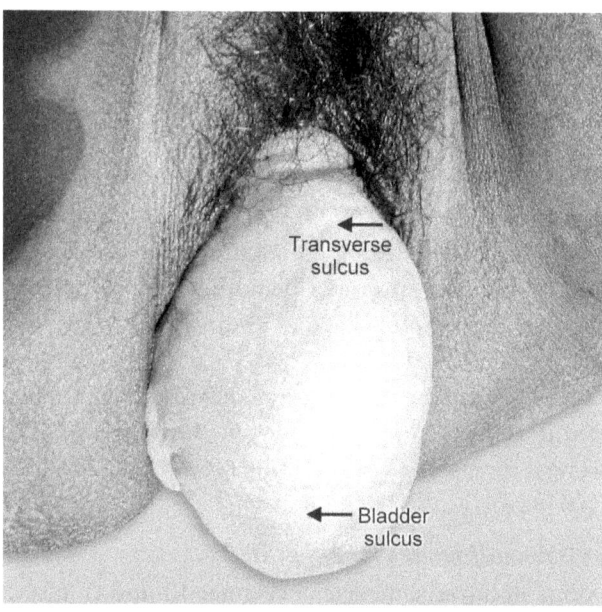

**Fig. 11.14:** Genitourinary prolapse. There are three sulci on the anterior vaginal wall. Transverse vaginal sulcus is situated at the junction of urethrocele above and the cystocele below. The bladder sulcus is at the level of attachment of anterior vaginal wall to the cervix. *See* also Figs. 11.15A and B.

**Q. What are the degrees of uterine prolapse?**

**Ans.** There are three degrees of prolapse (Figs. 11.15A and B).
  (i) *No prolapse (normal):* Cervix normally (anatomically) lies at the level of ischial spines.
  (ii) *First degree:* Slight uterine descent (from its normal anatomical position), but the external os remains inside the vagina.

(iii) *Second degree:* Cervix is outside but uterine body is inside the introitus.
(iv) *Third degree:* Uterine body remains outside the introitus.

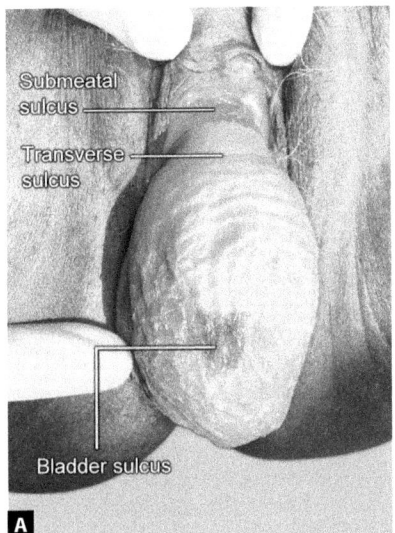 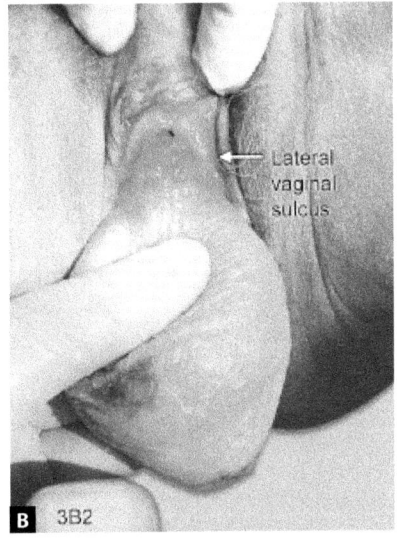

**Figs. 11.15A and B:** (A) Four sulci on the anterior vaginal wall are marked (pointers); (B) Examination procedure to differentiate second degree prolapse from procidentia.

**Q. Is there any other classification of genitourinary prolapse?**
**Ans.** The newer classification is POP-Q classification.

| Pelvic Organ Prolapse Quantitative (POP-Q) Scoring | |
|---|---|
| **Stage** | **Description** |
| 0 | No descent of pelvic organs |
| I | Leading edge of the prolapse remains 1 cm or more above the hymenal ring (≤1 cm). |
| II | Leading edge of the prolapse extends from 1 cm above to 1 cm below the hymenal ring (between −1 and +1 cm) |
| III | Extending from 1 cm beyond the hymenal ring but without complete vaginal eversion |
| IV | Essentially complete eversion of vagina |

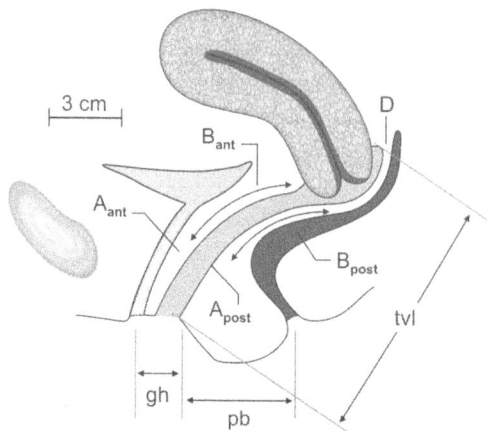

**Fig. 11.16:** Nine specific sites are considered. Hymen is taken as the fixed point. The plane of hymen is defined as the zero level. Leading point of prolapse may be above (proximal) or below (distal) to the plane of hymen. Prolapse measurements (cm) are recorded as negative (–ve) numbers when above and positive (+ve) numbers when lies below the plane of hymen. Organ prolapse is measured with a wooden Pap spatula with markings. The woman may be examined in lithotomy or standing position (or even under anesthesia). She may be asked to do some maneuvers (Valsalva) to demonstrate the prolapse maximally. TVL is measured after reducing the prolapse while rest of the measurements are done when the prolapse is seen maximally. Measurements are tabulated in the grid as shown below. POP-Q is considered as the objective, site specific and standard system for assessment of POP.

*(TVL: total vaginal length; POPQ: pelvic organ prolapse-quantification; POP: pelvic organ prolapse; gh, genital hiatus; pb: Perineal body).*

### Grid Used to Record Measurements in POP-Q System (Fig. 11.16)

| Aa<br>Anterior wall<br>(– 3 cm to + 3 cm) | Ba<br>Anterior wall<br>(– 3 cm to + tvl) | C<br>Cervix or vaginal cuff<br>(– tvl to + tvl) |
|---|---|---|
| gh<br>Genital hiatus<br>(2 cm) | pb<br>Perineal body<br>(3 cm) | tvl<br>Total vaginal length |
| Ap<br>Posterior wall<br>(– 3 cm to +3) | Bp<br>Posterior wall<br>(– 3 cm to + tvl) | D<br>Posterior fornix<br>(+/– tvl) |

### Table 11.1: Site-specific measurements in POP-Q system (Fig. 11.16)

| Site | Description | Range |
|---|---|---|
| Aa | Anterior vaginal wall, midline 3 cm proximal to the external urinary meatus | –3 cm to + 3 cm |
| Ba | Anterior vaginal wall, most dependent portion between Aa and anterior fornix | –3 cm to + tvl |
| C | Cervix or vaginal cuff | ± tvl |
| D | Posterior fornix or vaginal apex | ± tvl |
| Ap | Posterior vaginal wall, midline 3 cm proximal to hymen | –3 cm to + 3 cm |
| Bp | Posterior vaginal wall, most dependent portion, between Ap and posterior fornix | –3 cm to + tvl |
| gh | External urinary meatus to posterior hymenal ring | 2 cm |
| tvl | Point D to the hymenal ring | 10 cm |
| pb | Posterior hymen to mid-anal opening | 3 cm |

The other commonly used grading system is **Barden and Walker (1972)**:
- **Grade I** : Descent of any genital organ half-way to the hymen
- **Grade II** : Descent up to the hymen
- **Grade III** : Descent half-way past the hymen
- **Grade IV** : Complete eversion of vagina.

**Q. What are the urinary and other symptoms in a case of genitourinary prolapse?**

**Ans.**

| Urinary symptoms | Other gynecological symptoms |
|---|---|
| • Dysuria | • Vaginal fullness |
| • Incomplete evacuation | • Mass coming out of vagina |
| • Urgency and frequency | • Low backache |
| • Pain during voiding | • Bowel—incomplete evacuation/ Constipation |
| • Stress urinary incontinence | • Vaginal—discharge/bleeding |
| • Retention of urine—patient feels the need to push the prolapse mass manually up to pass urine | • Dyspareunia |

**Q. What other associated pathological conditions must be looked for during examination?**

**Ans.** Abdominal and pelvic examination for any pelvic mass, urinary incontinence, cystocele, rectocele, enterocele or decubitus ulcer.

**Q. What are the different types of anterior vaginal wall prolapse?**

**Ans.** (i) Upper 2/3rd: Cystocele
(ii) Lower 1/3rd: Urethrocele
(iii) Combined: Cystourethrocele.

**Q. What is a decubitus ulcer?**

**Ans.** It is a trophic ulcer found at the dependent part of the prolapsed mass lying outside the introitus.

**Q. How do you treat a case of decubitus ulcer?**

**Ans.** (a) Cervical cytology to exclude malignancy
(b) To reduce the prolapse mass with a vaginal pack using glycerine and acriflavine solution
(c) To use estrogen cream when tissues are atrophic due to menopause.

**Q. What is the change in the vaginal and in the supravaginal part of the cervix?**

**Ans. Vaginal part** of the cervix is congested and may become infected. It may be bulky (edematous). There may be some blood stained vaginal discharge (decubitus ulcer).

**Supravaginal part** becomes elongated due to the tug of war between the cardinal ligaments to pull the uterus up and the weight of the uterus that makes it fall down through the vaginal axis.

**Q. What are the anatomical changes in the urinary system in a case of genitourinary prolapse?**

**Ans.** (a) An angulation is developed between the urethra and the bladder. This may cause retention of urine.

(b) The ureters are dragged downwards. There may be hydroureteric changes.

**Q. What are the high-risk factors for the prolapse?**

**Ans.** (a) Repeated child birth trauma—too frequent, too many
(b) Traumatic delivery—prolonged and/or obstructed labor
(c) Injury to the supports of the uterus
(d) Menopause—tissue atrophy
(e) Chronic lung disease
(f) Multiparity

**Q. How you can clinically differentiate a third degree uterine prolapse from a second degree one?**

**Ans.** On inspection, in both the degrees of prolapse, the mass protrudes out through the introitus and the leading part of the mass is the external os. But to confirm a third degree prolapse, palpation is essential. The thumb of the left hand is placed anteriorly and the middle and the index fingers are placed posteriorly. The fingers should be placed above the mass and outside the introitus. If the fingers can be apposed, it is a third degree prolapse (Figs. 11.15A and B).

**Q. What is understood by rectocele, enterocele and the deficient perineum?**

**Ans. Rectocele:** It is the bulge in the middle third of the posterior vaginal wall due to the prolapse of anterior rectal wall.

**Enterocele:** It is the bulge in the upper third of the posterior vaginal wall due to the prolapse of the intestines.

**Deficient perineum:** It is due to deficiency of the tissues that bridges the distance between the introitus and the anal verge.

**Q. Who are the women that can be treated with pessary?**

**Ans.** Use of pessary gives temporary improvement of symptoms. The conditions are:
(i) Women not fit for surgery
(ii) Patient's unwillingness for operation
(iii) Women while waiting for operation
(iv) Prolapse in early pregnancy (up to 18 weeks)
(v) Prolapse in puerperium.

## Chapter 11 • Gynecology Case Discussion

**Q. Apart from pessary what other modes of conservative therapy could be suggested?**

Ans. (a) Weight reduction
(b) Improvement of chronic lung disease, treatment of constipation
(c) Pelvic floor exercise
(d) Lifestyle modification.

**Q. What are the different types of surgery, that can be done in a case with genitourinary prolapse?**

Ans. **Several factors** are considered before adopting any particular method of surgery. These are mainly:

(a) Age
(b) Parity
(c) Need of childbearing
(d) Type of prolapse
(e) Degree of prolapse. Other factors are women's health status and any other associated pathology (abnormal uterine bleeding, urinary incontinence) present or not.

**The different types of surgery that are commonly done are:**
(a) Anterior colporrhaphy
(b) Colpoperineorrhaphy
(c) Vaginal repair of enterocele with pelvic floor repair (PFR)
(d) McCall culdoplasty
(e) Paravaginal defect repair
(f) Fothergill's operation
(g) Repair of vault prolapse
(h) Vaginal hysterectomy with PFR.

**Q. What are the different routes for the correction of vault prolapse?**

Ans. (1) **Vaginal route:**
  (i) Sacrospinous colpopexy
  (ii) McCall's culdoplasty
  (iii) Colpocleisis.
(2) **Abdominal route:**
  (i) Sacral colpopexy
  (ii) Cervicopexy or sling operations.

**Q. What is a vault prolapse?**

Ans. Prolapse of the vaginal vault in a woman who had hysterectomy before, done either vaginally (common) or abdominally.

**Q. What are the different uterus preserving surgeries?**

Ans. (1) Fothergill's operation (Manchester operation)

(2) Abdominal sacrocolpopexy (laparotomy or by laparoscopy)

(3) Sling operations:

   (a) Purandare's sling

   (b) Shirodkar's sling

   (c) Khanna's sling.

**Q. What is the indication of Fothergill's operation?**

**Ans.** This is mainly done for a young woman where preservation of the uterus is desired either for reproductive function or for menstrual function. Where childbearing function is not needed (family completed), this operation may be combined with (vaginal/abdominal) sterilization procedure.

**Q. What are the composite steps of this Fothergill's operation?**

**Ans.** (a) Initial dilation and curettage

   (b) Amputation of cervix

   (c) Fixation of Mackenrodt's ligaments in front of the cervix

   (d) Anterior colporrhaphy

   (e) Colpoperineorrhaphy.

**Q. What is Fothergill's stitch?**

**Ans.** It is the stitch that fixes the Mackenrodt's ligament to the anterior surface of the cervix to make the uterus anteverted.

**Q. What are the complications of Fothergill's operation?**

**Ans.** Complications of Fothergill's operation (*see* table below):

| During operation | • Hemorrhage |
|---|---|
| | • Injury to the bladder and rectum |
| **Postoperative** | • Retention of urine or cystitis |
| | • Hemorrhage—primary or secondary |
| | • Infection |
| Late | • Dyspareunia     • Cervical stenosis—hematometra |
| | • Infertility     • Cervical incompetency |
| | • Cervical dystocia in labor |

**Q. What is the common operation for congenital or nulliparous prolapse?**

**Ans.** Cervicopexy or sling operation (Purandare's operation).

In this operation, the cervix is pulled up abdominally. Strips of rectus sheath or Marlex or Gore-tex (synthetic) tapes are used.

**Q. What are the complications of vaginal hysterectomy with pelvic floor repair operation?**

Ans. Complications may be:

(A) **During operation:** Hemorrhage, injury to bladder or rectum.

(B) **Postoperative (early):** Retention of urine, hemorrhage and urinary tract infection.

(C) **Late:** Dyspareunia, recurrence of prolapse.

**Q. What factors aggravate genitourinary prolapse?**

Ans. (a) Postmenopausal tissue atrophy

(b) Chronic cough and constipation

(c) Obesity (increased BMI)

(d) Under nutrition

(e) Obstetric factors: Repeated child birth trauma (multiparity).

**Q. What is congenital prolapse?**

Ans. Here the prolapse is due to congenital weakness of the supporting structures of the uterus. It is commonly seen in nulliparous women. Congenital prolapse is not associated with cystocele.

**Q. What are the important supports of the uterus?**

Ans. Supports of the uterus are described in a three tier system.

(A) **Upper tier: Indirect support** to maintain the anteverted position of the uterus.

Supporting structures are:
- Endopelvic fascia
- Round ligaments
- Broad ligaments with intervening pelvic cellular tissues.

(B) **Middle tier: Direct and strongest support**
- Endopelvic fascia
- Pericervical ring of fascia
- Mackenrodt's ligaments
- Uterosacral ligaments
- Pubocervical ligaments.

(C) **Inferior tier: Indirect support**
- Pelvic floor muscles (levator ani)
- Levator plate
- Perineal body
- Endopelvic fascia
- Urogenital diaphragm.

**Q. What important factors are generally considered for deciding the appropriate treatment for prolapse?**

**Ans.** (a) Age
(b) Parity
(c) Desire for future childbearing
(d) Associated pelvic pathology
(e) Degree of prolapse
(f) Presence of stress urinary incontinence
(g) Assessment of general health.

**Q. What treatment options should this woman be offered?**

**Ans.** For this patient (presented in the case), vaginal hysterectomy with repair of the pelvic floor would be appropriate. If she is unwilling or found unfit for surgery, she may be advised vaginal pessary.

**Q. What is levator plate and what is its function?**

**Ans.** It is a thick band of connective tissue formed by the medial fibers of the two levator ani muscles. It is the anococcygeal raphe extending from the anorectal junction to the coccyx. The anterior fibers encircle the anorectal junction and are inserted in the perineal body.

The levator plate forms a horizontal supportive shelf upon which the rectum, upper vagina and uterus rest. The levator plate thus prevents genital organ prolapse. When levator plate is damaged, the genital organs prolapse.

**Q. What are the types of prolapse?**

**Ans. Vaginal prolapse:**
(1) Anterior vaginal wall: Cystocele, urethrocele, cystourethrocele
(2) Posterior vaginal wall: Enterocele, rectocele, relaxed perineum

**Uterine prolapse:**
(1) Congenital: Nulliparous prolapsed
(2) Acquired (uterine descent): First degree, second degree, third degree

**Vault prolapse:**
(1) Primary: Enterocele
(2) Secondary: Following hysterectomy (abdominal/vaginal).

**Q. What is a compartment-wise classification of prolapse?**

**Ans.** (1) Anterior compartment: Cystocele, urethrocele
(2) Apical compartment: Uterine prolapse, vault prolapse
(3) Posterior compartment: Enterocele, rectocele, relaxed perineum

**Q. What is the difference between acquired and congenital uterine prolapse?**
Ans.

| Congenital prolapse | Acquired prolapse |
|---|---|
| Commonly seen in nulliparous women | Seen in multiparous women |
| Due to congenital weakness of support of uterus | Due to obstetric injury |
| Cystocele and rectocele are rare | Commonly associated with post-menopausal atrophy |
|  | Usually associated with cystocele and rectocele |

**Q. Differences between cystocele and Gartner's duct cyst.**
Ans.

| Cystocele | Gartner's duct cyst |
|---|---|
| Herniation of bladders | Retention cyst in the remnants of Wolffian duct |
| Through lax anterior vaginal wall<br>Situated in anterior vaginal wall | Situated in the anterolateral aspect of anterior vaginal wall |
| Diffuse margin | Well-defined margin |
| Rugosities present | Rugosities absent |
| Cough impulse present | Cough impulse absent |

**Q. What are the differential diagnosis of something coming down pervagina?**

Ans. (1) **Uterine prolapse:** Usually multiparous, elongation of supravaginal portion of cervix, vaginal fornices are shallow, associated with cystocele/cystourethrocele/rectocele.

(2) **Congenital elongation of cervix:**
   - Usually nulliparous
   - Vaginal portion of cervix is elongated
   - Vaginal fornices narrow and deep
   - Not associated with cystocele/cystourethrocele/rectocele.

(3) **Chronic inversion of uterus:**
   - External OS is not visible over the leading point of the protruding mass
   - P/V cervical rim may be felt at the top of the mass in complete inversion
   - P/R uterine body cannot be felt. A cup like depression is felt
   - Uterine sound cannot be passed (in complete inversion) or passed for a short distance only incomplete inversion).

(4) **Fibroid polyp:**
   (i) No external OS is visible. Broad shaggy mass is visible
   (ii) P/V pedicle can be felt coming out through the cervical canal
   (iii) P/R normal position and shape of the uterus
   (iv) Uterine sound can be introduced through normal length of uterus.

**Q. Why D and C done in Fothergill's operation?**
**Ans.** (A) Dilation done
   (a) To facilitate the passage of stitches through cervical canal.
   (b) It prevents cervical stenosis.
(B) Curettage done to remove and check the endometrium for any pathology and to delay next menstruation. This also avoids the confusion in the management of the patient in the postoperative phase. A woman who had D and C, and is having bleeding in the postoperative phase, is most likely due to the operation rather than the menstrual bleeding.

**Q. Make a management outline for different types of prolapse.**
**Ans.** (1) Anterior vaginal wall prolapse: Anterior colporrhaphy
(2) Posterior vaginal wall prolapse: Colpoperineorrhaphy
(3) Elderly women with family completed: Vaginal hysterectomy with repair of the pelvic floor
(4) Women desiring child bearing: Uterus preserving surgery (Fothergill's operation)
(5) Nulliparos prolapse:
   (i) Sling operation (Purendare, Shirodkar or Khanna's operation)
   (ii) Abdominal sacrocolpopexy
(6) Posthysterectomy vault prolapse:
   (i) Sacrospinous colpopexy
   (ii) McCall's culdoplasty
   (iii) Abdominal sacrocolpopexy (by laparotomy or laparoscopy)
(7) Prolapse in a elderly old woman with medical comorbidities—pessary may be the option till surgical fitness is obtained.

Woman having the symptoms of urinary incontinence: Prolapse surgery is combined with surgery for SUI.
(a) Abdominal: Burch colposuspension
(b) Vaginal: Tension free vaginal tape (TVT).

## CASE – 4 | GENITOURINARY FISTULA

### Case Summary

*Mrs LF, 26-year-old housewife, presented with continuous leakage of urine per vaginam. This, she noticed four days past her last childbirth at home. She stated that the labor was difficult and prolonged (2 days). She was delivered by local dais.*

**Q. What is most likely the diagnosis?**
**Ans.** Urinary incontinence most likely the vesicovaginal fistula (VVF).

**Q. What is a vesicovaginal fistula?**
**Ans.** It is an abnormal communication between the bladder and the vagina. Urine escapes through this passage into the vagina causing true incontinence.

**Q. What are the important causes of VVF?**
**Ans.** (A) Obstetric (most common: 80-90%):
- Ischemic
- Traumatic.

(B) Gynecological (10-20%).

**Q. What is the pathology of ischemic fistula?**
**Ans.** See below.

**Q. What are the different types of urinary incontinence?**
**Ans.** (i) **Urethral:**
(a) Stress incontinence (CSI)
(b) Detrusor instability (DI)
(c) Overflow
(d) Congenital (epispadias).

(ii) **Extraurethral:**
(a) Acquired fistulae
(b) Congenital ectopic ureter.

**Q. What are the different types of urinary fistula?**
**Ans. Bladder:** Vesicovaginal (most common), vesicouterine, vesicocervical.
**Urethra:** Urethrovaginal.
**Ureter:** Ureterovaginal (common), ureterouterine (rare).

**Q. What could be the possible cause in this case and what is the basic pathology?**
**Ans. Obstetric fistula** due to prolonged labor or obstructed labor. Prolonged compression of the bladder base between the fetal head and symphysis pubis → ischemic necrosis → infection → sloughing → fistula (this pathology usually takes about 3-5 days).

**Q. How do you confirm the diagnosis of a vesicovaginal fistula?**

**Ans.** Examination under anesthesia.
  (i) **Dye test:** Methylene blue dye is introduced into the bladder through a rubber catheter. Dye is seen to come out through the fistula site.
  (ii) **A metal catheter:** Passed through the urethra may be seen to come out through the fistula site (Fig. 11.17).
  (iii) **Three swab test** (*see* Dutta Gyne 7/e, p. 345).
  (iv) **Cystoscopy:** For detection of fistula site and to assess the proximity of the ureteric openings to the fistula site.
  (v) **IVP:** It may be needed to exclude ureterovaginal fistula and also in cases with recurrent urinary tract infection.

**Q. When should the repair be done? What are the different types of repair in a case of vesicovaginal fistula?**

**Ans.** Repair is done usually 3 months after the delivery.

Following are the different types of VVF repair:
- Local repair by flap splitting method is commonly done
- Edge paring and suturing may be done in a very small fistula
- Latzko repair (partial colpocleisis) is done for a fistula (VVF) which is small and situated high in the vagina (following hysterectomy)
- Sometimes, martius method of graft (bulbocavernosus muscle and fat) is used when the fistula is big.

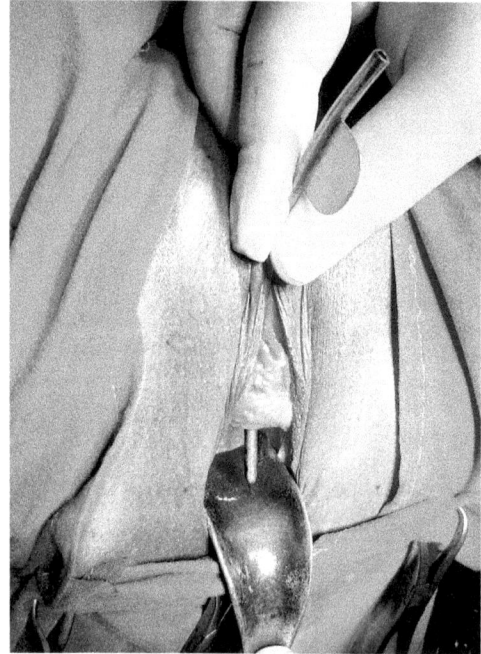

**Fig. 11.17:** Vesicovaginal fistula at the midvaginal level. The metal catheter is seen to come out through the vagina when introduced per the urethra.

**Q. Why is a three month delay important for repair?**

**Ans.** By this time, the local tissues are free from infection and the general health of the patient is improved. Further delay is unnecessary as it will produce more tissue fibrosis and also prolong the misery of the patient.

**Q. What are the principal steps of flap splitting method of repair?**

**Ans.** (i) Good exposure of the fistula site.
  (ii) Excision of the scar tissue from the margins of fistula.
  (iii) Mobilization of the bladder wall from the vagina.
  (iv) Suturing the bladder wall without tension in two layers (3-0 Vicryl-interrupted stitches). Bladder mucosa is excluded.
  (v) Apposition of the vaginal wall (1-0 Vicryl-interrupted stitches).
  (vi) Continuous bladder drainage for 10-14 days.

**Q. Mention some of the favorable factors for the successful repair of VVF.**

**Ans.** Favorable factors for successful repair are:
  (i) Fistula site easily accessible
  (ii) Site—midvaginal
  (iii) Size—not too big
  (iv) Margins—not too much fibrosis.

**Q. What preoperative assessment is needed before the actual repair?**

**Ans.**
- Assessment of patient's general health.
- Fistula status: Site, size, mobility, number, margin as well as the proximity with ureteric openings.

**Q. What postoperative care is important for the success of repair?**

**Ans.**
- Continuous bladder drainage for 10-14 days.
- Urinary antibiotics.
- Patient should pass urine frequently (say 2 hourly) following removal of the catheter.

**Q. What advice you would give her during the discharge?**

**Ans.**
- To avoid intercourse for at least 3 months
- To defer pregnancy for at least 2 years with the use of contraception
- Mandatory supervision and institutional delivery for the next pregnancy
- Delivery should be by elective cesarean section.

**Q. What is Sims' triad?**

**Ans.** **Marion Sims (1852) of New York** used to repair fistula by his own method using (*see* p. 550):
  (i) Sims' position (exaggerated left lateral position)
  (ii) Sims' speculum (*see* Fig. 16.2)
  (iii) Silver thread—to suture the fistula margins [currently replaced by Vicryl or PDS (polydioxanone) suture material].

## CASE – 5 URETERIC INJURY IN GYNECOLOGY

### Case summary

Mrs AC, 47-year-old lady underwent a difficult abdominal hysterectomy due to severe pelvic endometriosis. She observed leaking of urine through the vagina on the same day of the operation. She had the urge to pass urine and could pass urine normally also.

**Q. What is the most likely diagnosis?**

**Ans.** Ureterovaginal fistula.

**Q. How do you confirm the diagnosis?**

**Ans.** The diagnostic procedures used are:
   (i) IV indigocarmine test—dye is seen to leak through the vagina
   (ii) Cystoscopy and ureteric catheter introduction
   (iii) Excretory urography.

**Q. What are the common sites of ureteric injury during gynecological surgery?**

**Ans.** Ureteric injury may occur more commonly when pelvic anatomy is distorted. Due to the close proximity between the ureter and genital organs, ureteric injury results, especially in the presence of adhesions.
   (i) At the level of infundibulopelvic ligament.
   (ii) Below the level of ischial spine: Close to the uterosacral ligament.
   (iii) The site where the uterine artery crosses the ureter from above.
   (iv) Over the anterior vaginal fornix: Within the ureteric tunnel of Mackenrodt ligament.
   (v) Where ureter enters the bladder.
   (vi) Any congenital malformation of the ureter.

**Q. What are the different types of ureteric injury?**

**Ans.** Different types of ureteric injury are:
   (i) Kinking or angulation
   (ii) Ischemic injury due to damage of vascular supply
   (iii) Ligature incorporation
   (iv) Crushing by clamps
   (v) Transection
   (vi) Segmental resection
   (vii) Thermal injury—by diathermy or laser
   (viii) Injury by staplers (laparoscopic surgery).

**Q. What are the gynecological pathologies where ureteric injuries are more likely during operation?**

**Ans.** (i) Cervical fibroid
   (ii) Broad ligament tumor

(iii) Pelvic endometriosis
(iv) Gynecologic malignancy (carcinoma cervix and ovary)
(v) Pelvic hematoma
(vi) Tubo-ovarian mass.

**Q. Outline the management approach for a patient with ureteric injury in respect to the type.**

**Ans.** (1) Crushing (vascularity maintained): Placement of a ureteric stent (double J)

(2) Ligation: Deligation, remove the sutures

(3) Kinking/angulation: To release the adhesions, remove sutures causing angulation.

(4) Transaction:
   (a) At or below the pelvic brim:
      (i) Uretero-ureteric anastomosis
      (ii) Uretero-ileal interposition
      (iii) Trans uretero-uroteric anastomosis
   (b) Close to the bladder:
      (i) Ureteric mobilization—uretero-neocystostomy
      (ii) Psoas hitch procedure
   (c) Away from the bladder: Boari flap procedure and psoas hitch

**Q. What are the different methods of repair for ureteric injury?**

**Ans.** Repair could be done by:
(a) Ureteric mobilization and tension-free anastomosis (end to end) over an ureteric stent
(b) Ureteric implantation into the bladder or creating a bladder flap (Boari's flap).

**Q. What are the symptoms of urinary tract infections?**

**Ans** (a) Pain during micturition (dysuria)
(b) Frequency
(c) Pelvic pain
(d) Chill, rigor
(e) Urgency
(f) Backache
(g) Hematuria
(h) Fever
(i) Pain in the loins.

## CASE – 6  RECTOVAGINAL FISTULA

### Case Summary

*Mrs CL, 28-year-old housewife, presented with the complaints of leakage of flatus and feces into the vagina. She had a difficult forceps delivery during her last child birth 6 months ago. On rectovaginal examination, the findings are as shown in Figure 11.18.*

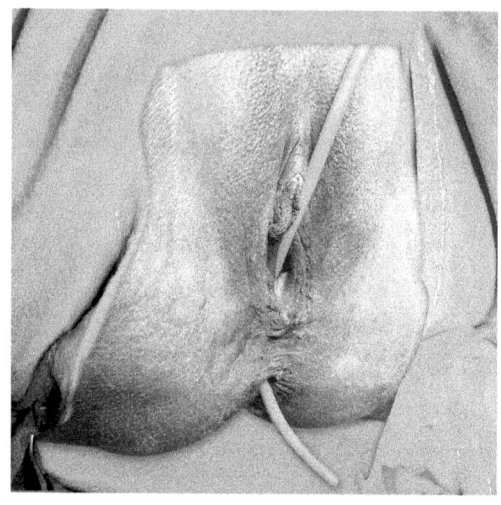

**Fig. 11.18:** Rectovaginal fistula following traumatic forceps delivery. The catheter is seen to come out through the anus when introduced through the fistula site in the vagina.

**Q. What is most likely the diagnosis?**

**Ans.** Rectovaginal fistula (RVF).

**Q. What are the common causes of rectovaginal fistula (RVF)?**

**Ans.** (A) Acquired and (B) Congenital

(A) *Acquired:*
- **Obstetrical:**
  - Unrepaired complete perineal tear (CPT)
  - Obstructed labor—where the sacrum is flat
  - Traumatic—during destructive operation.
- **Gynecological:**
  - Imperfect repair of complete perineal tear.
  - Trauma—perineorrhaphy, posterior colpotomy, vaginal reconstruction surgery.
  - Malignancy—vagina and cervix.
  - Radiation.

(B) *Congenital:* Anal canal may open into the vagina.

**Q. How do you repair a rectovaginal fistula?**

**Ans.** (A) Transvaginal method of repair is commonly done. Scar margin is excised. Vaginal wall is separated from the underlying rectal wall. Repair is done without any tension.

(B) High-up fistula: Initial colostomy is done. Local repair of fistula is done after 3 weeks, then after another 3 weeks, closure of colostomy is done.

## CASE – 7   OLD COMPLETE PERINEAL TEAR

### Case Summary

*Mrs LT, 27-year-old housewife, presented herself in the outpatient clinic for her inability to hold flatus and feces. She noticed this following her last childbirth that was nearly 4 months back at her home. Perineal examination revealed—see Figure 11.19.*

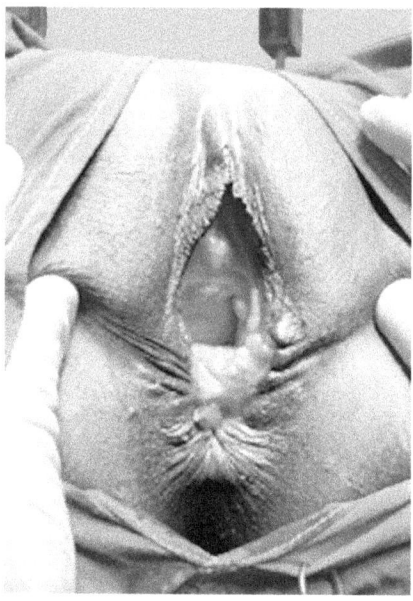

**Fig. 11.19:** Old complete perineal tear. Perineum is absent. The torn sphincter ends are seen.

**Q. What is most likely the diagnosis?**

**Ans.** Old complete perineal tear (both external and internal).

**Q. What do you mean by this?**

**Ans.** When there is tear of the perineal body involving the anal sphincter complex (both external and internal) with involvement of the anorectal mucosa. It is called old as because the duration is more than 3 months.

**Q. What are the different degrees of perineal tear?**

**Ans.** (a) **First degree:** Injury of the vaginal epithelium, perineal skin and fourchette. Perineal body remains intact.

(b) **Second degree:** Injury of the posterior vaginal wall and tear of the perineal body excluding the anal sphincter.

(c) **Third degree:** Injury of the posterior vaginal wall, tear of the perineal body including the anal sphincter complex (both the external and internal anal sphincters) without involvement of the anal canal or rectum.

3a: <50% EAS torn

3b: >50% EAS torn

3c: Both IAS and EAS are torn.

(d) **Fourth degree:** Injury to the perineum involving the perineal body, anal sphincter complex (EAS and IAS) and anal and rectal mucosa.

*Q. What are the important risk factors for complete perineal tear?*

**Ans.** Risk factors are:
- Primigravida
- Big baby (>3 kg)
- Midline episiotomy
- Forceps delivery
- Scar in the perineum.

*Q. What structures are torn in a case of complete perineal tear (CPT)?*

**Ans.** Posterior vaginal wall, perineal skin, perineal body with the sphincters (both external and internal anal) and anorectal mucous membrane (varying degree).

*Q. What are the preoperative preparations?*

**Ans.** She is admitted 3 days prior to surgery. Low residue diet (bread, milk) is given for 2 days. Intestinal antiseptics (metronidazole and neomycin) are given for 2 days. Lower bowel is cleared by giving enema for 2 days before the surgery.

*Q. What are the principal steps of the operation?*

**Ans.** Repair of CPT is done by flap method.
- Rectal wall is mobilized from the vaginal wall.
- Torn ends of the sphincter ani externus are mobilized.
- Rectal wall is repaired in two layers using interrupted sutures with 'O' Vicryl.
- Torn ends of the sphincter are approximated by interrupted sutures. 'O' Vicryl or PDS (polydioxanone) is used.
- Repair of the vaginal wall and skin.

*Q. What special postoperative care you will take for the patient?*

**Ans.**
- Nonresidual diet till the 5th postoperative day.
- Lactulose (stool softener) 10 mL twice daily from the 3rd postoperative day.

**Q. What advice you will give the patient on discharge?**

**Ans.**
- Mild laxative (lactulose) should be continued for few days more to keep stool soft
- Contraception to postpone immediate pregnancy.

**Q. What special precaution would be necessary during her next childbirth?**

**Ans.**
- Antenatal checkup during pregnancy and mandatory hospital delivery
- Liberal mediolateral episiotomy is a must.

**Q. What are the preventive measures that can avoid a CPT?**

**Ans.** Proper conduction of the second stage of labor: To maintain flexion of the fetal head, to deliver the head in between contractions, perineal guard (Ritzen's maneuver), episiotomy in time and care during delivery of the shoulders.

**Q. What are the complications following repair of a complete perineal tear?**

**Ans.**
(a) Complete dehiscence of the wound
(b) Incomplete dehiscence—leading to rectovaginal fistula
(c) Too much tightening of the sphincter causing difficulty in defecation
(d) Dyspareunia.

## CASE – 8  PELVIC INFECTIONS

### Case Summary

A 32-year-old parous woman presented with the complaints of (i) lower abdominal pain and (ii) abnormal vaginal discharge. On examination, there was raised oral temperature >101°F; pelvic examination revealed cervical motion tenderness, uterine and adnexal tenderness. Transvaginal sonography revealed tubo-ovarian mass, hydrosalpinx (Fig. 11.20) with hyperemia.

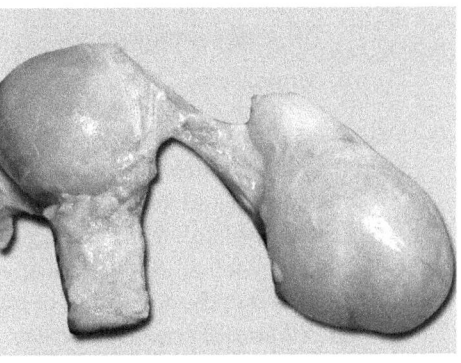

**Fig. 11.20:** Hydrosalpinx with huge dilatation of the tube (left) assuming the shape of a retort.

**Q. What is the most likely diagnosis?**

**Ans.** Pelvic inflammatory disease (PID). Hydrosalpinx with dilatation of the tube and formation of a tubo-ovarian mass.

**Q. What are the common organisms involved in pelvic infection?**

**Ans.** (1) Pyogenic (50%)
- Gram positive ⎫  Aerobic and
- Gram negative ⎭  Anaerobic

(2) Sexually transmitted diseases (STDs)
(3) Parasitic
(4) Fungal
(5) Viral
(6) Tubercular.

**Q. What are the modes of spread of gonococcus infection?**

**Ans.**
- Through continuity and contiguity
- Lymphatics and pelvic veins
- Bloodstream
- From adjacent extragenital organs.

**Q. What are the risk factors for PID?**

**Ans.** Women with:
(a) Multiple sexual partners
(b) Previous history of PID, are at risk of having PID.

**Q. What are the protective factors for PID?**
Ans. (i) Use of contraceptive measures:
- (a) Condoms
- (b) Oral contraceptives

(ii) Monogamy.

**Q. What is Fitz-Hugh Curtis syndrome?**
Ans. It is the sequelae of acute pelvic inflammatory disease. There is pain, discomfort and tenderness in the right hypochondrium due to perihepatitis. Presence of thin **'violin string'** adhesions around the liver and in the pelvis is observed following laparoscopy. The liver is involved due to transperitoneal or vascular dissemination of infection. The organisms commonly involved are *Chlamydia* or *Gonococcus*.

**Q. What are organisms involved in bacterial vaginosis (BV)?**
Ans. Organisms are: *Gardnerella vaginalis, Bacteroides, Peptococcus, Mobiluncus,* and *Mycoplasma hominis*.

**Q. How BV is diagnosed?**
Ans. Amsel's diagnostic criteria are:
(1) Homogeneous vaginal discharge
(2) Vaginal pH >4.5
(3) Positive Whiff's test: Fishy amine odor when the discharge is mixed with 10% KOH solution
(4) Presence of stippled epithelial cells in vaginal smear with Gram's stain: Presence of more *Gardnerella* and/or *Mobiluncus*.

**Q. How to treat the infection?**
Ans. Tablet metronidazole 200 mg, PO, TID × 7 days.

**Q. What are the clinical features of acute PID?**
Ans. (a) Fever ≥38°C
(b) Lower abdominal tenderness (bilateral)
(c) Vaginal discharge
(d) Deep dyspareunia.

**Q. What are the complications of pelvic inflammatory disease?**
Ans. **Immediate:**
(a) Pelvic peritonitis
(b) Septicemia—producing arthritis or myocarditis.

**Late:**
(a) Infertility
(b) Chronic pelvic pain
(c) Dyspareunia.

**Q. What are the indications of inpatient antibiotic therapy for a woman with PID?**

**Ans.** (a) Persistence of symptoms in spite of conservative management
   (b) Recurrence of acute attacks
   (c) Increase in size of the pelvic mass despite treatment.

**Q. What are the important causes of infertility in a woman with chronic PID?**

**Ans.**
- Loss of cilia (tubal damage)
- Loss of tubal peristalsis due to tubal thickening
- Cornual block
- Distortion of the tube due to peritubal adhesions
- Dyspareunia
- Chronic pelvic pain.

**Q. What are the indications of surgery in a woman with chronic PID?**

**Ans.** (a) Recurrence of acute attacks
   (b) Increasing size of pelvic mass
   (c) Infertility for adhesiolysis or restorative surgery.

**Q. What is the syndromic management of STIs and RTIs (WHO, UNAIDS – 1991)?**

**Ans.** Syndromic managements are based on epidemiological studies all over the world. Syndromic diagnosis and laboratory diagnosis have been found similar in terms of accuracy. Syndromic management has got many advantages.

   (i) It avoids delay in treatment where laboratory facilities are limited
   (ii) It avoids loss of follow up where referral system is not well-structured
   (iii) Transmission of infection is prevented
   (iv) Partner's counseling and management are the important steps of syndromic management
   (v) It is simple, rapid and inexpensive management of STIs and RTIs
   (vi) High cure rate is observed once treated appropriately.

## CASE – 9 | GENITAL TUBERCULOSIS

### Case Summary

*A 27-year-old woman presented with the complaints of: (a) chronic pelvic pain, (b) menstrual abnormality (oligomenorrhea and amenorrhea), (c) chronic ill health, and (d) inability to conceive. She gave the history of pulmonary tuberculosis for which she received complete treatment.*

**Q. Which genital organ is most commonly affected with tuberculosis?**
**Ans.** Fallopian tubes (100%).

**Q. What is the specific pathological change in the fallopian tube?**
**Ans.** Spread of infection: Hematogenous. Depending upon the site of infection, (A) **Interstitial** or (B) **Endosalpingeal**, the outcomes are:

| (A) **Interstitial salpingitis** | (B) **Endosalpingitis** |
|---|---|
| ⇩ | ⇩ |
| Destruction of muscles | Fimbriae are everted, abdominal ostium usually remains patent |
| ⇩ | ⇩ |
| Thickened calcified wall | "Tobacco pouch" appearance of the tube |

- **Salpingitis isthmica nodosa**: It is the nodular thickening of the tubes due to proliferation of tubal epithelium within the hypertrophied muscle layer. This is seen at the region of the isthmus. On HSG, it appears as a diverticulum. It may also be observed in pelvic endometriosis.

**Q. In genital tuberculosis, what is the pathological change in the uterus?**
**Ans.** Cornual ends are commonly affected (blocked). Endometrial ulceration → adhesion formation → synechiae (Asherman's syndrome).

**Q. What are the symptoms of genital tuberculosis?**
**Ans.** (i) **Infertility:** Due to tubal block, Asherman's syndrome (uterine synechiae) or ovarian dysfunction.

(ii) **Menstrual abnormality:**
  - Menorrhagia or irregular bleeding
  - Amenorrhea or oligomenorrhea.

(iii) **Others:** Chronic pelvic pain and vaginal discharge.

**Q. What are the contraindications of surgery in a case with genital tuberculosis?**
**Ans.** (i) Presence of active tuberculosis
(ii) When patient is responding to antitubercular therapy.

**Q. What is the regimen for antituberculous chemotherapy?**

**Ans. Revised National Tuberculosis Control Program (RNTCP) recommends:**

Category I (all new cases irrespective of smear positivity):

2H3 R3 Z3 E3 + 4H3 R3

Category II (smear positive cases with relapse, failure, default or others):

2H3 R3 Z3 E3 S3 + 1H3 R3 Z3 E3 + 5H3 R3 E3.

## CASE – 10  ABNORMAL UTERINE BLEEDING (AUB)

### Case Summary

*A 42-year-old parous woman presents with the problem of heavy and irregular menses for the last 6 months. She also experiences some amount of progressively increasing dysmenorrhea with it.*

**Q. What could be the possible type and reasons of this abnormality?**

**Ans.** Menstrual abnormality could be in the form of menorrhagia, dysfunctional uterine bleeding (DUB), metrorrhagia, polymenorrhea and dysmenorrhea. To know further about the type of menstrual abnormality and the cause, we need to know details of her menstrual history. This includes history of menarche, cycle regularity, length of the cycle, duration of period and the amount of bleeding. She needs a thorough clinical examination also.

**Q. What are the common causes of menorrhagia?**

**Ans.**
- Dysfunctional uterine bleeding
- Fibroid uterus
- Adenomyosis (Fig. 11.21)
- Pelvic endometriosis
- Chronic PID (tubo-ovarian mass)
- IUCD
- Hypothyroidism.

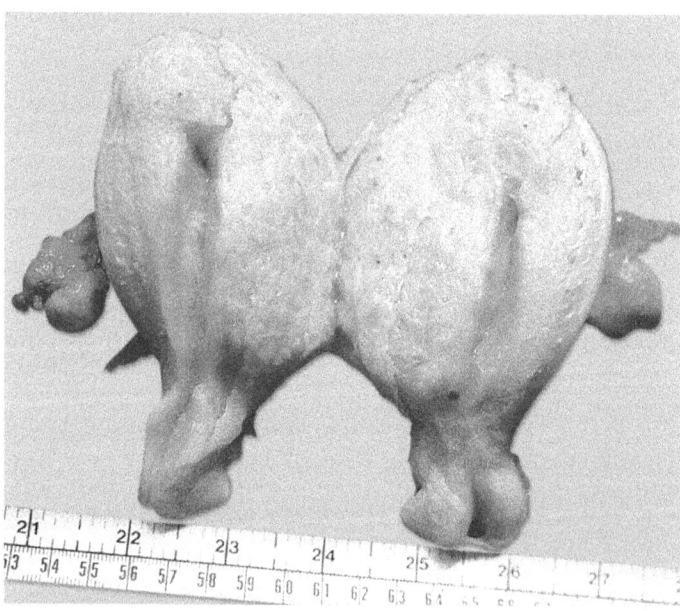

**Fig. 11.21:** Adenomyosis. The uterus is cut open to show thickened posterior wall. Dark hemorrhagic spots and cystic spaces are seen within the myometrium and there is no capsule.

## Chapter 11 • Gynecology Case Discussion

**Q. What are the important causes of contact bleeding?**

**Ans.**
- Carcinoma cervix
- Polyp of the cervix
- Vascular ectopy (erosion) of the cervix (pregnancy and pill use)
- Infections (chlamydial and tubercular)
- Cervical endometriosis (rare).

**Q. What are the important causes of oligomenorrhea?**

**Ans.** (a) Obesity
(b) Stress
(c) Women with PCOS.

**Q. How do you define dysfunctional uterine bleeding (DUB)?**

**Ans.** It is a state of abnormal uterine bleeding without any clinically detectable organic, systemic and iatrogenic cause (e.g. tumor, inflammation or pregnancy excluded).

**Q. What are the different types of uterine bleeding observed in DUB?**

**Ans.** (a) **Anovular bleeding (common):**
   (i) Menorrhagia

**(Cystic glandular hyperplasia/Metropathia hemorrhagica)**

**Slow rise in FSH**
⇩
Gradually increasing level of estrogen for a period of 6–8 weeks
⇩
With concomitant phase of amenorrhea 6–8 weeks
⇩
No ovulation
⇩
Endometrial thickness is increased as it is unopposed by progesterone.
⇩
**Break down of endometrial layer either due to fall in estrogen level or due to lack of endometrial stromal support**
⇩
Endometrial shedding
⇩
Heavy and prolonged bleeding.

**Uterus**: Myohyperplasia with symmetrical enlargement of about 8–10 weeks size.

**Endometrium**: Endometrial hyperplasia and cystic glandular hypertrophy.

(b) **Ovular bleeding (less common):**
   (i) Polymenorrhea/polymenorrhagia: Endometrium—secretory changes.
   (ii) Oligomenorrhea: Endometrium—secretory changes.
   (iii) Menorrhagia (rare):
   (iv) Others:
      (a) Irregular shedding of endometrium.
      (b) Irregular ripening of the endometrium.

**Q. How do you define abnormal uterine bleeding (AUB)?**

Ans. Any uterine bleeding outside the normal volume, duration, regularity or frequency is considered as AUB.

**Q. What are the common causes of AUB?**

Ans. (i) Organic pelvic pathologies are the common (uterine myomas)
(ii) Infections
(iii) Neoplasias
(iv) Hematological disorders
(v) Pregnancy complications
(vi) Endocrine dysfunctions

**Q. Describe the FIGO and ACOG classification of AUB.**

Ans. Abnormal uterine bleeding (AUB) according to FIGO, ACOG (2011) is classified with a newer system of terminology.

The newer classification is known by the acronym PALM-COEIN. It is based on the etiology:

| Classification Of AUB (FIGO–2011) | | | |
|---|---|---|---|
| **Structural causes (PALM)** | | **Nonstructural systemic causes (COEIN)** | |
| • Polyp | AUB–P | Coagulopathy | AUB–C |
| • Adenomyosis | AUB–A | Ovulatory dysfunction | AUB–O |
| • Leiomyoma (Fig. 11.22) | AUB–L | Endometrial | AUB–E |
| ▫ Submucosal myoma | AUB–L SM | Iatrogenic | AUB–I |
| ▫ Other myoma | AUB–LO | | |
| • Malignancy and hyperplasia | AUB–M | Not yet identified | AUB–N |

| | | |
|---|---|---|
| SM- Submucosal | 0 | Pedunculated intracavitary |
| | 1 | <50% intramural |
| | 2 | ≥50% intramural |
| O- Others | 3 | Contacts endometrium; 100% intramural |
| | 4 | Intramural |
| | 5 | Subserosal ≥50% intramural |
| | 6 | Subserosal <50% intramural |
| | 7 | Subserosal pedunculated |
| | 8 | Other (specify e.g. cervical, parasitic) |

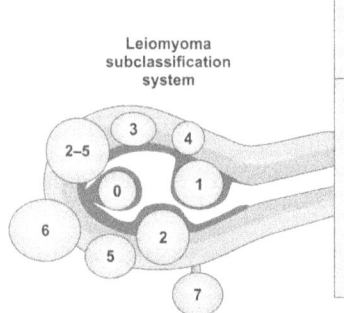

Leiomyoma subclassification system

**Fig. 11.22:** Leiomyoma subclassification system.

**Q. What special investigations are commonly done for the diagnosis of a case of abnormal uterine bleeding (AUB)?**

Ans. Investigations are designed to exclude any organic, systemic or pelvic pathology.

- Blood values: Complete hemogram (including platelet count, peripheral blood film and coagulation profile).
- Thyroid function tests: TSH, F T4, T3.
- Pelvic ultrasonography (transvaginal).
- Saline infusion sonography (SIS): Uterine cavitary pathology is better seen with the SIS than USG.
- Diagnostic uterine curettage (depending on age: Peri-or postmenopausal age group).
- Hysteroscopy: Visualization of the cavity and directed biopsy if needed.
- Laparoscopy: To see and treat any pelvic pathology (endometriosis).
- Hysterography to detect any filling defect (rarely done these days).

**Q. What is the purpose of doing D&C in the management?**

**Ans.** This is mainly done as a diagnostic procedure. We need to see any endometrial hyperplasia and neoplasia (diagnostic value). This may be due to anovulation or due to other causes of PCOS, or diabetes. This is also done to rule out endometrial malignancy specially in a postmenopausal woman. Dilatation and curettage may be helpful in a case with intractable uterine bleeding where medical treatment has failed (therapeutic value).

**Q. What is the medical management of AUB due to hormonal abnormalities?**

**Ans.** As majority of women respond well to conservative management.

Medications commonly used are:
(a) **Antifibrinolytic agents:** Tranexamic acid.
(b) **Prostaglandin synthetase inhibitors:** Mefenamic acid preparations.
(c) **Hormones:**
  (i) Medroxyprogesterone acetate
  (ii) Nonethisterone acetate.

**Q. What are the different types of surgery that can be done for the management of AUB?**

**Ans.** (i) Uterine curettage
(ii) Endometrial ablation or resection
(iii) Hysterectomy.

**Q. Make an outline of management of AUB keeping in mind the different age group of the women?**

**Ans.** All women, irrespective of the age, need to be investigated to detect the cause of AUB.

Common investigations done are:
(a) **Ultrasonography (TVS)**: Transvaginal sonography is superior to the transabdominal sonography in the diagnosis of abnormal uterine bleeding
(b) **Saline infusion sonography (SIS)**
(c) **Hysteroscopy and biopsy**
(d) **Endometrial sampling**
(e) **Dilatation and curettage**
(f) **Laparoscopy.**

**Q. Outline the actual management of such a patient with AUB.**

**Ans.** Management is done according to the pathology and the age of the women.

**Management depends on the following factors:**
(a) Age
(b) Desire of child bearing
(c) Severity of bleeding
(d) Associated pathology (thyroid dysfunction)
(e) Presence of organic pathology (myomas).

| Age group | Management |
|---|---|
| (a) **Pubertal or adolescent age (less than 20 years)** | ♦ **Medical therapy:**<br>– Mefenamic acid [prostaglandin synthetase inhibitor (PSI)]<br>– Tranexamic acid (antifibrinolytic agent)<br>– Hormones (progestogens-MPA, norethisterone), GnRH analogs<br>– Combined estrogen and progesterone. Progestogen therapy (commonly) is given |
| (b) **Reproductive age group (20–40 years)** | ♦ **Family not completed**<br>– Medical management: PSI, tranexamic acid<br>– Hormones<br>– LNG-IUS<br>♦ **Family completed:**<br>– Hormones<br>– LNG-IUS<br>– Endometrial resection/ablation<br>– Uterine artery embolization (UAE)<br>– Endometrial resection/hysterectomy |
| (c) **Perimenopausal age (>40 years)** | ♦ **Endometrial biopsy** (D/C, or endometrial sampling—Pipelle catheter) to exclude malignancy<br>♦ **Medical management**—progestins (benign pathology)<br>♦ **Hysterectomy** |
| (d) **Postmenopausal** | ♦ Exclude malignancy<br>♦ May need hysterectomy |

**Q. What are the general measures that are taken in the management of AUB?**

**Ans.** (A) **Improvement of anemia:**
   (i) Rest
   (ii) Oral/parenteral iron therapy
   (iii) Blood transfusion, if anemia is severe.

(B) **Others:**
   (i) Weight reduction in a obese woman
   (ii) Treatment of associated medical disorders (thyroid dysfunction).

**Q. How do you define heavy menstrual bleeding (HMB)?**

**Ans.** Any bleeding that interferes with woman's physical, emotional, social and material quality of life is defined as HMB.

Chapter 11 • Gynecology Case Discussion

## CASE – 11 | HYDATIDIFORM MOLE

### Case Summary

*Mrs CR, in her early pregnancy presented in the clinic with the complaints of vaginal bleeding and lower abdominal pain. She was investigated, diagnosed and advised for termination of pregnancy. This specimen has been removed following suction evacuation (Fig. 11.23).*

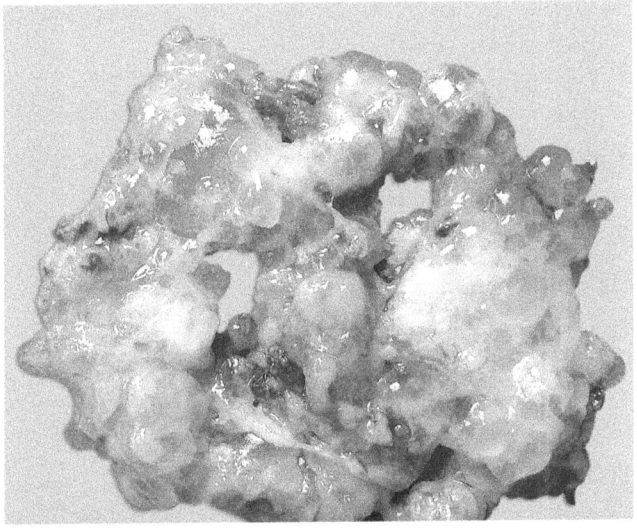

**Fig. 11.23:** Hydatidiform mole. Grape-like vesicles are seen.

**Q. What is the possible diagnosis?**

**Ans.** The specimen shows multiple grape-like vesicles of different sizes. This is the specimen of hydatidiform mole.

**Q. What are the characteristic microscopic changes in the molar tissue?**

**Ans.** (i) Marked proliferation of the syncytial and cytotrophoblastic epithelial cells

(ii) Thinning of the stromal tissue (hydropic degeneration)

(iii) Absence of blood vessels in the villi

(iv) The villus pattern is maintained.

**Q. What are the characteristic ovarian changes in molar pregnancy?**

**Ans.** Ovaries are enlarged due to formation of the theca lutein cysts. Ovarian changes may be unilateral or bilateral. It is present in about 25–50% of the cases.

**Q. What are the clinical features of molar pregnancy?**

**Ans.** • Vaginal bleeding
• Lower abdominal pain

- Constitutional symptoms: Vomiting, breathlessness and features of thyrotoxicosis
- Expulsion of grape-like vesicles (occasionally).

**On examination**

- **General examination:**
  - Pallor
  - Pre-eclampsia (early onset).
- **On abdominal examination:**
  - Uterine size: Usually more than the period of amenorrhea
  - Uterus feels: Doughy
  - Fetal parts: Not felt
  - FHS: Not heard.
- **On vaginal examination:**
  - No internal ballottement
  - Ovarian cyst (theca lutein cyst) may be palpable.

**Q. How to confirm the diagnosis of hydatidiform mole?**

**Ans.** (i) Sonography: **'snow storm'** appearance

(ii) Serum β-hCG raised (>100,000 IU/mL).

**Q. What are the complications of hydatidiform mole?**

**Ans.** (i) Early onset of pre-eclampsia

(ii) Hemorrhage

(iii) Shock

(iv) Sepsis

(v) Uterine perforation and internal hemorrhage

(vi) Respiratory distress

(vii) Choriocarcinoma (2–10%).

**Q. Who are the high-risk women to develop choriocarcinoma?**

**Ans.** (i) Woman's age is ≥39 years

(ii) Parity is ≥3

(iii) Serum hCG is ≥100,000 IU/mL

(iv) Uterine size is >20 weeks

(v) Previous history of molar pregnancy

(vi) Theca lutein cysts >6 cm.

**Q. What are the indications of prophylactic chemotherapy?**

**Ans.** This is an area of controversy. Prophylactic chemotherapy is considered for women at risk of developing gestational trophoblastic neoplasia (GTN).

The cases are:
(a) Age ≥35 years
(b) Initial level of serum hCG is ≥100,000 IU/mL
(c) hCG fails to become normal by 7–9 weeks' time or there is re-elevation
(d) Previous history of molar pregnancy
(e) Woman who is unreliable for follow-up
(f) Centers where follow-up facilities are not available.

**Q. What are the unfavorable manifestations during follow-up of a woman with molar pregnancy?**

**Ans.** (i) Persistent ill health
(ii) Irregular vaginal bleeding
(iii) Subinvolution of the uterus
(iv) hCG values remain elevated
(v) Chest radiograph—evidence of metastasis
(vi) Appearance of cough and hemoptysis.

**Q. How to differentiate a complete mole from a partial one?**

**Ans.** Complete mole can be differentiated from a partial mole by the following features:

**Complete mole:**
- Fetus is absent
- Hydropic changes of the villi are diffuse and not focal
- Uterine size is enlarged
- Levels of hCG is (>50,000) high; not so much high in a partial mole
- Risk of persistent GTN is high (20%). It is low in a partial mole.
- Karyotype:
  (a) Complete mole → 46 XX/XY
  (b) Partial mole → Triploid pattern ; 69XXX/69XXY/69XYY

**Q. What is persistent gestational trophoblastic neoplasia (GTN) and how is it treated?**

**Ans.** Persistent GTN is a condition where there is persistence of trophoblastic activity following evacuation of molar pregnancy. This is clinically diagnosed when the patient presents with:
(a) Irregular vaginal bleeding
(b) Subinvolution of the uterus
(c) Persistence of theca lutein cysts
(d) Levels of hCG either plateaus or re-elevates after an initial fall.

**Q. How is the workup done for the treatment of GTN?**

**Ans:** Patients are evaluated and then scored according to WHO prognostic scoring system. Depending upon the score, woman is treated either with single agent (WHO score <7) and the cases with WHO score ≥7 with multiagent chemotherapy. Surgery is reserved for selected cases.

**Q. How should this patient be followed up and for how long?**

**Ans.** Serial urinary β-hCG estimation weekly till negative. Usually, it becomes negative by 4–6 weeks time. Once negative, she is followed up at every month with serum hCG report for 6 months to 1 year.

**Q. What precautionary measures she should be advised while on follow-up?**

**Ans.** She should avoid pregnancy for at least 6 months to 1 year. For contraception, she can use barrier methods. Combined oral pills (low dose) may be used following normalization of β-hCG.

**Q. What are the reasons that the patient needs to be followed up following initial treatment?**

**Ans.** • Detection of cases with persistent trophoblastic disease
- Early detection of choriocarcinoma.

**Q. What is her prospect of future pregnancy and chance of recurrence of the problem?**

**Ans.** Prospect of future successful pregnancy is high, provided she is followed up. The risk of recurrence is less than 5%.

**Q. What is the karyotype pattern of a complete hydatidiform mole and that of a partial mole?**

**Ans.** In complete moles—karyotype pattern in majority is normal—46XX (90%). There is fertilization of 'an empty ovum' by a single sperm carrying 23 chromosomes. The usual 46XX chromosome pattern is the result of doubling of the paternal set of chromosomes (Fig. 11.24).

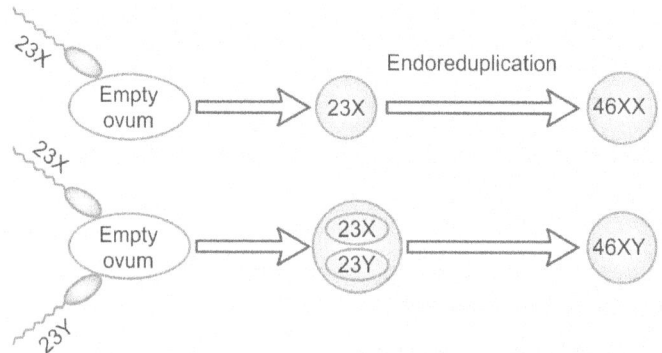

**Fig. 11.24:** Karyotype pattern of a complete mole—genome is entirely paternal in origin.

In about 10% cases, an empty ovum is fertilized by two sperm (dispermy), one carrying X and the other carrying Y chromosome. The chromosomal pattern is 46XY. All the chromosomes are derived paternally.

Partial moles (Fig. 11.25) consist of both the placenta and the fetus. Partial moles usually (90%) have triploid karyotype (Fig. 11.26). A normal ovum is fertilized by double sperm (dispermy), resulting in 69 chromosomes with sex chromosome configuration of 69XXX, 69XXY and 69XYY. The extra haploid set of chromosomes usually is derived from the father. The fetus is usually triploid, dies in the first trimester or is growth retarded with multiple malformations (syndactyly, hydrocephaly) (*see* Dutta's Textbook of Obstetrics, 9th edition, p. 230).

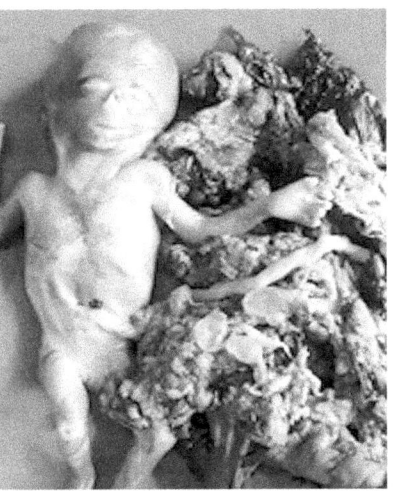

**Fig. 11.25:** Partial mole with a stillborn baby.
*Courtesy:* Dr S Mitra, Professor, Department of Obstetrics and Gynecology, India.

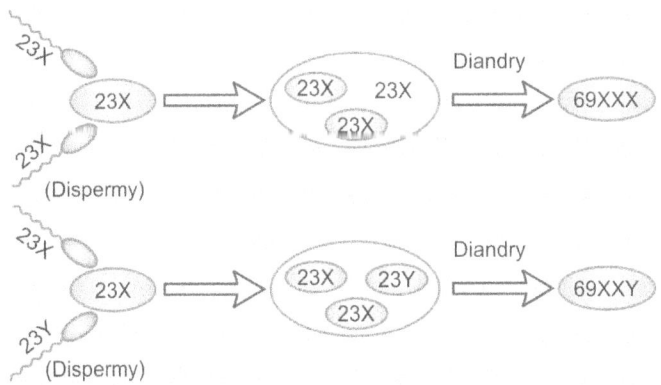

**Fig. 11.26:** Triploid chromosomal pattern of a partial mole. Genome is both paternal and maternal in origin.

**Q. How to manage a case of hydatidiform mole ?**

**Ans.** Principles of management are:
(a) Supportive therapy (blood transfusion)
(b) Suction evacuation of the uterus
(c) Follow up of the patient to prevent the complications.

## CASE – 12  UTERINE POLYP

*This specimen with the tumor (Fig. 11.27) had been removed from a 45-year-old lady.*

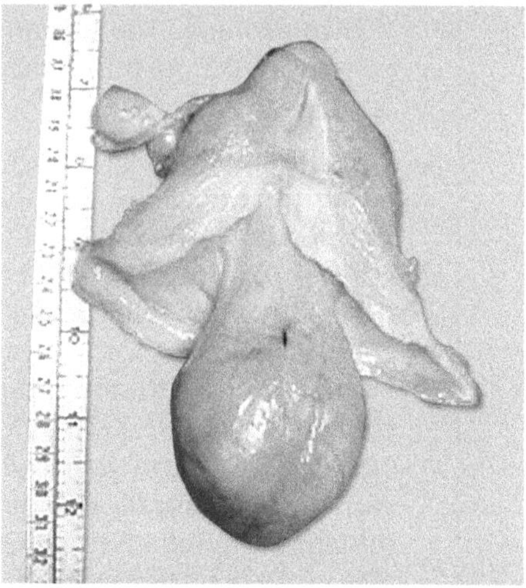

**Q. What is the diagnosis?**

**Ans. Uterine polyp:** The uterus is cut open to show a huge pedunculated polyp arising from the fundus. It is protruding out of the external os of the cervix. Cervix is seen to be thinned out.

**Q. What was her clinical presentation?**

**Ans.** Vaginal discharge, irregular bleeding, intermenstrual bleeding, pain in lower abdomen.

*Others:* There is enlargement of the uterus, at times the polyp is seen to protrude out of the cervix. The cervix is effaced (thinned out).

**Fig. 11.27:** Huge fibroid polyp with a thick pedicle arising from the fundus. Cervix is seen thin and effaced.

**Q. How a polyp could be diagnosed?**

**Ans.** Diagnosis could be made by:
  (a) Transvaginal ultrasonography
  (b) Saline infusion sonography (SIS)
  (c) Hysteroscopy
  (d) Hysterography (HSG).

**Q. What could be the complications of this tumor if not treated?**

**Ans.** Infection, ulceration, bleeding, sarcomatous change (rarely).

**Q. What treatment has been done on her?**

**Ans.** Total abdominal hysterectomy with bilateral salpingo-oophorectomy.

**Q. What could be the alternative method of treatment in such a case?**

**Ans.** Polypectomy (removal of the polyp only).

**Q. How could you differentiate a fibroid polyp from inversion of the uterus?**

**Ans. Sound test:** A uterine sound can be passed all around the pedicle and the dilating cervical canal whereas in a case with chronic inversion, the sound cannot be passed.

**Q. How is a polyp treated?**

**Ans.**
- Endometrial polyp can be removed by hysteroscopy and resection under direct vision.
- Big fibroid polyp lying in the vagina is removed in piecemeal. The pedicle is then transfixed.

**Q. What alternative treatment could have been done for her?**

**Ans.** Polypectomy could have been the alternative procedure. Polypectomy could be done by hysteroscopically. It takes less time and is safe.

**Q. How a case of endometrial polyp presents?**

**Ans.** Characteristic features of presentations are:
  (i) **Age:** It may be at any age
  (ii) **Type:** May be sessile or pedunculated
  (iii) **Symptoms:** May remain asymptomatic, otherwise the symptoms are—intermenstrual bleeding, menorrhagia
  (iv) **Signs:** Uterus may be normal or enlarged in size
  (V) **Diagnosis:** Hysteroscopy or SIS is useful
  (vi) **Management:** depending upon the factors mentioned above. Biopsy must be done before making the final decision. Polypectomy is commonly done.

## CASE – 13  INFERTILITY

### Case Summary

*Mrs VP, 26-year-old, married for 3 years is seen in the gynecology clinic with the problem of her inability to conceive. She is living with her husband with regular conjugal relationship.*

**Q. What is the diagnosis?**

**Ans.** Primary infertility.

**Q. What are the common causes of male infertility?**

**Ans.** (a) **Pretesticular:**

(i) Thyroid dysfunction

(ii) Hyperprolactinemia

(iii) Psychosexual

(iv) Drugs (antipsychotics).

(b) **Testicular:** Cryptorchidism, mumps orchitis, genetic (46 XXY) and testicular failure.

(c) **Post-testicular:** Obstruction of vas deferens (infection and trauma).

**Q. How much proportion of infertility each partner is responsible for?**

**Ans.** **Male** = 30–40%

**Female** = 40–50%

**Both** = 10%

**Unexplained** = 10%.

**Q. What is understood by primary and secondary infertility?**

**Ans.** Primary infertility is a condition in which the woman had never been pregnant despite more than 1 year of unprotected intercourse.

A woman who had been pregnant before (live born, ectopic pregnancy or abortion), yet is currently unable to conceive after 1 year of unprotected intercourse is called **secondary infertility**.

**Q. What are the important causes of female infertility?**

**Ans.** (a) Ovarian factors (15–20%)

(b) Tubal and peritoneal factors (25–35%)

(c) Endometriosis (1–10%)

(d) Uterine and cervical factors.

**Ovarian factors for infertility are:**

(i) Anovulation/oligo-ovulation

(ii) Luteal phase defect (LPD)

(iii) Luteinized unruptured follicle (LUF) syndrome.

## Chapter 11 • Gynecology Case Discussion

**Q. What are the possible causes of anovulation?**

**Ans.** Obesity, PCOS, endocrine dysfunction, like hypothyroidism and raised prolactin level.

**Q. What are the important tubal factors?**

**Ans.** Tubal block may be due to infection and/or adhesions.

**Q. What are the normal values of semen analysis?**

**Ans.** Normal semen volume: $\geq 2$ mL; Normal sperm concentration is 20 million/mL (15 million/mL); Sperm motility: $\geq 50\%$ having progressive forward motility; Sperm morphology: $\geq 15\%$ normal form; Viability: $\geq 75\%$ living (WHO—2010).

**Q. How do you detect ovulation?**

**Ans.**
(i) **Women having regular normal menstruation** are usually ovulating.
(ii) **Biphasic pattern of BBT** suggests ovulation.
(iii) **Cervical mucus study:** Disappearance of fern pattern after 22nd day of the cycle, which was present before, indicates ovulation.
(iv) **Serum progesterone:** Increased value from D8 ($\leq 1$ ng/mL) to D21 ($>6$ ng/mL) suggests ovulation.
(v) **Serum LH:** Detection of midcycle LH surge indicates impending ovulation by next 10-12 hours.
(vi) **Serum estradiol** reaches its peak level 24 hours prior to LH surge.
(vii) **Endometrial biopsy (sampling):** Evidence of secretory endometrium in the second half of the cycle suggests ovulation.
(viii) **Sonography:** Cervical sonography (TVS) to detect growth and development of follicle and subsequently collapsed follicle and fluid in the pouch of Douglas suggests ovulation.

**Q. How do you interpret BBT chart?**

**Ans.** Biphasic pattern of BBT, suggests ovulation, as progesterone is thermogenic.

**Q. Which day of the menstrual cycle endometrial biopsy is done to detect ovulation?**

**Ans.** Biopsy is done on 21st-23rd days of the cycle.

**Q. How can serum progesterone estimation be helpful?**

**Ans.** See above.

**Q. How do you assess the anatomical patency of the tubes?**

**Ans.** (a) **Insufflation test:** It is done 2 days after stoppage of menstrual bleeding. Air or $CO_2$ is pushed transcervically into the peritoneal cavity which is heard as a hissing sound on auscultation at either of the iliac fossa.

(b) **Hysterosalpingography:** Principle of this method is the same as that of dilatation and insufflation. A radiopaque dye is used instead of air or $CO_2$. It is more precise as it can detect the side as well as the site of tubal block. It is done between D7 and D10 of the cycle.

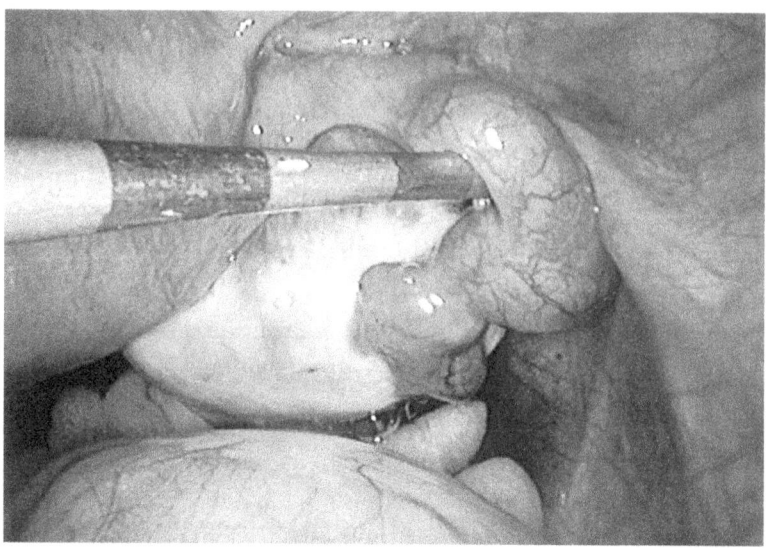

**Fig. 11.28:** Laparoscopic chromopertubation. Dye is seen coming out from the abdominal ostium of the tube.

(c) **Laparoscopy and chromopertubation (Fig. 11.28):** It is the gold standard method. A dye (methylene blue) is pushed transcervically. When the dye is seen to be spilled in the peritoneal cavity through the abdominal ostium, tubes are noted as patent. Laparoscopic method has other advantages also. Tubal block (its side, site) and other pelvic pathology (PCOS or pelvic endometriosis), can be detected simultaneously.

**Other methods are:**
(i) Falloposcopy
(ii) Salpingoscopy.

**Q. How do you treat a woman with anovulatory infertility?**

**Ans.** Ovulation induction is to be done. Commonly used drug are: Letrozole or clomiphene citrate. Clomiphene citrate is given in a dose of 50 mg twice daily for 5 days (D3 to D7). It enhances gonadotropic secretion due to its antiestrogenic property. Letrozole is given in a dose of 2.5 mg twice daily for 5 days (D3 to D7). It acts as an aromatase inhibitor (*see* p. 645).

**Q. What is the place of adjuvant therapy?**

**Ans.** Some women need adjuvant therapy:
(a) Women with hyperinsulinemia: Metformin therapy
(b) Hypothyroidism: Thyroxin replacement
(c) Hyperprolactinemia: Dopamine agonist.

# CHAPTER 12

# Special Topics

## Chapter Objectives
**To demonstrate the knowledge and understanding of:**
- Physiology and endocrinology of menstruation, puberty, reproduction, ovulation, including infertility
- Pathological conditions related to endocrine abnormalities (PCOS, amenorrhea)
- Principles in the management of benign diseases of the reproductive organs

| | | |
|---|---|---|
| ❖ | 1. Physiology of Menstruation | 434 |
| ❖ | 2. Polycystic Ovarian Syndrome | 440 |
| ❖ | 3. Ovulation Induction | 442 |
| ❖ | 4. Endometriosis | 445 |
| ❖ | 5. Cervical Intraepithelial Neoplasia | 449 |
| ❖ | 6. Amenorrhea | 453 |

# 1: PHYSIOLOGY OF MENSTRUATION

**Q. What is menarche?**

Ans. Onset of *first menstruation* in a girl's life is called menarche.

**Q. What is the mean age of menarche?**

Ans. Menarche may occur any time between 10–16 years of age. The mean age of menarche is 12.7 years.

**Q. How do you define normal menstruation?**

Ans. **Normal menstruation** is defined as the visible manifestation of cyclic and physiological uterine bleeding due to shedding of the endometrium. It is the ultimate expression of the invisible interplay of different hormones over the endometrium acting mainly through the hypothalamus-pituitary-ovarian axis.

**Q. What is a menstrual cycle? What is its usual duration and interval?**

Ans. Menstrual cycle begins from the first day of a period to the beginning (D1) of the next one. **Duration** of menstruation is about 4–5 days. Normal menstruation occurs at an **interval** of 21–35 days with a mean of 28 days.

**Q. What is the usual amount of blood loss in a normal menstrual cycle?**

Ans. It is a estimated to be 20–80 mL with an average of 35 mL.

**Q. What are the different layers of endometrium and what is their hormonal responsiveness?**

Ans. The **basal layer**: Usually unresponsive to hormonal stimulation and is not shed out during menstruation.

The **functional layer:** Responsive to hormonal stimulation. It is subdivided into **stratum compactum and spongiosum**. Most of this layer is lost during menstruation.

**Q. What are germ cells? When and how are the germ cells populated in genital ridge?**

Ans. Germ cells are derived from the endoderm of the yolk sac in the region of the hindgut. Germ cells migrate to the genital ridge along the dorsal mesentery of the hindgut. The migration of germ cells occurs at 5 and 6 weeks of embryonic life.

**Q. How many germ cells are there in the fetal, neonatal and pubertal ovary?**

Ans. The germ cells undergo rapid mitotic division and some enter into the prophase of the first meiotic division. These are called primary oocytes. The total number of oocytes vary at different phases of life are as shown below:

| Period of life | Total number of germ cells |
|---|---|
| A. 20 weeks of fetal life | 6–7 million |
| B. Birth | 2 million |
| C. Puberty | 4,00,000 |
| D. Entire reproductive period | About 400 ovulates |
| Majority of germ cells undergo degeneration | |

## Chapter 12 • Special Topics

**Q. What is a primordial follicle?**

**Ans.** Primordial follicle consists of an oocyte which is surrounded by a single layer of flattened granulosa cells. Its growth is not dependent upon gonadotropins. This oocyte is arrested in the prophase of the first meiotic division (diplotene phase).

**Q. What is a preantral follicle?**

**Ans.** An oocyte surrounded by the zona pellucida with several layers of granulosa cells and a theca layer, is a preantral follicle. Growth of preantral follicle is independent of gonadotropins.

**Q. What is an ovarian cycle of a normal menstruation cycle?**

**Ans.** An ovarian cycle consists of:
   (a) Recruitment of group of follicles
   (b) Selection of dominant follicle
   (c) Ovulation
   (d) Formation of corpus luteum
   (e) Demise of corpus luteum.

**Q. How does recruitment of follicles occur?**

**Ans.** Follicular-stimulating hormone (FSH) is the essential hormone for follicular recruitment. Estrogen acts synergistically with FSH to increase the numbers of FSH receptors on the granulosa cells. It also increases the mitotic activity of granulosa cells and increases the number of granulosa cells. FSH begins to increase in the late luteal phase of the previous cycles.

**Q. How is the dominant follicle selected?**

**Ans.** As early as D5–D7, one out of several follicles, become dominant and undergoes further maturation. The follicle having highest antral concentration of estrogen and lowest concentration of androgen and whose granulosa cells contain the maximum number of FSH receptors, becomes the dominant follicle. The rest of the follicles undergo atresia.

**Q. Which hormones are necessary for progressive follicular growth and development?**

**Ans.** FSH initiates follicular recruitment. FSH is responsible for induction of LH receptors in the follicle. LH stimulates the theca cells to produce androgens. These androgens percolate in the granulosa cells. Granulosa cells secrete the enzyme aromatase. The enzyme aromatase in granulosa cells is essential for conversion of androgen to estrogen within the developing follicle.

**Q. What are the different cell layers of a mature Graafian follicle?**

**Ans.** The cell layers from outside inwards are:
   (a) Theca externa
   (b) Theca interna

(c) Membrana granulosa

(d) Granulosa cell layers

(e) Discus proligerus—containing the ovum which is surrounded by radially arranged cells (corona radiata)

(f) Antrum-containing fluid.

**Q. How long is ovarian cycle?**

**Ans.** An ovarian cycle takes about 85 days and it spreads over 3 menstrual cycles.

**Q. What is the two-cell and two-gonadotropin concept of ovarian steroidogenesis?**

**Ans. Two cells** are—theca cells and granulosa cells

**Two gonadotropins** are—FSH and LH

During the follicular phase, LH stimulates theca cells to produce androgens (androstenedione, dehydroepiandrosterone and testosterone). These androgens diffuse into the granulosa cells where they are aromatized under the influence of FSH to estrogen (estradiol).

**Q. What are the main features of proliferative phase?**

**Ans.** (a) Duration: First 14 days of the menstrual cycle—D1 to D14.

(b) Important events: Ovarian changes—follicular growth and maturation. This ultimately leads to ovulation.

(c) Endometrial changes: Proliferative changes—characterized by dilatation and elongation of the glands; endometrial cells are columnar and pseudostratified.

(d) Endometrial thickness: Increased 4 to 6 mm.

(e) Main hormone: Estrogen (E2).

**Q. What are the main features of secretary phase?**

**Ans.** (a) Duration: Last 14 days of the menstrual cycle—D15 to D28

(b) Important events: Ovarian changes—ovulation and formation of the corpus luteum

(c) Endometrial changes: Secretory changes—characterized by secretion in the glands, stromal edema leukocyte infiltration; endometrial cells are short columnar with subnuclear vacuolation

(d) Endometrial thickness: 8 to 10 mm

(e) Main hormone: Progesterone.

**Q. What factors are detrimental for follicular growth and maturation?**

**Ans.** (a) The preantral follicles that are not rescued by FSH, undergo atresia.

(b) The antral follicles that have the dominant androgenic follicular microenvironment instead of estrogenic microenvironment, undergo atresia.

(c) Premature increase in the levels of LH decrease mitogenic activity of granulosa cells. This causes follicular atresia.

(d) As the levels of estrogen secreted from the dominant follicle increase, FSH is inhibited by negative feedback effect. This causes withdrawal of gonadotropin support of poorly developed follicles. Less developed follicles have got less number of FSH receptors and they undergo atresia.

(e) Dominant follicle plays two important roles in this regard : (a) It optimizes its own growth by maintaining dominant estrogenic microenvironment, with maximum FSH receptors and (b) suppresses the growth of other follicles by creating negative feedback to FSH.

**Q. What are the functions of LH surge?**

Ans. (a) Completion of first meiotic division with extrusion of the first polar body which is pushed to the perivitelline space.

(b) Physiological act ovulation—release of ovum.

(c) Luteinization of granulosa cells.

(d) Formation and maintenance of corpus luteum.

(e) Synthesis of progesterone and prostaglandins.

**Q. What is the important predictor of ovulation?**

Ans. Ovulation occurs approximate 34–36 hours after the start of LH surge or 10–12 hours after the peak of the LH surge.

**Q. What are the important hormonal events that precede ovulation?**

Ans. (1) Optimum serum levels of estradiol (E2) ≥200 pg/mL and it is to be sustained for 48 hours.

(2) Peak and sustained level of E2 exerts a positive feedback action on LH.

(3) LH surge generally persists for 24 hours.

(4) Ovulation occurs approximately 10–12 hours after the peak of LH surge or 24–36 hours after the peak estradiol level.

**Q. What causes extrusion of the oocyte from the follicle (ovulation)?**

Ans. It is the passive stretching following necrobiosis of the overlying follicular wall due to the effect of combined LH and FSH. There is enzymatic activation of plasminogen and hyaluronidase. It is more likely that there are degenerative changes in follicular wall with enzymatic destruction of collagen which allows passive expansion and ultimate rupture of the follicle. Though there is increase in antral fluid volume, the follicular fluid hydrostatic pressure is not increased.

**Q. What is the corpus luteum (CL)?**

Ans. Following ovulation, the ruptured Graafian follicle develops into the corpus luteum.

**Q. What are the different stages of the growth of CL?**

Ans. There are four stages of the growth of CL:

(1) Proliferation

(2) Vascularization
(3) Maturation
(4) Regression.

**Q. Which hormones are necessary for the formation and maintenance of CL?**
**Ans.** (a) Normal luteal function requires adequate follicular development. This needs adequate FSH stimulation of the dominant follicle.
(b) Midcycle LH surge causes ovulation, luteinization of the granulosa cells and optimum secretion of progesterone.
(c) LH secretion must be continued for function of CL, failing which the CL will regress. Therefore, life span and steroidogenic capacity of CL are dependent on continued tonic secretion of LH.

**Q. What is the life span of CL in a nonconception cycle?**
**Ans.** CL has a life span of about 12–14 days. $PGF_{2\alpha}$ liberated from the ovary is luteolytic.

**Q. When does the level of progesterone reach the peak in the luteal phase?**
**Ans.** Progesterone level peaks approximately on the D-8 after the LH surge. This causes secretory changes in the endometrium and also suppresses new follicular growth.

**Q. When is the implantation likely to occur?**
**Ans.** The implantation window in a normal cycle menstrual cycle is between $D_{20}$–$D_{24}$.

**Q. What changes occur in a corpus luteum of pregnancy?**
**Ans.** There is marked hyperplasia in all the layers between $D_{23}$ and $D_{28}$ of the cycle. This is due to human chorionic gonadotropin (hCG) secreted by the trophoblastic cells. Progesterone secretion is continued from the CL of pregnancy.

**Q. What is luteal placental shift?**
**Ans.** This shift is the taking over of function of CL by the developing placenta. This turnover of function from the CL of pregnancy to placenta is called **luteal placental shift**. This transition period continues between 7 and 10 weeks.

**Q. What is a luteal phase defect?**
**Ans.** Deficient function of CL with diminished secretion of progesterone, is called luteal phase defect. The role of luteal phase defect as an etiology of infertility is not clearly understood. Diagnosis and management of luteal phase defects are discussed (*see* Dutta Gyne 7/e, p. 194, 201).

**Q. What is the endometrial cycle of normal menstruating women?**
**Ans.** It is the sequence of endometrial changes in response to ovarian cycle. Normal endometrium has a **basal zone** (nonresponsive to hormones) and a **functional zone**, responsive to cyclic ovarian hormones.

***Q. What are the different phases of endometrium during a menstrual cycle?***

**Ans.** The four phases are as follows:

(1) **Phase of regeneration**: D2–D3, regeneration of blood vessels, glands, stroma and surface epithelium starts even before menstruation ceases.

(2) **Phase of proliferation**: Growth of endometrial glands takes place. Glands become tubular, surface epithelial cells are columnar type. The cell nucleus is placed at the base of the cell. Spindle-shaped stromal cells proliferate with evidences of mitosis. Blood vessels continue to grow unbranched up to the level of surface epithelium. The endometrium becomes 3–4 mm thick, proliferative changes are due to ovarian estrogens.

(3) **Phase of secretory endometrium**: The endometrial changes are due to progesterone. However, progesterone can only act on the endometrium previously primed by estrogen. Presence of subnuclear vacuolation is the earliest evidence of progesterone effect (ovulation). The endometrium becomes 6–8 mm thick.

(4) **Menstrual phase:** This is described below.

***Q. What is the menstrual phase?***

**Ans.** It is essentially the phase of degeneration and shedding off the endometrium. Regression of the corpus luteal function and its demise causes fall in the level of estrogen and progesterone. This is an inevitable physiological change in a nonconceptual cycle. As a result of the withdrawal of hormonal support, the endometrium is casted off. It normally lasts for 5–6 days.

## 2: POLYCYSTIC OVARIAN SYNDROME

**Q. What is polycystic ovarian syndrome?**

**Ans.** PCOS is a multifactorial heterogeneous condition.

**Diagnosis** is based upon the presence of any two of the following three features (ASRM/ESHERE-2003):

(1) Oligo-ovulation and/or anovulation.

(2) Hyperandrogenemia (clinical and/biochemical)

(3) Polycystic changes of the ovaries: The ovaries are enlarged in volume ($\geq 10$ cm$^3$), with presence of multiple ($\geq 12$) follicular cysts around the ovarian cortex.

**Q. What are the common presenting features of PCOS?**

**Ans. Symptoms:**
- Infertility (due to anovulation)
- Menstrual abnormalities: Amenorrhea, oligomenorrhea, menorrhagia, irregular cycles
- Dysfunctional uterine bleeding
- Obesity
- Acne, alopecia
- Hirsutism
- Acanthosis nigricans (skin changes)
- HAIR-AN syndrome [hyperandrogenism (HA), insulin resistance (IR) and acanthosis nigricans (AN)].

**Q. What are the biochemical abnormalities associated with PCOS?**

**Ans.**
- Hyperandrogenemia (increased levels of testosterone and DHEA)
- Hyperinsulinemia
- Insulin resistance (mutations in the insulin receptor gene of tissues)
- High levels of serum estrogen (E1 and E2)
- Hyperprolactinemia
- Hypersecretion of LH
- Low FSH
- Low serum SHBG levels
- Hyperlipidemia
- Abnormal glucose tolerance (increased risk of diabetes mellitus (25–30%).

**Q. What are the important management options of a woman with PCOS?**

**Ans.** (a) **Weight reduction in obese women, is the first line management:**
  – Body mass index (BMI) <25 improves obesity, menstrual abnormality, infertility, insulin resistance and hyperandrogenemia.

(b) **When fertility is not desired**:
- Combined oral contraceptive pills is the other option. It reduces excess androgen levels. At the same time, it makes the menstrual cycle regular.
- Hirsutism: Antiandrogens (cyproterone acetate and flutamide), may be used.

**Q.** *What is your management approach of a married woman with PCOS who is interested to have a baby.*

**Ans.** Women with PCOS often suffer from anovulation. This woman needs to be investigated to identify the husband factor, tubal factor and ovulatory factors of conception. Once she is found to suffer from anovulation, induction of ovulation should be considered for her.

**Q.** *What are the common drugs used for induction of ovulation?*

**Ans.**
- Clomiphene citrate
- Letrozole (aromatase inhibitor)
- Gonadotropins (FSH and LH)

(**Also see:** Ovulation induction: Topic 3).

**Q.** *What are the long-term sequelae of PCOS?*

**Ans.** Possible adverse effects are the development of:
- Type II diabetes mellitus (DM)
- Endometrial carcinoma
- Hypertension, cardiovascular disease
- Coronary artery disease (heart attack)
- Dyslipidemia (abnormal lipid metabolism: ↑triglycerides and LDL)
- Sleep apnea.

## 3: OVULATION INDUCTION

**Q. What are the common causes of anovulation?**

**Ans.** Common causes are:
(a) Polycystic ovarian syndrome
(b) Hypo/hyperthyroidism
(c) Hyperprolactinemia
(d) Hypothalamic causes (stress and weight loss)
(e) Premature ovarian failure
(f) Dysgenetic gonads (45 XO, 46 XX).

**Q. What is ovulation induction?**

**Ans.** It is the method to stimulate the ovaries to produce eggs using medications. Commonly used medications are of four types:
(1) Clomiphene citrate
(2) Letrozole (aromatase inhibitor)
(3) Gonadotropins (FSH/LH)
(4) GnRH.

**Q. When is clomiphene citrate indicated and how is it prescribed?**

**Ans.** It is used for induction of ovulation primarily in cases with PCOS. It is prescribed on days 3–7 of the menstrual cycle. The starting dose is usually 50 mg twice a day.

**Q. How does clomiphene citrate (CC) work?**

**Ans.** Clomiphene citrate works as an antiestrogen as well as weak estrogen at the level of hypothalamus. It binds with the estrogen receptors and blocks the receptors for a long time. This causes increased GnRH pulse amplitude resulting in increased gonadotropin secretion from the pituitary. This ultimately results in increased secretion of FSH by the anterior pituitary. High levels of FSH cause increased follicular growth and maturation.

**Q. What is the overall result of clomiphene therapy?**

**Ans.** Successful induction rate is about 80%. However, cumulative pregnancy rate is about 70%.

**Q. What should be the management option when the woman fails to ovulate with CC?**

**Ans.** In such a case, the dose of CC may be increased up to a maximum of 200 mg/day for 5 days. If the woman does not respond even with this, she may be considered for gonadotropin therapy provided she has got good ovarian reserve.

**Q. What is the place of metformin as an adjuvant therapy?**

**Ans.** Women with PCOS with obesity (BMI ≥25) are insulin resistant. Treatment with metformin are found to reduce hyperandrogenemia and hyperinsulinemia. Combined treatment with metformin and clomiphene increases ovulation rate.

**Q. What is metformin?**

**Ans.** Metformin is:
- An oral biguanide and an antihyperglycemic drug
- Used for treatment of non-insulin dependent diabetes
- Category B drug for pregnant women.

**Q. How metformin works?**

**Ans.** The functions of metformin are:
  (a) **Metformin lowers blood glucose by:**
    - Inhibiting hepatic glucose-production
    - Decreasing intestinal glucose uptake
    - Inhibiting lipolysis, decreases FFA levels
    - Decreasing hepatic neoglucogenesis
    - Enhancing peripheral glucose uptake
    - Enhancing insulin sensitivity at the post receptor level
    - Stimulating insulin mediated glucose disposal.
  (b) **Other functions of metformin are:**
    - Increases insulin sensitivity
    - Decreases weight and BMI
    - Decreases LDL cholesterol
    - Decreases blood pressure
    - Decreases CRP levels.

**Q. What is the place of letrozole in ovulation induction?**

**Ans.** Letrozole is an aromatase inhibitor. This inhibits enzyme aromatase which prevents the conversion of androgens to estrogens. Letrozole is the most widely used aromatase inhibitor to induce ovulation. It is used orally and is relatively less expensive. Compared to CC, it is associated with higher pregnancy rates. When used in combination with gonadotropins, the need of gonadotropins is less. Letrozole has pregnancy rates comparable to gonadotropin treatment alone. Side effects are minor. The usual dose is 2.5 mg to 5 mg orally daily for 5 days. It is commonly used from D3 to D7 of the cycle. Another aromatase inhibitor used is anastrozole.

**Q. What are the risks of ovulation induction?**

**Ans.** (a) Multiple pregnancies
  (b) Ovarian hyperstimulation.

**Q. What is ovarian hyperstimulation syndrome (OHSS)?**

**Ans.** OHSS is the development of multiple follicles with enlargement of the ovaries following hCG stimulation. It is observed in 1-2% of cases following induction of ovulation with gonadotropins.

**Q. Can OHSS occur with CC therapy?**

**Ans.** It may occur but is very rare.

**Q. How does a woman with OHSS present?**

**Ans.** Presenting features are nausea, vomiting, abdominal enlargement due to ascites. There is ovarian enlargement, ascites, severe fluid and electrolyte imbalance, hemoconcentration, oliguria and rarely thromboembolism. Patient needs hospitalization when the features are moderate to severe.

## 4: ENDOMETRIOSIS

**Q. What is endometriosis?**

**Ans.** It is the functioning endometrium situated in sites other than uterine mucosa.

**Q. What is adenomyosis?**

**Ans.** When the ectopic endometrial tissues are found to grow within the layers of myometrium, it is called endometriosis interna or adenomyosis.

**Q. What are the common sites of endometriosis?**

**Ans.** Common sites are:
- Ovaries
- Uterosacral ligaments
- Pelvic peritoneum
- Pouch of Douglas
- Rectovaginal septum
- Sigmoid colon
- Umbilicus (bleeding) (Fig. 12.1).

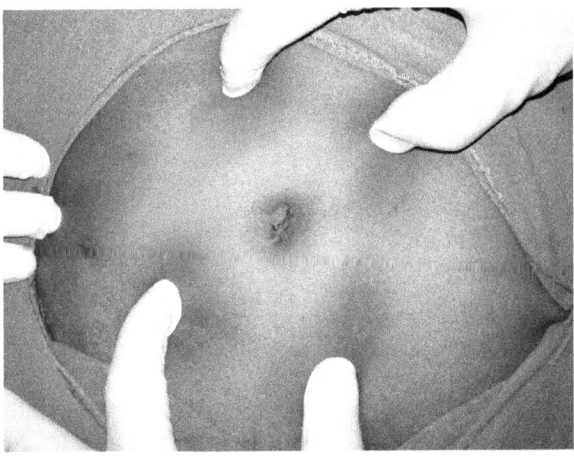

**Fig. 12.1:** Endometriosis in a umbilicus. This is relatively an uncommon site for endometriosis.

**Q. How does pelvic endometriosis appear on clinical examination?**

**Ans.** They appear as small black dots on uterosacral ligaments and pouch of Douglas. These also appear as **'Powder Burns'**.

Other appearances are: Red flame-shaped areas and yellow-brown patches.

**Q. How does a woman with pelvic endometriosis present?**

**Ans.** Common presenting features are:
  (i) Woman's age between 25–45 years
  (ii) Parity: Mostly nulliparous

(iii) Dysmenorrhea (70%); it is gradually increasing
(iv) Menstrual abnormality: Menorrhagia
(v) Infertility (40–60%)
(vi) Dyspareunia
(vii) Chronic pelvic pain
(viii) Other rare symptoms may be backache, hematuria, and painful defecation.

**Abdominal and pelvic examination:**
(a) Chocolate cysts may be felt on abdominal examination.
(b) Pelvic examination reveals nodules in the pouch of Douglas and tenderness.

However some women may remain asymptomatic.

**Q. How can pelvic endometriosis be diagnosed?**
Ans. (a) Clinical: As discussed above
(b) Ultrasonography: Ovarian endometrioma
(c) Laparoscopy is the gold standard. It can confirm the diagnosis.

**Q. What are the different treatment options for pelvic endometriosis?**
Ans. (a) Expectant management (observation only)
(b) Medical therapy:
   (i) Hormones
   (ii) Others
(c) Surgery (Figs. 12.2 and 12.3):
   (i) Conservative
   (ii) Definitive
(d) Combined therapy.

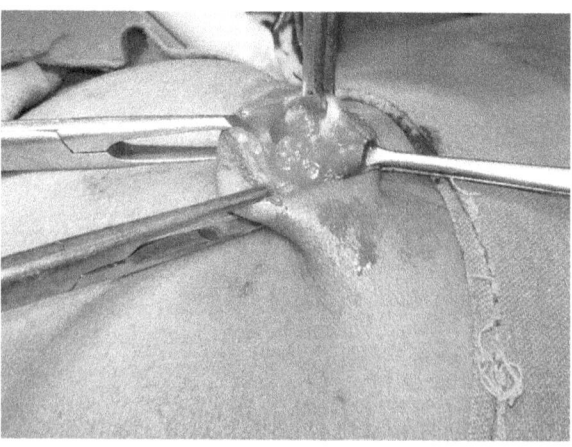

Fig. 12.2: Dissection for excision of endometriotic nodule in the umbilicus.

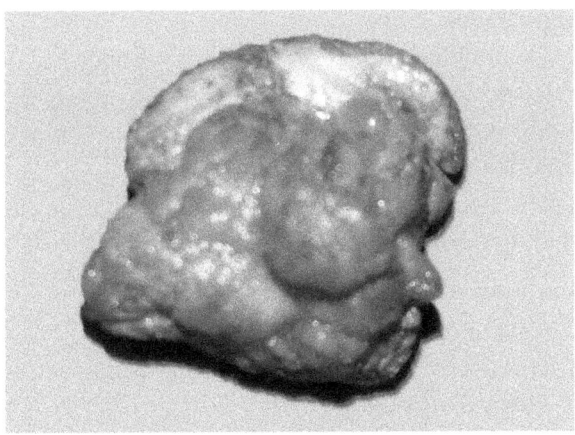

**Fig. 12.3:** Endometriotic nodule dissected out. Histopathology confirmed endometriosis.

**Medical therapy:** It is done mainly to suppress the growth of endometriotic implants. The endometriotic tissues gradually become atrophic.

Hormones commonly used are:

(a) Combined estrogen and progesterone (oral pill) for 6–9 months

(b) Progestogens: Medroxyprogesterone acetate 10 mg thrice daily for 6 months; it can also be given as 150 mg 3 monthly intramuscular (IM) injections. Depo-SubQ provera 104 is also effective.

(c) Levonorgestrel releasing IUCD has been found helpful.

(d) Dienogest is a 19 nortestosterone derivative progestin. It reduces endometriosis-related pain effectively. It is given in a dose of 2 mg daily. It is very effective for deep infiltrating endometriosis (DIE). It is thought to be equivalent to that of GnRH agonists.

(e) Danazol.

(f) GnRh analogs.

(g) Aromatase inhibitors (AIs): Anastrozole, letrozole are used to create hypoestrogenic condition. Progestins or COCs are combined to reduce the side effects due to hypoestrogenemia.

(h) Selective progesterone receptor modulators (SPRMs): Mifepristone and ulipristal are commonly used drugs. However, long-term safety report of these drugs is awaited.

(i) Gestrinone is an antiprogestogenic agent used for endometriosis. It has antiprogesterone, antiestrogenic and androgenic effects. It is given orally, 2.5 to 10 mg a week in three divided doses.

**Conservative surgical management**

(a) **Conservative surgery:**
  (i) Laparoscopic
  (ii) Laparotomy.

(b) **Surgeries are:**
  (i) Electrofulguration of endometriotic lesions
  (ii) Laser vaporization
  (iii) Ovarian cystectomy.
(c) **Definitive surgery**
  Hysterectomy and bilateral salpingo-oophorectomy in women who are elderly and have completed their family.

*Q. How does a women with adenomyosis present?*

**Ans.** (a) **Clinical features:**
  (i) Women are usually parous with age usually ≥40 years
  (ii) Menorrhagia (70%)
  (iii) Dysmenorrhea (30%)
  (iv) Women in their reproductive age group often suffer from infertility.
(b) **On examination:**
  (i) Mass may be felt in the hypogastrium
  (ii) On pelvic examination—uterus is found uniformly enlarged and it is often tender
  (iii) Ultrasonography reveals hypoechoic myometrium with multiple small cysts in the myometrium
  (iv) Magnetic resonance imaging (MRI) is more specific to the diagnosis. Low signal intensity and junctional zone (JZ) ≤8 mm excludes the disease. JZ thickening ≥12 mm is suggestive of adenomyosis.

*Q. What are the management options available for adenomyosis of the uterus?*

**Ans.** (a) Medical therapy (hormones and others) is usually not effective
(b) LNG-IUS is found to be helpful
(c) Surgical treatment commonly done:
  (i) Adenomyomectomy or
  (ii) Hysterectomy (in parous and elderly women).

## 5: CERVICAL INTRAEPITHELIAL NEOPLASIA

*Q. What is CIN?*

Ans. **Cervical intraepithelial neoplasia (CIN):** It is a condition where cervical squamous epithelium is replaced by cells with varying degree of atypia.

*Q. What is the site of origin for CIN?*

Ans. CIN arises in the area of metaplasia which is located in the transformation zone of the squamocolumnar junction (SCJ).

*Q. What is the significance of detection of CIN?*

Ans. Most CIN-1 and some CIN-2 regress spontaneously. But CIN may progress to invasive cervical carcinoma over a period of 10–15 years. CIN is caused mainly by human papilloma virus (HPV) infection. Over 99.7% of patients with CIN and invasive cancer are found to be positive with HPV-DNA.

*Q. What important types of HPV are of concern?*

Ans. Types of HPV that cause 90% of CIN and invasive cancers are: HPV 16, 18, 31, 33, 39, 45, 51, 56, 58, 59, 68.

- Type 16 is the most common (47%).
- Type 18 is present in about 23% of the cases with invasive cancers.
- Usually HPV infection does not persist for a long time.
- In vast majority, the infection will clear in 9–15 months.
- Persistent, high-risk HPV infection increases the risk of CIN 3 and invasive cancer.

*Q. How do you diagnose a case with CIN?*

Ans. **Cervical cytology screening:** Pap test reduced cervical cancer by 79% and the mortality by 70%. Pap test errors could be due to several reasons in sampling, smear preparation, fixation (two thick, two thin or bloody smear) or even in interpretation.

False-negative rate of Pap smear—up to 25%. To reduce false-negative errors of Pap test, liquid-based cytology (LBC) is used. Screening of cervical cytology by automated microscope with digital camera and review by expert cytopathologist is done. These methods can reduce the false negative rate by 32%.

**Bethesda system** of cervical cytology reporting is uniform.

**Q. What is the current recommendation for cervical cytology screening (ACOG, 2011)?**

**Ans.** Cervical cancer screening guidelines:
- Women between ages
  - **21 to 29 years:** Pap testing every 3 years, no HPV testing
  - **30 to 65 years:** Co-testing with Pap and HPV every 5 years (preferred) or Pap testing alone every 3 years
- Screening is not recommended for women >65 years, who had 3 consecutive negative Pap test or 2 consecutive negative HPV test, provided they have had no history of CIN-2 or CIN-3 or cancer (CIN-2+) in the past 20 years
- Women aged 65 years or older who have no previous screening should undergo Pap and HPV testing
- Screening with Pap test or HPV testing is not recommended for women who have had a hysterectomy with removal of the cervix and who do not have a history of CIN-2+

**Currently, primary HPV testing alone is gaining acceptance.** WHO recommends HPV testing as the preferred screening method in countries where Pap testing is not feasible and HPV testing is available (WHO 2015).

**Q. Describe the procedure of cytology testing.**

**Ans.** Cusco's vaginal speculum is introduced. Spatula and cytobrush are used for collecting cells from the transformation zone, where cervical cancer begins. Collected sample is placed on a glass slide and fixed with alcohol (*see* Pap test; p. 548). Cytology sample is currently collected in a liquid medium for transport to laboratory where the slide is prepared. This liquid based approach can also be used for HPV DNA testing.

**Q. What are the recommendations for a woman to be tested for HPV-DNA?**

**Ans.** **HPV-DNA** testing may be combined with cervical cytology for women older than 30 years of age. For women having both the test results negative, the test interval can be increased by more than 3 years. The negative predictive value of a double negative test exceeds 99%.

**Q. What are the recommendations for a woman to be referred to colposcopy clinic?**

**Ans.** (1) Any woman with **cytology screening suggestive of HSIL**, should be referred for colposcopy and directed biopsy.
(2) Persistent CIN-1.
(3) Positive results for HPV-DNA.
(4) Visual inspection with acetic acid (VIA): Acetowhite lesions are considered for colposcopic examinations and/or biopsy.

**Q. What are the abnormal findings on colposcopy?**

**Ans.** Abnormal colposcopic findings are:
  (a) White epithelium
  (b) Acetowhite epithelium
  (c) Punctuation
  (d) Mosaic
  (e) Atypical blood vessels
  (f) Irregular surface contour (ulceration, fragility).

**Q. What can are the alternatives when colposcopy is not available?**

**Ans.** Schiller's test is done and biopsy is taken from the Schiller's unstained area (positive).

Endocervical curettage is mandatory.

**Q. When is conization of cervix done?**

**Ans.** Diagnostic conization may be done in cases where:
  (a) Entire limits of the lesion is not visible even with colposcopy.
  (b) Transformation zone (SCJ) is not seen.
  (c) Normal colposcopic finding but there is abnormal cytology.
  (d) Cases with CIS or microinvasion on biopsy, to exclude invasive cancer.
  (e) Endocervical curettage (ECC) is positive for CIN-2 or CIN-3.
  (f) Cases with atypical glandular cells.

**Q. What are the treatment options for CIN?**

**Ans.** **1. CIN-I:** Spontaneous regression rate of CIN-1 is 60% to 80%. Patients may be followed up with Pap testing at 6 and 12 months interval or HPV-DNA testing at 12 months.

  **Results are analyzed:**
  (a) Both the results negative → Routine screening yearly is done.
  (b) Persistent CIN 1 (LSIL) after 2 years → Expectant management and follow-up cytology or ablative therapy (Cryo) or excisional procedures like LLETZ or LEEP is done.

  **2. CIN-2 and 3:** Excisional methods → LLETZ/LEEP (*see* p. 525).

  **Follow-up:** Women need to be followed up at 6 months interval with cytology, colposcopy or HPV-DNA. Recurrence risk may be up to 10%.

**Q. What are the different methods of ablative therapy available?**

**Ans.** Methods are:
  (i) Cryotherapy
  (ii) Electrodiathermy
  (iii) Laser vaporization
  (iv) Cold coagulation.

**Q. What are the different excisional methods?**

**Ans.** Excisional methods are:
  (i) Large loop excision of the transformation zone (LLETZ) or loop electrosurgical excision procedure (LEEP)
  (ii) Conization
  (iii) Hysterectomy in a selected case.

**Q. What are the conditions where ablative therapy could be done?**

**Ans.** (a) No evidence of microinvasive or invasive disease
  (b) The lesion is on the ectocervix and is seen entirely
  (c) No involvement of endocervix.

**Q. What are the indications of hysterectomy for cases with CIN?**

**Ans.** (i) Elderly women with persistent CIN-2 or CIN-3
  (ii) Cases with microinvasion
  (iii) Presence of other gynecological problems (fibroids, PID and AUB) needing hysterectomy
  (iv) Poor compliance for follow up.

**Q. What are the different vaccines available to prevent cancer cervix?**

**Ans.** Three prophylactic HPV vaccines are currently available in many countries for use in females and males from the age of 9 years. It is given for the prevention of premalignant lesions and cancers affecting the cervix, vulva, vagina, and anus caused by high-risk HPV types:

**Preparations available are :**
  (i) A bivalent vaccine targeting HPV16 and HPV18
  (ii) A quadrivalent vaccine targeting HPV6 and HPV11 in addition to HPV16 and HPV 18
  (iii) A nonavalent vaccine targeting HPV types 31, 33, 45, 52, and 58 in addition to HPV 6, 11, 16, and 18.

The last two vaccines target anogenital warts caused by HPV 6 and 11 in addition to the above-mentioned malignant and premalignant lesions. All the vaccines are recombinant vaccines composed of virus-like particles (VLPs) and are not infectious since they do not contain viral DNA.

For girls and boys aged 9–14 years, a two-dose schedule (0.5 mL at 0 and 5–13 months) is recommended. If the second vaccine dose is administered earlier than 5 months after the first dose, a third dose is recommended. For those aged 15 years and above, and for immunocompromised patients irrespective of age, the recommendation is for three doses (0.5 mL at 0, 1, 6 months). WHO has reviewed the latest data and concluded that there is no safety concern regarding the HPV vaccines.

There is some evidence of cross-protection from nonvaccine types also. Recent observational studies have reported evidence for effectiveness in preventing high-risk HPV infections following a single dose vaccine.

However, further long-term follow-up will clarify the role of one dose in preventing cervical neoplasia.

## 6: AMENORRHEA

**Q. What is amenorrhea?**

Ans. Amenorrhea literally means absence of menstruation.

**Q. How do you define primary amenorrhea?**

Ans. A young girl who has not menstruated by 16 years of age (16th birth day) is considered primary amenorrhea.

**Q. What are the common causes of amenorrhea?**

Ans. Amenorrhea may be: (a) Physiological and (b) Pathological

(a) Physiological:
  (i) Before puberty
  (ii) Following menopause
  (iii) During pregnancy
  (iv) During lactation.
(b) Pathological:
  (i) Cryptomenorrhea
  (ii) Primary amenorrhea
  (iii) Secondary amenorrhea.

## PRIMARY AMENORRHEA

**Q. What are the common causes of primary amenorrhea?**

Ans. (a) **Hypogonadotropic hypogonadism:**
  (i) Delayed puberty due to delayed GnRH pulse reactivation.
  (ii) Hypothalamic pituitary dysfunction: Stress, weight loss, anorexia nervosa, chronic illness (tuberculosis), Kallmann's syndrome (deficiency of GnRH).
(b) **Hypergonadotropic hypogonadism:**
  (a) Primary ovarian failure
  (b) Galactosemia.
(c) **Abnormal chromosomal pattern:**
  (i) Turner's syndrome (45 XO)
  (ii) Pure gonadal dysgenesis (46XX or 46YY)
  (iii) Androgen insensitivity syndrome (testicular feminization syndrome), 46 XY.
(d) **Developmental defect:**
  (i) Imperforate hymen
  (ii) Transverse vaginal septum
  (iii) Absence of uterus in **MRKH syndrome.**
(e) **Others:**
  (i) Cretinism
  (ii) Tuberculosis
  (iii) Malnutrition.

## SECONDARY AMENORRHEA

**Q. How do you define secondary amenorrhea?**

**Ans.** Absence of menstruation for 6 months or more in a woman who has menstruated normally in the past.

**Q. What are the common causes of secondary amenorrhea?**

**Ans.** Common causes of secondary amenorrhea are:

(1) **Uterine factors**:
  (a) Synechiae (tuberculosis)
  (b) Hysterectomy.

(2) **Ovarian factors**:
  (i) Polycystic ovarian syndrome
  (ii) Premature ovarian failure
  (iii) Pelvic radiation
  (iv) Bilateral oophorectomy.

(3) **Pituitary factors**:
  (i) Adenoma (prolactinoma)
  (ii) Sheehan's syndrome (pituitary ischemia causing destruction).

(4) **Hypothalamic factors**:
  (i) Stress
  (ii) Trauma—accidents
  (iii) Infection (tuberculosis)
  (iv) Tumor.

(5) **Adrenal**: Adrenal tumor/hyperplasia—causing excess androgen production.

(6) **Thyroid:** Hypothyroid state.

(7) **Medical illness:** Tuberculosis.

(8) **Iatrogenic drugs**: Antihypertensives (reserpine), psychotropic (phenothiazines), tricyclic antidepressants.

   **Other drugs:** Metoclopramide and opiates.

**Q. What most common cause should be excluded in the diagnosis of amenorrhea?**

**Ans.** A thorough history taking and physical examination is needed. Very often this will lead to the correct diagnosis. History of sexual contact is important. **Pregnancy is the most common cause of amenorrhea in a woman of reproductive age.**

**Q. What is cryptomenorrhea?**

**Ans.** When there is periodic shedding of endometrium and bleeding but menstrual blood fails to come out from the genital tract due to obstruction in the passage.

**Q. What are the common causes of cryptomenorrhea?**

**Ans.** Causes may be: (a) Congenital and (b) Acquired

(a) **Congenital**
   (i) Imperforate hymen
   (ii) Transverse vaginal septum
   (iii) Agenesis of upper part of vagina and the cervix.

(b) **Acquired**
   (i) Cervical stenosis following amputation, conization or cauterization
   (ii) Vaginal atresia following traumatic and difficult vaginal delivery (forceps).

**Q. What is progesterone challenge test?**

**Ans.** The test is performed by giving tablet medroxyprogesterone acetate 10 mg twice daily orally for 5 days. A positive test means bleeding (even spotting) within 10 days of the test.

**Q. What is the significance of positive progesterone challenge test?**

**Ans.** Positive progesterone challenge test means:
(a) Intact hypothalamo-pituitary ovarian axis
(b) Serum level of estrogen ($E_2$) is ≥40 pg/mL
(c) Anatomical patency of the outflow tract
(d) Endometrium is responsive.

**Q. What should be the next step when progesterone challenge is negative?**

**Ans.** Combined estrogen-progesterone challenge test.

**Q. What is the significance when withdrawal bleeding occurs following estrogen–progesterone challenge test?**

**Ans.** It indicates presence of responsive endometrium but the level of endometrium estrogen is inadequate. The underlying defect may be in the ovary or in the pituitary gland.

**Q. What is the significance of negative result of estrogen-progesterone challenge test?**

**Ans.** A negative estrogen-progesterone challenge test suggests:

Local endometrial pathology like:
(i) Complete destruction of endometrium as in uterine synechiae.
(ii) Endometrial fibrosis, severe endometritis.
(iii) Outflow tract obstruction: Cervical stenosis, uterine agenesis or transverse vaginal septum.

**Q. What other tests should be performed for a woman with amenorrhea (with normal anatomical tract), who had no bleeding on progesterone challenge test?**

Ans. Evaluation of thyroid function (serum TSH), and serum levels of prolactin, FSH and LH.

**Q. What is the significance of performing FSH and LH estimation?**

Ans. This test will differentiate between the cause of low estrogen levels.
   (a) If the serum FSH level is low (<5 mIU/mL), it indicates hypothalamo-pituitary level of dysfunction (hypogonadotropic hypogonadism).
   (b) High levels of FSH (>40 mIU/mL) suggest ovarian failure (hypergonadotropic hypogonadism).
   (c) When the levels of LH ≥10 mIU, and/or LH:FSH is >3, it suggests polycystic ovarian syndrome (PCOS).

# CHAPTER 13

# Gynecology Short Questions

**Chapter Objectives**

**Short Questions:** Model answers are provided to develop the art of writing in a concise way with important and updated information. Presentation needs to be focused.

❖ Gynecology Short Questions with Answers  458

## Q. 1 — All pregnant women should be offered screening for HIV infection in early pregnancy—discuss.

**Ans.** Human immunodeficiency virus (HIV) infection which leads to acquired immunodeficiency syndrome (AIDS) is an incurable disease. The prevalence of HIV infection (seropositivity) among Asian pregnant women is less than 0.5%. In India, it varies from one zone to the other.

The main modes of transmission of HIV are:
(i) Sexual contact
(ii) Transplacental
(iii) Exposure to infected blood or tissue fluid and
(iv) Through breast milk.

Once the mother is infected, perinatal transmission is high. Vertical transmission is about 14–25%. Transplacental transmission occurs in early pregnancy. But majority (40–80%) occurs during the labor. Breastfeeding increases transmission by 14%.

**Prevention of parent to child transmission (PPTCT) or mother-to-child transmission (MTCT)** of HIV infection is a major step against the spread of the AIDS. Therefore, all pregnant women attending the prenatal (antenatal) clinic should be counseled and offered screening for HIV infection in early pregnancy. Presently integrated counseling and testing (ICT) in the antenatal clinic (ANC), to all pregnant women with an 'Opt out' approach is offered. The woman is counseled with the risk of HIV transmission to the fetus, and termination of pregnancy is offered.

However, if the woman is found seropositive and desires to continue pregnancy, several steps are taken to minimize the spread of the infection to the fetus, neonate and the others in the society (healthcare staff).

(i) Use of highly active antiretroviral therapy (HAART)
(ii) Elective cesarean delivery
(iii) Avoidance of breastfeeding can reduce the risk of vertical transmission to only 2%. WHO recommends breastfeeding in developing countries until the replacement feeding is safe. Further to this, the neonate is treated with zidovndine or nevirapine syrup. Barrier methods of contraception are prescribed to prevent further HIV transmission.

HAART is started from 14 weeks onwards till the intrapartum period (Cesarean delivery). Baby is screened for HIV and treated accordingly.

All the measures against the spread of infection (PPTCT) can only be adopted once the woman is adequately counseled and offered the screening. Therefore, it is the screening that is important. However, health awareness programs and practice of safer sex are the other important steps. Considering these benefits, all pregnant woman should be counseled and offered the screening for HIV in early pregnancy to prevent the spread of this serious infection.

### Q. 2  Hormone replacement therapy should be advised in all post menopausal women—discuss.

**Ans.** Menopause is often associated with **a number of symptoms**. These are **vasomotor** (hot flush, sweating), **genital and urinary symptoms** (atrophic changes, dyspareunia and dysuria), **psychological** (anxiety, mood swing, insomnia, irritability, depression), **osteoporosis** and **fracture** of bones, **cardiovascular** (coronary artery disease) and **cerebrovascular** disease. All these lead to significant morbidity and mortality in post-menopausal women. These are mainly due to deficiency of estrogen with the onset of menopause. Menopause may be either natural (normal) with age or abnormal:

(i) Premature
(ii) Artificial—surgical or radiation induced.

Hormone replacement therapy (HRT) can improve these symptoms which are often distressing to the woman. There are certain benefits of HRT that are evidence-based. These are improvement of vasomotor symptoms, urogenital atrophy and bone mineral density. HRT reduces the risk of vertebral and hip fractures.

There are several preparations used for HRT namely—estrogen, combined estrogen and progestin and others. Selection of HRT should be made depending upon the need of the woman and also whether her uterus is intact or has been removed (hysterectomy). On one side, there are certain benefits of HRT but at the same time, there are **some risks**. The risks are breast cancer, endometrial cancer, venous thromboembolism, coronary artery disease and altered lipid metabolism.

There are also certain **contraindications of HRT**. These are undiagnosed genital tract bleeding, estrogen dependent neoplasm in the body, active liver and gallbladder disease and history of thromboembolism. But there are **women who are most benefitted with the use of HRT provided they do not have any high-risk factor or any contraindication**. This group includes women with premature ovarian failure, gonadal dysgenesis and women with surgical or radiation menopause. HRT is really helpful to:

(i) Relieve the menopausal symptoms
(ii) Prevent osteoporosis
(iii) Maintain the quality of life in the menopausal years.

However, there are many nonhormonal methods of treatment that can be used for the problems of menopause. Currently, there are some changes in the knowledge and management of menopause. Changes in lifestyle, exercise, intake of calcium and vitamin D are found beneficial in the management of menopause. Considering all these, **there are selective women who are really benefitted with HRT rather than all**. But, it is imperative that every individual woman should be given **informed choice of HRT** based on the current knowledge of benefits and risks.

**Current recommendation is to prescribe HRT to control the symptoms of the woman. It is given in the lowest dose and for a short period only.**

## Q. 3 Laparoscopy is complementary to hysterosalpingography in evaluation of female infertility—discuss.

**Ans.** In the evaluation of female infertility, both laparoscopy and hysterosalpingography (HSG) are used primarily for the detection of the patency of the fallopian tubes.

**Hysterosalpingography** can detect any block in the fallopian tube specifically with regard to the side and site. This information is essential from the management point of view. Besides the tubal patency, HSG can give **many useful information** like detection of uterine malformation (septate or subseptate uterus), cervical incompetence, uterine synechiae, any submucous polyp or fibroid. Appearance of the tube on HSG also gives information regarding the pathology (hydrosalpinx, tubal diverticula and beaded appearance).

**It is a noninvasive test and is relatively simple.** However, it has got certain **contraindications** (pelvic infection) and **complications** (pelvic pain and infection).

On the other hand, laparoscopy has got certain **advantages over and above that of HSG.** It can diagnose **peritubal adhesions**, and pelvic **endometriosis**. It can detect **ovarian pathology** (PCOS changes and endometriosis). Chromopertubation is helpful to study the nature of tubal motility besides tubal patency. Therefore **laparoscopy helps to evaluate the pelvic, ovarian and the peritoneal factors for infertility besides that of tubal patency.** These pathologies are often considered as the important female factors for infertility.

**Laparoscopy is also useful for the treatment of such pathologies.** Laparoscopic **ovarian drilling** for PCOS and **salpingolysis** for peritubal adhesions are helpful to improve fertility. Laparoscopic electrofulguration of pelvic endometriotic implants is done to improve fertility as well as to improve the symptoms of pelvic pain in women. However, laparoscopy cannot evaluate the uterocervical factors that can be diagnosed with HSG. Laparoscopy is an **invasive procedure** and needs general anesthesia. It is expensive compared to HSG and it needs specialized training. Considering the benefits and limitations, the two procedures (HSG and laparoscopy) are regarded as complementary to each other.

## Q. 4 Chemotherapy is the mainstay of treatment in choriocarcinoma—discuss.

**Ans.** Choriocarcinoma is a highly malignant tumor arising from the chorionic epithelium. It is not a tumor of the uterus and uterus is involved secondarily. About 3–5% of all patients with molar pregnancies develop choriocarcinoma.

**Chemotherapy is the mainstay in the treatment as it is found to be highly effective. Depending upon the risk factors, either single drug or multidrug regimen is used.**

In general, patients with nonmetastatic (low-risk) and good prognosis (score <7) disease are treated with single drug (methotrexate or actinomycin). Methotrexate is an antimetabolite and acts as folic acid antagonist. Methotrexate has many side effects affecting the gastrointestinal, hemopoietic and other systems. Folinic acid is combined with methotrexate to minimize the side effects.

On the other hand, patients with poor prognosis and metastatic **(score ≥7) disease are treated with multidrug regimen (EMA-CO).** Drugs combined in this protocol are etoposide, methotrexate, actinomycin D, cyclophosphamide, vincristine and folinic acid. During the course of chemotherapy, serum hCG levels should be estimated at 1 week interval. Chemotherapy should be changed if there is no fall in hCG by at least 25% after each treatment cycle. Usually, 1–3 additional cycles of chemotherapy are given following normalization of serum hCG level. This is done to prevent recurrence of disease.

Prognosis with this regimen of chemotherapy is found satisfactory. **Cure rate is almost 100% in low-risk and about 70% in high-risk metastatic groups.** Young women can get pregnant in 1 year after the successful completion of chemotherapy. Chemotherapy has got no adverse effect on the fetus. **Primary hysterectomy has got a limited scope unless the tumor is found resistant to chemotherapy.** Considering all the benefits and its high efficacy, chemotherapy is considered the mainstay in the treatment of choriocarcinoma.

## Q. 5 Early diagnosis of ovarian cancer is still not possible—discuss.

**Ans.** Ovaries are deep seated organs. Unlike cervix, ovaries are not easily accessible by clinical evaluation (inspection, palpation or bimanual examination). Epithelial ovarian cancers are common. Unlike cervical intraepithelial neoplasia (CIN), **ovarian cancer has got no preinvasive stage**. No age is specific to ovarian cancer. The disease has got **no specific symptoms**. It remains **asymptomatic in about 15–20% of cases**. Duration of **symptoms** has got no correlation with the stage of the disease. Even with symptoms of short duration, the disease may have extensive spread and may be in advanced stage. **The tumor size** also does not have any correlation with the stage of the disease. A big tumor may remain benign, whereas a small tumor may be malignant with advanced stage. Unlike cancer cervix, there is **no effective screening procedure for ovarian malignancy.** Tumor markers like CA-125, HE4, OVXI, HER-2 neu and inhibin are extensively studied. The commonly tested tumor marker for epithelial ovarian cancer is CA-125, value ≥35 U/mL is suggestive of epithelial ovarian cancer. **Unfortunately, the tumor marker is nonspecific**. There are several other conditions where the level of CA-125 is found raised (normal woman, endometriosis, peritonitis, carcinoma of breast, colon and endometrium).

Early diagnosis of ovarian cancer with ultrasound imaging has been attempted. Transvaginal ultrasound with color Doppler imaging has been found helpful to differentiate a malignant ovarian tumor from a benign one. Currently, three-dimensional contrast enhanced power Doppler sonography is being done for more information.

**Risk of malignancy index (RMI)** has been evaluated. **High value of RMI (>250)** correlates **with high-risk of ovarian cancer (75%). Inspite of all these progresses in the screening methods, improvement in early detection of ovarian cancer has not yet been possible**. There are few high-risk cases for epithelial ovarian cancer like women of age ≥40 years, familial cancer (breast and ovary) and history of induction ovulation. **Inspite of all these risk evaluation, screening and detection procedures, diagnosis of ovarian cancer is late and often in the advanced stage**.

**Unless detected early and at a curable stage, survival of women with ovarian cancer is poor.** Because of these reasons, the 5 years survival rate of ovarian cancer has remained the same (35%) over the last 3 decades.

## Q. 6 Justify the place of HSG in the work-up protocol of female infertility.

**Ans.** Work-up protocol of female infertility needs evaluation of the following parameters:
  (i) Ovulatory factors (30–40%)
  (ii) Tubal and peritoneal factors (25–35%)
  (iii) Endometriosis (1–10%), uterine and cervical factors (15–20%).

Of all these different factors responsible for female infertility, hysterosalpingography can detect the tubal, uterine and cervical factors.

**HSG is a noninvasive procedure** that can assess the cervical canal, uterine cavity and the lumen of the tube including tubal patency. Compared to laparoscopy, it is less expensive. HSG can be done in the work-up protocol of female infertility **for the following information:**
  (i) Patency of the fallopian tubes.
  (ii) Uterine malformation (bicornuate and septate uterus) in cases with recurrent miscarriages.
  (iii) To detect cervical incompetency (midtrimester recurrent miscarriages).
  (iv) To diagnose uterine synechiae.
  (v) To detect any submucous fibroid or polyp.
  (vi) Tubal outline in HSG can be helpful to detect the type of pathology (hydrosalpinx due to infection or beaded appearance due to tuberculosis).
  (vii) HSG can demonstrate the side and site of tubal block.

However, HSG has to be done aseptically to avoid the **risk of infection. It should not be done** in cases with pelvic infection.

So HSG is an important tool in the work-up protocol of female infertility when done carefully and selectively.

## Q. 7 Selection of cases must be meticulous before prescribing HRT—discuss.

**Ans.** Women with symptoms of **estrogen deficiency** are the cases for prescribing HRT. **Generally, the postmenopausal women** are the main group who often suffer from the hazards of estrogen deficiency.

**Health hazards** are due to vasomotor instability, urogenital atrophy, osteoporosis and fracture, cardiovascular disease, cerebrovascular disease, psychological changes and changes in skin, collagen tissue and hair. However, not all the postmenopausal women suffer from these hazards. **Therefore, HRT should not be prescribed as a routine. Besides HRT, many women may be benefitted** with dietary changes (calcium and vitamin D supplementation), exercise and other nonhormonal methods (bisphosphonates). HRT includes many preparations and they can be used by different routes (oral, subdermal implants, skin patches and skin or vaginal cream). The **selection of HRT** for an individual woman is different depending on whether her uterus is intact or removed (hysterectomy). This is also important depending on her lifestyle and severity of symptoms.

Generally, there are women who are **benefitted with HRT**. They are women with menopausal symptoms, osteoporosis and women who wish to improve quality of life in the menopausal years. However, other group of women are premature ovarian failure, gonadal dysgenesis and women with surgical or radiation menopause.

But there are certain **definite contraindications to the use of HRT**. These are undiagnosed genital tract bleeding, estrogen-dependent neoplasm in the body, history of venous thromboembolism, active liver disease, gallbladder disease.

One should be very careful to exclude these women before prescribing HRT. Again there are **certain risks of HRT**—these include endometrial cancer, breast cancer, venous thromboembolism, coronary artery disease, abnormal lipid metabolism and dementia.

Women having all these risk factors already present should be counseled before prescribing HRT. Women should be informed about the other nonhormonal (calcium and SERMs) methods of management. Therefore, **women should be counseled not only with the benefits of HRT but also with the risks involved in it and other alternatives including nonhormonal methods of management**. Compliance during the therapy and regular follow-up is also important and women should be counseled about the same. Considering all these points, selection of cases must be meticulous before prescribing HRT.

## Q. 8  Staging of ovarian cancer is essentially surgicopathological one—discuss.

**Ans.** Clinical diagnosis of ovarian cancer is very imprecise. **The reasons for difficulties in clinical diagnosis are:**

(a) No specific symptoms
(b) Severity of symptoms and the duration of symptoms has no correlation with the spread or extent of the disease
(c) Tumor size assessed clinically has no correlation with the stage or spread of the disease.

There are several ancillary aids for the diagnosis like:

(i) Detection of malignant cells on abdominal paracentesis
(ii) Diagnosis of malignancy with noninvasive methods like sonography, MRI or CT scan, and
(iii) Estimation of serum CA-125.

However, these methods are also ineffective to confirm the diagnosis of malignancy and to assess the actual spread or stage of the disease.

**Correct staging of ovarian cancer can only be made by a systematic exploration on laparotomy** and confirmation by biopsy (histology).

**Presence of tumor limited to pelvis or spreading to para-aortic lymph nodes, liver and under surface of diaphragm has got different prognostic outcome.** Therefore, presence of tumor metastasis to different sites are grouped into different stages of the disease by FIGO.

The practical guideline for surgical procedures includes a systematic exploration (visual and manual) of all pelvic and abdominal viscera for any metastatic deposit and lymph nodes (pelvic and para-aortic) involvement. All these areas of spread need cytological and/or histological confirmation.

**There are several prognostic factors for survival outcome of ovarian malignancy.** These are:

(i) Spread of the disease (surgical stage)
(ii) Histological type
(iii) Histological grade
(iv) Peritoneal cytology
(v) Presence of ascites
(vi) Presence of metastatic disease
(vii) Volume of residual tumor after primary surgery
(viii) Ploidy status
(ix) The degree of oncogene expression.

This information can only be obtained by a combined approach of a systematic surgical exploration and pathological confirmation by taking biopsy.

**Moreover only with accurate staging, the prognostic outcome and the comparison of results following different modalities of therapy is possible.**

Hence, staging of ovarian carcinoma is essentially a surgicopathological one.

### Q. 9 Laparoscopy is an important diagnostic tool in gynecology—discuss.

**Ans.** Laparoscopy is an operative procedure for visualization of peritoneal and pelvic cavity by means of a fiberoptic endoscope introduced through the abdominal wall. It gives an opportunity of **seeing pelvic and abdominal organs and their pathology directly**. It is also possible to take tissue for biopsy. Moreover, it is also useful **to treat many such pathologies** at the same time. Diagnosis of many pelvic pathologies may not be possible only clinically or even when combined with other diagnostic aids like sonography. **In these situations, laparoscopy is superior to others.**

There are many conditions when **diagnostic laparoscopy may be of immense value**. Some of the conditions are:

(a) **Infertility work-up:** Detection of tubal patency, peritubal adhesions, ovulation stigma on the ovary and assessment of the tubes before reversal of sterilization operation.

(b) **Pelvic endometriosis:** Diagnosis (minimal or mild disease) and stage of the disease.

(c) **Chronic pelvic pain:** It is done in women where pathology is not detected clinically.

(d) **Acute pelvic lesion:** For exclusion of ectopic pregnancy and acute appendicitis.

(e) **Suspected mullerian abnormalities:** Uterine and ovarian pathologies (PCOS, endometrioma).

(f) **Detection of uterine perforation:** Accidental during dilation and curettage.

(g) **Amenorrhea for detection of pathology:** Uterine, ovarian or pelvic pathology (tuberculosis).

(h) **Follow-up following pelvic surgery:** Tuboplasty, ovarian malignancy (second look) and pelvic endometriosis.

(i) **Differentiation** of a clinically palpable pelvic mass (fibroid and ovarian cyst).

However, laparoscopy is an **invasive procedure**. It needs specialized training on the part of the surgical team. It is done under anesthesia.

Laparoscopy has got **few contraindications** :

(i) Severe cardiopulmonary disease
(ii) Hemodynamically unstable patient
(iii) Generalized peritonitis
(iv) Intestinal obstruction
(v) Large pelvic tumor or pregnancy >16 weeks
(vi) Previous periumbilical surgery (relative)
(vii) Extreme obesity.

There are certain situations where laparoscopy has a **complementary role** (e.g. HSG and laparoscopic chromopertubation). Considering all these benefits laparoscopy is regarded as an important diagnostic tool in gynecology.

## Q. 10 Combined oral contraceptive is the ideal method of contraception for a newly married woman—discuss.

**Ans.** Contraception for a newly married woman should be safe, effective, reversible, simple to use and without any significant side effects. Such a contraceptive method should not have any adverse effect on the woman on her future pregnancy. Usually, a newly married woman needs the contraception for a short period of time (usually 1–2 years) only.

Considering all the points mentioned above, combined oral contraceptive (COC) is ideal one. Moreover compared to other available methods (barriers, IUCD and injectables). **COC is user friendly, safe and failure rate is minimum (0.1 per 100 women years).**

**Barrier methods** have got high failure rates. Barrier methods (condoms) may not be liked by the young couple due to lack of satisfaction. **IUCD** runs the risk of pelvic infection. **Progestin only pills, injectables (DMPA) and implants are expensive and have many side effects** including menstrual abnormalities.

Currently used low dose pills with lipid-friendly progestin has got very **minimal side effects**. The **absolute contraindications of COCs (WHO) are only few. It has been proved that potential benefits of COC are greater compared to the risks in a well-selected individual.**

Above all, use of COC has got **many noncontraceptive benefits also. Some of these are:**
  (i) **Improvement** of menstrual abnormalities.
  (ii) **Improvement of** anemia.
  (iii) **Protection against** pelvic infections, ectopic pregnancy, endometriosis, functional ovarian cysts and hirsutism.
  (iv) **Protection against** the risk of ovarian cancer (50%), endometrial cancer (50%) and colorectal cancer compared to the nonusers.
  (v) **Long-term metabolic effect** is not significant on the health of the woman.
  (vi) **Prospect of future pregnancy** following stoppage of drug is quick.
  (vii) **Inadvertent intake of COC** during early pregnancy does not increase the risk of fetal congenital malformation.

However, the woman needs to be under follow-up for any problem that she faces.

Considering all the above reasons, COCs are considered the ideal method of contraception for a newly married woman.

## Q. 11 Cervical screening programs can reduce deaths from cancer cervix—discuss.

**Ans.** Cancer cervix is the second common cause of cancer death in female throughout the world. Nearly 80% of the deaths are in the developing world. In the developed world, incidence of cancer cervix has declined significantly as a result of effective population screening programs. Cancer cervix has a premalignant (CIN) state and also a microinvasive stage after which it becomes an invasive disease. **Duration from CIN to invasive cancer is about 10–15 years**. If the state of CIN or even the microinvasive stage is diagnosed, death from cervical cancer can be prevented entirely.

Early detection of CIN, CIS or microinvasive cancer is possible with different methods of screening and conducting various tests. **There are several screening methods for detection of premalignant state of the cervix. These are:**

(a) **Exfoliative cytology (Pap test) screening:** It is highly effective. False negative rate of Pap smear is 10% and false-positive rate is about 15–20%. To reduce the false-negative and the false-positive rates of Pap smear, liquid-based cytology (LBC) has been recommended (NICE). Cytology screening has reduced incidence of cancer cervix by nearly 80% and cervical cancer death by 70%.

(b) **Colposcopy:** Cases with abnormal cytology (moderate-to-severe dyskaryotic smear) are referred to for colposcopic evaluation and directed biopsy.

(c) **Visual inspection with acetic acid (VIA)** is a method where acetowhite area of the cervix is considered abnormal. Biopsy is taken from abnormal area.

(d) **Lugol's iodine** (5%) use and cervical biopsy from the unstained areas is an alternative method to colposcopic directed biopsy.

(e) **Human papilloma virus (HPV)** is currently considered the etiologic agent of cancer cervix. **Over 99.7% of women with CIN and cancer cervix are found to be positive with HPV-DNA.** Detection of HPV-DNA in cervical discharge is possible by **hybrid capture** technique and **using polymerase chain reaction (PCR)**. HPV-DNA testing is accepted as an important method of screening for cancer cervix. **Vaccines have been developed against the high risk group of HPV 16 and 18. Vaccines are effective against the development of cancer cervix.**

Cervical pathology once detected by any screening method in the cervical intraepithelial neoplasia (CIN) state or even in the microinvasive stage, can be cured completely. Different modalities of treatment are available for CIN (local excisional methods or electrodiathermy). In view of the above reasons, cervical screening programs are effective in reducing death from cancer cervix.

## Q. 12 Misoprostol has almost replaced the other methods for termination of pregnancy—discuss.

**Ans. Misoprostol is** a synthetic prostaglandin analogue ($PGE_1$). Currently, misoprostol is most commonly used for medical termination in the first as well as in the second trimesters of pregnancy. It **stimulates myometrial receptors to cause strong myometrial contractions**. It also **causes cervical softening and dilatation**. As a result there is expulsion of the products of conception.

In the first trimester, it may be used either alone or in combination with other drugs like mifepristone (200–600 mg) or methotrexate (50 mg/$M^2$). Standard drug regimen includes 1 tab (200 mg) mifepristone on day-1 followed by misoprostol 400 µg either oral or vaginal on day-3. Efficacy of this regimen is up to 95–98% when used with gestation ≤49 days.

**Combipack** (1 tablet mifepristone 200 mg and 4 tab misoprostol 200 µg each) is approved up to 63 days of pregnancy (DGHS-2008). In 50% cases, expulsion occurs within 4–5 hours of misoprostol intake.

Other evidence-based regimen has shown that **lower dose mifepristone** (200 mg) and **higher dose misoprostol** (800 µg vaginal or sublingual) increases the efficacy of abortion (95%) up to 63 days of pregnancy.

For **second trimester pregnancy termination,** the commonly used regimen is misoprostol 400 µg intravaginally every 6 hours. **Vaginal route misoprostol is more effective than oral administration.** When used in the second trimester, success rate of vaginal misoprostol is 86% within 24 hours.

Misoprostol has been found highly effective and safe in many clinical trials for medical termination of pregnancy (MTP). It is acceptable and privacy is maintained.

The **common side effects are:** Vaginal bleeding, cramping abdominal pain and nausea. The woman should be counseled and explained about the side effects. She should be assured of medical help in case of any emergency.

**Complications** of misoprostol induced abortion are rare (0.5%). Incomplete abortion occurs in 3% of cases. This can be managed by giving additional misoprostol or by suction curettage. Risk of endometritis is rare (0.09%). The maternal death rates remain 1 woman per 100,000 use.

**Benefits of misoprostol compared to surgical methods:** No risk of injury to cervix, uterine perforation, anesthetic reaction, hemorrhage, infection (endometritis), Asherman syndrome, infertility, chronic PID or psychological problems.

Considering all the safety, efficacy and benefits, misoprostol has almost replaced the other methods for termination of pregnancy.

### Q. 13 Phenotypically females are not always genetically females—discuss.

**Ans.** The development and differentiation of male and female external and internal genital organs are dependent on several factors that start working as early as 6–7 weeks of embryonic life.

**Differentiation of a bipotential gonad to testis needs the active drive of SRY gene present on the short arm of Y chromosome.** Absence of SRY gene leads to the development of ovary in a passive way.

**Regarding the development and differentiation of Wolffian duct and regression of Müllerian duct, the secretion of testosterone (from Leydig cells) and anti-Müllerian hormone (from Sertoli cells) are essential.** Conversion of testosterone to dihydrotestosterone is the factor for development of male external genitalia. On the other hand, absence of testosterone and AMH leads to the development of Müllerian duct, regression of Wolffian duct and development of female external genitalia. Therefore for an individual with absent SRY gene, though the chromosomal complement is 46 XY, the gonadal and ductal development is towards female (XY gonadal dysgenesis).

Many developmental anomalies of the external genitalia and ambiguity of sex are usually genetic in origin.

Individuals with gonadal dysgenesis, though phenotypically female, are chromosomally male (46 XY). Individuals with androgen insensitivity syndrome are phenotypically female due to the inability of end organs to respond to androgens though chromosomally they are males (46 XY). It is also true for individuals of Klinefelter's syndrome (46 XXY) and those with true hermaphroditism (46 XY).

Therefore, it is justified to say that not all phenotypical females are genetically females.

## Q. 14 Laparoscopic tubectomy has many advantages—discuss.

Laparoscopic tubal sterilization is a very popular method throughout the world. Compared to open methods (laparotomy), laparoscopic procedure has got many advantages.

This procedure can be done in the interval period, concurrent with vaginal termination of pregnancy (S/E) or 6 weeks following delivery (postpartum). It can be done either with single or double puncture technique. The tubes can be occluded by a silastic ring (Falope ring), Filshie clip or by electrosurgical methods (diathermy or laser).

In India, laparoscopic tubectomy is commonly done with the use of Falope ring or Filshie clip (less used).

**The advantages are:**

(1) **Like any endoscopic surgery,** it has all the advantages:
  (a) Rapid recovery
  (b) Shorter hospital stay (day care basis)
  (c) Quicker resumption of day-to-day activity
  (d) Less adhesion formation and
  (e) Minimal abdominal scar.

(2) **Failure rate:** When the procedure is done using Falope ring or by Filshie clip, it is only 0.1%. Electrosurgical method has got higher failure rate.

(3) **Reversibility:** Only about 2–3 cm of the tube is destroyed when Falope ring is used or 4 mm of the tube is destroyed when Filshie clip is used. So the chances of reversibility are high.

However, since the laparoscopic equipments are expensive, the surgeon must be specially trained and the case must be well-selected to achieve the benefits because the procedure has a few complications too.

## Q. 15 All adolescent girls should be given HPV vaccine—discuss.

**Ans.** Cancer of the cervix is the most common gynecological cancer in women of the developing countries. **It is an important cause of cancer death in India.** This is because screening facilities are inadequate. Cervical cancer is a preventable disease as the screening procedures like cytology and HPV-DNA detection are effective. There is significant reduction in death from cervical cancer in all the developed countries due to effective screening, early detection and treatment in the preinvasive stage. The diagnostic and therapeutic procedures for early disease is also very effective. It has a long (10-14 years) precancer phase (CIN) which once detected can be treated effectively and the disease is cured entirely.

Over 99% of patients with CIN and invasive cancer are found to be positive with HPV-DNA. HPV has been considered the causative agent of cancer cervix. Worldwide prevalence of HPV infection among healthy woman is 11.7%. HPV vaccine is found to be effective when given prophylactically to all school girls (9-15 years) and women (16-25 years). This vaccine is recommended as a primary measure of prevention against cervical cancer.

**The reasons that adolescent girls should be given the vaccine are:**
(i) Adolescent girls (9-14 years) are usually not sexually active.
(ii) Vaccine when given at this age, confers immunity by the time the adolescent becomes sexually active.
(iii) The impact of vaccine is greatest when given in women who are not infected with HPV.

There are three types of vaccines available now:
(i) The **bivalent vaccine** (Cervarix) gives protection against HPV types 16 and 18 which are responsible for 70% of all cervical cancers.
(ii) The **quadrivalent vaccine** (Gardasil) works against HPV types 16, 18, as well as 6 and 11. The HPV types 6 and 11 are responsible for anogenital warts.
(iii) **Nonavalent vaccine is currently available.** It targets HPV types: 31, 33, 45, 52, 58 in addition to 6,11,16,18.

**The vaccines offer some cross protection to other types also.**

The vaccines are type specific and they work when given prophylactically. The vaccines are given IM (over the deltoid muscle) in three doses with a schedule of 0-1 and 6 months (Cervarix) or 0-2 and 6 months (Gardasil). Once a complete course is given the immunity lasts for more than 6 years. Vaccines are safe and well-tolerated with no evidence of teratogenicity. There is no such recommendation for booster dose as yet. However, the woman should undergo routine cytology screening even if she is immunized with HPV vaccine. The vaccine works by increasing the levels of antibodies (IgG and IgA) locally in the cervical secretion. These antibodies prevent the attachment of HPV virus to the cells at the transformation zone. Therefore, the vaccine should be given to the adolescent girls as a primary measure of prevention against cancer cervix.

## Q. 16 Medical methods of termination of pregnancy (TOP) should be the method of choice—discuss.

**Ans.** Medical methods of TOP is a nonsurgical procedure using a combination of drugs. The commonly use drugs are:

(1) Mifepristone (RU 486)
(2) Misoprostol (PGE$_1$)
(3) Methotrexate (less used).

Mifepristone is a progesterone antagonist and it binds the progesterone receptors in the endometrium and decidua resulting in necrosis and detachment of products of conception. It also softens the cervix and sensitizes the uterus to the effect of prostaglandins. The different protocols of medical methods are given in the table below:

| | Pregnancy (weeks) | Day of therapy | Drug | Dose | Route | Efficacy |
|---|---|---|---|---|---|---|
| **PROTOCOLS FOR USE OF MIFEPRISTONE AND MISOPROSTOL FOR MEDICAL TOP** ||||||||
| A | Up to 7 weeks (49 days) | D1<br>D3 | Mifepristone (RU 486)<br>Misoprostol (PGE$_1$) | 200 mg<br>400 µg<br>(2 tab 200 µg each) | Oral<br>Oral/<br>vaginal | 95–98% |
| B | Up to 12 weeks | D1<br>D3 | Mifepristone<br>Misoprostol | 200 mg<br>800 µg<br>(4 tab 200 µg each) | Oral<br>Vaginal/<br>oral | 97% |
| **Combipack (mifepristone 200 mg + misoprostol 800 µg) has been approved for medical TOP up to 63 days (Director General of Health Services, Government of India — 2008)** ||||||||
| C | Up to 13–20 weeks | D1<br>D3 | Mifepristone<br>Misoprostol | 200 mg<br>400 µg every 3–6 up to total 5 doses | Oral<br>Vaginal/<br>Oral/<br>Sublingual | 97% |
| **When mifepristone is not available, misoprostol alone can be used with an efficacy of 84%.** ||||||||

Misoprostol is a prostaglandin (PGE$_1$) which stimulates strong myometrial contractions and causes cervical softening and dilatation. It causes expulsion of the conceptus from the uterus due to its combined effect on the myometrium and the cervix.

## ADVANTAGES OF MEDICAL METHODS OF TOP WHEN COMPARED TO SURGICAL METHODS (SE OR D and E)

1. It is a simple, safe and highly effective (95–98%) method.
2. Needs minimal or no technical assistance as regard to instruments, operation theater, anesthesia or hospital stay.
3. No effect on future fertility.
4. Complications are rare (0.5%). No risk of cervical injury, uterine perforation, anesthetic reaction, hemorrhage, infection, Asherman syndrome, chronic PID or infertility.

## DISADVANTAGES OF MEDICAL METHODS OF TOP

1. Unpredictable outcome in a small percentage of cases.
2. Whole process may take longer time.
3. Surgical method may be needed in a case of failure or incomplete expulsion.
4. There is risk of fetal malformation in a case of failure.

Considering all the above issues medical methods of the TOP should be the method of choice.

# CHAPTER 14

# Viva-Voce in Gynecology

## Chapter Objectives
- A wide range of topics (as models) have been discussed with questions of different levels of hardness
- The information is presented in a concise and as much as in simpler language
- The answers provide the up-to-date information

❖ Gynecology Questions and Answers 476

# GYNECOLOGY QUESTIONS AND ANSWERS

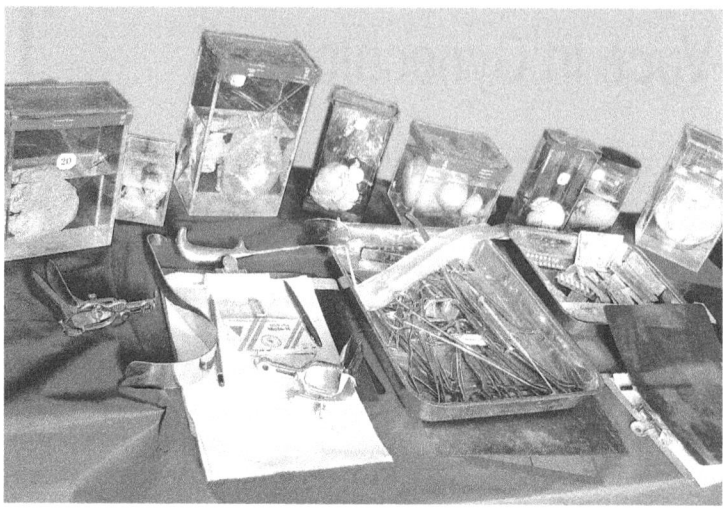

Viva table in gynecology. Candidate is expected to be familiar with all the items

## 1. HYSTEROSALPINGOGRAPH

**Q. Describe the skiagram shown in Figure 14.1.**

**Ans.** It is a hysterosalpingographic plate showing the cervical canal, uterine cavity, both the tubes. The HSG cannula is in situ. There is bilateral spillage of dye in the peritoneal cavity.

**Q. What is your inference with this HSG?**

**Ans.** Both the tubes are patent.

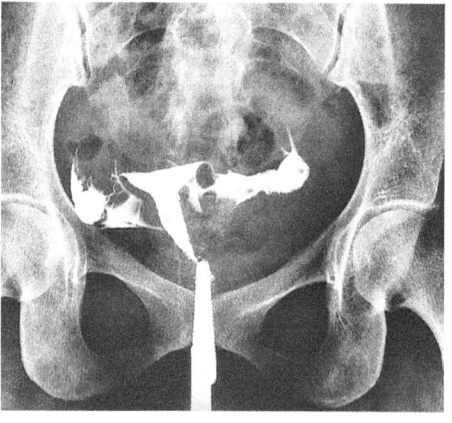

Fig. 14.1: Hysterosalpingogram with bilateral peritoneal spillage.

**Q. What are the indications of HSG?**

**Ans.** (a) To assess tubal patency in a woman with infertility (Figs. 14.2 and 14.3).
(b) To detect uterine malformations (unicornuate uterus).
(c) Diagnosis of cervical incompetence.
(d) Diagnosis of submucous fibroid.
(e) Diagnosis of uterine synechiae.
(f) Evaluation of a case with recurrent miscarriage.

**Q. In which phase of the menstrual cycle HSG is done?**

**Ans.** In the first half of the cycle (proliferative phase) between D7 and D10. It is avoided in the secretory phase, as there is risk of pregnancy interference by chance the woman has conceived in that cycle.

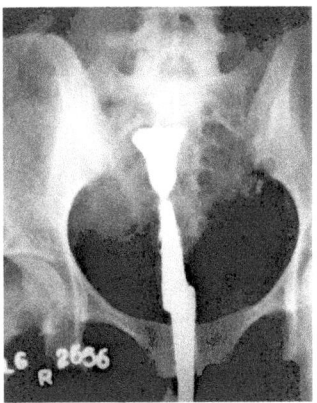

**Fig. 14.2:** Hysterosalpingogram showing bilateral cornual block. She had a history of MTP.

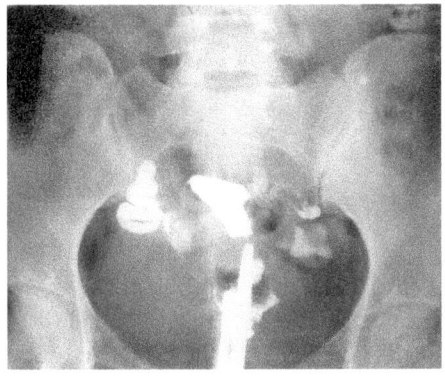

**Fig. 14.3:** Hysterosalpingogram showing bilateral fimbrial block. Bilateral salpingostomy was done. Thereafter, she suffered an ectopic pregnancy.

**Q. What are the advantages of laparoscopy over HSG?**

**Ans.** SAQ-3, p. 460.

**Q. What are the other methods for assessment of tubal patency?**

**Ans.** Laparoscopy and dye test, sonohysterosalpingography, insufflation test, salpingoscopy and falloposcopy.

**Q. What is sonohysterosalpingography?**

**Ans.** Normal saline is pushed within the uterine cavity with a pediatric Foley catheter. Thereafter ultrasonography of the uterus, tubes are done. The procedure can detect uterine malformations, synechiae or polyps. This is a noninvasive procedure and without the hazard of radiation.

**Q. What is the management if tubes are found normal?**

**Ans.** To evaluate the male factor (semen analysis) and ovarian factor (ovulation) for infertility.

**Q. What other information can be obtained from HSG?**

**Ans.** Detection of intrauterine adhesions, submucous fibroids, uterine malformations (bicornuate or septate uterus) (Fig. 14.4).

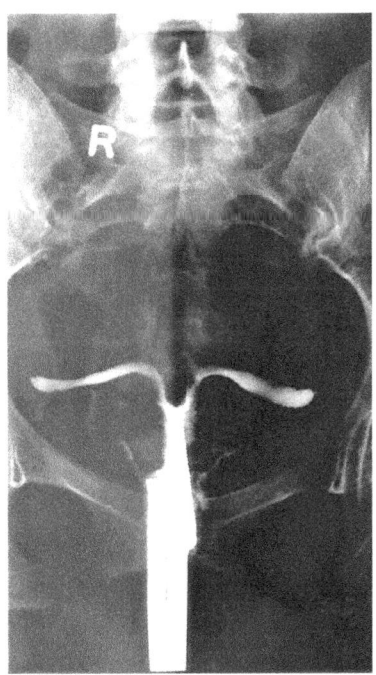

**Fig. 14.4:** Hysterosalpingogram showing bicornuate uterus. Metroplasty was done for recurrent midtrimester abortion. Subsequently, she had LSCS at 39 weeks and a live baby girl was delivered.

**Q. How septate uterus could be differentiated from a bicornuate uterus?**

**Ans.** The common differentiating features are:
   (a) The angle between horns: In septate uterus: Acute angle (<80°); in bicornuate >105°.
   (b) The intercornual distance is <4 cm, where as it is >4 cm in bicornuate uterus.
   (c) MRI can delineate clearly both the horns (bicornuate uterus) and the septum (septate uterus). However, HSG should not be used for differentiation. Hysteroscopy combined with laparoscopy is commonly used for diagnosis and management.

**Q. What are the advantages of aqueous-based media used in HSG?**

**Ans.** Compared to the oil-based media the differences are:
   (i) Risk of embolism is less
   (ii) No risk of granuloma formation
   (iii) Time for the procedure is less
   (iv) Risk of acute flare of pelvic infections are less
   (v) However, the outline of the uterus is less well demarcated compared to the oil-based media.

**Q. What are the common contraindications of HSG?**

**Ans.** (a) Presence of pelvic inflammatory disease
   (b) Uterine bleeding
   (c) Presence of pelvic mass with tenderness
   (d) Drug allergy.

**Q. What is the management of a bicornuate uterus?**

**Ans.** It is difficult. Metroplasty or unification (Strassman or Tompkins) operation has been recommended.

## 2. CERVICAL SMEAR, CYTOLOGY AND CERVICAL INTRAEPITHELIAL NEOPLASIA

**Q. How to take cervical smear?**

**Ans.** Cervix is exposed with a Cusco's bivalve speculum (Fig. 14.8, p. 482) without any lubricant. Prior bimanual examination should not be done. The cells are collected from the ectocervix using the Ayre's spatula (Fig. 14.5) and from the endocervix with the cytobrush (Fig. 14.5).

**Methods of slide preparation and fixation:** The material so collected is immediately spread over a slide. Fixative (95% ether and ethyl alcohol) is then spread over it. Once the slide is dried up, the slide is then stained (in the laboratory) either with Papanicolaou or Sorr's method. It is then examined under the microscope by a cytopathologist.

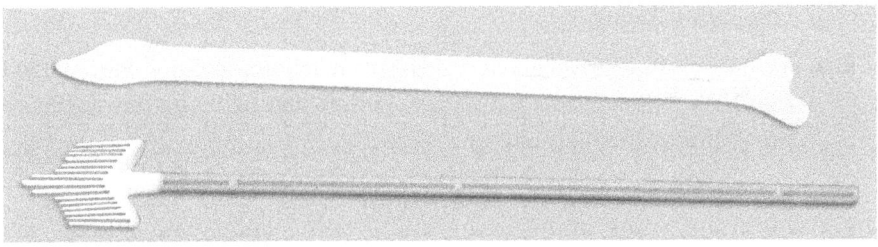

**Fig. 14.5:** Ayre's spatula (top) and cytobrush (bottom).

**Q. Which group of women are at risk and require cervical cytology screening?**

**Ans.** Any sexually active women between 21 years and 65 years of age.

**Others:**
- Multiple sexual partners
- HPV infection
- HIV positive (immune-compromised) women
- Oral pill users.

**Q. What is the grading of Papanicolaou's smear?**

**Ans.** Gradings are total five:
(i) Normal
(ii) Infective
(iii) Suspicious
(iv) Few malignant cells
(v) Plenty of malignant cells.

However, Bethesda system of classification is currently followed (For details see Dutta Gyne 7/e, p. 91).

**Q. What is a dyskaryotic smear? What are the different types of dyskaryotic smear?**

**Ans.** Dyskaryosis is the presence of morphological abnormalities of the nucleus.

**Nuclear abnormalities may be:**
(i) Increase in number and size
(ii) Irregular in outline (shape)
(iii) Multinucleation
(iv) Hyperchromasia.

**Dyskaryotic smear may be graded as:**
(i) Mild
(ii) Moderate
(iii) Severe.

**Q. What is a koilocyte?**

**Ans.** It is an abnormal cell characterized by nuclear abnormalities due to infection with HPV. The typical changes are: Perinuclear halo, nuclear irregularity, hyperchromasia and multinucleation.

**Q. What is CIN? How do you diagnose CIN?**

**Ans.** It is the histological abnormality where part or whole of thickness of cervical squamous epithelium is replaced by cells with varying degree of atypia. Basement membrane remains intact.

**Diagnosis of CIN is made by:**
(i) Cytology
(ii) Visual inspection with acetic acid (VIA)
(iii) Colposcopy
(iv) Cervicography
(v) Biopsy
(vi) Conization of cervix.

**Q. How do you manage a case of CIN?**

**Ans.** CIN can be managed by (*see* p. 451)
(i) Local ablative methods
(ii) Excisional methods or by
(iii) Hysterectomy.

## 3. RETENTION OF URINE IN GYNECOLOGY (Fig. 14.6)

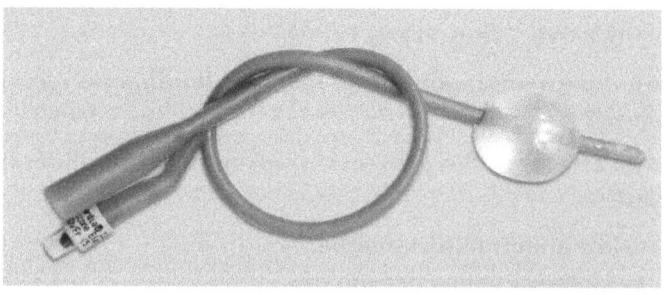

**Fig. 14.6:** Foleys catheter with inflated bulb.

**Q. What are the causes of acute and chronic retention of urine?**

**Ans.** (i) Postoperative (common)
(ii) Obstructive (due to growth, vaginal packing)
(iii) Failure of detrusor contraction (epidural anesthesia)
(iv) External sphincter spasm (perineal injuries)
(v) Others.

**Q. What are the menstrual abnormalities that may manifest with retention of urine?**

Ans. (a) Primary amenorrhea, cryptomenorrhea

(Hematocolpos) ⟶

(b) Secondary amenorrhea

(Retroverted gravid uterus) ⟶

(c) Menorrhagia

(Impacted uterine fibroid in the POD) ⟶

(d) Irregular bleeding and pain

(Pelvic hematocele and pelvic abscess) ⟶

(e) No menstrual abnormality

(Impacted ovarian tumor and cervical fibroid) ⟶

RETENTION OF URINE

## 4. VAGINAL SPECULUM

**Q. What are the types of vaginal specula used in gynecology?**

Ans. (i) Cusco's self-retaining vaginal speculum
(ii) Sim's posterior vaginal speculum.
(iii) Auvard's self-retaining posterior vaginal speculum.
(iv) Huffman-Graves self-retaining speculum.

**Q. What is Huffman-Graves speculum and where it is used (Fig. 14.7)?**

Ans. Huffman-Graves speculum is also a self-retaining speculum. Blades are narrow and long. It is designed for the adolescents in whom the introitus is narrow. It helps in easy inspection of the cervix in adolescents. It is also known as Duckbill speculum.

**Q. What are the advantages of Cusco's speculum (Fig. 14.8)?**

Ans. (i) It is self-retaining—so no assistant is required to hold the speculum as in Sims' posterior vaginal speculum.

(ii) It makes complete visualization of the cervix.

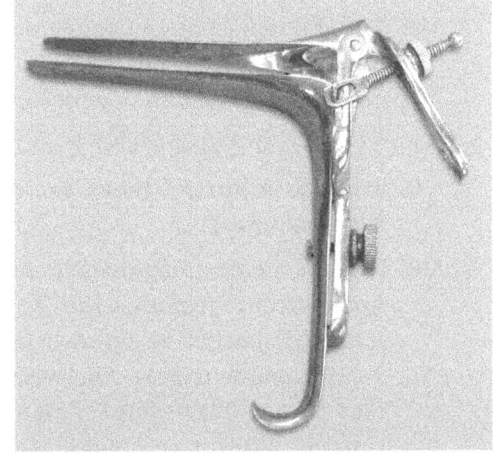

Fig. 14.7: Huffman-Graves speculum.

In Sims' speculum the anterior vaginal wall is to be pushed up with an anterior vaginal wall retractor.

(iii) Procedures like cervical smear, colposcopy, cervical biopsy and swabs can be performed simultaneously.

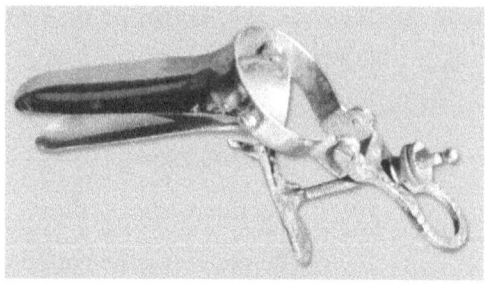

Fig. 14.8: Cusco's speculum.

**Q. How is it introduced?**

Ans. The patient is brought to the edge of the table. The speculum is introduced with blades closed and keeping the blades parallel to the vaginal introitus. The gloved left hand fingers (thumb and the index) are used to keep the labia apart. The speculum, smeared with a lubricant, is introduced gently. Once inside the vagina, it is rotated at right angle keeping handle downwards. The blades are now opened up and the screw is tightened.

**Q. What are the disadvantages of using this speculum?**

Ans. The anterior and the posterior walls of the vagina cannot be seen as they are covered up by the blades.

**Q. How can you get the benefit of using Cusco's speculum while using the Sims' posterior vaginal speculum?**

Ans. Anterior vaginal wall is to be pushed up using an anterior vaginal wall retractor when Sims' speculum is used. Hence, one assistant is needed.

**Q. What is cervical ectopy?**

Ans. It is the replacement of squamous epithelium of the ectocervix by columnar epithelium of endocervix by the process of metaplasia.

**Q. What is a polyp? What are the different types?**

Ans. Polyp is a protruding tissue growth from mucous membrane (Fig. 14.9). It may be attached by a pedicle (Fig. 14.9) (pedunculated) otherwise it may be sessile. It may be benign (mucus, fibroid or placental) or malignant.

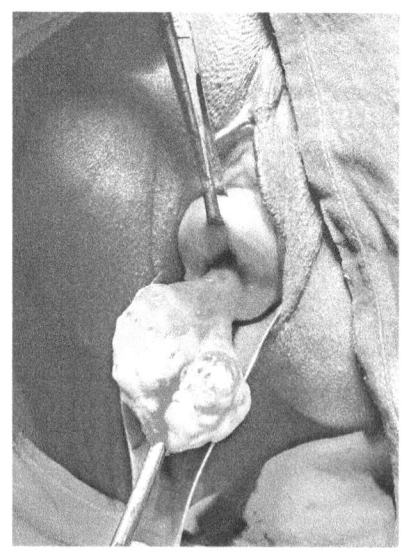

Fig. 14.9: A large cervical polyp with a pedicle seen to arise from the endocervix.

## 5. SHARMAN'S CURETTE (Fig. 14.10)

**Q. What are the advantages of this curette over the sharp and blunt curette?**

**Ans.** It is thin and narrow. There is no need of dilatation of the cervical canal. It can be introduced after the introduction of the uterine sound. It causes minimal trauma. Adequate tissue is obtained for endometrial histology.

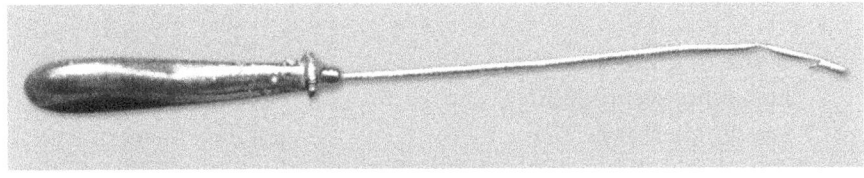

Fig. 14.10: Sharman's curette.

**Q. What is the purpose of doing endometrial biopsy in a woman with infertility?**

**Ans.** To detect evidence of ovulation—by seeing the secretory changes in the endometrium.

**Q. On which day of the menstrual cycle is endometrial biopsy usually done?**

**Ans.** Biopsy should be done on 21-23rd day when the cycle is regular. When the cycles are irregular, it is done within 24 hours of menstruation.

**Q. In the endometrial biopsy, what is the earliest evidence of ovulation?**

**Ans.** Subnuclear vacuolation is the earliest evidence appearing within 36-48 hours of ovulation.

**Q. What are other methods of diagnosis of ovulation?**

**Ans.** Basal body temperature (BBT), cervical mucus study, vaginal cytology, estimation of serum progesterone, LH and estradiol, sonography and laparoscopy.

**Q. What are the ovarian causes of infertility?**

**Ans.** Anovulation, luteal phase defect (LPD) and Luteiniz unruptured follicle (LUF).

## 6. CHORIOCARCINOMA (Fig. 14.11)

**Q. What are the common sites of metastasis?**

**Ans.** (a) Lungs (80%)

(b) Anterior vaginal wall (30%)

(c) Brain (10%)

(d) Liver (10%).

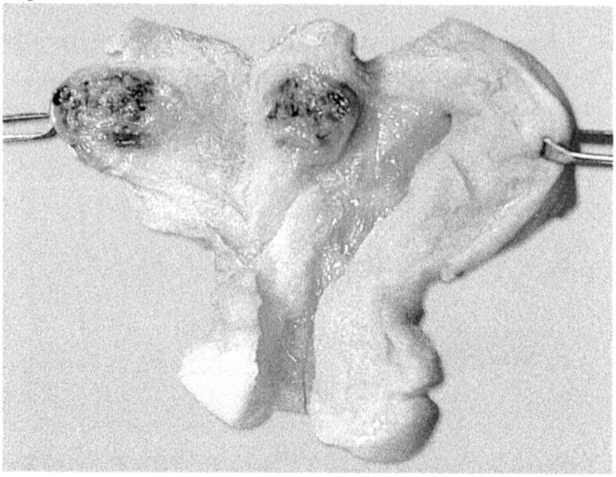

**Q. What are the important parameters in WHO scoring system of GTD?**

**Ans.** The important parameters in WHO scoring system are: Age, antecedent pregnancy, interval, pretreatment hCG, largest tumor size (cm), site of metastasis, number of metastasis and previous chemotherapy.

**Fig. 14.11:** Mrs LD, a 43 years old parous lady was admitted for her problems of repeated episodes of irregular vaginal bleeding. She had a prior history of miscarriage for which she underwent dilatation and evacuation operation. Examination revealed: Uterus of 12 weeks size, ovaries were enlarged. USG Doppler study revealed enlarged uterus with a highly vascular growth at the region of the uterine fundus. Serum β-hCG was 2,09,755 mIU/mL. She scored in the high-risk group. She received multi-agent chemotherapy. (WHO) Hysterectomy specimen, cut opened to show the hemorrhagic growth within the myometrium—histology confirmed a case of choriocarcinoma.

**Q. How do you score the risk factors?**

**Ans.** According to WHO (modified by FIGO) scoring system:

Score <6 = Low-risk.

Total score ≥7 = High-risk.

**Q. What is the significance of scoring?**

**Ans.** Single agent chemotherapy is usually given for low-risk women.

Women with high-risk need multimodal therapy (surgery and radiation therapy). Multiple agent chemotherapy are used for women with high-risk disease (score ≥7), (see p. 425). Radiation (brain and liver) therapy may have to be given.

**Q. Make a brief outline of management for a case with choriocarcinoma.**

**Ans.** (1) Most cases are treated with chemotherapy.

(A) Low-risk GTN (WHO):

(a) Single agent: Methotrexate—dose—50 mg/M$^2$: IM/IV

(b) Dactinomycin—less commonly used.

(B) High-risk GTN: Multiagent chemotherapy—EMA-CO regimen is commonly used. It is well-tolerated and highly effective.

(2) Surgery: Hysterectomy is needed in few cases:
   (a) Cases resistant to chemotherapy
   (b) Cases with intractable bleeding (vaginal or abdominal)
   (c) Cases with placental site trophoblastic tumor (PSTT)
   (d) Epithelioid trophoblastic tumors
   (e) Craniotomy for cases with cerebral metastasis presenting with seizures
   (f) Thoracotomy for cases with lung metastasis not responding to therapy.
(3) Radiotherapy for cases with brain or chest metastasis.

## 7. FIBROID UTERUS

**Q. Describe the specimen shown in figure 14.12.**

**Ans.** It is a specimen of uterus with the cervix, ovaries and tubes of both the sides. The uterus is enlarged in size and irregular in shape due to multiple fibroids of different sizes. One of the fibroids is huge in size. It has invaded within the leaves of the broad ligament (pseudobroad ligament fibroid— *see* p. 375, Fig. 11.3). So, it is a specimen of multiple fibroid uterus.

**Q. What is the operation done here?**

**Ans.** Total abdominal hysterectomy and bilateral salpingo-oophorectomy.

**Q. What could be the possible clinical presentation for this women?**

**Ans.** Menorrhagia, metrorrhagia, dysmenorrhea, pain abdomen, abdominal lump and pressure symptoms.

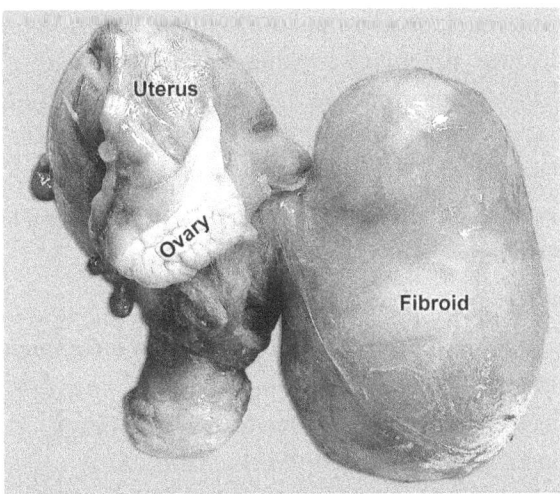

Fig. 14.12: Multiple fibroid (pseudobroad ligament fibroid) uterus. Majority are subserous in variety. This huge size fibroid invaded the broad ligament. Total hysterectomy with bilateral salpingo-oophorectomy done.

**Q. Describe the specimen shown in figure 14.13.**

**Ans.** It is the specimen of uterus, cervix, tubes and ovaries of both the sides. The uterus is cut open to show a big interstitial myoma in the region of the fundus. There is a submucous myoma at the fundus also. There are also few small seedling myomas. The tubes, ovaries and the cervix are apparently normal. So, it is a specimen of fibroid uterus.

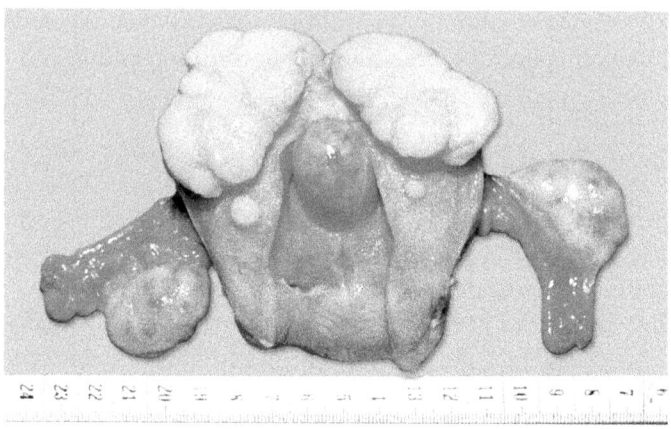

**Fig. 14.13:** Fibroid uterus — interstitial and submucous variety.

**Q. What operation has been done in this case?**

**Ans.** Total abdominal hysterectomy with bilateral salpingo-oophorectomy.

**Q. What could be the presenting symptoms of this woman?**

**Ans.** Commonly such women present with: Menorrhagia, metrorrhagia, dysmenorrhea, abdominal swelling or pelvic heaviness.

**NB** *With this specimen of hysterectomy (Figs. 14.12 and 14.13), the women are unlikely to suffer from infertility. Her probable age would be 40 years, or above as bilateral oophorectomy had been done.*

**Q. What are the indications, conditions to be fulfilled, and contraindications of myomectomy?**

**Ans.** See p. 516.

**Q. How do you differentiate fibroid uterus from adenomyosis?**

**Ans.**
- Adenomyosis is commonly seen in elderly women (>40 years)
- Uterus is enlarged diffusely due to myohyperplasia
- Uterine size is around 12–16 weeks of pregnancy
- On TVS: There are cystic spaces seen in the myometrium
- MRI is diagnostic: Absence of endometrial-myometrial junctional zone
- On cut section: Capsule is absent (present in a fibroid uterus).

## 8. TUMORS OF THE OVARY (Fig. 14.14)

**Q. What are the common tumors of the ovary?**

**Ans.** Common tumors of the ovary are as follows:

### A. Epithelial ovarian tumors (60–70%)
- Serous cystadenoma
- Mucinous cystadenoma
- Endometrioid tumor.

### B. Germ cell tumors (20–25%)
- Dysgerminoma
- Mature teratoma (dermoid cyst)
- Endodermal sinus cell tumor (yolk sac tumor)
- Choriocarcinoma
- Immature teratoma.

### C. Sex cord stromal tumors (6–10%)
- Granulosa cell tumors
- Theca cell tumors
- Sertoli-Leydig cell tumors
- Fibroma.

### D. Other unclassified tumors

### E. Secondary metastatic tumor (Krukenberg tumor).

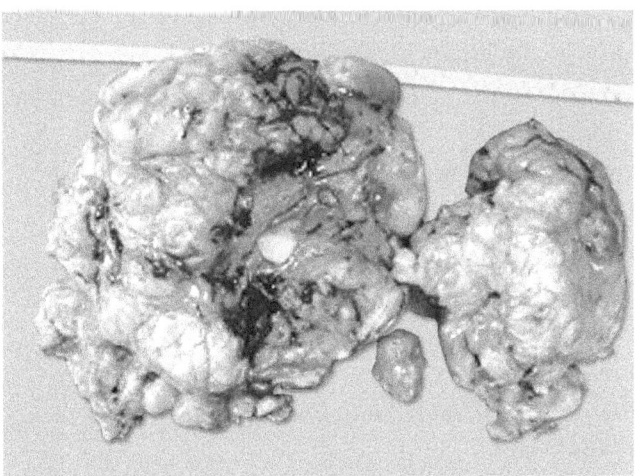

**Fig. 14.14:** Bilateral malignant epithelial tumors of the ovary. Specimen shows solid nodular masses with areas of hemorrhage and necrosis.

**Q. What are the common malignant tumors of the ovary?**

**Ans.** (A) **Epithelial ovarian tumors** often undergo malignant changes:
- Serous cyst adenocarcinoma
- Mucinous cyst adenocarcinoma
- Malignant endometrioid (rare).

(B) **Germ cells tumors** as mentioned above are malignant. Dermoid cyst is mostly benign. Risk of malignancy in a dermoid is very low (1-2%).

(C) **Sex cord stromal tumors** may be benign, but they are potentially malignant.

**Q. Mention some of the clinical features of a malignant ovarian tumor.**

**Ans.** Malignant ovarian tumors may remain asymptomatic.

**Common symptoms are:** Abdominal distension and discomfort, dyspepsia, loss of appetite, dull aching lower abdominal pain, weight loss and respiratory distress due to ascites or pleural effusion.

**Important signs are:** Cachexia, anemia, edema legs, jaundice.

**Abdominal examination:** A mass in the hypogastrium with features of malignancy.

**Per vaginal examination:** Nodules in the POD.

**Q. What are the high-risk as well as the protective factors for ovarian malignancy?**

**Ans. High-risk factors for ovarian malignancy:**

(a) Age: 40–60 years

(b) Familial cancers: Breast, endometrial and ovarian

(c) Postmenopausal palpable ovary (volume >8 cc)

(d) History of infertility.

(e) Obesity

(f) Endometriosis.

**Protective factors for ovarian malignancy are:**

(a) Combined oral contraceptives

(b) Pregnancy

(c) Tubal ligation

(d) Salpingectomy

(e) Breastfeeding.

**Q. What are the principles (guidelines) of surgical approach in a malignant ovarian tumor?**

**Ans. Surgery is the keystone in the management of ovarian cancers.**

Practical guidelines for surgery are:

(1) Incision—vertical.

(2) To collect ascitic fluid for cytology.

(3) A systematic exploration of the pelvic and abdominal cavity to detect metastasis and enlarged lymph nodes.

(4) Biopsy from any metastatic deposit or from the peritoneum when no metastasis is observed.

(5) Risk of malignancy index (RMI): RMI ≥250, the risk of cancer is 75% (see below).

**Q. What is the place of prophylactic oophorectomy during hysterectomy?**

**Ans.** Prophylactic oophorectomy during hysterectomy may be considered in women who are at high-risk for ovarian malignancy.

**Q. What is the surgical treatment of malignant ovarian tumor?**

**Ans.** (A) **Early stage disease (stage IA, G1, G2)**

Young woman<br>⇩<br>Unilateral oophorectomy (fertility conserving surgery)<br>⇩<br>Routine follow-up<br>⇩<br>Once family completed<br>⇩<br>Removal of uterus and other ovary.

- Elderly woman—hysterectomy and bilateral salpingo-oophorectomy
- In stage Ia, G3 and rest of stage I—hysterectomy, bilateral salpingo-oophorectomy, omentectomy and chemotherapy.

(B) **Advanced stage disease**

(a) Cytoreductive surgery or debulking procedure

(b) Adjuvant chemotherapy.

**Q. What are screening methods for ovarian malignancy?**

**Ans.** Clinical, biochemical (tumor markers) and biophysical (sonography including color Doppler) methods are commonly used.
- Clinical examination: Neither sensitive nor specific
- Tumor markers; Raised CA-125, HE4, M-CSF—nonspecific
- USG, Doppler study: Presence of increased vascularity
- Risk of malignancy index (RMI): U (Ultrasonographic features) × M (Menopausal status) × CA-125 (measured in units) = RMI. If RMI ≥250: Risk of malignancy is 75%.

**Q. How can a benign ovarian tumor can be differentiated from a malignant one clinically?**

**Ans.** Benign ovarian tumor has the following clinical features: It is usually:
(a) Unilateral
(b) Mobile
(c) Cystic feel
(d) Smooth surface

(e) No ascites

(f) Slow growing.

**Q. How can laparotomy findings be helpful to differentiate a benign tumor from a malignant one?**

Ans. A malignant ovarian can be differentiated from a benign one on laparotomy by the following features:

(a) **Ascites**—present and often it is hemorrhagic.

(b) **Tumor growth** is present on the surface.

(c) **Cut section** of the tumor shows solid and hemorrhagic areas.

(d) **Adhesions** and peritoneal nodules are present.

(e) **Metastatic** deposits may be present on liver surface para-aortic nodes may be palpable.

**Q. What are psammoma bodies?**

Ans. These are tiny, calcified bodies observed in cases with serous cyst adenoma of the ovary. It found in areas of cellular degeneration.

**Q. What are the complications of a benign ovarian tumor?**

Ans. (a) Torsion

(b) Intracystic hemorrhage

(c) Infection

(d) Rupture

(e) Pseudomyxoma peritonei

(f) Malignancy.

**Q. Discuss the differential diagnosis of a pelvic abdominal lump.**

Ans. (a) Pregnancy

(b) Fibroid uterus

(c) Chocolate cyst of the ovary

(d) Encysted tuberculosis

(e) Adenomyosis uteri

(f) Full bladder.

**Q. Mention the features of functional ovarian cysts.**

Ans. The important feature of the functional cysts of the ovary are:

(a) It is due to temporary hormonal disorders

(b) Usually 6–8 cm in diameter

(c) Usually asymptomatic

(d) Unilocular

(e) Regresses spontaneously

(f) Contains clear fluid.

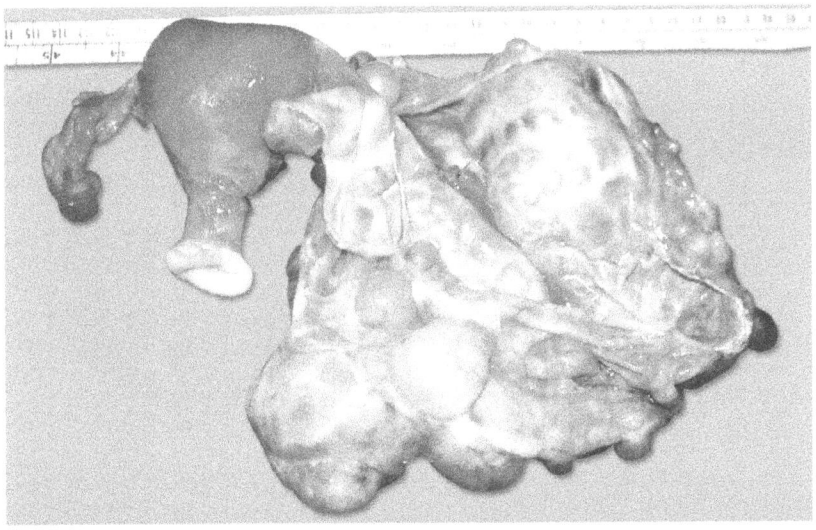

**Fig. 14.15:** Serous cystadenoma (gross appearance on cut specimen).

***Q. Outline the management of a benign ovarian tumor.***

**Ans. Laparotomy:** Incision → vertical — exploration of pelvic organs and the abdominal cavity.

**Benign**

(i) Young woman—ovarian cystectomy or ovariotomy,

(ii) Parous women 40 years or above; total hysterectomy with bilateral salpingo-oophorectomy.

***Q. What are the common malignant ovarian tumors?***

**Ans.** **(a) Epithelial cell carcinomas**

(i) Serous cyst adenocarcinoma (Fig. 14.15)

(ii) Mucinous cyst adenocarcinoma.

**(b) Germ cell carcinomas**

(i) Dysgerminoma

(ii) Endodermal sinus tumor.

***Q. What adjuvant chemotherapy is commonly used in the management of carcinoma ovary following surgery?***

**Ans.** Adjuvant chemotherapy with carboplatin and paclitaxel for six cycles is used.

***Q. Mention the difficulties in the management of ovarian cancers.***

**Ans.** Diagnosis is often late as many patients remain asymptomatic for a long time. Unlike cervix, there is no effective screening procedure. There is no premalignant stage for ovarian cancer.

## 9. PELVIC INFECTION (Fig. 14.16)

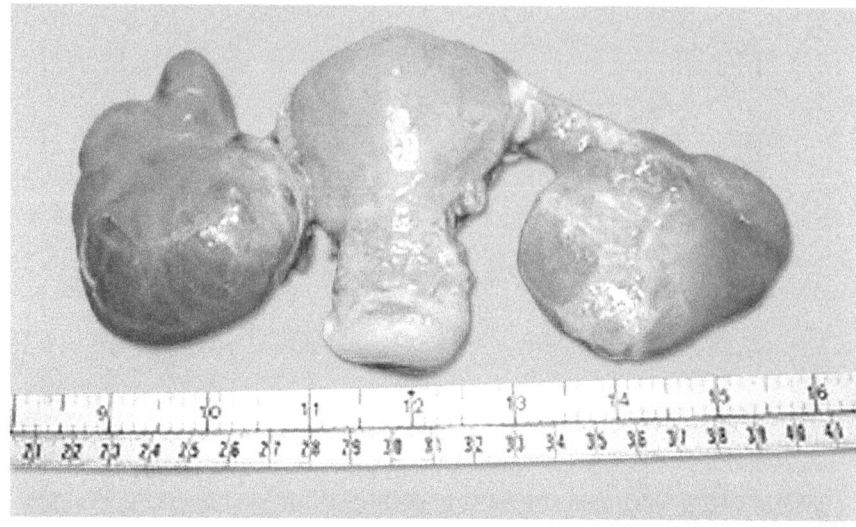

**Fig. 14.16:** Specimen of bilateral pyosalpinx. There is marked distension of the tubes at the ampullary region. The isthmic region distends less as it is more muscular and thick. As the mesosalpinx is fixed, the tubes look 'retort' shaped.

**Q. How infertility and menstrual abnormalities could be explained with genital tuberculosis.?**

Ans. *See* p. 416

**Q. What organs are commonly affected with chlamydial infection and how the infection is treated?**

Ans.
- Chlamydial infection affect the columnar and transitional epithelium of the genitourinary tract.
- Urethritis, bartholinitis, cervicitis, endometritis and salpingitis are common.
- Recommended drugs for chlamydial infection are azithromycin 1 g, PO. Single dose or doxycycline 100 mg, PO BID for 7 days.
- Husband should also be treated simultaneously.

**Q. What are the clinical features of bacterial vaginosis? How can the infection be diagnosed and how is it treated?**

Ans. **A. Clinical features:**
  (i) Smelly vaginal discharge
  (ii) Discharge grayish-white in color.

**B. Diagnosis:**
  (i) **Whiff test:** Fishy (amine) odor when a drop of discharge is mixed with 10% solution of KOH.

(ii) **Clue cells:** Vaginal epithelial cells appear granular when seen under a microscope.

C. **Treatment:** Metronidazole 200 mg orally thrice daily for 7 days is effective. Husband (sexual partner) should also treated simultaneously.

**Q. What is HIV? What is the immunopathogenesis of this infection? What is the current recommendation for the treatment of HIV?**

**Ans.** Human immunodeficiency virus (HIV) is a retrovirus having the enzyme reverse transcriptase. There is progressive depletion of CD4+ cells. This results in immunodeficiency of the infected person. AIDS is considered when the count of CD4+ are <200 cells/mm$^3$.

Current recommendation for treatment for highly active antiretroviral therapy (HAART) are: Two drugs from nucleoside reverse transcriptase inhibitors (NRTI) plus one drug from non-nucleoside reverse transcriptase inhibitors (NNRTI).

**Q. What is hydrosalpinx and how is it formed?**

**Ans.** It is the collection of watery secretion within the fallopian tube. It is the end result of mild endosalpingitis by pyogenic infection.

Pyogenic infection
⇩
Endosalpingitis
⇩
Inflammation of the fimbriae
⇩
Adhesion formation
⇩
Closure of abdominal ostium
⇩
Secretion (pus) is pent up
⇩
Distension of the tube markedly at the ampulla
(muscular isthmus is rigid and there is minimal distension).

**The distended tube is curled (as the mesosalpinx is fixed) and takes 'retort' shaped** (*see* Fig. 11.17). The pus (pyosalpinx) is gradually liquefied and settles down with clear fluid above (hydrosalpinx).

As the uterine ostium is not closed anatomically, there may be repeated infections. There is also intermittent passage of fluid into the uterine cavity and vagina. This is known as **intermittent hydrosalpinx or hydrops tubal profluens.**

**Q. What are the different causes of pelvic abscess?**

**Ans.** (a) Postabortal, puerperal sepsis
(b) Acute salpingitis
(c) Perforation of an infected uterus
(d) Irritant peritonitis (following HSG).

**Q. What are the different types of surgery for the management of a case with pelvic abscess?**

**Ans.** To start systemic antibiotics to cover both aerobic and anaerobic micro-organisms.

Abscess is to be drained thereafter by:
(a) Posterior colpotomy
(b) Laparotomy.

Pus should be sent from culture and antibiotic sensitivity.

**Q. How do you diagnose genital tuberculosis?**

**Ans.**
- **Clinical presentation** is similar to any other patient with tuberculosis.
- Important gynecological symptoms are:
  - Weakness, low-grade fever, anemia
  - Infertility (tubal blockage)
  - Menstrual abnormality (amenorrhea, dysmenorrhea)
  - Chronic pelvic pain.
- On examination:
  - Ascites may be present
  - Per vaginum—adnexal mass may be felt
- Investigations:
  - General investigation: Complete hemogram, Mantoux test, X-ray chest
  - Diagnostic uterine curettage: Endometrium is tested for:
    (a) Histopathological examination
    (b) Culture in Löwenstein-Jensen media
    (c) AFB—microscopy (Ziehl-Neelsen's stain)
    (d) PCR—for nucleic acid (DNA) amplification
  - Hysterosalpingography
  - Laparoscopic biopsy and/or aspiration of fluid for AFB culture.

**Q. What are the features of the tube on HSG when affected with tuberculosis?**

**Ans.** The following features on HSG are suggestive of tuberculosis. However, in a proved case of tuberculosis, HSG is contraindicated.
- Vascular or lymphatic extravasation of dye.
- Rigid (lead-pipe) tubes with nodulations at places.
- 'Tobacco pouch' appearance with blocked fimbrial end.
- Beaded appearance of the tube with variable filling density.

- Distal tube obstruction.
- Coiling of the tubes or calcified shadow at places.
- Bilateral cornual block.
- Tubal diverticula and/or fluffiness of tubal outline.
- Uterine cavity—irregular outline, honeycomb appearance or presence of uterine synechiae.

**Q. What are the indications of surgery in a woman with pelvic tuberculosis?**

**Ans.** (a) Patient not responding to antitubercular therapy
(b) Formation of tubercular pyosalpinx, abscess or pyometra
(c) Persistent chronic pelvic pain.

**Q. What is the result of treatment in terms of reproduction in a woman with genital tuberculosis?**

**Ans.** The prognosis is mostly unfavorable. Pregnancy is rare (5–10%). Abortion and ectopic pregnancy are common.

# Operative Gynecology

CHAPTER

15

## Chapter Objectives

**Operative gynecology:**

Core knowledge and understanding with:

- Surgical anatomy of abdomen and pelvis and pelvic floor muscles
- Outlines of common surgical procedures
- Case selection (indications of surgery) based on pathology
- Principles of homeostasis and hemostasis
- Postoperative care
- Surgical complications
- Follow-up procedures

**Gynecologic oncology:**

- **Basic knowledge of:** Principles of surgery, chemotherapy, radiotherapy and follow-up
- Advances in gynecologic surgery including laparoscopy, hysteroscopy, robotics

---

- ❖ 1. Dilatation and Curettage — 498
- ❖ 2. Dilatation of Cervix — 501
- ❖ 3. Dilatation and Insufflation (Rubin's Test) — 501
- ❖ 4. Hysterosalpingography — 502
- ❖ 5. Cervical Biopsy — 503
- ❖ 6. Thermal Cauterization of the Cervix — 504
- ❖ 7. Marsupialization of a Bartholin's Cyst — 504
- ❖ 8. Female Sterilization (Tubectomy) — 505
- ❖ 9. Amputation of Cervix — 507

- 10. Fothergill's Operation — 508
- 11. Operations on the Ovary — 509
- 12. Abdominal Hysterectomy — 509
- 13. Myomectomy — 516
- 14. Vaginal Hysterectomy — 519
- 15. Anterior Colporrhaphy — 523
- 16. Colpoperineorrhaphy — 523
- 17. Large Loop Excision of Transformation Zone — 525
- 18. Radical Hysterectomy — 526
- 19. Endoscopic Surgery in Gynecology — 528
  - Laparoscopy — 530
  - Hysteroscopy — 536
  - Laparoscopic Tubal Sterilization — 541
- 20. Robotics in Gynecology — 545

# 1. DILATATION AND CURETTAGE

### Indications

(A) *Diagnostic*:
  (i) Infertility
  (ii) Dysfunctional uterine bleeding (DUB)
  (iii) Endometrial tuberculosis
  (iv) Endometrial carcinoma
  (v) Postmenopausal bleeding.

(B) *Therapeutic*:
  (i) DUB
  (ii) Endometrial polyp
  (iii) Removal of IUCD.

### Instrument Trolley for Dilatation and Curettage Operation (Fig. 15.1)

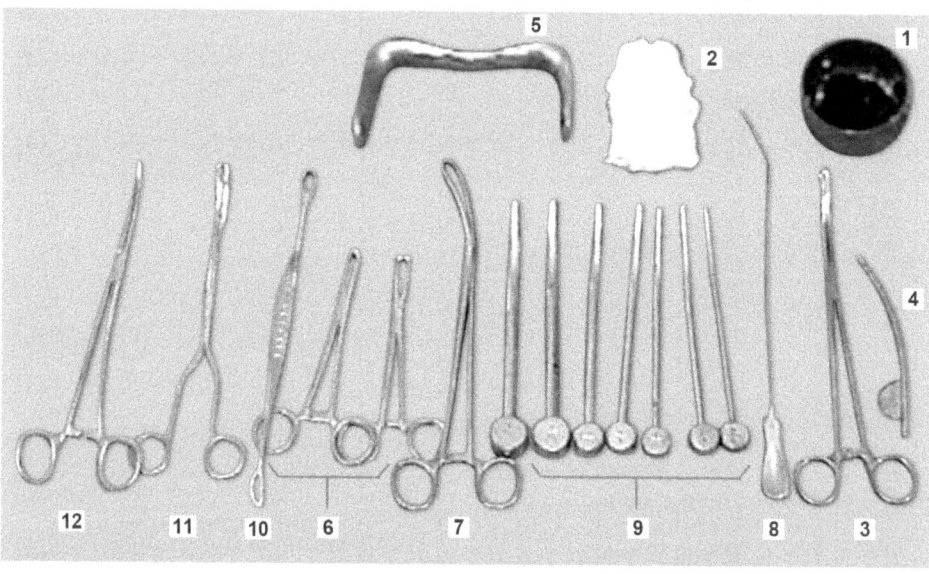

**Fig. 15.1:** (1) Bowl with antiseptic lotion (Povidine iodine), (2) Gauze pieces, (3) Sponge holding forceps, (4) Female metal catheter, (5) Sim's posterior vaginal speculum, (6) Allis tissue forceps, (7) Vulsellum, (8) Uterine sound, (9) Hawkin-Ambler dilators (different sizes), (10) Sharp and blunt curette, (11) Ovum forceps, and (12) Uterine dressing forceps.

### Steps of operation

Principal steps are mentioned here.
  (1) The woman is to empty her bladder (before coming to the operation theater).
  (2) General anesthesia or sedation is used.
  (3) Lithotomy position.
  (4) Antiseptic cleaning and draping.
  (5) Catheterization of the bladder (if not passed urine before coming to the theater) (Fig. 15.1, instrument—4)
  (6) Bimanual examination is done.
  (7) Posterior vaginal speculum (Sim's) is introduced (Fig. 15.1, instrument—5).

(8) Anterior lip of the cervix is held with an Allis tissue forceps or with a vulsellum. (Fig. 15.1, instrument—6/7).
(9) An uterine sound is introduced to confirm the position and the length of the uterine cavity (Fig. 15.1, instrument-8).
(10) Cervical canal is dilated with graduated dilators (Hegar's or Hawkin-Ambler's) (Fig. 15.3).
(11) After the desired dilatation, the uterine cavity is curetted by a uterine curette. Thorough but gentle curettage is usually done (Fig. 15.1, instrument—10).
(12) At the end, Allis tissue forceps and the speculum are withdrawn (Fig. 15.5).
(13) The curetted material is preserved in 10% formol saline or normal saline (in case of tuberculosis) and sent for histopathological or bacteriological examination (Fig. 15.6).

## Complications
*Immediate*:
 (i) Injury to the cervix
 (ii) Uterine perforation
(iii) Infection
(iv) Injury to the gut (following perforation)
 (v) Hemorrhage.

*Remote*:
 (i) Cervical incompetence
(ii) Uterine synechiae.

**Q.** *Pick up the instruments as in sequence to the steps of the operation.*
**Ans.** Instruments number and the names are as below:
 (a) No. 3: Sponge holding forceps
 (b) No. 4: Female metal catheter
 (c) No. 5: Sim's posterior vaginal speculum
 (d) No. 6: Allis tissue forceps or
 (e) No. 7: Multiple toothed vulsellum
 (f) No. 8: Uterine sound
 (g) No. 9: Cervical dilators (Hawkins ambler type)
 (h) No. 10: Sharp and blunt curette
 (i) No. 11: Ovum holding forceps
 (j) No. 12: Uterine dressing forceps.

## Important Figures of Dilatation and Curettage

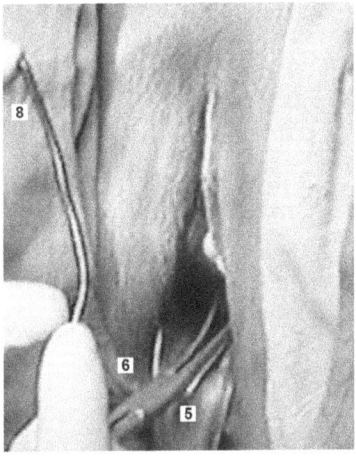

**Fig. 15.2:** Antiseptic cleaning and drapings; catheterization, bimanual examination—all done. Sim's posterior vaginal speculum is applied. Anterior lip of the cervix is grasped with an Allis tissue forceps. Uterine sound is passed and the uterocervical canal length is measured (see fingers).

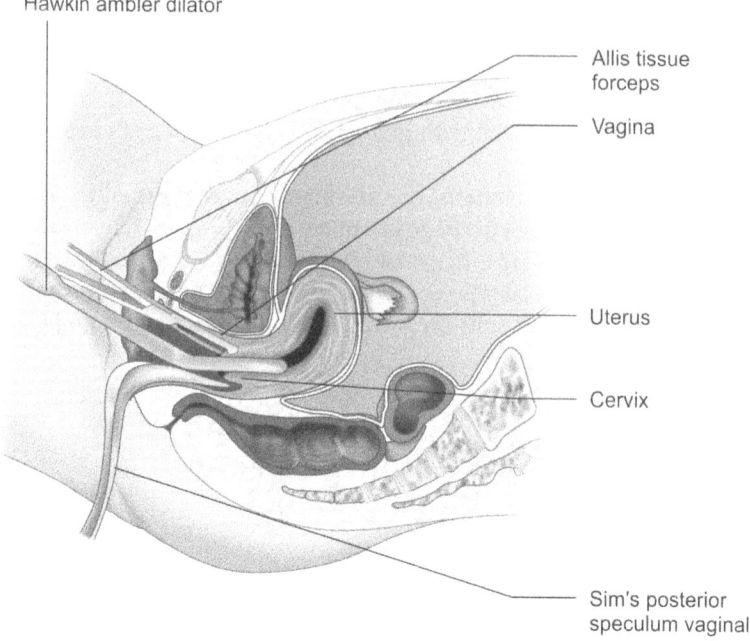

**Fig. 15.3:** Cervical canal is dilated with Hawkin-Ambler's dilator.

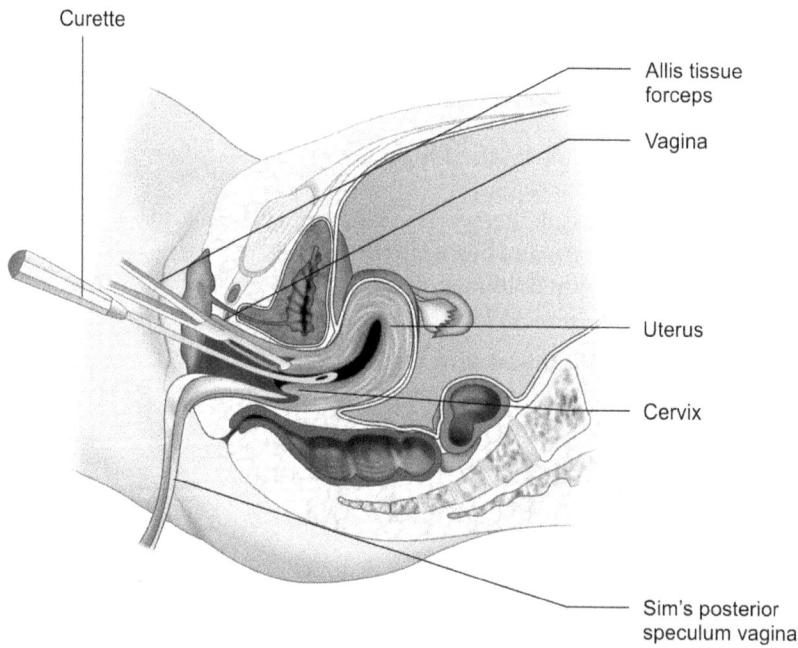

**Fig. 15.4:** Endometrium is being curetted. The curette is seen.

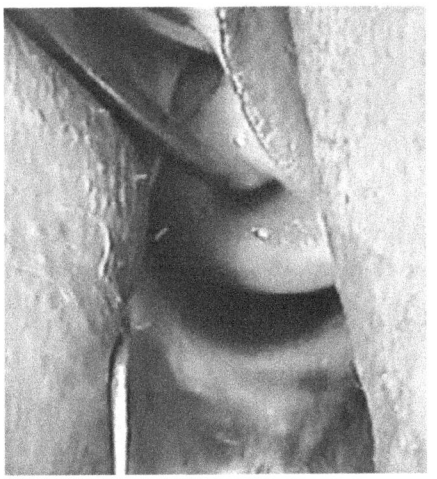

**Fig. 15.5:** End of the procedure. Cervix is seen without any bleeding.

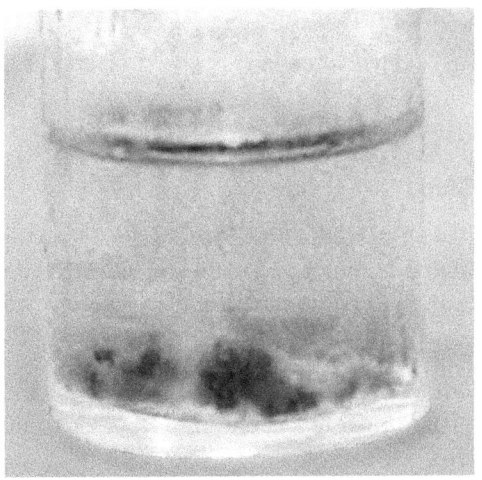

**Fig. 15.6:** Curetted endometrium is taken in a bottle dipped in formol saline. It is to be sent for histopathology examination.

## 2. DILATATION OF CERVIX

(a) Preliminaries: As mentioned in dilatation and curettage till point 8 on p. 499.
(b) Uterine sound is introduced to measure the uterocervical length. It acts as a first dilator.
(c) Dilatation of the cervical canal is thereafter done gradually by using cervical dilators (graduated) (see Figs. 16.8A and B).

**Indications**

(i) Prior to amputation of cervix
(ii) Prior to hysteroscopy
(iii) For drainage of pyometra or hematometra
(iv) Prior introduction of uterine curette, insertion of IUCD, laminaria tent or radium
(v) Spasmodic dysmenorrhea.

## 3. DILATATION AND INSUFFLATION (RUBIN'S TEST)

*Q. What are the indications of this procedure?*
**Ans. Indications:** To note the patency of the fallopian tubes in:
(i) Investigation of infertility
(ii) Following tuboplasty operation.

*Q. When is this test done?*
**Ans.** It is usually done between the 8th and 12th day of the cycle.

### Contraindications

(i) Pelvic infection
(ii) Vaginal bleeding
(iii) Pregnancy.

### Steps

Not commonly done these days. This is due to the availability of better alternative methods. Major part of the procedure is similar to D and C. Media used for insufflation is air or $CO_2$ into the uterine cavity.

### Complications

*Immediate:*
(i) Similar to faced during D + C operation
(ii) Air embolism
(iii) Rupture of the tube
(iv) Flaring up of the pre-existing pelvic infection.

*Remote:* Pelvic endometriosis.

## 4. HYSTEROSALPINGOGRAPHY

### Indications

- To note tubal patency in a case with infertility
- To detect uterine malformations
- To diagnose uterine synechiae
- Incidental diagnosis of uterine submucous fibroid or polyp or hydrosalpinx.

### Steps

**Important steps of the procedure:**
- Steps 1 to 7 as discussed in dilatation and curettage operation are the same except that this procedure is done in the radiology department and without anesthesia
- HSG cannula (Fig. 15.7), fitted with syringe containing the radio-opaque dye is pushed slowly inside the uterine cavity
- Two radiographic images are generally taken
  - The first one to show the filling of the uterine cavity
  - The second one after 10 to 12 minutes to show the tubal findings.
- Tubal patency is diagnosed by peritoneal spillage.

### Contraindications

(i) Presence of pelvic infection
(ii) Pregnancy
(iii) Vaginal bleeding.

### Complications

(i) Peritoneal irritation and pelvic pain
(ii) Vasovagal attack
(iii) Intravasation of dye
(iv) Flaring up of pelvic infection.

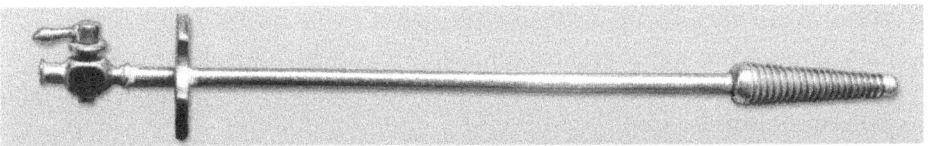

**Fig. 15.7:** Hysterosalpingography cannula (Leech Wilkinson variety).

## 5. CERVICAL BIOPSY

### Types
- Surface biopsy (cervical smear)
- Punch (Fig. 15.8)
- Wedge
- Ring
- Cone
- Four quadrant biopsy
- Colposcopy guided biopsy
- Large loop excision (LLETZ) and biopsy (*see* p. 525).

### Indications
(i) When the cervix appears suspicious clinically
(ii) When there is presence of any growth or ulcer on the cervix
(iii) Surface biopsy (smear) is done as a routine.

### Procedure for Individual Biopsy

### Cone biopsy (conization)
Cone-shaped tissue of the cervix including the squamocolumnar junction is removed.

### Indications
*Diagnostic:*
- Unsatisfactory colposcopic examination.
- Inconsistent findings: Colposcopy, cytology and directed biopsy.
- Endocervical curettage: Positive.
- When biopsy shows CIS or microinvasion to exclude invasive carcinoma.

*Therapeutic:*
- CIN
- CIS in a young woman

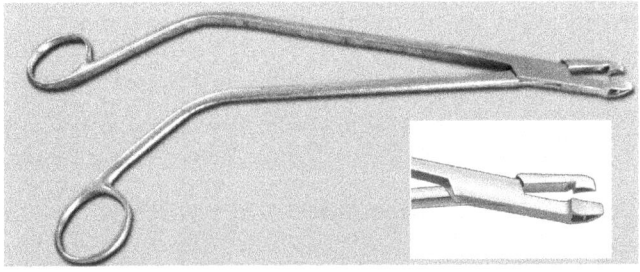

**Fig. 15.8:** Punch biopsy forceps.

- Invasive carcinoma (<1 mm stromal invasion)
- Carcinoma cervix stage 1a (in exceptional cases where childbearing is desired and where the patient is strongly motivated for long-term follow up. Surgical margins must be free of disease).

**Complications**

- Secondary hemorrhage
- Cervical stenosis
- Cervical incompetence
- Infertility
- Diminished cervical mucus
- Midtrimester abortion (recurrent) or preterm labor.

## 6. THERMAL CAUTERIZATION OF THE CERVIX

**Indications**

- Cervical ectopy (*see* p. 482)
- CIN—selected cases (to destroy tissues up to depth of 8–10 mm) (*see* p. 451).

**Procedures**

- Generally, the operation is done under general anesthesia.
    - Initial steps are the same as in D and C (*see* p. 499).
    - Cervical canal is dilated by one or two small dilators.
    - The whole of the eroded area is cauterized by radial strokes of the cautery (Fig. 15.9). The strokes are made at least 2 mm deep and at a distance of 1 cm.
    - The area is smeared with antibiotic ointment (metrogyl and povidone iodine or tri-sulpha cream).

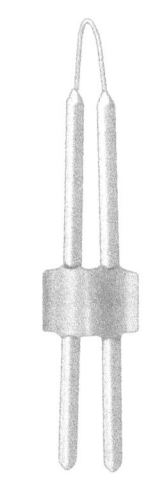

Fig. 15.9: Thermal cautery.

> *Q. How does the ectopy heal?*
> Ans. It takes 2–3 weeks for sloughing off the burnt area. Complete epithelialization by squamous epithelium occurs by 6–8 weeks.

> *Q. What advice is given to the patient on discharge?*
> There may be serosanguinous or even blood-stained discharge for 2–3 weeks till there is complete regrowth of epithelium. Rarely, there may be secondary hemorrhage when she needs to be admitted and treated.

## 7. MARSUPIALIZATION OF A BARTHOLIN'S CYST (FIG. 15.10)

It is commonly done under general anesthesia.

**Actual Steps**

Lithotomy position, antiseptic cleaning of the vulva, vagina and drapings are done. An incision is made on the inner side of the labium minus just outside the hymenal ring.

The cut margins are trimmed off to make an elliptical opening of about 1 cm in diameter. The pus is allowed to drain. The edges of the vaginal and the cyst walls are sutured by interrupted catgut stitches, thus leaving behind an opening for drainage.

> **Q. What are the advantages of marsupialization over the traditional incision and drainage?**
>
> **Ans.** (i) Simple procedure
> (ii) Can be done under local anesthesia
> (iii) Shorter hospital stay (24 hours)
> (iv) Postoperative complications are less
> (v) Gland function (lubricant) remains intact
> (vi) Risk of recurrence is minimal.

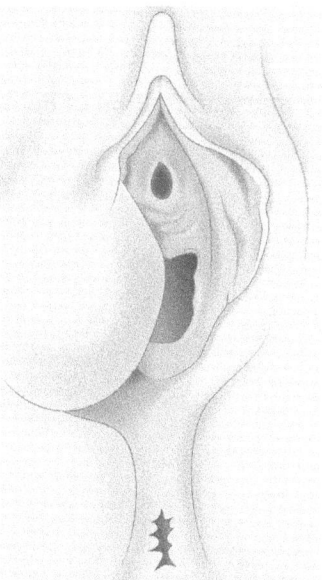

Fig. 15.10: Right-sided Bartholin's cyst.

## 8. FEMALE STERILIZATION (TUBECTOMY)

This operation can be done either by:
(a) Abdominal (common)
(b) Vaginal route.

**Abdominal route:** It may be by:
(a) Conventional—laparotomy
(b) Minilaparotomy (Mini-Lap) procedure
(c) Laparoscopic method (*see* p. 541).

**Time of operation:**
(a) **During puerperium**
(b) **Interval:** About 6–8 weeks following delivery or abortion
(c) **Concurrent** with MTP or cesarean section.

### Steps of Operation

**Anesthesia:** General or spinal or local.

**Site of skin incision: In puerperal cases:** Two fingers breadth (1″) below the fundus. **In interval cases,** 2 fingers breadth above the symphysis pubis. The incision may be transverse or midline. It is usually $1/2$″ to 1″ in length.

**Delivery of the tube:** The tube is hooked out with the index finger. The finger is passed along the posterior uterine surface then to the posterior leaf of the broad ligament to reach the tube. The tube is identified by the fimbrial end.

**Technique: In Pomeroy's method** (Figs. 15.10 to 15.15), a loop of the tube [at the level of the isthmus (mainly) and part of the ampulla] is held by an Allis tissue forceps. Both the limbs of the tube are then tied firmly together using No. 'O' chromic catgut. About 1–1.5 cm of the segment of the loop distal to the ligature is excised. The same procedure is repeated on the other side. The excised segment of the tube should be inspected and may be sent for histology.

It is a safe and effective procedure.

**Failure rate** is 0.1–0.5%.

### Important Figures of Female Sterilization (Tubectomy) (Figs. 15.11 to 15.15)

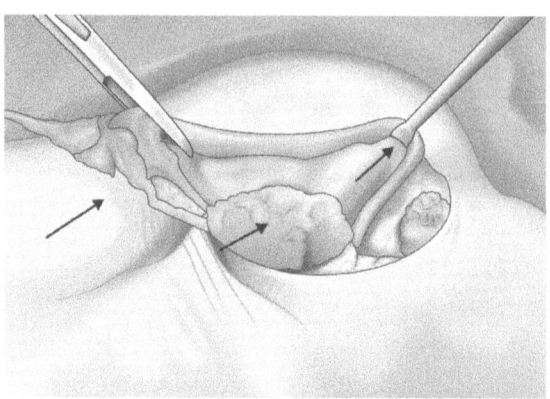

Fig. 15.11: Left tube is delivered through the incision margins. Fimbrial end is seen (arrow). Ovary is seen behind (arrow). The tube and the mesosalpinx are stretched out. A loop of the tube is made (arrow).

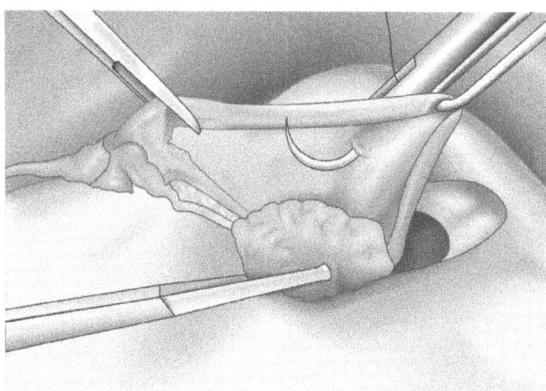

Fig. 15.12: The needle is passed through the avascular part of the mesosalpinx.

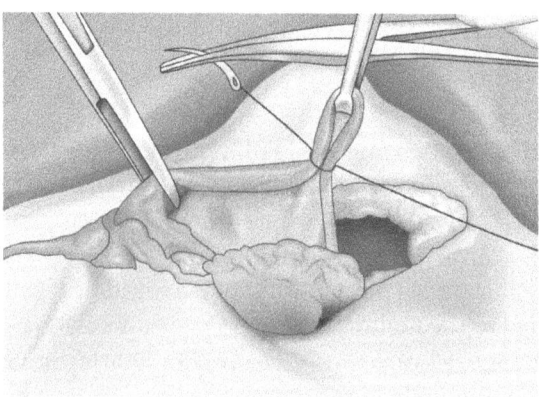

Fig. 15.13: Both the limbs of the loop are tied firmly together with chromic catgut. About 2 cm of the loop segment is seen distal to the ligature.

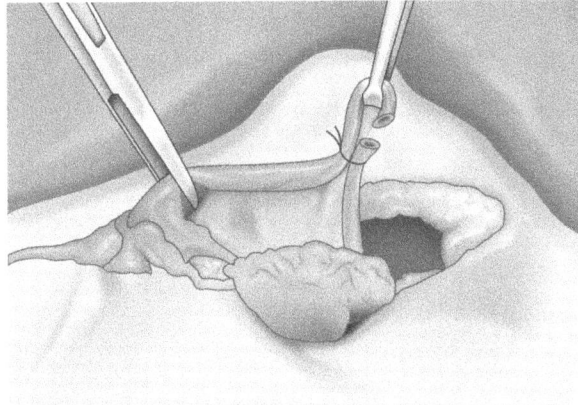

**Fig. 15.14:** About 1.5 cm of the loop distal to the ligature is excised.

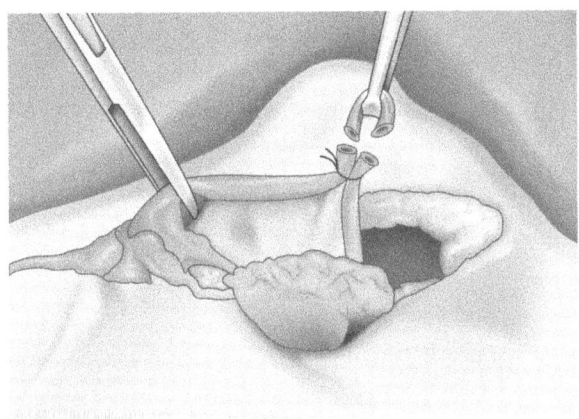

**Fig. 15.15:** The stump of the tubal ends are inspected to ensure that the tube is cut completely and there is no bleeding.

# 9. AMPUTATION OF CERVIX

### Indications

- Congenital elongation of cervix.
- As a component of Fothergill's operation (see below)
- Chronic hypertrophy and elongation of cervix.

### Principal steps

See Dutta Gyne 7/e, p. 489.

### Complications

***Immediate:*** ▪ Hemorrhage: Both primary and secondary.
▪ Sepsis.

*Remote:*
- Cervical stenosis leading to hematometra.
- Cervical incompetency leading to midtrimester (recurrent) miscarriage.
- During labor: Secondary cervical dystocia.

## 10. FOTHERGILL'S OPERATION

**Q. What are the composite steps of Fothergill's operation?**

**Ans.** (1) Preliminary dilatation and curettage

(2) Amputation of cervix

(3) Plication of Mackenrodt's ligament in front of the cervix

(4) Anterior colporrhaphy

(5) Colpoperineorrhaphy.

**Q. What is Sturmdorf suture?**

**Ans.** It is the procedure of covering the posterior lip of the amputated cervix by using the vaginal flap.

**Q. What is Fothergill's stitch?**

**Ans.** This stitch passes through the following tissues in sequence.

Vaginal skin at the level of the Fothergill's lateral point
⇩
Mackenrodt's ligament
⇩
Through the cervical tissue from outside inwards
⇩
Cervical tissue from inside outwards
⇩
Mackenrodt's ligament of the other side
⇩
Vaginal skin (Fothergill's lateral point) of the other side.
This stitch is used to make the uterus anteverted.

**Q. What are the complications of Fothergill's operation?**

**Ans.** (a) Hemorrhage primary and secondary

(b) Injury to the bladder and rectum

(c) Retention of urine cystitis

(d) Cervical stenosis

(e) Infertility

(f) Cervical incompetence

## 11. OPERATIONS ON THE OVARY

(a) **Oophorectomy:** Removal of healthy ovarian tissue (unilateral or bilateral).

(b) **Ovarian cystectomy:** Removal of the ovarian cyst (tumor) leaving behind the healthy ovarian tissue.

(c) **Ovariotomy:** Removal of the tumor along with healthy ovarian tissue. This is better termed as oophorectomy.

### Steps

(i) **Laterally:** Paired clamps are placed on the infundibulopelvic ligament.

(ii) **Medially:** Paired clamps are placed by the side of the uterus containing the fallopian tube and the ovarian ligament (salpingo-oophorectomy). If the tube is to be preserved, the clamp to be placed on the mesovarium lateral to the tube.

Pedicles are cut
⇩
In between the clamps
⇩
Ovarian tumor is removed
⇩
Clamps are replaced by transfixation sutures.

(c) **Wedge resection of the ovary:** A wedge of ovarian tissue is removed. It was done in the past in PCOS cases.

(e) **Laparoscopic ovarian drilling:** Done by monopolar or bipolar cautery or by laser, done in PCOS cases.

(f) **Ovarian biopsy:** Sometimes done for the problem of intersexuality.

## 12. ABDOMINAL HYSTERECTOMY

### Types

(A) **Total:** When the entire uterus (including the cervix) is removed.

(B) **Subtotal:** Removal of the body or corpus leaving behind the cervix.

(C) **Hysterectomy with bilateral salpingo-oophorectomy (pan-hysterectomy).**

(D) **Extended hysterectomy:** Type 'C' plus removal of the vaginal cuff.

(E) **Radical hysterectomy:** Removal of uterus, tubes, ovaries of both the sides, upper one-third of vagina, adjacent parametrium and the draining pelvic lymph nodes.

*Q. What are the common indications of abdominal hysterectomy?*

**Ans.** Common indications are:

(1) Fibroid uterus
(2) Abnormal uterine bleeding (AUB)
(3) Endometriosis

(4) Adenomyosis
(5) Carcinoma: (a) Endometrium, (b) Cervix, (c) Ovary.
(6) Obstetrics: Atonic PPH.

**Trolly with All the Instruments for Abdominal Hysterectomy Operation (Fig. 15.16)**

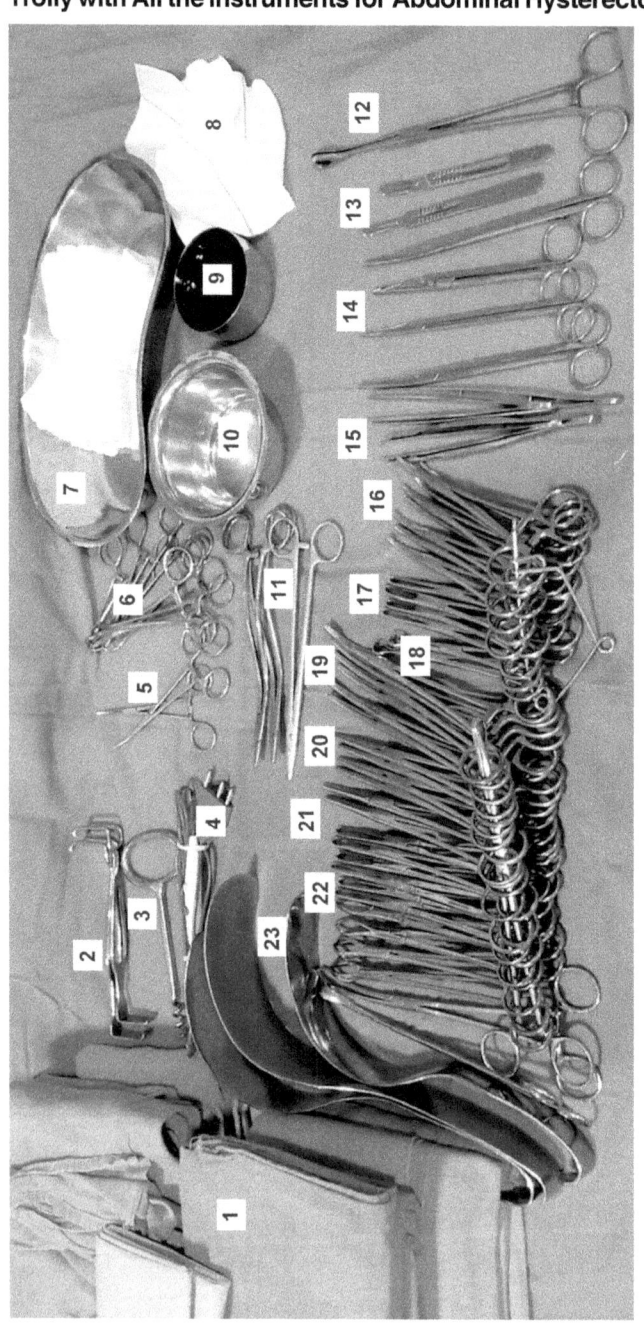

**Fig. 15.16:** Operation trolley for abdominal hysterectomy.

**Key:** (1) Large towels for drapings, (2) Skin retractors (Langenback's and Czerney's retractors), (3) Myoma screw, (4) Electrodiathermy set, (5) Hemostatic forceps, (6) Towel clips, (7) Kidney dish with large swabs (mops), (8) Gauze pieces (small), (9) Bowl containing povidone iodine, (10) Empty bowl, (11) Needle holders (straight and curved varieties), (12) Sponge holding forceps, (13) Knives (two), (14) Scissors (tissue cutting and dissecting-4), (15) Dissecting forceps (plane and toothed/short and long varieties), (16) Haemostatic forceps (straight and curved varieties), (17) Allis tissue forceps (short), (18) Babcock tissue forceps, (19) Clamps for hysterectomy (straight and curved varieties), (20) Allis tissue forceps (long), (21) Lens tissue forceps, (22) Multiple toothed vulsellum (2), and (23) Langenback's and Ezlery's retractors (different Sizes -3).

**Q. What are the steps of abdominal hysterectomy?**

**Ans** Abdomen is opened either by a low transverse incision (common) or by a infraumbilical paramedian or midline incision. The uterus is pulled up either by using a vulsellum or by placing long artery forceps one on either side at the cornu of the uterus. Clamps are placed on one side first. Similar steps are repeated on the other side.

**Q. What are the important sites for placing the clamps?**

**Ans** **If the ovaries are to be preserved: The first pair of clamps** (two long straight artery forceps) (Fig. 15.16) are placed at the cornu of the uterus to include:
 (a) Fallopian tube
 (b) Mesosalpinx containing utero-ovarian vessels
 (c) Ovarian ligament: Structures are cut in between the clamps → replaced by transfixation sutures (Fig. 15.18). Similar steps are done on the other side.

**When the ovaries are to be removed:**
 (i) **First pair of clamps** are placed in the infundibulopelvic ligament. The tissues in between are cut and replaced by transfixation sutures (Vicryl-0 or chromic catgut-1) (Fig. 15.19). Similar steps are done on the other side.
 (ii) **Second pair of clamps**→ on the round ligament → cut → replaced by transfixation sutures (Fig. 15.20).

 The loose peritoneum of the uterovesical pouch is incised and the bladder is pushed down. This minimizes the injury to the bladder (Figs. 15.21A and B).
 (iii) **Third pair of clamps** are placed on the parametrium containing ascending branch of uterine artery → cut → replaced by transfixation sutures (Fig. 15.22).
 (iv) **Fourth pair of clamps** are placed on the uterosacral ligaments → cut → replaced by transfixation sutures (Fig. 15.23).
 (v) **Fifth pair of clamps** are placed on the Mackenrodt's ligament containing the descending cervical artery → cut → transfixation sutures (Fig. 15.24).
 (vi) **The vault of the vagina** is opened→ the cervix is transected from vagina entirely (Fig. 15.25).

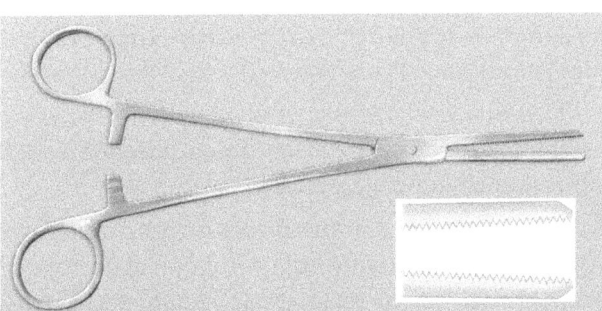

Fig. 15.17: Long straight hemostatic forceps (Spencer Wells).

(vii) **The lateral angles of the vagina** are closed by transfixation sutures (Fig. 15.26) and the vaginal vault is closed by interrupted sutures (Figs. 15.27A and B). Pelvic peritonization may be done.

(viii) Hemostasis is rechecked, counting done and satisfied, abdomen closed in layers.

**Q. What are the important complications of total abdominal hysterectomy?**

**Ans.** Complications are: (a) Immediate and (b) Remote

(a) ***Immediate:***

- **During operation:**
  - Hemorrhage (primary)
  - Injury (bladder, ureter and bowel)
  - Anesthetic hazards

- **Postoperative:**
  - Hemorrhage (secondary) and shock.
  - Urinary retention and cystitis
  - *Pyrexia* and *sepsis*

(b) ***Remote:*** Vault granuloma, vault prolapse, incisional hernia.

| Advantages of vaginal over abdominal hysterectomy | Advantages of abdominal over vaginal hysterectomy |
|---|---|
| (i) Less postoperative pain and less need of analgesia | (i) Thorough exploration of the abdominopelvic organs can be done |
| (ii) No abdominal incision and scar | (ii) Tubo-ovarian pathology (TO mass) can be managed simultaneously |
| (iii) Less postoperative morbidity and mortality | (iii) Associated ovarian tumor or larger uterus (fibroid) are best managed abdominally |
| (iv) Less hospital stay | (iv) Woman with associated pelvic adhesions or previous history of laparotomy are best managed by abdominal route |
| (v) Early resumption to work | (v) Indicated in cases where pelvic and abdominal (para-aortic) lymph nodes are to be palpated and sampled |
| (vi) Convenient in obese patients | |

**Q. What are the common complications of abdominal wound?**

**Ans.** Wound infection, discharge, wound dehiscence or burst abdomen.

**Q. What are wound dehiscence and burst abdomen? How are they managed?**

**Ans. Wound dehiscence:** When the separation of the layers of abdominal wound is up to the peritoneum—it is called as complete dehiscence.

If the intestines come out of the wound, it is called **evisceration or burst abdomen**. Burst abdomen usually occurs between 7 and 10 days of the operation.

**Predisposing factors** for burst abdomen are malnutrition, infection, cough due to chronic lung disease or abdominal distension.

**Management:** In the operation theater, under general anesthesia, necrotic tissues and clots are removed. The bowel is cleaned thoroughly with warm normal saline and placed back in the abdominal cavity. Through and through nylon (No. 2) sutures are passed 2 cm apart and about 3 cm from the skin margins to close the wound. Sutures are left in place for 3 weeks. Antibiotic (broad spectrum) is started and modified according to the culture and sensitivity report. Predisposing factors are to be taken care of.

## Important Figures of Abdominal Hysterectomy Operation (Figs. 15.18 to 15.27)

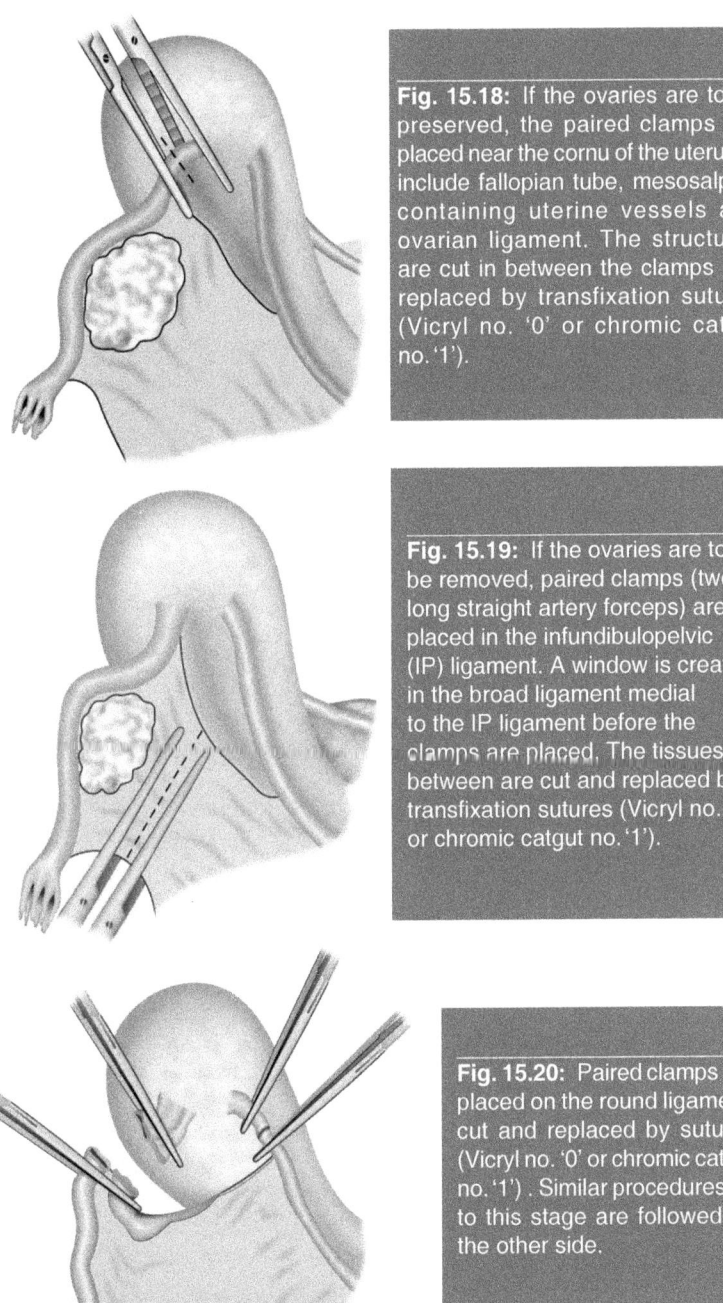

**Fig. 15.18:** If the ovaries are to be preserved, the paired clamps are placed near the cornu of the uterus to include fallopian tube, mesosalpinx containing uterine vessels and ovarian ligament. The structures are cut in between the clamps and replaced by transfixation sutures (Vicryl no. '0' or chromic catgut no. '1').

**Fig. 15.19:** If the ovaries are to be removed, paired clamps (two long straight artery forceps) are placed in the infundibulopelvic (IP) ligament. A window is created in the broad ligament medial to the IP ligament before the clamps are placed. The tissues in between are cut and replaced by transfixation sutures (Vicryl no. '0' or chromic catgut no. '1').

**Fig. 15.20:** Paired clamps are placed on the round ligament, cut and replaced by sutures (Vicryl no. '0' or chromic catgut no. '1'). Similar procedures up to this stage are followed on the other side.

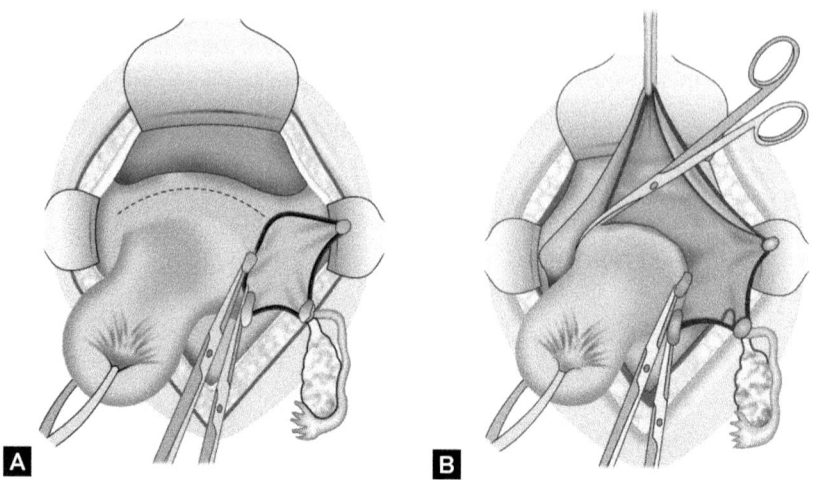

**Figs. 15.21A and B:** Loose peritoneum of the uterovesical fold is cut and extended from one divided round ligament to the other. The bladder is pushed down and out with gauze added with scissors stripping till the anterior vaginal wall is reached. This will minimize injury to the bladder and ureters in subsequent steps of operation.

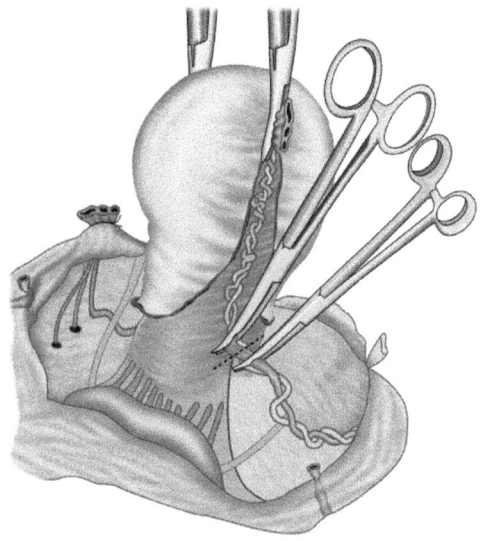

**Fig. 15.22:** Paired clamps are placed on the parametrium containing ascending branch of the uterine artery, close to the uterus at the level of internal os. The tissues in between are cut with the scalpel and replaced by ligature (Vicryl no. '0' or catgut no. '1'). Similar step is followed on the other side.

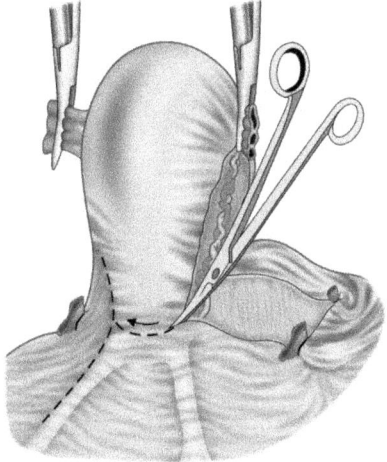

**Fig. 15.23:** The uterus is now pulled forwards to make the uterosacral ligaments prominent. Clamps are placed over the uterosacral ligaments as close to the cervix. The ligaments are cut. The peritoneum in between the ligaments is dissected down with scissors and finger. The clamps are replaced by sutures (same suture material).

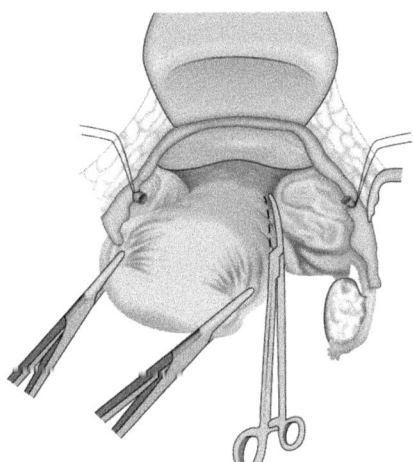

**Fig. 15.24:** Clamps are placed close to the cervix on the paracervical tissue (Mackenrodt's) containing descending cervical artery, cut and replaced by ligature (same suture material). Similar step is followed to the other side.

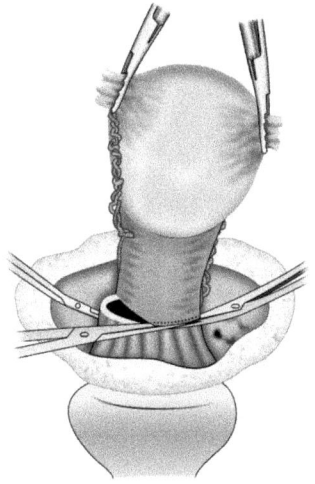

**Fig. 15.25:** Vault of the vagina is opened by a stab incision with a scalpel at the cervicovaginal junction. The remaining vault of the vagina is cut while traction is given with a single toothed vulsellum on the cervix.

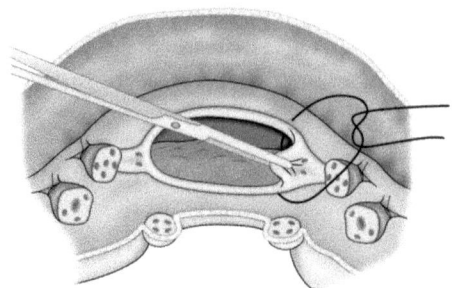

**Fig. 15.26:** The edges of the cut vaginal vault are grasped by Allis forceps. Lateral vaginal angles are closed by transfixation suture.

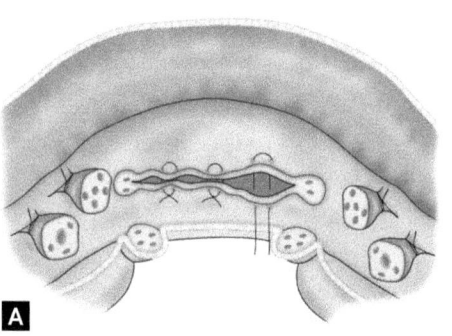
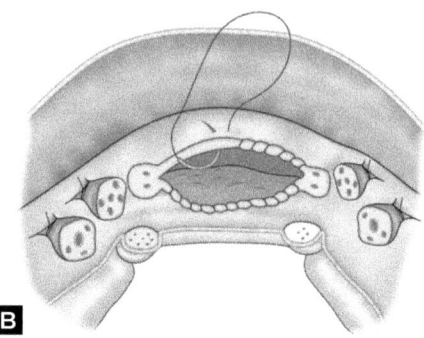

**Figs. 15.27A and B:** (A) Vault is closed by interrupted sutures; or (B) The free vaginal margin is reefed with a continuous locking suture.

## 13. MYOMECTOMY

**Q. What are the indications of myomectomy?**

**Ans.** (a) Persistent uterine bleeding in spite of medical therapy
(b) Excessive pain or pressure symptoms
(c) Rapidly growing myoma
(d) Infertility due to fibroid (Fig. 15.28).

**Q. Mention the contraindications of myomectomy?**

**Ans.** (a) Infected fibroid
(b) Suspected malignant change
(c) Growth of myoma during menopause.

**Q. What are the principal steps of myomectomy?**

**Ans.** (i) A single incision is made (preferably) in the midline on the anterior wall. It is deepened through the myometrium and through the capsule till the myoma is reached (Fig. 15.29).

(ii) The myoma is grasped with a single toothed vulsellum (Fig. 15.30) and the myoma is enucleated from its bed by sharp and blunt dissection (Fig. 15.31).

(iii) The myoma bed (deep space) is obliterated by interrupted mattress or figure of eight sutures. Sometimes layers of sutures (tier stitch) may be required to approximate the myometrium.

**Q. What are the complications of myomectomy?**

**Ans. (A)** *Immediate:*
   (a) Hemorrhage
   (b) Visceral injury (bladder, uterine tube)
   (c) Others (anesthetic complications).

**(B)** *Remote:*
   (a) Risk of recurrence of myoma (30-50%)
   (b) Persistence of menorrhagia (1-5%)
   (c) Risk of relaparotomy (20-25%).

**Q. How can you control hemorrhage during myomectomy?**

**Ans.** Measures to control blood loss during myomectomy are:
   (a) Preoperative treatment with GnRH analog.
   (b) Use of vasoactive agents: Injection vasopressin in the myometrium over the fibroids.
   (c) Use of tourniquets to occlude uterine vessels.
   (d) Use of Victor Bonney's clamp.

**Q. What are the long-term results of myomectomy in respect of recurrence and others?**

**Ans.** (a) Recurrence of myoma (30-50%)
   (b) Persistence of menorrhagia (1-5%)
   (c) Risk of relaparotomy (20-25%).

## Important Figures of Myomectomy (Figs. 15.28 to 15.31)

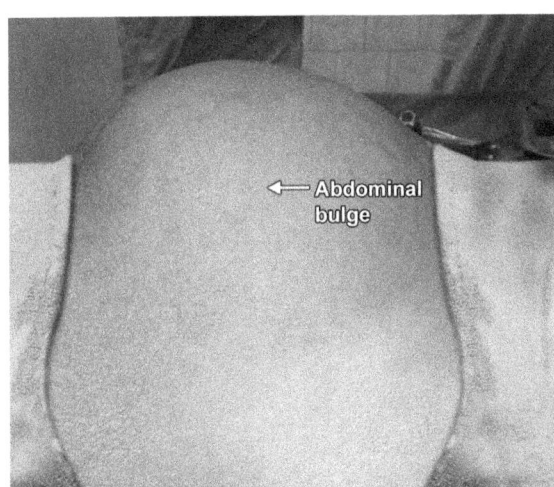

**Fig. 15.28:** Lateral view of a huge pelvic abdominal mass (fibroid uterus).

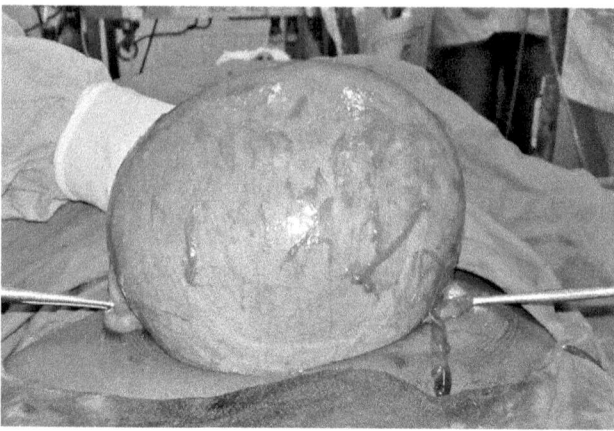

**Fig. 15.29:** The huge uterine mass (fibroid uterus) is delivered through the abdominal incision.

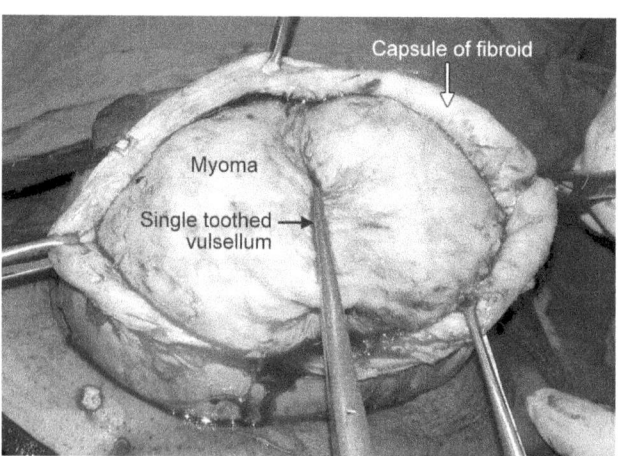

**Fig. 15.30:** A midline vertical incision is made. It is deepened to reach the myoma. The capsule of the fibroid is seen dissected out. Traction is given on the myoma with a single toothed vulsellum.

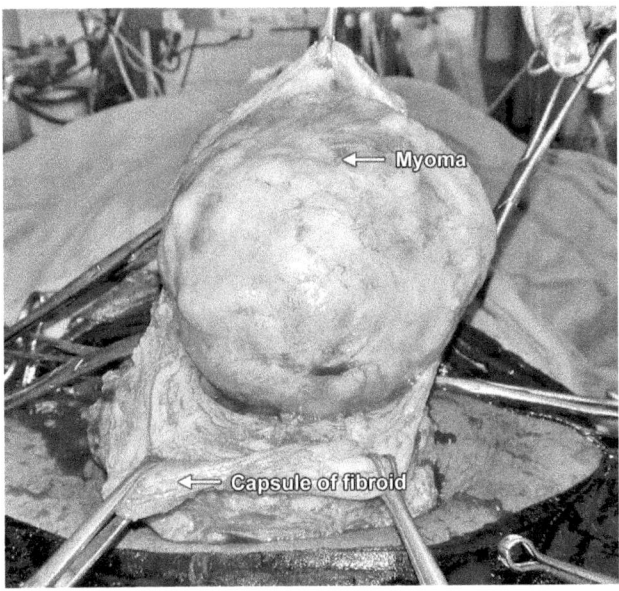

**Fig. 15.31:** The fibroid is enucleated from its bed by sharp and blunt dissection.

## 14. VAGINAL HYSTERECTOMY

**Preliminaries**

- Under general or epidural anesthesia, patient is placed in lithotomy position.
- Antiseptic cleaning and drapings are done.
- Bladder is evacuated by a metal catheter.
- Vaginal examination is done.
- Sim's posterior vaginal speculum is introduced. Anterior lip of the cervix is held and pulled down by a multiple toothed vulsellum (Fig. 15.32).
- A metal catheter is introduced to know the lower limit of the bladder.
- An inverted T-shaped incision is made on the anterior vaginal wall. The horizontal incision is made below the bladder and the vertical incision is made starting from the midpoint of the transverse incision up to a point about 1.5 cm below the external urethral meatus.
- The triangular vaginal flaps including the fascia on either sides are dissected off by knife and gauze dissection.
- The vesicocervical ligaments are dissected out and divided. The bladder is then pushed up by gauze covered finger till the peritoneum of the uterovesical pouch is visible.

**Actual steps**

- The U-V pouch peritoneum is cut open. Landon's retractor is introduced to push up the bladder (Fig. 15.33).

- The posterior vaginal wall is cut at the level of the cervicovaginal junction (Fig. 15.34A). The vaginal wall is dissected down till the pouch of Douglas (POD) is reached. The peritoneum of the POD is cut open (Fig. 15.34B).

- **First clamp** is now placed. This clamp includes: Uterosacral ligament, Mackenrodt's ligament and the descending cervical artery. The tissues are cut close to the cervix. The clamp is replaced by vicryl '0' or chromic catgut No. 1 suture. Similar steps are done on the other side (Fig. 15.35).

- **Second clamp** includes the uterine artery. Tissues are cut → clamp is replaced by ligature as above. Similar steps are repeagted on the other side (Fig. 15.36).

- The fundus of the uterus is brought out through the anterior pouch by a pair of Allis tissue forceps (Fig. 15.37).

- **Third clamp** includes round ligament, fallopian tube, mesosalpinx and the ligament of ovary. Structures are cut and replaced by ligature as above. Similar steps are repeated on the other side. The uterus is removed (Fig. 15.37).

- **The peritoneum** is closed by a pursestring suture (Fig. 15.38).

- The sutures of the pedicle containing the uterosacral, Mackenrodt ligaments are passed through the vaginal vault cross-wise and are held temporarily.

- Steps of anterior colporrhaphy are now followed.

- Redundant vaginal flaps are excised and the margins are approximated by interrupted sutures.

- **The cross-wise passed sutures** of the lowermost pedicles are now tied, thus fixing the ligaments with the vaginal vault.

- Colpoperineorrhaphy is done (described above).

- Vaginal packing may be done (see above).

- Self-retaining catheter is introduced.

**Q. What are the complications of vaginal hysterectomy and PFR?**

Ans.

| Operative | Postoperative | Late |
|---|---|---|
| Hemorrhage | Urinary retention | Vault prolapse |
| Trauma to bladder and rectum | VVF and RVF | Recurrence of primary, secondary prolapse |
| VVF, RVF | Hemorrhage | • Infection<br>• Pelvic abscess |

## Important Figures of Vaginal Hysterectomy (Figs. 15.32 to 15.38)

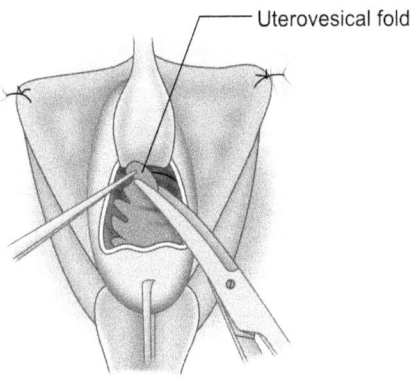

**Fig. 15.32:** Sims' posterior vaginal speculum is introduced and the anterior lip of the cervix is held by multiple toothed vulsellum and firmly brought down by assistant. The triangular vaginal flaps including the fascia on either sides are separated from the endopelvic fascia covering the bladder by knife and gauze dissection. The vesicocervical ligament is held up with Allis tissue or toothed dissecting forceps and divided. The bladder is then pushed up by gauze covered finger till the peritoneum of the uterovesical pouch is visible.

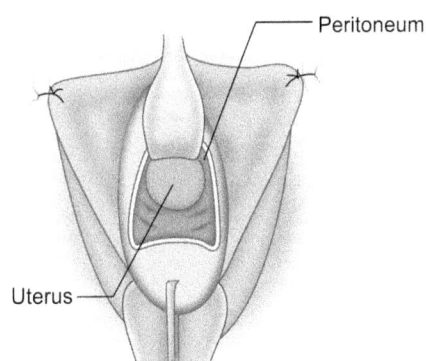

**Fig. 15.33:** The uterovesical peritoneum is cut open. Landon's retractor is introduced and to be held by an assistant.

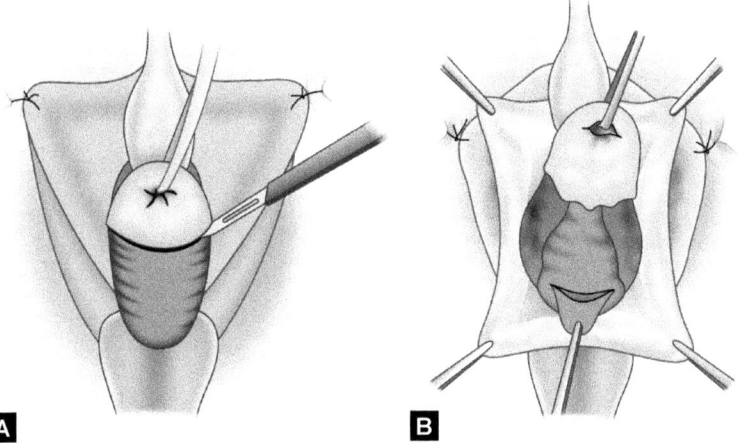

**Figs. 15.34A and B:** (A) The posterior vaginal wall along the cervicovaginal junction is cut; (B) The vaginal wall is dissected down till the pouch of Douglas is reached. The peritoneum is cut open.

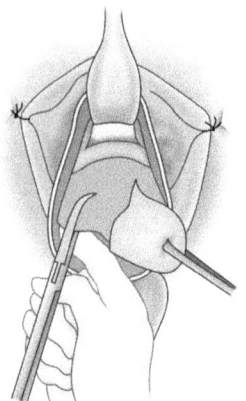

**Fig. 15.35:** First clamp is placed which includes uterosacral ligament, Mackenrodt's ligament and descending cervical artery. The tissues are cut as close to the cervix and replaced by Vicryl No. 1. Similar procedures are followed on the other side.

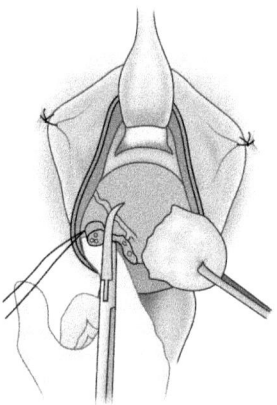

**Fig. 15.36:** Second clamp includes uterine artery and base of the broad ligament. The structures are cut as close to the uterus and replaced by ligature (Vicryl No. 1). Same procedures are followed on the other side.

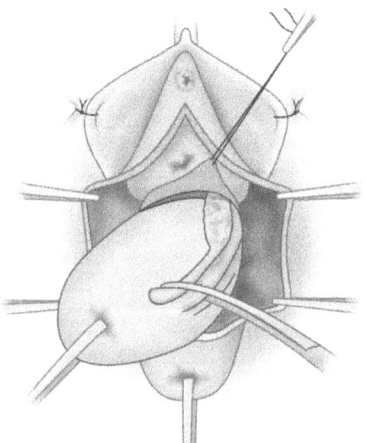

**Fig. 15.37:** The fundus is now brought out through the anterior pouch by a pair of Allis tissue forceps. The third clamp includes round ligament, fallopian tube, mesosalpinx and ligament of the ovary. The structures are cut and replaced by transfixing suture (Vicryl No. 1). Same procedures are carried out on the other side. The uterus is removed.

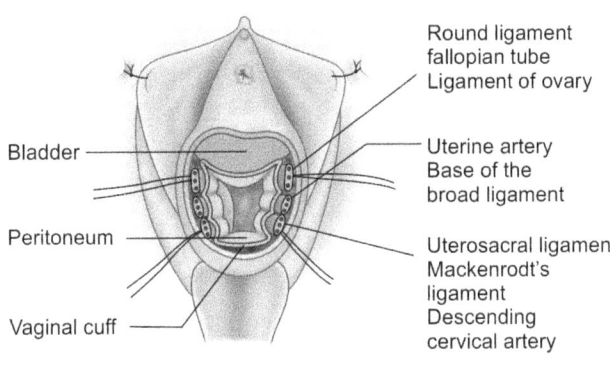

**Fig. 15.38:** Peritoneum is closed by a purse-string suture.

## 15. ANTERIOR COLPORRHAPHY

### Indications

Repair of:
 (i) Cystocele
 (ii) Urethrocele and as a part
 (iii) Vaginal hysterectomy and repair of pelvic floor (PFR).

### Preliminaries

Preliminaries are the same as in vaginal hysterectomy.

### Important steps

- To proceed the steps as that of vaginal hysterectomy, up to pushing up the bladder and to see the peritoneum of the uterovesical (U-V) pouch (*see* p. 519).
- The pubocervical fascia is plicated by interrupted sutures with No. '0'. Chromic catgut using atraumatic needle.
- The redundant portion of the vaginal mucosa is excised on either side.
- The cut margins of the vagina are apposed by interrupted sutures with No. '0' Chromic catgut using atraumatic needle.
- The metal catheter is introduced once again to be sure that bladder is not injured.
- Cleaning of the vagina is done.
- Vagina may be packed with a roller gauze smeared with antiseptic cream.
- A self-retaining catheter is introduced.

## 16. COLPOPERINEORRHAPHY

### Indications

Repair of:
 (i) Relaxed perineum
 (ii) Rectocele
 (iii) Enterocele and as a part in the operation
 (iv) Vaginal hysterectomy and repair of pelvic floor (PFR).

## Preliminaries

Preliminaries are the same as in vaginal hysterectomy (*see* p. 519).

## Principal steps

- A pair of Allis tissue forceps are placed one on each side at the lower end of the labium minus and a third of Allis forceps is placed on the posterior vaginal wall in the midline well above the rectocele bulge (Fig. 15.39).
- A horizontal incision is made on the mucocutaneous junction joining the two Allis tissue forceps below.
- Through the midpoint of this incision, another vertical incision is made up to the third Allis tissue forceps of the apex.
- Two triangular vaginal flaps are dissected off laterally from the perineal body and the rectum. The rectum and the levator ani muscles are exposed (Fig. 15.40).
- The redundant vaginal flaps are excised.
- The rectocele is corrected by suturing the pararectal fascia.
- Two or three interrupted sutures are passed through the levator ani using No. '1' chromic catgut. The knots are to be made at a later stage.
- The cut margins of the posterior vaginal walls are approximated starting from the apex. No. '0' chromic catgut stitches are used. When the sutures reach the perineal body, the knots for the sutures of the levator ani muscles are placed.
- The rest of posterior vaginal wall and the skin margins are apposed using interrupted sutures.
- Cleaning of the vagina is done.
- Vaginal pack, soaked with antiseptic lotion (betadine) may be used.

## Important Figures of Colpoperineorrhaphy (Figs. 15.39 and 15.40)

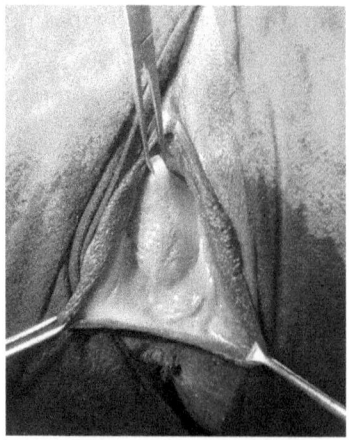

Fig. 15.39: Allis tissue forceps are placed on the posterior vaginal wall. The midline bulge of the rectocele is seen.

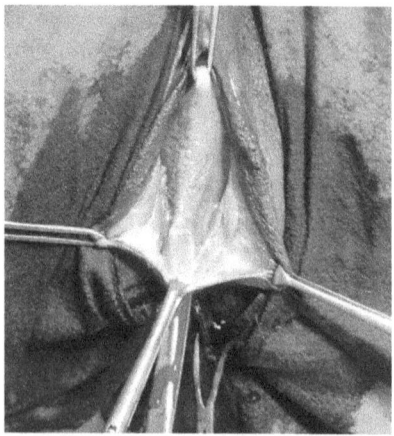

Fig. 15.40: The posterior vaginal wall is dissected off from the perineal body and the rectum to expose the levator ani muscles.

## 17. LARGE LOOP EXCISION OF TRANSFORMATION ZONE

**Q. What is LLETZ?**

Ans. Large loop excision of transformation zone (LLETZ) is a simple procedure with minimal complications. A thin stainless steel wire is used (Fig. 15.41) for excision of the TZ. Tissue up to 10 mm thick can be removed with the procedure.

**Q. What are the advantages of LLETZ?**

Ans. Abnormal area of the cervix could be removed with LLETZ and the excised tissue material could be sent for histology (Fig. 15.42).

**Q. How this LLETZ works?**

Ans. LLETZ works on tissue effects of electricity. Tissue cutting and coagulation effects are present (blended) at the same time. Sometimes, a rollerball is used for electrocoagulation of the bleeding sites.

**Q. What are the complications of LLETZ procedure?**

Ans. Complications are less. Bleeding, infection and vaginal discharge are common. Increased risks of preterm labor has been mentioned.

**Q. What are the contraindications of LLETZ?**

Ans. (a) Evidence of microinvasive or invasive disease on cytology, colposcopy or biopsy.

(b) Lesion is not seen entirely.

(c) Endocervical glandular involvement on endocervical curettage.

**Important Figures of LLETZ**

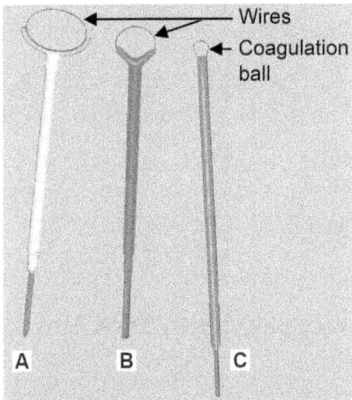

Fig. 15.41: Loops for LLETZ procedure.
Loops (A & B) for tissue excision and (C) Ball electrode: It is used to coagulate the bleeding points following the excision (LLETZ) procedure.

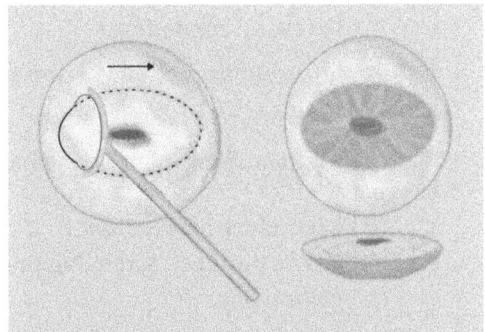

Fig. 15.42: Procedure of loop excision. The entire abnormal area on the cervix is removed by a single pass. Tissue excised, is to be sent for histology examination.

# 18. RADICAL HYSTERECTOMY

**Q. What are the tissues removed in radical hysterectomy?**

**Ans.** (i) Uterus and cervix

(ii) The tubes and the ovaries (may be preserved in a young woman)

(iii) Wide parametrial tissues

(iv) Superior vesical artery

(v) Cardinal and uterosacral ligaments

(vi) Upper three-fourth of vagina

(vii) Pelvic lymph nodes (external, internal, common iliac and obturator nodes)

(viii) Para-aortic lymph node sampling is done if found enlarged.

**Q. What are the complications of radical hysterectomy?**

**Ans.** Complications:

(a) As observed following abdominal hysterectomy (*see* p. 512)

(b) Ureteric fistula

(c) Vesicovaginal fistula

(d) Urinary tract infection

(e) Bladder dysfunction

(f) Lymphocyst formation.

**Q. Preventive measures for carcinoma cervix—primary and secondary prevention.**

**Ans.** **(A) Primary prevention:**

(a) Prophylactic HPV vaccination

(b) Use of condom

(c) Avoiding multiple partners

(d) Removal of cervix during hysterectomy

(e) Identifying 'high risk' female and males.

**(B) Secondary prevention**

Cervical cancer, screening procedures (cytology), HPV-DNA, VIA and colposcopy.

**Q. What is the role of human papillomavirus (HPV) in cancer cervix?**

**Ans.** Infection with high oncogenic risk types of HPV (Types 16, 18, 31, 33, 35, 45, 56) is mainly responsible for cervical cancer. Over 99% of patients with CIN and invasive cancer are found to be positive with HPV-DNA.

**Q. What is the pathogenesis of HPV infection in cancer cervix?**

**Ans.**

High-risk HPV (Types 16, 18, 31, 33) infection of cervical epithelium
⇩
Expression of E6 and E7 oncoproteins
⇩
HPV-induced neoplastic transformation of cervical epithelium
⇩
CIN
⇩
Invasive cancer.

**Q. Causes of death in carcinoma cervix.**

**Ans.** Patients of cancer cervix die of complications when left untreated:

(a) Uremia due to ureteric obstruction

(b) Sepsis

(c) Cachexia

(d) Metastasis (lung and lymph nodes).

**Q. Differential diagnosis of carcinoma cervix.**

**Ans.** Cervical tuberculosis, fibroid polyp, syphilitic ulcer, products of conception in incomplete abortion.

# 19. ENDOSCOPIC SURGERY IN GYNECOLOGY

**Synonym: Minimally Invasive Surgery (MIS)**

Introduction of endoscopic surgery (laparoscopy and hysteroscopy) has mostly replaced the traditional laparotomy in gynecology these days. It is possible to visualize the abdominal cavity with laparoscopy and the uterine cavity by doing hysteroscopy. Laparoscopy and hysteroscopy can be done both for the purpose of diagnosis as well as for surgical procedures.

**Q. Discuss briefly the pneumoperitoneum:**

**Ans:** Pneumoperitoneum is created with a especially designed needle called Veress needle. It is introduced into the peritoneal cavity making a small incision (1.25 cm) below the umbilicus. Abdomen is inflated with about 1–4 L of carbon dioxide gas. Intraperitoneal pressure should not increase >20 mm Hg.

**Q. Why $CO_2$ is preferred for the creation of pneumoperitoneum?**

**Ans:** (a) $CO_2$ is a gas soluble in blood and is rapidly absorbed

(b) Risk of embolism is less

(c) It does not support combustion when electrodiathermy is used inside.

**Q. How the correct placement of Veress needle is ascertained?**

**Ans:** Different methods are there to ascertain the correct placement of the needle:

(a) Hanging drop method.

(b) Syringe barrel test: Aspiration is done to exclude inadvertent injury to any organ (e.g. blood from vessel puncture, urine from bladder puncture and fecal matter from bowel puncture).

(c) Low intra-abdominal pressure (<10 mm Hg) on correct placement of the needle.

(d) Obliteration of liver dullness on percussion when there is free flow of $CO_2$ inside the abdominal cavity.

**Q. What are the different methods of hemostasis used during laparoscopic surgery?**

**Ans.** (1) Electrocoagulation:

    (a) Monopolar electrosurgery

    (b) Bipolar electrosurgery.

(2) Laser coagulation (using $CO_2$, KTP-532 a Nd-YAG lasers)

(3) Ligasure—to cut and seal blood vessels

(4) Enseal vessels fusion where tissues are desiccated and cut

(5) Mechanical clips and staples (titanium clips and staples)

(6) Sutures as used in open surgery.

**Q. What are the complications of laparoscopic surgery?**

**Ans:** Complications may be specific to laparoscopic surgery.

These are:

(a) Extraperitoneal insufflations leading to surgical emphysema.

(b) Cardiac arrhythmias due to $CO_2$ absorption.

(c) Injury to blood vessels (mesenteric, inferior epigastric vessels).

(d) Injury to viscera: Bowel, bladder.

(e) Complications due to electrosurgical methods: Thermal injury to bowel, bladder and ureter.

(f) Other complications are: Due to anesthesia, infections, hemorrhage, etc.

**Q. What are the contraindications of laparoscopy?**

**Ans.** (a) Severe cardiopulmonary disease

(b) Patient hemodynamically unstable

(c) Extensive peritoneal adhesions

(d) Generalized peritonitis.

**Q. What is hysteroscopy?**

**Ans.** Endoscopic visualization of the cervical canal as well as the uterine cavity, is known as hysteroscopy. Hysteroscopy may be done for diagnostic as well as therapeutic purposes.

**Q. What is the distension media used in hysteroscopy?**

**Ans.** (a) $CO_2$

(b) Normal saline

(c) Glycine (1.5%)

(d) Mannitol (5%).

**Q. What are the contraindications of hysteroscopy?**

**Ans.** (a) Pelvic infection

(b) Pregnancy

(c) Cervical cancer

(d) Cardiopulmonary disorders.

# LAPAROSCOPY

It is the visualization of peritoneal cavity using a telescope with cold light and fiber optics. Abdominal cavity is distended using a gas ($CO_2$ is commonly used). Diagnostic laparoscopy does not need much of instruments and electrosurgical energy source. Imaging system includes a telescope (Fig. 15.43A), light source, fiberoptic cord, camera units and monitors.

**Laparoscopic surgical procedures** need basic instruments (graspers, scissors, aspirator, irrigator, morcellator, uterine manipulator and electrosurgical energy sources) and the imaging system (Figs. 15.43A to C).

## Advantages of Laparoscopy Over Laparotomy

- No large abdominal incisions
- Less blood loss
- Rapid postoperative recovery
- Less postoperative pain and reduced need of postoperative analgesia
- Shorter hospital stay and reduced concomitant cost
- Quicker resumption of day-to-day activity
- Less adhesion formation
- Minimal abdominal scars (cosmetic value)
- Reduced risk of incisional hernia
- Increased patient satisfaction.

## Indications of Laparoscopy

### A. Diagnostic Laparoscopy

- Infertility work up (chromopertubation)
- Chronic/acute pelvic pain (adhesions and endometriosis)
- Pelvic mass: Fibroid and ovarian cyst
- Ectopic pregnancy
- Amenorrhea
- Suspected Müllerian abnormalities.

### B. Operative Laparoscopy

- Tubal sterilization
- Ovarian surgery (cystectomy/biopsy)
- Ectopic pregnancy (salpingostomy)
- Hysterectomy
- Adhesiolysis
- Endometriosis
- Myomectomy
- Retroperitoneal lymphadenectomy

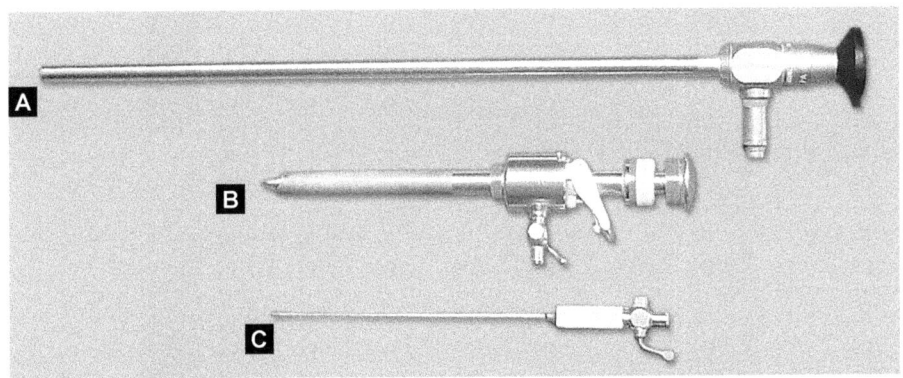

**Figs. 15.43A to C:** Laparoscopic instruments: (A)Telescope; (B) Trocar and cannula; and (C) Veress needle.

## Complications of Laparoscopy

Complications may be at different levels:

(A) ♦ **Veress needle** (Fig. 15.43C): Injury to bowel, blood vessels, bladder and surgical emphysema.

♦ **Trocar and cannula** (Fig. 15.43B): Same as above.

♦ **Electrosurgical complications:** Thermal injury.

♦ **Pneumoperitoneum:** Gas ($CO_2$) embolism and arrhythmia.

(B) ♦ **Anesthetic complications:**

♦ Hypercarbia, acidosis and basal lung atelectasis.

(C) ♦ **Common to any surgery:**

- Hemorrhage
- Infection
- Postsite hernia.

## Laparoscopic View of Pelvic Organs in Health and Disease

**Q.** *What are the structures attached at the cornu of the uterus?*

**Ans.** From anterior to posterior, structures are:

(a) Round ligament (*arrow in* Figure 15.44) in front
(b) Fallopian tube (*middle*)
(c) Ligament of ovary (*posteriorly*).

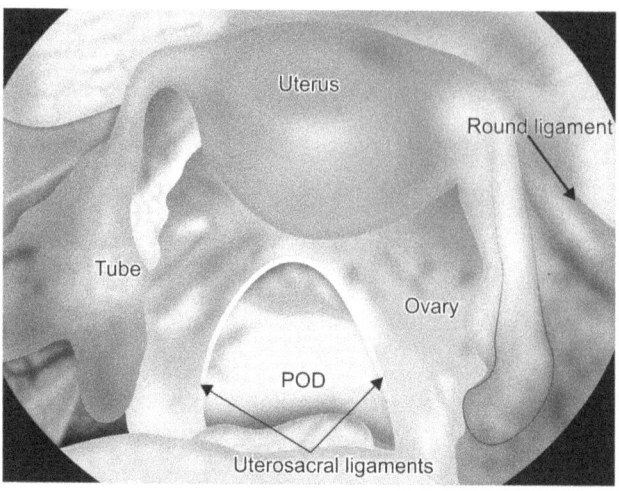

**Fig. 15.44:** Laparoscopic view of normal pelvis showing uterus, tubes, ovaries, round ligament (right), uterosacral ligaments and the pouch of Douglas.

**Q. What is the best method to diagnose pelvic endometriosis?**

**Ans.** Double puncture laparoscopy is considered the 'gold standard' for the diagnosis of pelvic endometriosis.

**Benefits of laparoscopy are:**

(a) Confirmation of diagnosis

(b) Staging the disease

(c) Biopsy if needed

(d) Treatment at the same time.

**Q. What is the classic appearance of endometriotic lesions on laparoscopy?**

**Ans.** Lesions may appear

(a) Black dots—powder burns

(b) Red—flame-shaped areas

(c) Red—polypoid areas

(d) Yellow—brown patches

(e) White—peritoneal areas

(f) Circular—peritoneal defects

(g) Ovarian endometriomas—chocolate cysts (Fig. 15.45)

(h) Pelvic adhesions (Fig. 15.45).

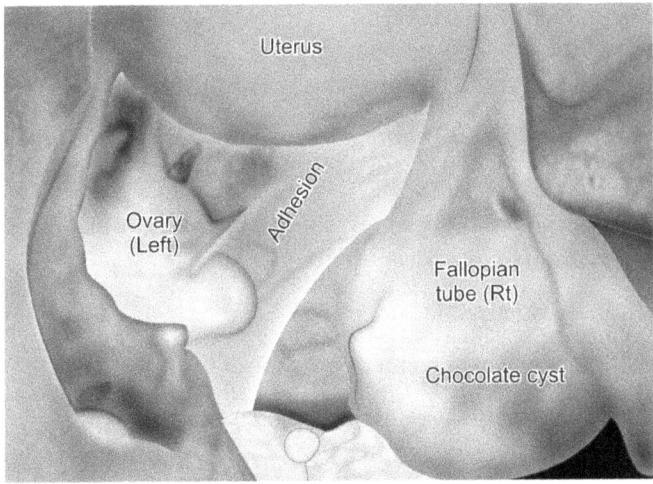

**Fig. 15.45:** Laparoscopic view of pelvic endometriosis. Right-sided chocolate cyst with enlarged ovaries. There are adhesions in the POD and the left ovary.

***Q. How laparoscopy could be helpful in the diagnosis and management of unruptured tubal ectopic pregnancy?***

**Ans.** Women in reproductive age with features suggestive of ectopic pregnancy (delayed period, lower abdominal pain, lower level of β-hCG value and empty uterine cavity on transvaginal sonography) should have the benefit of laparoscopy (Fig. 15.46).

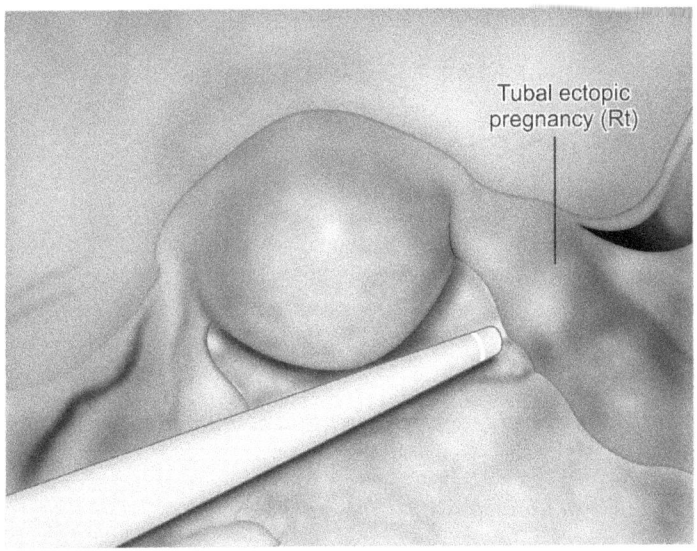

**Fig. 15.46:** Laparoscopic view of uterus, both the tube and ovaries showing right-sided unruptured tubal ectopic pregnancy.

**Advantages are:**
(a) Confirmation of diagnosis
(b) Treatment could be done at the same time.

**Q. What are the different management options for unruptured tubal ectopic pregnancy?**

**Ans.** (A) Expectant management: Only observation hoping spontaneous resolution.

(B) Conservative management:

(i) Medical management (methotrexate and KCl)

(ii) Surgical management (salpingostomy).

(C) Salpingectomy.

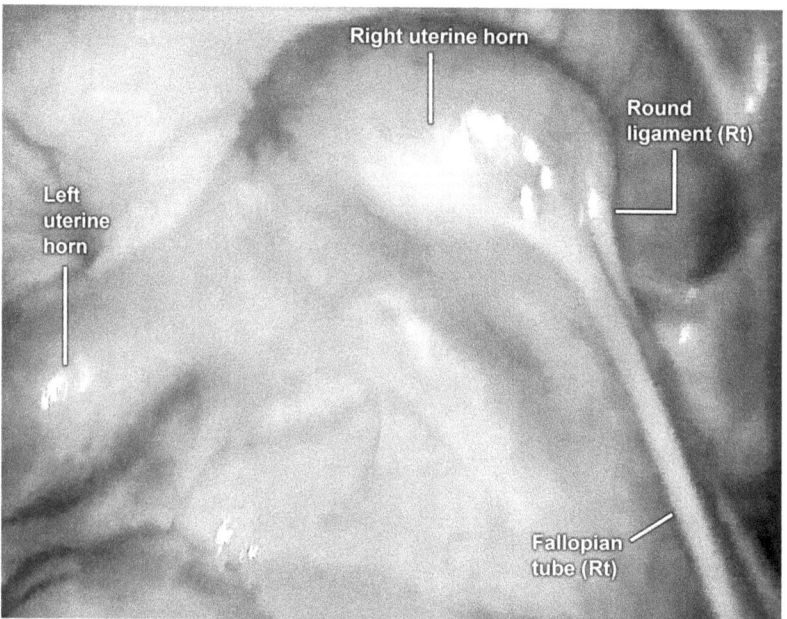

**Fig. 15.47:** Laparoscopic view of a bicornuate uterus. Both the horns are seen. Left-sided horn is seen smaller compared to the right one. Patient suffered recurrent fetal loss (P0+3+4+0)

**Q. What is the risk of recurrence of tubal ectopic in subsequent pregnancy?**
**Ans.** About 10–12%.

**Q. What type of abnormality is this one?**

**Ans.** It is the maldevelopment of the uterus (Fig. 15.47). It is due to failure of fusion of two Müllerian ducts. According to American Fertility Society (AFS) classification of Müllerian anomalies, it belongs to class IV.

**Q. What is the clinical presentation of a woman with this abnormality?**

**Ans.** The woman may not have any symptoms. But in some, clinical presentation may be with gynecological and/or obstetrical symptoms.

(A) **Gynecological**
- Dysmenorrhea
- Menstrual disorders—menorrhagia
- Infertility.

(B) **Obstetrical**
- Miscarriage (recurrent)
- Cornual pregnancy
- Preterm labor
- Malpresentation
- Intrauterine growth restriction (IUGR) and intrauterine fetal death (IUFD).

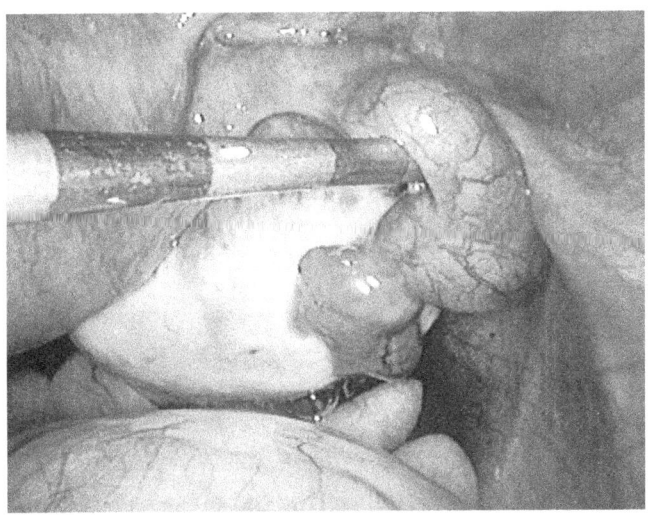

**Fig. 15.48:** Laparoscopic chromopertubation. Methylene blue dye is seen to come out of the abdominal ostium of the right fallopian tube.

**Q. What are the advantages of laparoscopic chromopertubation over hysterosalpingography?**

**Ans.** *See* SAQ 3 on p. 382 (Figs. 15.48 and 15.49).

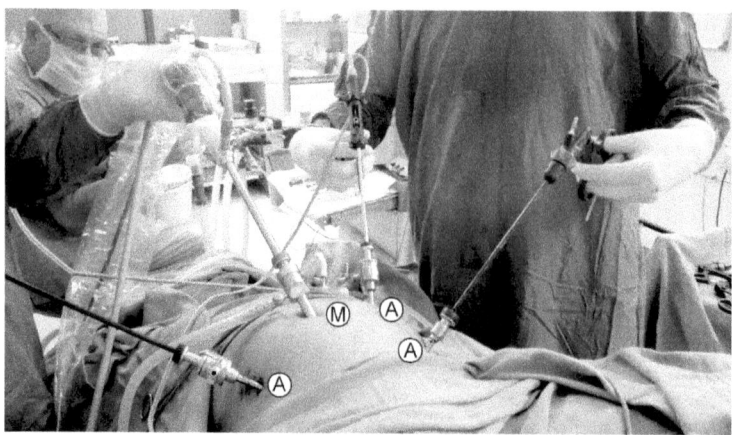

**Fig. 15.49:** Operative laparoscopic procedure in progress. Optimal placement of ports shown. Ipsilateral surgical procedures done. The ports are shown; M: Umbilical port or the main port for the telescope, A: Accessory ports.

## HYSTEROSCOPY

Hysteroscopy is a procedure that allows visualization of the endocervical canal and the uterine cavity. It is used both for the purpose of diagnosis and therapy.

**Basic instruments and equipment for hysteroscopy are (Figs. 15.50 to 15.52):**

(a) Telescope (Fig. 15.50)

(b) Distending media (gas $CO_2$ or liquid media—normal saline or glycine 1.5%)

(c) Working elements for operative procedures: Resectoscope (Fig. 15.52), cutting loop electrode, ball electrode, scissors and biopsy forceps.

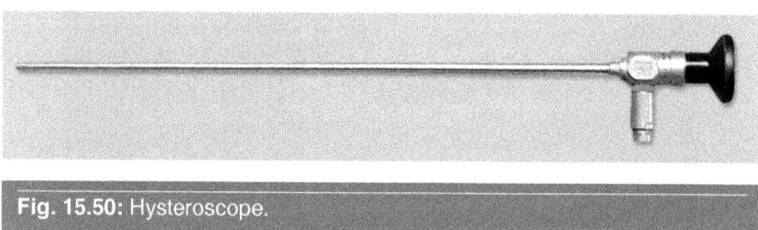

**Fig. 15.50:** Hysteroscope.

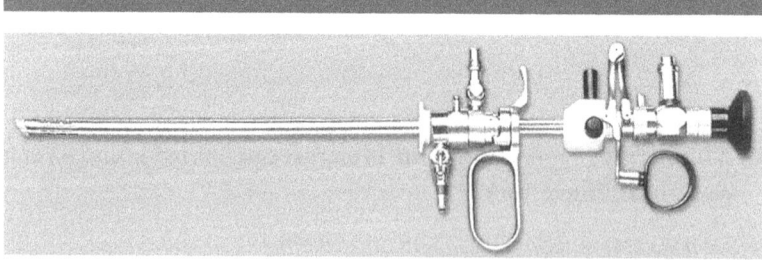

**Fig. 15.51:** Hysteroscope with working element for operative interventions (outer diameter: 8 mm).

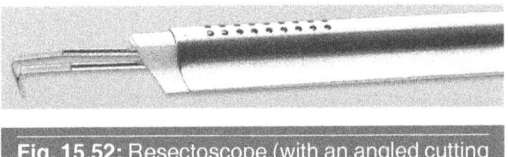

**Fig. 15.52:** Resectoscope (with an angled cutting loop).

Imaging system is similar to that of laparoscopy.

## Indications of Hysteroscopy

### Diagnostic

(A) **Abnormal uterine bleeding**
 - Endometrial polyp
 - Submucous fibroid
 - Postmenopausal bleeding
 - Missing IUCD
 - Endometrial cancer.

(B) **Infertility work up**
 - Uterine synechiae
 - Filling defect on HSG
 - Uterine septum

(C) **Müllerian anomalies**
 - Subseptate, septate, bicornuate uterus or uterus didelphys can be diagnosed. This procedure is combined with laparoscopy for confirmation.

(D) **Recurrent miscarriage:** Intrauterine pathology (Asherman's syndrome, fibroids and polyps) for diagnosis and treatment.

(E) **Misplaced IUCD** (for diagnosis and removal).

### Operative Hysteroscopy

(A) **Polypectomy and myomectomy**
(B) **Endometrial ablation/resection**
(C) **Metroplasty (resection of uterine septum)**
(D) **Release of intrauterine adhesions (synechiolysis)**
(E) **Removal of intrauterine foreign body (IUCD)**
(F) **Endometrial biopsy under direct vision (endometrial cancer)**
(G) **Tubal cannulation**
(H) **Tubal sterilization (essure).**

## Complications of Hysteroscopy

Complications may be due to any of the following factors:

(A) **Distension media**
- Fluid overload (due to absorption)
- Pulmonary edema and cerebral edema
- Electrolyte imbalance
- Embolism.

(B) **Operative procedures**
- Uterine perforation
- Hemorrhage—during or after the operation
- Injury to intra-abdominal organs.

(C) **Electrosurgical**: Thermal injury to intra-abdominal organs.

(D) **Others**: Infection and anesthetic complications.

### Hysteroscopic View of the Uterine Cavity (Fig. 15.53)

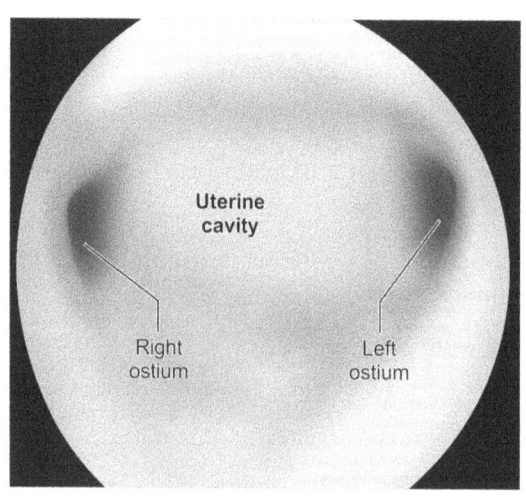

**Fig. 15.53:** Hysteroscopic view of normal uterine cavity. Both the ostia are seen.

*Q. What is the place of hysteroscopy for the purpose of infertility work up?*
**Ans.** See p. 537.

*Q. What are the common causes of Asherman's syndrome?*
**Ans.** Overzealous curettage in postabortal or puerperal phase is often responsible. It may be due to tuberculous endometritis also (Fig. 15.54).

*Q. How does a woman with Asherman's syndrome usually present?*
**Ans.** Menstrual abnormality in the form of hypomenorrhea, oligomenorrhea or amenorrhea depending upon the extent of adhesions (partial or total).

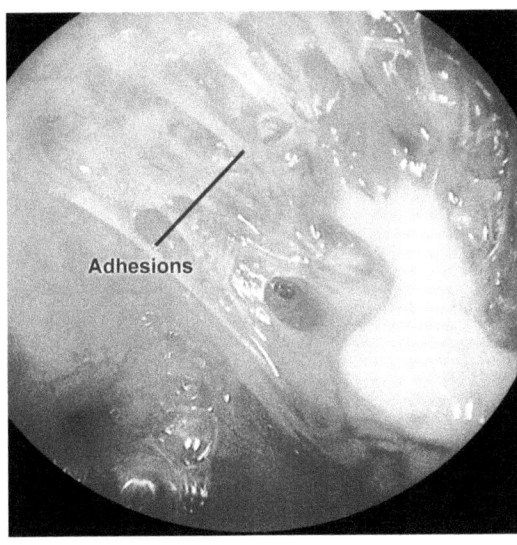

Fig. 15.54: Hysteroscopic view of intrauterine adhesions (*Asherman's syndrome*).

*Q. How the condition is treated?*
**Ans.** Hysteroscopic adhesiolysis followed by insertion of an IUCD is usually effective.

*Q. What could be the symptoms of this woman?*
**Ans.** (a) Menorrhagia
(b) Metrorrhagia
(c) Dysmenorrhea
(d) Infertility
(e) Recurrent miscarriage.

*Q. What is the management option for this patient?*
**Ans.** (a) Hysteroscopic resection of the fibroid (Fig. 15.55) using the resectoscope.
(b) Hysterectomy may be the other option.

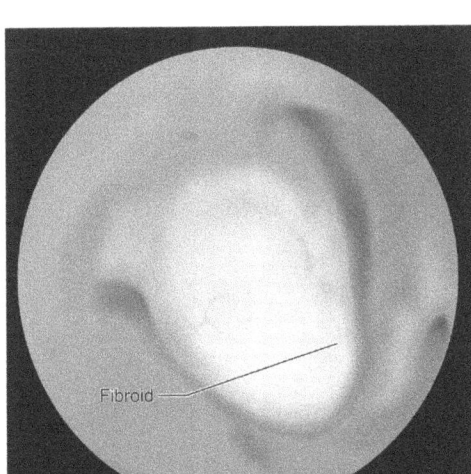

Fig. 15.55: Hysteroscopic view of a submucous fibroid polyp (Grade – 0).

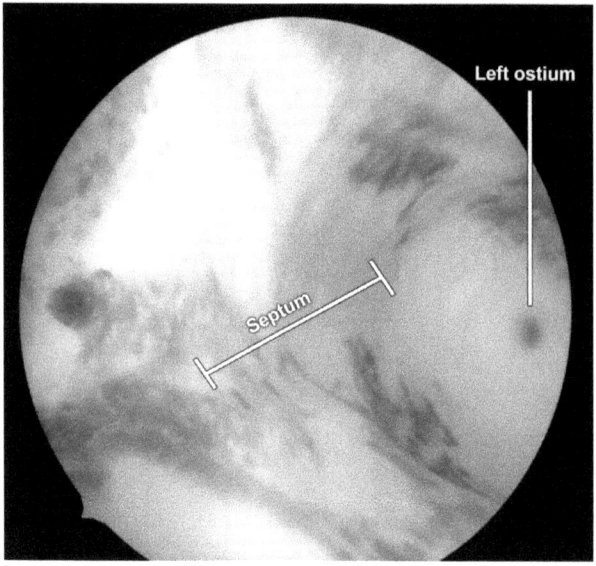

Fig. 15.56: Septate uterus. Left-sided uterine ostium is seen at a depth.
Common complications associated with a septate uterus are: (A) In gynecology: Infertility, recurrent miscarriage, (B) In obstetrics: Malpresentation, preterm labor.

Mrs Murthy, a 27-year-old lady presented with history of recurrent miscarriage (P0+0+5+0). Thorough investigation with laparoscopy and hysteroscopy revealed a complete uterine septum (Figs. 15.56 and 15.57).

**Q. What type of abnormality is this one?**

**Ans.** The two Müllerian ducts have partially fused together, but there is the persistence of the septum in between the two. This septal persistence may be complete (Fig. 15.57) or incomplete.

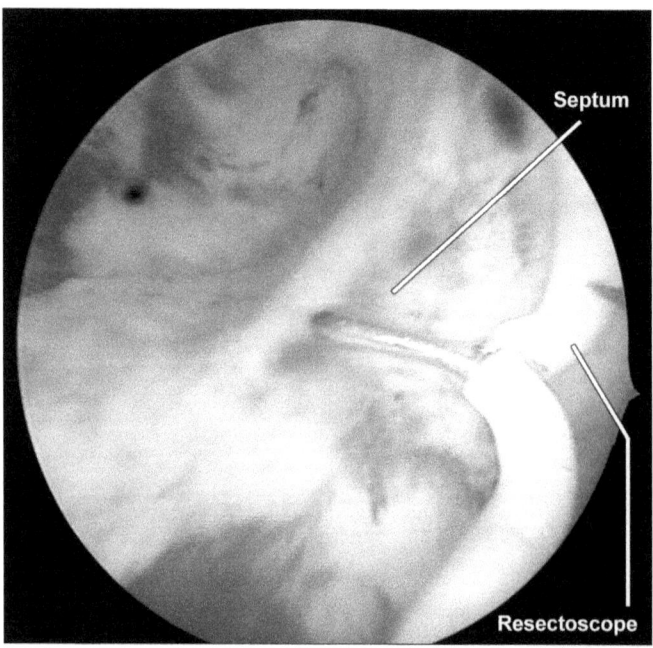

Fig. 15.57: Same patient with complete septum. Resection of the septum is being done using the resectoscope. Presently, she is under supervision for her sixth pregnancy (following septum resection).

**Q. What are the benefits of hysteroscopic metroplasty?**

**Ans.** (a) High success rate (80-89%)

(b) Reduced postoperative morbidity

(c) Short hospital stay (2-3 days)

(d) Successful pregnancy

(e) High chance of vaginal delivery.

**Q. What are the complications of operative hysteroscopy?**

**Ans.** *See* p. 538 (Fig. 15.58).

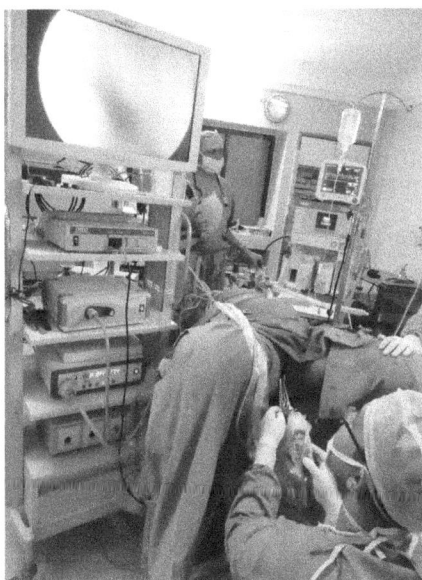

**Fig. 15.58:** Operative hysteroscopic procedure in progress.

## LAPAROSCOPIC TUBAL STERILIZATION

**Q. What are the different methods of tubal sterilization?**

**Ans.** Methods are:
- **(A) Open surgical**
    - (i) Minilaparotomy (commonly done)
    - (ii) Laparotomy procedure (ligation of the tubes using sutures, *see* p. 505)
- **(B) Laparoscopic methods for tubal occlusion** using rings or clips
    - (i) Fallope ring method (commonly used in India)
    - (ii) Filshie clip method (titanium lined with silicon rubber)
    - (iii) Hulka Clemens clip (spring loaded).
- **(C) Laparoscopic methods using electrodiathermy** (less commonly done)\
    - (i) Bipolar electrocautery
    - (ii) Monopolar electrocautery

(D) **Hysteroscopic method** of tubal block
   (i) Essure (microcoil) inserted within the tubes
   (ii) Insertion of quinacrine pellets
   (iii) Adiana-procedure of blocking the tube using radiofrequency energy and also with silicon palette.

**Q. When should ideally the laparoscopic tubal sterilization be done?**

**Ans.** It is best done in the interval period or 6 weeks following delivery or termination of pregnancy.

**Q. What are the other laparoscopic procedures that can be done for tubal sterilization?**

**Ans.** (a) Filshie clip
  (b) Hulka-Clemens spring clip
  (c) Electrosurgical methods (monopolar, bipolar or laser photocoagulation of the tube).

**Q. What is the Falope ring made of?**

**Ans.** It is a silastic ring made of silicon rubber with 5% barium sulfate (*see* Fig. 15.59, p. 543).

**Q. How much length of the tube is destroyed in this procedure?**

**Ans.** About 2.5 cm.

**Q. What is the failure rate of the procedure?**

**Ans.** About 0.1%, if done correctly and by a trained person.

**Q. What are the advantages of laparoscopic tubectomy?**

**Ans.** (a) Simple surgical steps
  (b) Easier (trained person) to perform
  (c) Effective
  (d) Minimal damage to the tube (4 mm)
  (e) Low failure rate (0.2–0.6%)
  (f) Less hospital stay (3–4 hours)
  (g) Early resumption of day-to-day work.

**Q. What method is superior in terms of tubal reversal (recanalization) with higher success rate?**

**Ans.** It depends upon the extent of tubal damage and the fibrosis within the tube after the procedure. Filshie clip is superior to all other methods. However, Fallope ring is better compared to pomeroy method.

## Instruments Used for Laparoscopic Sterilization (Figures 15.59 to 15.64)

**Description and Use:** This is a silicon rubber ring having its inner diameter 1 mm and outer diameter of 3 mm. Its thickness is 2 mm. The rings are loaded over a ring applicator using the loader and pusher. To maintain the rings effective elastic memory, the ring should not be stretched more than 6 mm for a period not more than 3 minutes. It occludes a segment of the fallopian tube including the mesosalpingeal blood vessels. The segment of the tube undergoes avascular necrosis and falls off.

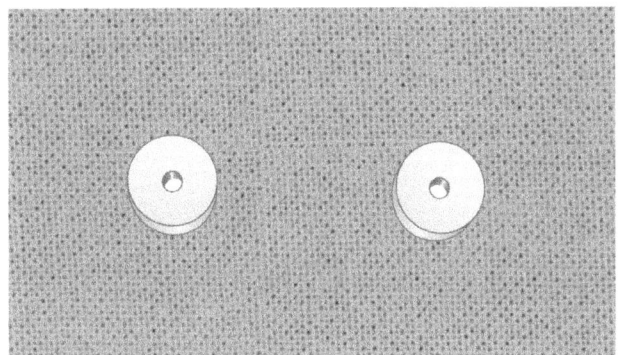

Fig. 15.59: Fallope rings used for laparoscopic sterilization.

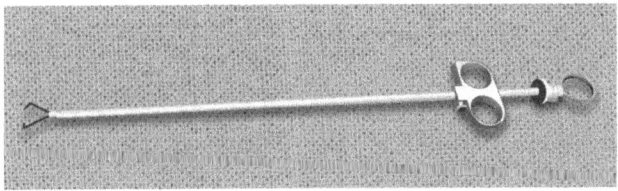

Fig. 15.60: Fallope ring applicator with two ends; (a) One end showing the tongs to grasp the fallopian tube.

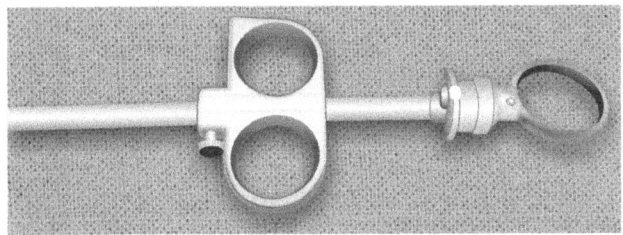

Fig. 15.61: The upper end of the Fallope ring applicator. It has got three rings. The middle and the index fingers go within the lower two rings and the thumb through the upper ring. This end maneuvers the instrument to grasp the tube and to release the Fallope rings.

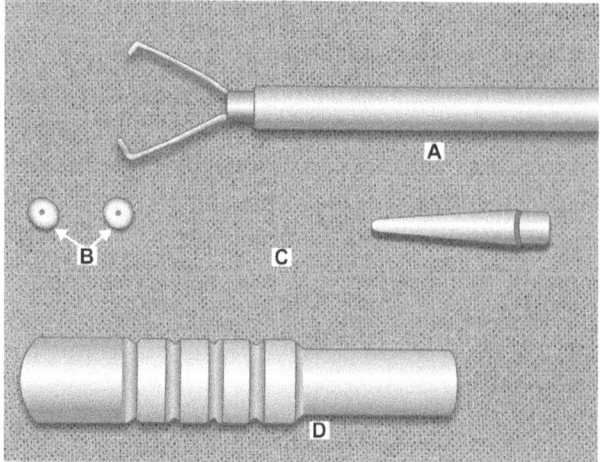

**Fig. 15.62:**
A. Lower end of the Fallope ring applicator. This end shows the tongs to grasp the fallopian tube. It has got a slot to accommodate the Fallope rings
B. Fallope rings
C. Ring loader
D. Ring pusher.

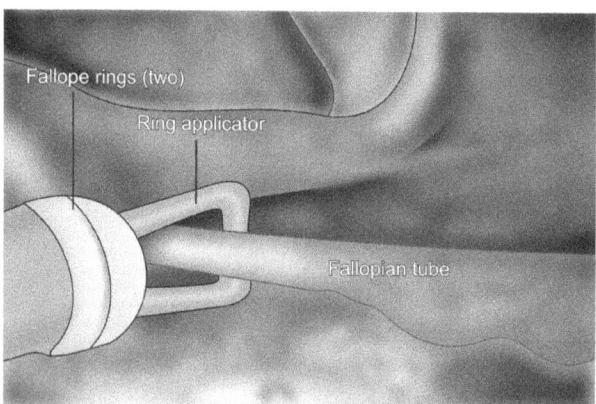

**Fig. 15.63:** Laparoscopic procedure for tubal sterilization using Fallope ring. Ring-loaded applicator is seen to grasp the right tube.

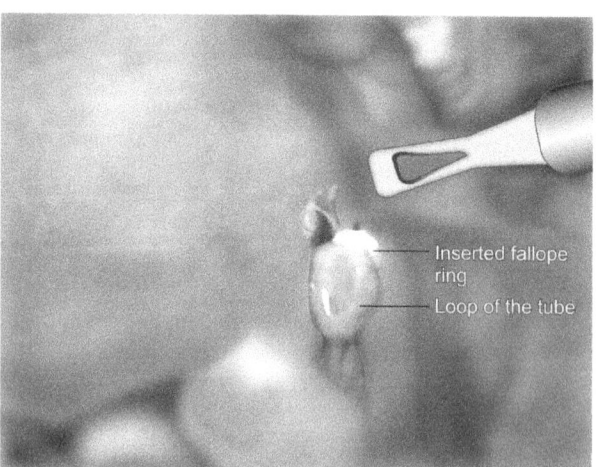

**Fig. 15.64:** Laparoscopic view of tubal sterilization. Fallope ring had been inserted and the loop of the fallopian tube is seen blanched.

## 20. ROBOTICS IN GYNECOLOGY

***Robotic surgery:*** It is facilitated laparoscopy having a computerized interface between the patient and the surgeon. Similar to laparoscopy most gynecological surgical procedures can be done with this robotic technique.

From technological point of view, robotic surgery in superior to laparoscopy especially in terms of accuracy, dexterity, time (suturing), and overall performance. Surgeon's fatigue is less. Robotic surgery is found to have less number of surgical complications compared to laparoscopy.

Robotic movements are intuitive where the tip of the instrument minimics the movements of the surgeon's hands (Figs. 15.65A and B). Whereas in laparoscopy the movements of the tip of the instruments are counter intuitive, opposite to the movements of the surgeon's hands. The instruments in robotic surgery allows complex maneuvers within a small space with seven degrees of freedom compared to four degrees in laparoscopy.

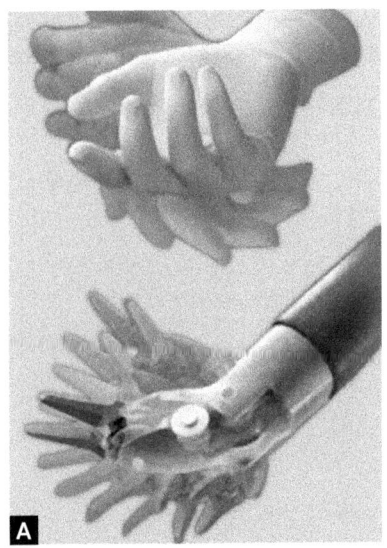
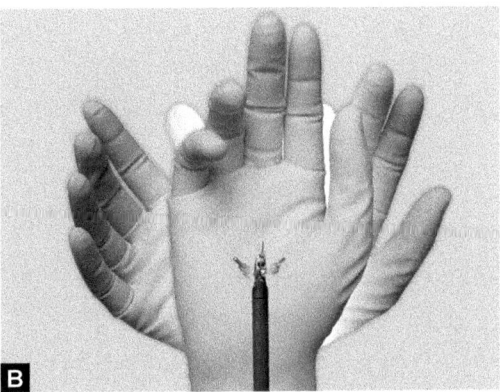

**Figs. 15.65A and B:** Hand movements versus robotic movements.

Robotic surgery permits three-dimensional view. This helps surgeon to have a greater depth of field to dissect tissues. This is especially important in delicate areas (major vessels, ureter) to dissect tissues. The robotics increase surgical accuracy and reduces complications. The learning curve for robotic surgery is not long especially for those who are conversant with advanced laparoscopic surgery.

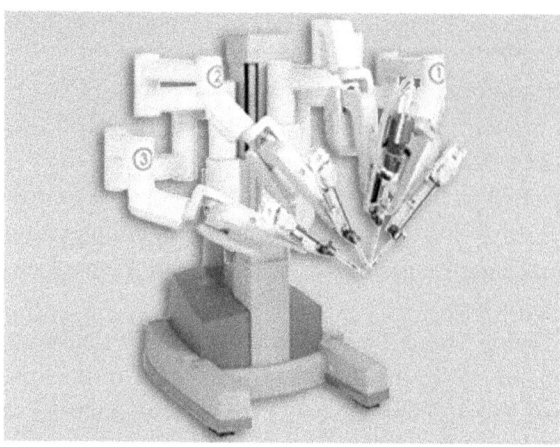

Fig. 15.66: The four armed surgical robotic system.

***Disadvantages***:
- Tactile feel is absent with robotic surgery
- Equipments are expensive (Fig. 15.66)
- Initial setup time needed for each case is long besides the surgeon's training cost.

# CHAPTER 16

# Practical Gynecology

- 16A. Gynecology Instruments — 548
- 16B. Specimens — 592
- 16C. Imaging Studies in Gynecology — 626
    - Hysterosalpingogram — 626
    - Ultrasonography — 633
    - X-ray — 640
    - CT scan — 642
    - MRI — 643
- 16D. Drugs in Gynecology
    - Clomiphene Citrate — 645
    - Letrozole — 645
    - Danazol — 645
    - Progesterone — 646
    - Combined (Estrogen and Progesterone) Oral Contraceptive Preparations — 646
    - Tranexamic Acid — 648
    - Mifepristone — 648
    - Metformin — 649
    - Methotrexate — 649
    - Cisplatin/Carboplatin — 649

# 16A. GYNECOLOGY INSTRUMENTS

**Chapter Objectives**
Basic knowledge and understanding of:
- Identification of the instrument
- Uses
- Related surgical procedures with its use (gynecology)
- Principal steps in surgery
- Complications out of the surgical procedures

## SPATULA AND CYTOBRUSH (FIG. 16.1)

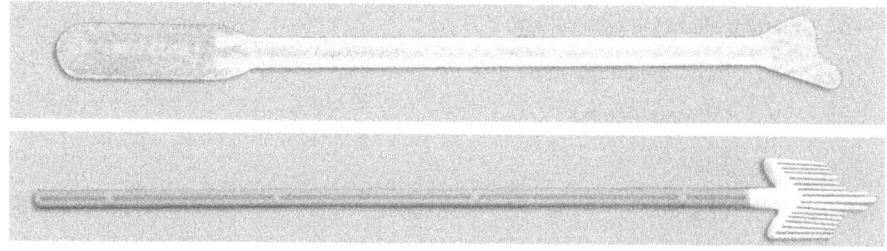

**Fig. 16.1:** Spatula (top) and cytobrush (bottom).

**History:** *Papanicolaou, George Nicholas (1883-1962), worked in New York hospital on exfoliative cytology for the diagnosis of cancer of the female genital tract. In collaboration with Dr Herbert Trout, he published their landmark work in 1941. Later, in 1947, JAMES IRE simplified cell collection procedure with a wooden spatula. This is currently being used. In 1961, Papanicolaou became the director of the Miami Cancer Institute.*

Ayre's spatula (wooden or plastic) and the endocervical brush are used for **collection of cells for cytology screening**.

**Uses**

- For cervical cells—projected end of the spatula goes within the external os. The spatula is rotated 360° to collect cells from the entire ectocervix.
- For endocervical cells—the cytobrush goes within the cervical canal and is rotated to collect cells.
- For cytohormonal study, the rounded end of the spatula is used.

**Methods of slide preparation and fixation:** The cervix is exposed with a Cusco's self retaining vaginal speculum (*see* Fig. 16.3). The material collected (as described above) is immediately spread over a slide. Fixative (95% ethyl alcohol) or cytology fixative aerosol (ethyl alcohol with polyethylene glycol) is spread over it. Once dried up, the slide is then stained (in the laboratory) either with Papanicolaou or Sor's method. It is examined under the microscope by a cytopathologist.

**Self-assessment:**

**Q. Who are the women (at risk) that need cervical cytology screening?**

Ans. 
- Any sexually active women between 21 years and 65 years of age.
- Others (*See* p. 450).

**Q. What is the grading of Papanicolaou's smear?**

Ans. Gradings are total five—normal, infective, suspicious, few malignant cells and plenty of malignant cells. Bethesda system of classification is also followed (*see* p. 553).

**Q. What is a dyskaryotic smear? What are the different types of dyskaryotic smear?**

Ans. Smear showing morphological abnormalities of the nucleus is called as dyskaryotic smear. The important morphological nuclear abnormalities are:
(a) Disproportionate nuclear enlargement
(b) Abnormalities of the nucleus in number, size and shape
(c) Hyperchromasia
(d) Condensation of chromatin material.

**Types are:**
(a) Mild
(b) Moderate
(c) Severe, depending on severity.

**Q. What is Koilocytosis?**

Ans. It is the nuclear abnormalities of a cell, seen in HPV infection. The typical changes are—perinuclear halo, nuclear irregularity, hyperchromasia and multinucleation.

**Q. What is CIN? How do you diagnose CIN?**

Ans. It is the histological observation where part or whole of thickness of cervical squamous epithelium is replaced by cells with varying degrees of atypia. Basement membrane remains intact.

Diagnosis of CIN is made by:
(i) Cytology
(ii) Visual inspection with acetic acid
(iii) Colposcopy
(iv) Cervicography
(v) Biopsy
(vi) Conization of cervix.

**Q. How do you manage a case of CIN?**

Ans. (a) Local ablative methods
(b) Excisional methods or by
(c) Hysterectomy (*see* p. 451).

**Q. How to take cervical smear?**

**Ans.** Cervix is exposed with a Cusco's bivalve speculum without any lubricant. Prior bimanual examination should not be done. Cells are obtained from the squamocolumnar junction of cervix using Ayre's spatula. Endocervical cells are collected with the cytobrush. The collected materials are spread over a slide, fixed with 95% ethyl alcohol. A cytology fixative spray is also used to create a fine mist over the slide for fixation of cells and to reduce air drying. The slide is then stained. It is then examined by a cytopathologist.

**Q. How HPV infection and CIN are related and how it could be prevented?**

**Ans.** High oncogenic risk HPV (types 16, 18, 31, 33, 35, 45, 56) are responsible in the etiopathogenesis of CIN and invasive cancer cervix. 99.7% of cases with CIN and invasive cancer are found to be positive with HPV-DNA. Vaccines (cervarix, gardasil) are approved to all school girls (9-15 years) and women (16-26 years). Vaccine is found to be very effective in preventing HPV infection. Vaccines are type specific and effective only when used prophylactically (*see* p. 452).

## SIMS' DOUBLE-BLADED POSTERIOR VAGINAL SPECULUM (FIG. 16.2)

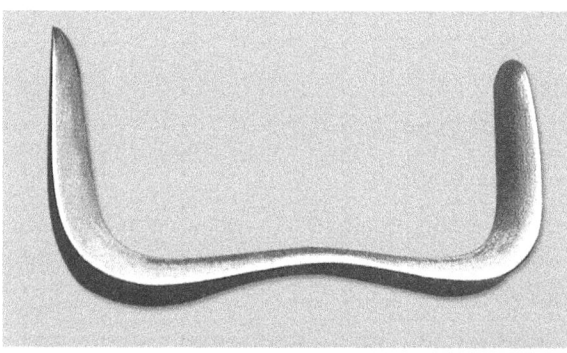

**Fig. 16.2:** Sims' double-bladed posterior vaginal speculum.

**History: Sims, James Marion** *(1813-1883)—Sims worked in Women's Hospital, New York. There he treated nearly 250 vesicovaginal fistula patients, a year with 75% cure rate. He designed this* **speculum.** *He used* **silver thread** *for repair of VVF.* **Sims' position**—*the left lateral semiprone position goes by his name. Sims made many contributions to surgery and gynecology. In 1880, Sims became the President of American Gynecological Society. Sims relentless surgical work on VVF was recognized almost a century later by* **John Chassar Moir,** *who later became the master of surgery on VVF. A bronze statue of Marion Sims stands in the Central Park, New York.*

The instrument was designed by Marion Sims. The blades are of unequal breadth. For description of an instrument see section (Section-1, Chapter-8, p. 283).

## Uses

- It is commonly used in vaginal operations, such as D + C, D + E, anterior colporrhaphy, vaginal hysterectomy, etc. to retract the posterior vaginal wall.
- To visualize the cervix and inspect the abnormalities in the anterior vaginal wall like cystocele, VVF or Gartner's cyst after placing the patient in Sims' position.
- To collect the materials from the vaginal pool for cytology or Gram stain and culture.

*Self-assessment:*

**Q. What is Sims' position?**
**Ans.** *See* p. 550

**Q. What is Sims' triad?**
**Ans.** *See* p. 405

**Q. How is Sims' speculum Introduced?**
**Ans.** (*See* p. 550)

**Q. What are the indications of dilatation and curettage (D + C)?**
**Ans.** (A) **Diagnostic:**
- Infertility
- Dysfunctional uterine bleeding (DUB)
- Endometrial tuberculosis
- Postmenopausal bleeding

(B) **Therapeutic:**
- Endometrial polyp.
- Removal of IUCD
- DUB (occasional).

**Q. Mention the important steps of dilatation and curettage (D + C).**
**Ans. Important steps are:**
   (a) Patient to empty her bladder.
   (b) The operation is done under general anesthesia or under diazepam sedation.
   (c) Lithotomy position.
   (d) Antiseptic cleaning and drapings.
   (e) Bimanual examination.
   (f) Sims' posterior vaginal speculum is placed.
   (g) Anterior lip of the cervix is grasped with an Allis's tissue forceps.
   (h) A uterine sound is introduced.
   (i) Cervical canal is dilated with dilators of gradually increasing size.
   (j) Uterine curette is introduced and the uterine cavity is curetted gently but thoroughly.
   (k) Curette is removed and curetted material is collected.
   (l) The vulsellum/Allis's tissue forceps and the speculum are removed.

(m) The endometrium is preserved (10% formaline) in a vial, labeled and sent for HPE.

(n) The patient is observed for another 2-3 hours and may be discharged.

**Q. Why are the blades of unequal sizes?**

**Ans.** This is to facilitate its introduction into the vagina. Narrow blade in nulliparous and the wider blade in parous women where more space is available.

**Q. What are the lesions in the vaginal wall?**

**Ans. Ulcers:** Syphilitic, tubercular, chancroid and malignant.

**Others:** Gartner's duct cyst, inclusion cyst.

## CUSCO'S BIVALVE ADJUSTABLE SELF-RETAINING VAGINAL SPECULUM (FIG. 16.3)

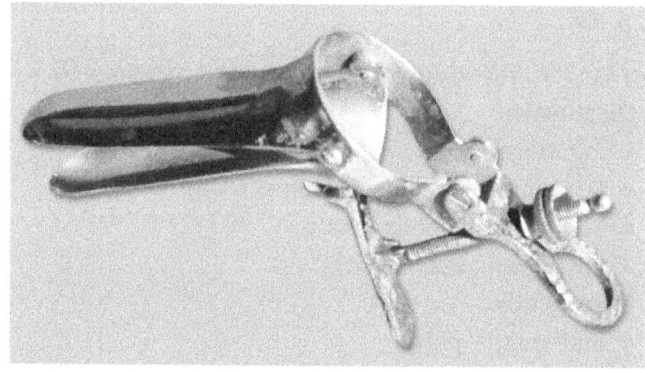

Fig. 16.3: Cusco's bivalve adjustable self-retaining vaginal speculum.

The valves are to retract the anterior and posterior vaginal wall so as to have a good look to the cervix.

A light source from behind is essential. It is commonly used in the OPD.

**Uses**

- To visualize the cervix and vaginal fornices.
- To collect vaginal pool materials and cervical smear for cytologic screening.
- To have cervicovaginal swabs for Gram stain and culture.
- To insert or to remove IUCD or to check the threads.
- To perform minor operations like punch biopsy, surface cauterization or snipping a small polyp.

**Self-assessment:**

**Q. Describe the use of two blades**

**Ans.** See above.

**Q. What are the lesions in the cervix?**

**Ans.** Common lesions are:

(a) Lesions with infection, e.g. trichomoniasis, ectopy
(b) Lesions with ulcer, e.g. Tubercular ulcer
(c) Lesions with growth, e.g. Ca cervix.

**Q. Disscuss the procedures of taking materials for Pap smear.**
**Ans.** See p. 478

**Q. Mention the Bethesda classification system of cytology.**
**Ans.**
- **Sample adequacy**
  - Satisfactory
  - Unsatisfactory.
- **Squamous cell abnormalities**
- **Atypical squamous cells (ASC)**
  - ASC of undetermined significance (ASC-US)
  - ASC cannot exclude high-grade lesion (ASC-H)
- **Low-grade squamous intraepithelial lesion (LGIL)**
- **High-grade squamous intraepithelial lesion (HSIL)**
- **Squamous cell carcinoma**
- **Glandular cell abnormalities**
- **Other cancers (lymphoma, sarcoma).**

**Q. What is cervical ectopy?**
**Ans.** It is the replacement of squamous epithelium of the ectocervix by columnar epithelium of endocervix by the process of metaplasia.

**Q. What are the different types of polyps?**
**Ans.** Polyps may be benign (mucous, fibroid or placental) or malignant. It may be sessile or pedunculated. (*see* p. 428).

## AUVARD'S SELF-RETAINING POSTERIOR VAGINAL SPECULUM (FIG. 16.4)

### Uses
- It is used as posterior vaginal wall retractor in operations like anterior colporrhaphy, vaginal hysterectomy, etc.
- It should be used only when the operation is done under general or regional anesthesia as the instrument is heavy. It requires no assistant.

### Disadvantage
Prolonged use may cause perineal pain in the postoperative period.

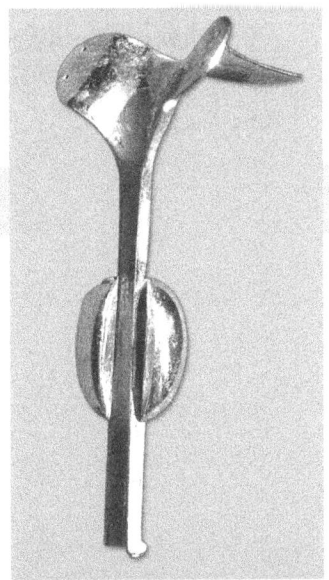

Fig. 16.4: Auvard's self-retaining posterior vaginal speculum.

## FEMALE RUBBER CATHETER (FIG. 16.5)

**Uses**

- To empty the bladder for retention of urine.
- To administer oxygen.
- To use as a tourniquet in myomectomy operation as an alternative to myomectomy clamp.

*Self-assessment:*

**Q. Describe the procedure of catheterization.**

**Ans.** The vestibule is cleaned with a betadine swab from above downwards. The catheter is held away from the tip. It is then introduced through the external urinary meatus.

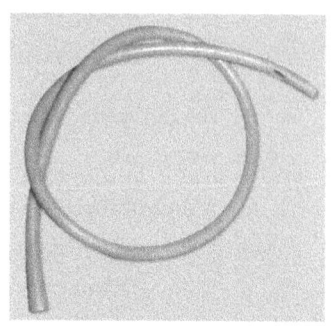

Fig. 16.5: Female rubber catheter.

**Q. What are the causes of acute and chronic retention of urine?**

**Ans.** (i) Postoperative (common due to pain)
(ii) Obstructive (vaginal packing)
(iii) Failure of detrusor contraction (epidural analgesia)
(iv) External sphincter spasm (perineal operation)
(v) Others (*see* page 480).

**Q. What are the different causes of urinary incontinence?**

**Ans.** (a) Urinary fistulae (vesical, urethral and ureteral).
(b) Urethral sphincter incompetence (stress urinary incontinence).
(c) Detrusor overactivity (overactive bladder).

**Q. What are the different menstrual abnormalities that can manifest with retention of urine?**

**Ans.** *See* p. 481.

## FEMALE METAL CATHETER (FIG. 16.6)

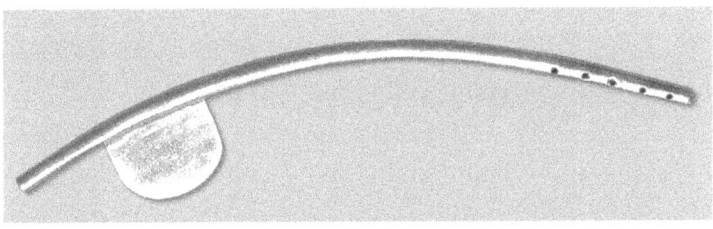

Fig. 16.6: Female metal catheter.

**Uses**
- To empty the bladder prior to major vaginal operations. Not only it facilitates the operation but minimizes the injury to the bladder.
- To confirm the diagnosis of Gartner's cyst from cystocele.
- It is not used in obstetrics as it may cause trauma.

**Use in Pelvic Floor Repair**
- To empty the bladder prior to the operation
- To note the lower limit of the bladder before making the incision on the vagina
- Prior to cutting the vesicocervical ligament
- At the end of the operation to make sure about absence of any injury.

*Self-assessment:*

Q. *What is the length of female urethra?*
Ans. It measures about 4 cm.

Q. *How Gartner's duct cyst could be differentiated from cystocele?*
Ans. Gartner's duct cyst is situated in the anterolateral vaginal wall. Margins are well-defined as it is not reducible. The metal catheter tip introduced per urethra could not be easily palpated through the vaginal mucosa. On the other hand, the urinary bladder is situated in midplane of the anterior vaginal wall. The cystocele bulge is reducible. The catheter tip could be palpated through the cystocele bulge.

Q. *How do you manage an injury to the bladder during surgery?*
Ans. Bladder mucosa is apposed with 3-0 delayed absorbable suture (vicryl) as a continuous layer. A second layer of (musculofascial) suture with the same material is used to reinforce the first layer. Continuous bladder drainage is maintained for 10 days.

## FOLEY'S CATHETER (FIG. 16.7)

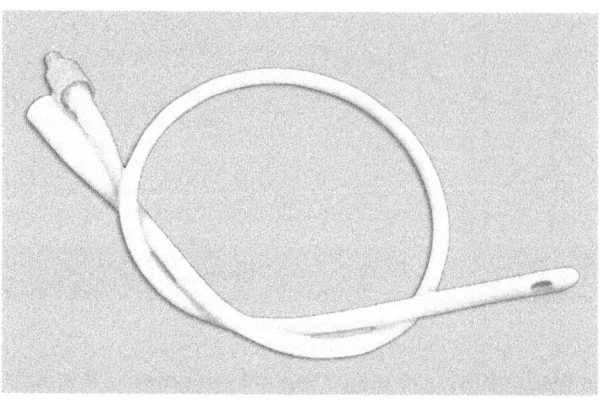

Fig. 16.7: Foley's catheter.

**History:** *Foley, Frederick Eugene Basil (1891-1966)—Frederick Foley was a urologist in St Paul's Hospital, Minnesota. He devised a 'hemostatic bag' catheter, to provide hemostatic tamponade to the excised prostatic bed and for continuous drainage of bladder. It was originally a soft rubber catheter with a balloon sleeve of rubber around the shaft below the eye of the catheter. Currently, the catheter is made of latex which is less irritating to urethral mucosa. Frederick Foley died of lung cancer in 1966.*

### Use in Gynecology

(a) For continuous drainage of bladder—common indications are:
   (a) Vaginal/abdominal hysterectomy
   (b) Pelvic floor repair
   (c) Following repair of VVF
   (d) Urinary retention due to pelvic tumor
   (e) Following radical hysterectomy.
(b) During hysterosalpingography, sonohysterosalpingography, the catheter is introduced into the uterocervical canal (transcervically), balloon is inflated to occlude the canal and then the medium (dye/saline) is pushed.
(c) To assess the patency of the fallopian tube during laparotomy, catheter is introduced in the uterocervical canal (vaginally) and the balloon is inflated then dye is pushed.

## CERVICAL DILATORS (FIGS. 16.8A AND B)

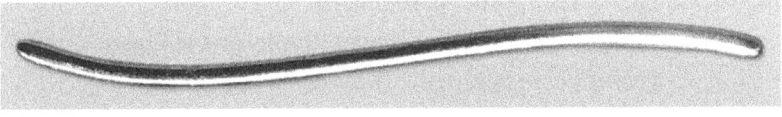

Fig. 16.8A: Hegar's dilator.

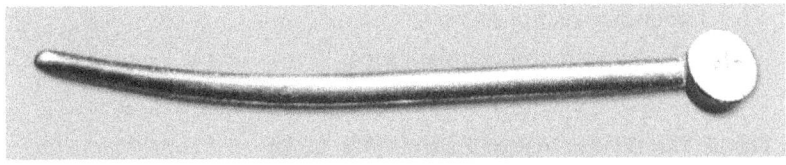

Fig. 16.8B: Hawkin—ambler dilator.

**Varieties**

- Hegar's (Fig. 16.8A)—there are 12 sets, the smallest one is of 1-2 mm. This is used mainly in gynecological operations.
- Hawkin-Ambler—there are 16 sets starting from 3/6 and ending with 18/21 (Fig. 16.8B).
- Das's dilator (named after Sir Kedarnath Das) (Fig. 16.8A).

**Uses**

- To dilate the cervix to facilitate intrauterine introduction of instruments (curette) or devices (IUCD) or hysteroscope or radium.
- To dilate the cervix to facilitate drainage of intrauterine collection—pyometra, hematometra or lochiometra.
- To confirm patency of cervical canal after amputation of cervix.
- To dilate the urethra in urethral stricture.

*Self-assessment:*

Q. *What are the indications of dilatation of the cervix only?*

Ans. (a) Prior to amputation of the cervix
  (b) Drainage of pyometra or hematometra
  (c) Prior to hysteroscopy.

Q. *What are the complications of dilatation operation?*

Ans. (a) Injury to the cervix
  (b) Uterine perforation
  (c) Bowel injury (rare)
  (d) Infection
  (e) Hemorrhage.

**Q. What are the indications of amputation of cervix?**
**Ans:** (a) Congenital elongation of the cervix
(b) Chronic cervicitis leading to hypertrophy and elongation of the cervix
(c) As a component part of the Fothergill's operation.

**Q. What are the causes of pyometra?**
**Ans:** (a) Senile endometritis
(b) Endocervical carcinoma
(c) Tubercular endometritis
(d) Infected lochiometra (obstetrical).

## MULTIPLE TOOTHED VULSELLUM (FIG. 16.9)

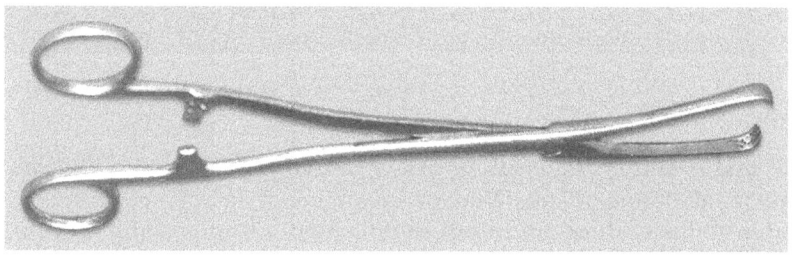

**Fig. 16.9:** Multiple toothed vulsellum.

### Uses

- To hold the parous cervical lip in operations like D + C, anterior colporrhaphy or vaginal hysterectomy. Its function is to make the cervix steady by traction.
- To remove a polyp by twisting as an alternative to Lane's tissue forceps.
- To hold the fundus of the uterus and to give traction while the clamps are placed during total abdominal hysterectomy for benign lesion.

*Self-assessment:*

**Q. Which cervical lip is held?**
**Ans.** Usually, the anterior lip is held in conditions like D and C, D and E, but in some conditions, the posterior lip is to be held.

**Q. Indications of holding the posterior lip of the cervix.**
**Ans.** Usually, the anterior lip is held but in some conditions, the posterior lip is to be held. Such conditions are:
(a) During amputation of cervix or vaginal hysterectomy when the posterior cervicovaginal mucous membrane is incised.
(b) During posterior colpotomy for drainage of pus collected in the POD.
(c) During ligation of tubes done vaginally.
(d) When there is growth in the anterior lip of cervix.
(e) Culdocentesis to aspirate through the pouch of Douglas as in a case of pelvic abscess.

# SINGLE-TOOTHED VULSELLUM (FIG. 16.10)

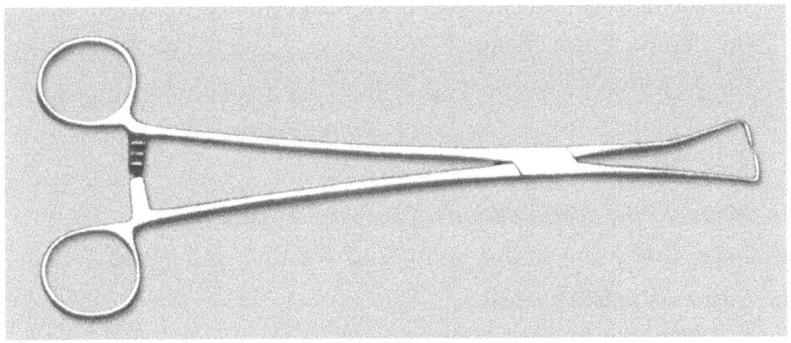

**Fig. 16.10:** Single-toothed vulsellum.

## Uses

- To hold the cervix after opening the vault of vagina and to give traction while the remaining vault is being cut in total abdominal hysterectomy.
- To hold the new cervical stump after amputation of the cervix and Fothergill's operation.
- To hold the cervical stump left after subtotal hysterectomy.
- Sometimes to hold the anterior lip of nulliparous cervix in operation of D + C. (Allis' tissue forceps preferred).

*Self-assessment:*

**Q. What are the indications of amputation of cervix?**

**Ans.** See p. 507

**Q. What are the indications of subtotal hysterectomy?**

**Ans.** Subtotal hysterectomy is done in certain situations where total hysterectomy is found to be difficult or time-consuming. This is done particularly where there is risk of injury to the other viscera like urinary bladder, rectum or ureters.

**Indications are:**

(1) Difficult tubo-ovarian mass with obliteration of the anterior and posterior pouches.
(2) Pelvic endometriosis with involvement of the rectovaginal septum.
(3) Emergency hysterectomy (rupture uterus in obstetrics).

**Q. What are the common indications of abdominal hysterectomy?**
**Ans.** See p. 509

**Q. What are the indications of vaginal hysterectomy?**
**Ans.** (a) Uterine prolapse in postmenopausal women
(b) Uterine prolapse in perimenopausal age group with uterine pathology (DUB).
(c) In nondescent uterus vaginal hysterectomy may be done as an alternative to laparoscopic hysterectomy.

**Q. What are the indications of Fothergill's operation?**
Ans. Uterine prolapse where preservation of uterus of desired for:
  (a) Reproductive function
  (b) Menstrual function (*see* p. 398).

**Q. Mention the principal steps of Fothergill's operation.**
Ans. *See* p. 508.

**Q. What are the complications of Fothergill's operation?**
Ans. *See* p. 508.

**Q. Causes of pelvic abscess.**
Ans.
  - Postabortal/puerperal sepsis
  - Postoperative pelvic peritonitis
  - Infection of pelvic hematocele.

## ANTERIOR VAGINAL WALL RETRACTOR (FIG. 16.11)

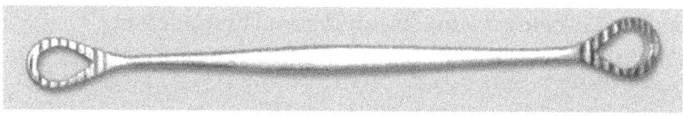

Fig. 16.11: Anterior vaginal wall retractor.

**Use**

To retract the sagging anterior vaginal wall, to have a good look on the cervix while retracting the posterior vaginal wall by the Sims' speculum.

## OLIVE POINTED MALLEABLE GRADUATED METALLIC UTERINE SOUND (FIG. 16.12)

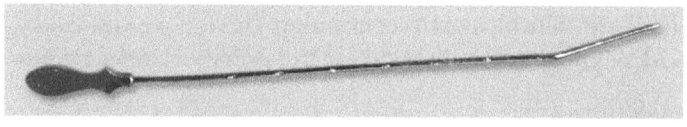

Fig. 16.12: Olive pointed malleable graduated metallic uterine sound.

**Uses**
- To confirm the position of the uterus
- To note the length of the uterocervical canal
- It acts as a first dilator
- To sound the uterine cavity in a case of IUCD with missing threads
- To differentiate a polyp from inversion of uterus.

*Self-assessment:*

**Q. What is the normal position of the uterus and length of the uterocervical canal.**

Ans. The normal position is of anteversion and anteflexion. The uterocervical canal measures 7.5 cm.

*Q. Mention the conditions where the length of the uterocervical canal is increased.*

**Ans.**
- Fibroid uterus
- Elongation of cervix
- Endometrial carcinoma.

## UTERINE CURETTE (FIGS. 16.13A TO C)

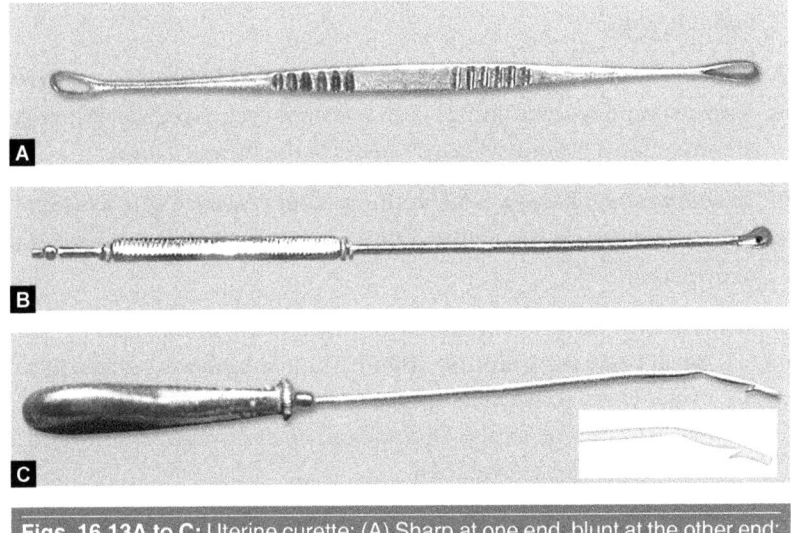

**Figs. 16.13A to C:** Uterine curette: (A) Sharp at one end, blunt at the other end; (B) Flushing curette; (C) Sharman's curette.

### Types
- Sharp at one end, blunt at the other (Fig. 16.13A)
- Sharp or blunt at both ends
- Handle with only sharp at one end
- Flushing curette (blunt) (Fig. 16.13B)
- Sharman's curette (Fig. 16.13C).

### Uses

**Sharp curette (Fig. 16.13A)**
- Infertility
- DUB
- Tubercular endometritis.

**Blunt curette**
- Suspected choriocarcinoma
- Suspected endometrial carcinoma.

**Flushing curette (Fig. 16.13B)**

Following D + E.

**Sharman's curette (Fig. 16.13C)**

Infertility workup where only a strip of endometrium is enough to study the hormonal reflection. It is done as an outpatient procedure and without anesthesia.

*Self-assessment:*

- **Q. What is the purpose of doing endometrial biopsy in a woman with infertility?**
  **Ans.** To detect evidence of ovulation—by seeing the secretory changes in the endometrium.

- **Q. Which day of the menstrual cycle endometrial biopsy is usually done?**
  **Ans.** Biopsy should be done on D21–D23 when the cycle is regular. When the cycles are irregular, it is done within 24 hours of the menstruation.

- **Q. In endometrial biopsy, what is the earliest evidence of ovulation?**
  **Ans.** Subnuclear vacuolation is the earliest evidence appearing within 36–48 hours of ovulation.

- **Q. What are the different methods for detection of ovulation?**
  **Ans:** (1) **Basal body temperature (BBT):** There is biphasic pattern in ovulatory cycle. There is rise in temperature following ovulation.
  (2) **Cervical mucus study:** Disappearance of fern pattern beyond 22nd of the cycle suggests ovulation.
  (3) **Vaginal cytology:** Maturation index shifts to the left due to the effect of progesterone.
  (4) **Serum progesterone:** A rise in serum levels of progesterone in the secretory phase of the cycle (D21) when compared to D8 of the cycle suggests ovulation.
  (5) **Serum LH:** Mid cycle LH surge may predict ovulation.
  (6) **Sonography:** Serial sonography—to defect Graafian follicle (18–20 mm) and subsequently collapsed follicle and fluid in the POD suggests ovulation.
  (7) **Laparoscopy:** Direct visualization of recent corpus luteum.
  (8) **Endometrial biopsy**—secretory changes in the endometrium is diagnostic, appearance of subnuclear vacuolation is the earliest evidence of ovulation (<48 hours).

- **Q. What are the ovarian causes of infertility?**
  **Ans.** (a) Anovulation
  (b) Decreased ovarian reserve
  (c) Luteal phase defect (LPD)
  (d) Luteinized unruptured follicle syndrome (LUF).

## UTERINE DRESSING FORCEPS (FIG. 16.14)

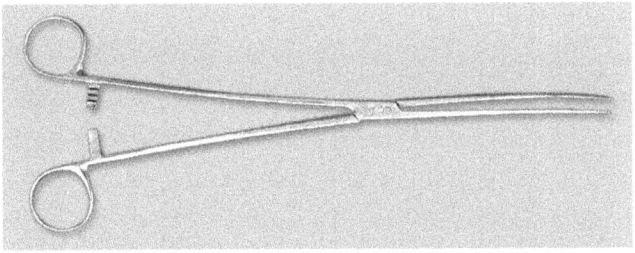

Fig. 16.14: Uterine dressing forceps.

The instrument is often confused with laminaria tent introducing forceps. The blades are transversely serrated while in the latter, there is a groove on either blade.

**Uses**
- To swab the uterine cavity following D+E operation with a small gauze piece.
- To dilate the cervix in lochiometra or pyometra.
- To plug the uterine cavity with gauze twigs in continued bleeding after removal of polyp.

*Self-assessment:*
 Q. *What are the causes of pyometra?*
 Ans. *See* Dutta Gyne 7/e, p. 138.

 Q. *Discuss uterine polyps.*
 Ans. *See* p. 428.

## SPONGE HOLDING FORCEPS (FIG. 16.15)

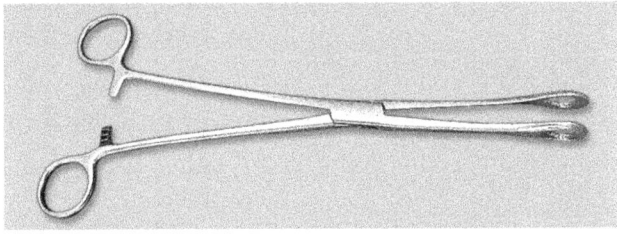

Fig. 16.15: Sponge holding forceps.

**Uses**
- Antiseptic dressing before any abdominal or vaginal operation
- To clean the vagina with gauze pieces before and after vaginal operations
- To hold the cervix in cerclage operation during pregnancy.

*Self-assessment:*
 Q. *Name a few common abdominal operations.*
 Ans. Abdominal hysterectomy, myomectomy, ovariotomy.

 Q. *Name a few common vaginal operations.*
 Ans. Pelvic floor repair, vaginal hysterectomy, Fothergill's operation.

## OVUM FORCEPS (FIG. 16.16)

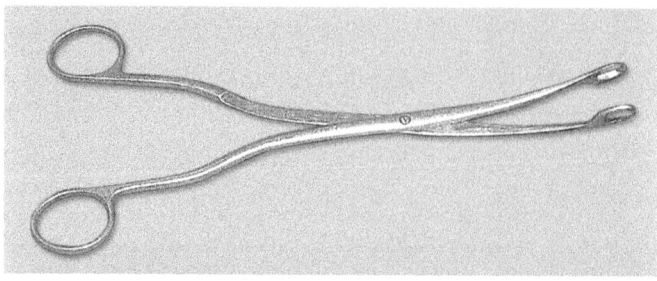

Fig. 16.16: Ovum forceps.

It is often confused with sponge holding forceps, but it has no ratchet. As such, it minimizes trauma to the uterine wall if accidentally caught and also it has got no crushing effect on the conceptus.

### Uses

- To remove the products of conception in D and E after its separation partially or completely.
- To remove molar tissue in hydatidiform mole.
- To remove uterine polyp (small).

**Methods:** The cervical canal is dilated first. The instrument is introduced with the blades closed and opened inside the cavity. The products are caught and then with twisting movements and simultaneous traction, the products are removed.

**Dangers:** It may produce injury to the uterine wall to the extent of even perforation. Not infrequently, a segment of intestine or omentum may even be pulled out through the rent.

## ALLI'S TISSUE FORCEPS (FIG. 16.17)

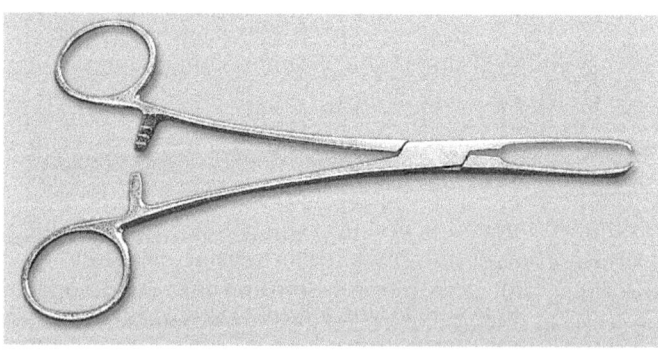

Fig. 16.17: Allis tissue forceps.

**History:** *Allis Oscar Huntington (1836–1921) was a surgeon at Presbyterian Hospital, Philadelphia, USA.*

This forceps is used to hold soft tissues for a long time with minimal tissue damage. Using the ratchet it can be locked and can be used to give gentle traction.

**Uses**

- To hold the margins of the vaginal flaps in colporrhaphy operation
- To hold the peritoneum or rectus sheath during repair of the abdominal wall
- To hold the margins of the vagina in abdominal hysterectomy
- To hold the anterior lip of the cervix in D and C operation when vulsellum is not available
- To catch the torn ends of the sphincter ani externus in complete perineal tear repair
- To remove a small polyp
- To take out the tissue in wedge biopsy.

*Self-assessment:*

**Q. What are the common symptoms associated with genital prolapse?**

**Ans.** Woman may remain asymptomatic if the prolapse is mild. The common symptoms are:
- Genital organs protruding out of the vaginal opening
- Difficulty in walking, sitting, urination or defecation
- Prolapse may interfere with sexual intercourse or may cause vaginal bleeding due to ulceration of mucosa.
- It may cause incontinence of urine
- Pelvic pressure or backache.

# LITTLE WOOD'S FORCEPS (FIG. 16.18)

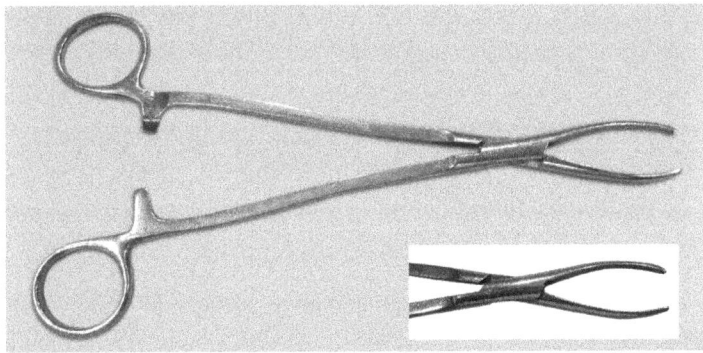

**Fig. 16.18:** Little Wood's Forceps.

This instrument is designed similar to Allis tissue forceps except that the blades have a smooth curvature with its concavity inwards. It has the catches at the handle. The tip has got teeth.

**Use**

- Uses are similar to that of Allis tissue forceps

## LANES TISSUE FORCEPS (FIG. 16.19)

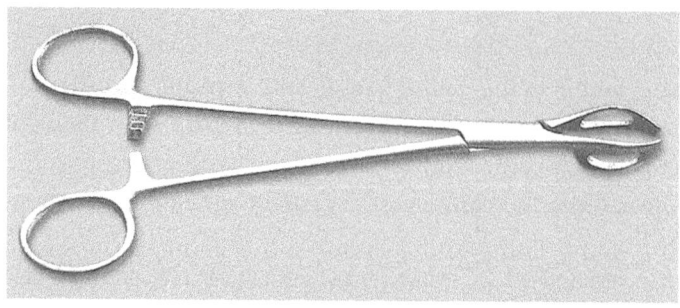

Fig. 16.19: Lanes tissue forceps.

### Uses

- To hold parietal wall (bulk of tough tissues) for retraction during abdominal operations with transverse incision.
- To hold the polyp or fibroid in polypectomy or myomectomy operation.
- To hold the towel during draping.

## UTERUS HOLDING FORCEPS (FIG. 16.20)

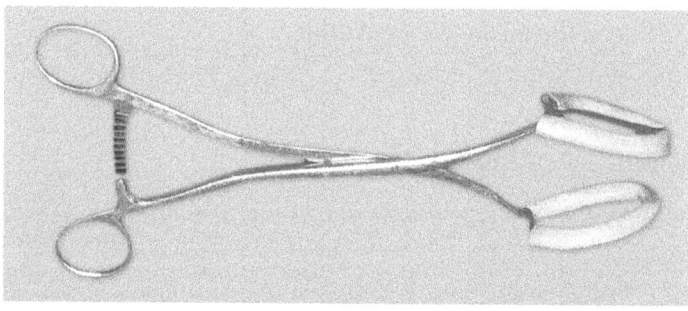

Fig. 16.20: Uterus holding forceps.

The blades are protected with rubber tubes to minimize trauma to the uterus.

### Use

To fix and steady the uterus when conservative surgery is done on the adnexae (tuboplasty operation).

*Self-assessment:*

> **Q. What are the different surgical procedures for proximal and distal tubal disease?**
> **Ans.** Procedures are:
> (1) **Proximal tubal block:** Hysteroscopic cannulation.
> (2) **Distal tubal block:** Fimbrioplasty, fimbriolysis, or neosalpingostomy.

## CERVICAL OCCLUSION CLAMP (FIG. 16.21)

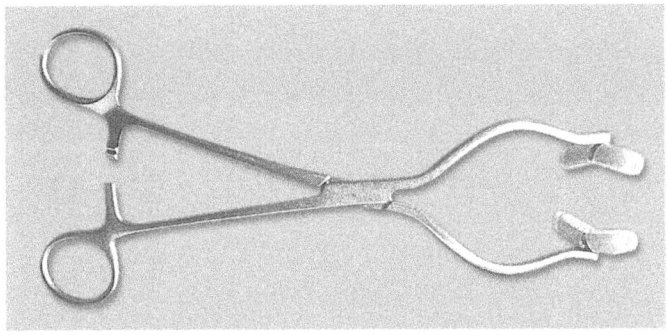

**Fig. 16.21:** Cervical occlusion clamp.

The blades are guarded with rubber tubes to avoid trauma to tissues.

**Uses**

Evaluation of tubal patency during laparotomy (following tuboplasty). Cervix is occluded with the instrument and methylene blue dye is injected into the uterine cavity through the fundus using a syringe and a needle.

*Self-assessment:*

Q. *What are the different methods to assess tubal patency?*

Ans.
- Dilatation and insufflation text (D and I) not commonly done
- Hysterosalpingography (HSG)
- Laparoscopy and chromopertubation
- Sonohysterosalpingography
- Falloposcopy ⎤ not usually done
- Salpingoscopy ⎦

Q. *What are the different types of tubal reconstructive surgery?*

Ans. **Types of tuboplasty operations are:**
(1) Adhesiolysis
(2) Fimbrioplasty
(3) Salpingostomy
(4) Tubotubal anastomosis
(5) Tubocornual anastomosis.

## MYOMA SCREW (FIG. 16.22)

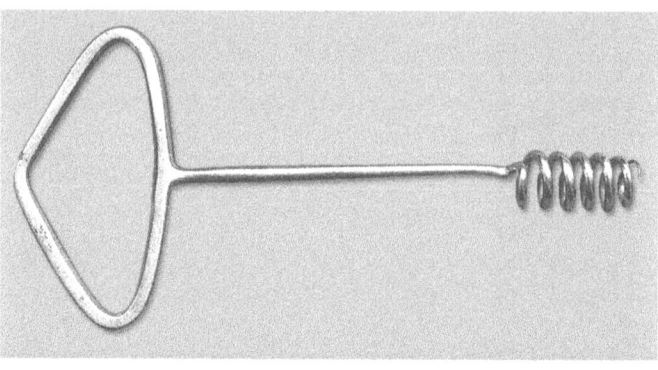

Fig. 16.22: Bonney's myoma screw.

**Uses**

- To fix the myoma after the capsule is cut open and to give traction while the myoma is enucleated out of its bed (myomectomy).
- To give traction in a big uterus (multiple fibroid) requiring hysterectomy while the clamps are placed.

*Self-assessment:*

   **Q. Discuss the principles of myomectomy.**

   **Ans.** It is the enucleation of myoma from within the capsule of the fibroid. The fibroid bed is then closed. The uterus is preserved for future reproductive or menstrual function.

   **Q. What are the complications of myomectomy?**

   **Ans.** (See p. 517).

   **Q. Mention the important considerations before myomectomy (prerequisites of myomectomy).**

   **Ans.** Submucosal polyp, submucous fibroid, any tubal block or endometrial carcinoma should be excluded before performing myomectomy.

**History:** *Bonney, William Francis Victor (1872-1953)*—gynecologist at the Middlesex and Chelsea Hospitals, London. He is mostly remembered for his conservative surgery for fibroids (myomectomy). His contributions in gynecology are many. The significant ones are:

(a) Bonney's myomectomy screw (see Fig. 16.22)
(b) Bonney's myomectomy clamp (see Fig. 16.23)
(c) Bonney's hood myomectomy (see Dutta Gyne 7/e, p. 498)
(d) Bonney's test: Elevation of bladder neck during vaginal examination (not currently practised)
(e) Bonney's gynecology surgery: Textbook on operative gynecology

Unfortunately before he pioneered myomectomy, his wife had subtotal hysterectomy due to fibroid uterus.

## BONNEY'S MYOMECTOMY CLAMP (FIG. 16.23)

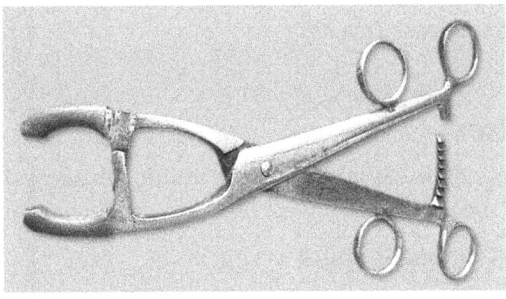

Fig. 16.23: Bonney's myomectomy clamp.

**Uses**

- The clamp is used in myomectomy operation. It curtails the blood supply to the uterus temporarily, thereby minimizing the blood loss during operation. Simultaneous, bilateral clamping of the infundibulopelvic ligaments by rubber-guarded sponge holding forceps may be employed.
- This clamp is seldom used nowadays and is being replaced by—
  (a) Preoperative use of GnRH analogue. (*see* p. 517)
  (b) Intraoperative use of tourniquets (*see* p. 517)
  (c) Vasoconstrictive agents (vasopressin).
- The instrument is placed at the level of internal os with the concavity fitting with the convexity of the symphysis pubis. The round ligaments of both sides are included inside the clamp to prevent slipping of the instrument and preventing the uterus from falling back. The clamp is removed after suturing the myoma bed but before closing the peritoneal layers.

## HYSTEROSALPINGOGRAPHY CANNULA (LEECH WILKINSON VARIETY) (FIG. 16.24)

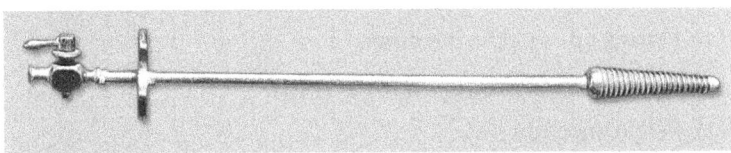

Fig. 16.24: Hysterosalpingography cannula (Leech Wilkinson variety).

In HSG, a syringe is required to push the dye. Iodine-containing radio-opaque dye (urograffin) is used. It is done in the radiology department without anesthesia.

**Uses**

- Hysterosalpingography
- It is also used for hydrotubation.

**Hydrotubation**—Medicated solution is pushed transcervically in conditions, such as following tuboplasty operation, to restore tubal patency or in cases with suspected flimsy adhesions in the tubal lumen or in the fimbria. The drugs instilled are—dexamethasone 4 mg with gentamicin 80 mg in 10 mL normal saline. It should be instilled in the proliferative phase for at least 3 cycles.

*Self-assessment:*

**Q. What is HSG?**

**Ans.** It is a radiographic study to assess the interior anatomy of the uterus, cervical canal and the tube.

**Q. When HSG should be done?**

**Ans.** HSG is done between D7 and D10 of the cycle.

**Q. What are the advantages of HSG over laparoscopy?**

**Ans.** (see SAQ-3 on p. 460).

**Q. How do you compare the oil-based versus water-based media used in HSG?**

**Ans.** Water-based media is commonly used. It causes less cramping pain and discomfort. Oil-based media gives better image and has higher pregnancy rates. Granuloma is more with oil-based media. Embolization is minimal with either media.

**Q. What are the indication of HSG?**

**Ans.** To assess tubal patency.

**Q. Advantages of HSG over laparoscopy.**

**Ans.** (a) To detect uterine malformation.
(b) To detect uterine synechiae.

**Q. What are the complications of HSG?**

**Ans.** (1) Pelvic pain
(2) Vasovagal attack
(3) Dye intravasation within the venous or lymphatic channel
(4) Flaring up of pelvic infection.

**Q. What are the contraindications of HSG?**

**Ans.** (1) Pelvic infection
(2) Presence of adnexal mass (PID)
(3) Pelvic tenderness on pelvic examination.

**Q. What are the other alternatives to HSG?**

**Ans.** Diagnostic laparoscopy and dye test; sonohysterosalpingography and insufflation test (see p. 477).

**Q. What is sonohysterosalpingography?**

**Ans.** It involves instillation of saline in the uterine cavity to study the uterine cavity and the tubes with transvaginal sonography. Uterine polyp and submucous fibroid are better diagnosed with this method.

## KOCHER'S ARTERY FORCEPS (FIG. 16.25)

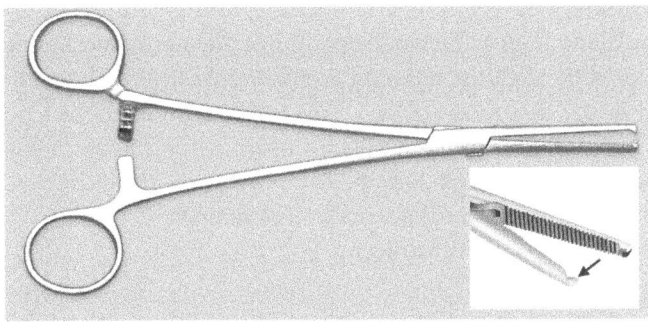

Fig. 16.25: Kocher's artery forceps. **Inset:** Tooth of Kocher's artery forceps.

**Use**

To use as a clamp in hysterectomy operation.

*Self-assessment:*

**Q.** *What added advantage it has got?*

**Ans.** Due to the presence of tooth, it gives a firm grip to the pedicle hold.

**Q.** *What are the indications of abdominal hysterectomy?*

**Ans.** See p. 509.

**Q.** *Mention the different sites where the clamps are placed in total abdominal hysterectomy*

**Ans.** See p. 511.

**Q.** *Mention the principal steps of Fothergill's operation.*

**Ans.** See p. 508.

**Q.** *What are the complications of Fothergill's operation?*

**Ans.** See p. 508.

## LANDON'S BLADDER RETRACTOR (FIG. 16.26)

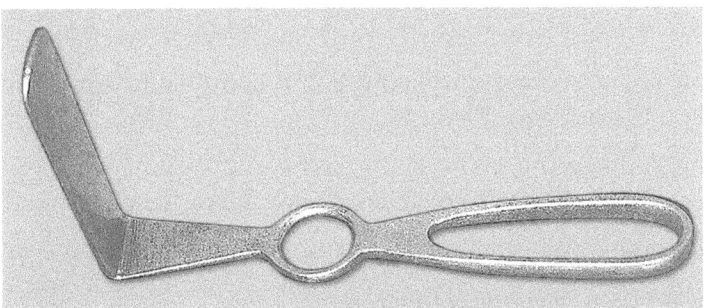

Fig. 16.26: Landon's bladder retractor.

## Uses

- In vaginal hysterectomy.
- To keep the bladder up, to facilitate opening of the uterovesical peritoneum.
- To introduce it through the opening of the uterovesical pouch and to retract the bladder while the clamps are placed. This prevents injury to the bladder.
- To inspect the suture lines after completion of vaginal plastic operations by retracting the anterior or posterior vaginal wall.
- Intravaginal plugging can be done under its guidance.
- To use as lateral vaginal wall retractor.

*Self-assessment:*

Q. **What are the nonsurgical treatments of prolapse?**

Ans. **Conservative treatments include:**
   (i) To avoid aggravating factors (obesity, chronic cough, constipation)
   (ii) Pelvic floor exercise
   (iii) Estrogen replacement therapy
   (iv) Pessary in some cases.

Q. **Mention the different sites where the clamps placed during vaginal hysterectomy.**

Ans. *See* p. 520.

Q. **Important postoperative complications following vaginal hysterectomy with PFR.**

Ans. *See* p. 520.

## INSUFFLATION CANNULA (FIG. 16.27)

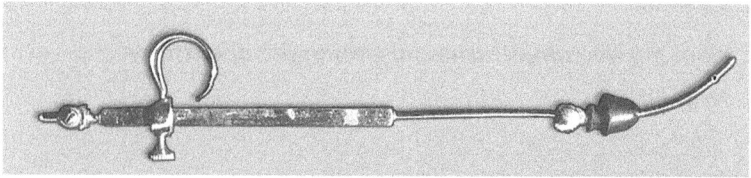

Fig. 16.27: Insufflation cannula.

The instrument is not complete. It requires a 'Y' rubber tube. One end is attached to a bulb and the other end to a manometer.

### Use

To know the patency of the tubes in infertility investigation or following tuboplasty.

*Self-assessment:*

Q. **What is the ideal time of operation?**

Ans. It is done in the early proliferative phase usually 2 days after the menstrual bleeding stops.

**Q. What are the complications of the procedure?**
Ans. ▪ Flaring up of pelvic infection
▪ Shoulder pain.

**Q. What are the advantages of HSG over D and I?**
Ans: (i) HSG can precisely detect the side and the site of block in the tube
(ii) Additionally it can reveal any abnormality in the uterus
(iii) D and I can be false-negative also.

## ABDOMINAL RETRACTORS (FIGS. 16.28A TO C)

Retractors are used to retract tissues out of the operative field. This is needed for better exposure during surgery. Retractors are held in place either by an assistant (**manual retractor**) or by counter pressure with some device (**self-retaining retractor**). Manual retractor can be used alone or in combination with a self-retaining retractor. A pack may be placed between the viscera and the retractor to avoid direct trauma to the viscera.

**Doyen's retractor (Fig. 16.28A)**

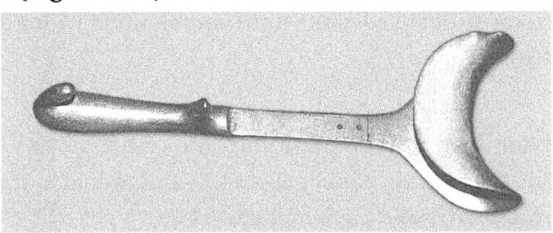

Fig. 16.28A: Doyen's abdominal retractor.

**Uses**
- To retract the abdominal wall in abdominopelvic surgery to expose the field of operation.
- As an alternative, self-retaining retractor may be used.

**Balfour self-retaining retractor (Fig. 16.28B)**

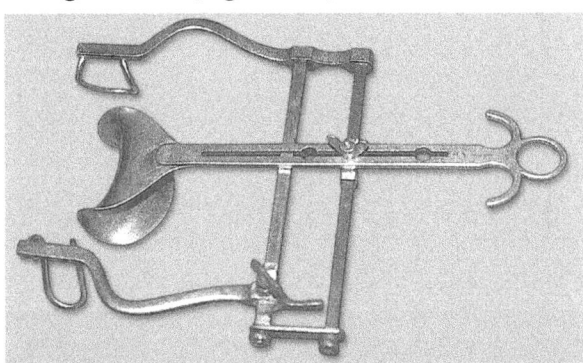

Fig. 16.28B: Balfour self-retaining retractor.

Two lateral blades and an additional (third) blade. All the blades are detachable and may be of different sizes.

## Uses
- To retract the abdominal wall all around.
- To expose the field of operation widely (no assistant is needed for manual retraction).

### Deaver's retractor (Fig. 16.28C)

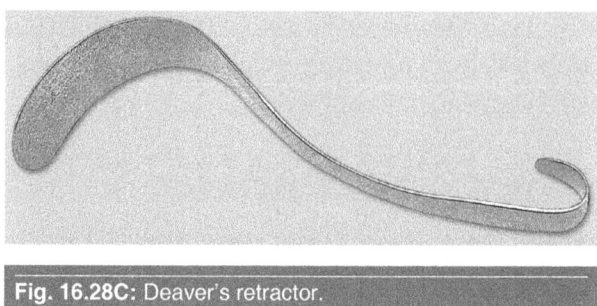

Fig. 16.28C: Deaver's retractor.

**History:** *Deaver John Blair (1855-1931) was Professor of Surgery at University of Pennsylvania Medical School, Philadelphia, USA.*

It is a manual retractor either used alone or in combination with a self-retaining one. It has got different sizes.

## Uses
- It is used in abdominal operation to retract the viscera as and when required in order to facilitate the operative procedures like abdominal hysterectomy. For that purpose, it may also be used as a lateral retractor.
- To retract the parietal wall during abdominopelvic surgery (hysterectomy).
- To retract the bladder and intestines during the surgery.

## LONG STRAIGHT HEMOSTATIC FORCEPS (SPENCER WELL'S CLAMPS) (FIG. 16.29)

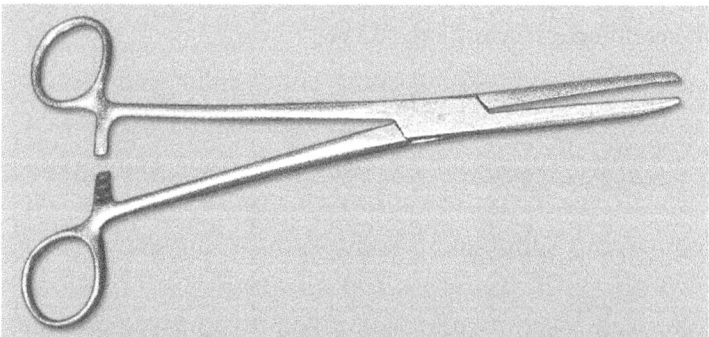

Fig. 16.29: Long straight hemostatic forceps (Spencer Well's Clamps).

**History:** *Sir Spencer Wells Thomas (1818–1897) was a Surgeon at the Samaritan Free Hospital for Women and Children, London (UK). He devised the clamp to place across the ovarian pedicles. He established himself as the most prolific ovariotomist of his era. In 1884, he was elected the President of Royal College of Surgeons.*

## Uses

- It is used as a clamp in hysterectomy, salpingectomy or salpingo-oophorectomy operation.
- To catch a bleeding vessel for hemostasis deep into the pelvis.

*Self-assessment:*

**Q. What are the pedicles held in total abdominal hysterectomy?**
**Ans.** *See* p. 511.

**Q. What are the indications of salpingectomy?**
**Ans.** (i) Tubal ectopic pregnanc
(ii) Hydrosalpinx
(iii) Pyosalpinx.

**Q. What is salpingo-oophorectomy?**
**Ans.** It is the surgical procedure of removing the tube and the ovary.

**Q. How is the procedure done?**
**Ans.** Paired clamps are placed on the infundibulopelvic ligament on the lateral side and another paired clamps are placed medially over the medial end of the fallopian tube including the ovarian ligament and the mesosalpinx. The clamp tips are to be approximated. The pedicles are cut in between the clamps. The clamps are replaced by transfixation sutures. Long straight spencer Well's Clamps are commonly used.

**Q. What are the pedicles held in vaginal hysterectomy?**
**Ans.** *See* p. 520.

**Q. What are the pedicles held during salpingo-oophorectomy?**
**Ans.** *See* p. 511.

**Q. What are the complications of total abdominal hysterectomy?**
**Ans.** *See* p. 512.

## BABCOCK'S FORCEPS (FIG. 16.30)

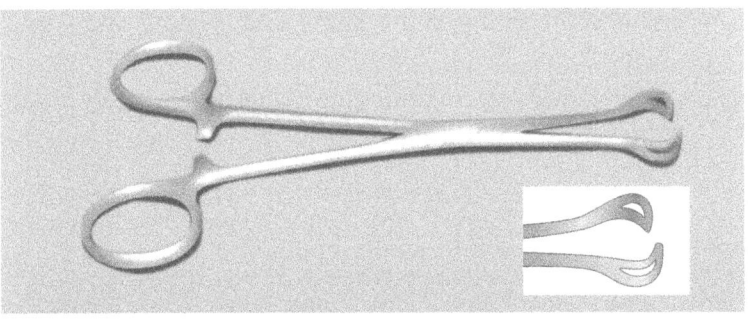

**Fig. 16.30:** Babcock's forceps.

## Uses

- To hold the fallopian tube in tuboplasty operation.
- To hold lymph glands during dissection in radical hysterectomy (lymphadenectomy).
- To hold the appendix during appendicectomy.

# NEEDLE HOLDER (FIG. 16.31)

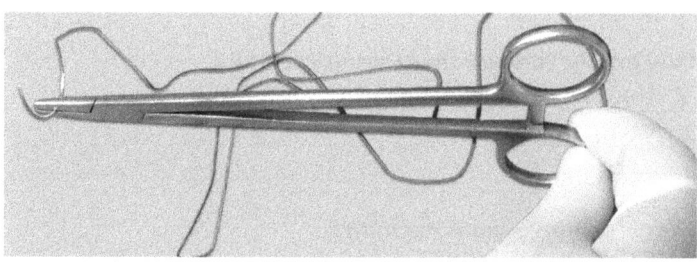

Fig. 16.31: Needle holder with needle and suture.

## Uses

- It may be straight or curved variety.
- To catch-hold the needle. The needle should be caught at the junction of anterior 2/3rd and posterior 1/3rd.

# BARKELAY BONNEY VAGINAL CLAMP (FIG. 16.32)

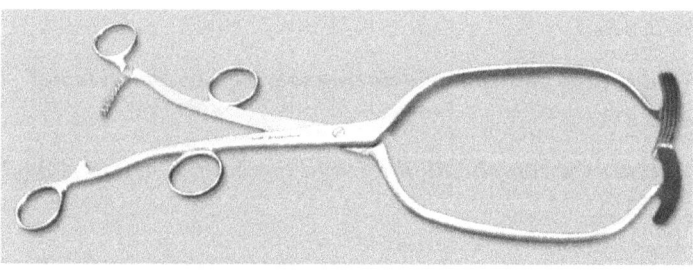

Fig. 16.32: Barkelay Bonney vaginal clamp.

## Use

To occlude the vaginal canal prior to cutting the vagina in Wertheim's hysterectomy.

# PUNCH BIOPSY FORCEPS (FIG. 16.33)

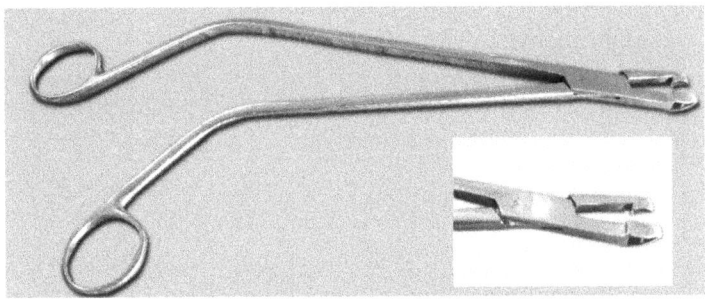

**Fig. 16.33:** Punch biopsy forceps.

**Uses**

- To take biopsy from the cervix.
- The biopsy is taken as an outdoor procedure without anesthesia. The site of biopsy is either from the suspected area or Schiller's iodine or colposcopic directed.

*Self-assessment:*

**Q. What are the different types of cervical biopsy?**

**Ans.** Types are:
(a) Surface biopsy (smear)
(b) Punch biopsy.

**Other biopsies are:**
(a) Wedge biopsy
(b) Ring biopsy
(c) Cone biopsy.

**Q. How to send the tissue for histology?.**
**Ans.** This tissue is sent for HPE in a container with normal saline labeled properly.

**Q. What is Schiller's test?**
**Ans.** Cervical biopsy is taken following application of Schiller's (0.3%) iodine solution. Punch biopsy is taken from the unstained area.

**Q. What is VIA?**
**Ans.** Visual inspection (of the cervix) following application of acetic acid. Women having acetowhite areas on the cervix are considered for colposcopic examination and/or biopsy.

**Q. What are the different histological types of carcinoma cervix?**
**Ans.** (a) Commonest—squamous cell carcinoma (80–90%)
(b) Adenocarcinoma (10–15%)
(c) Remaining are—clear cell, adenosquamous, neuroendocrine tumors or sarcomas.

**Q. What are the complications of cervical biopsy?**

**Ans.** (a) Hemorrhage (primary or secondary). Cone biopsy has got more complications.
(b) Cervical incompetence.
(c) Infertility.
(d) Cervical stenosis.
(e) Vaginal discharge.
(f) Infection.

## DISSECTING FORCEPS (FIGS. 16.34A AND B)

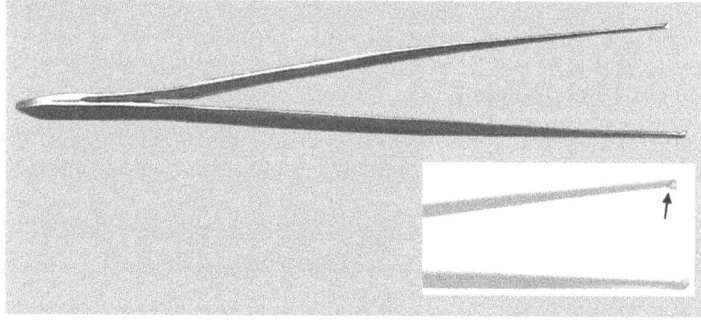

Fig. 16.34A: Toothed dissecting forceps, **Inset:** Tooth of dissecting forceps.

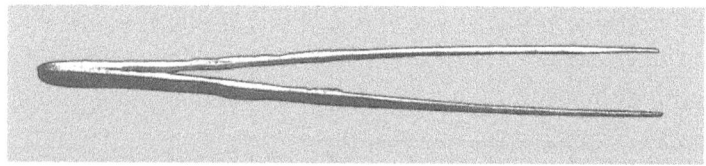

Fig. 16.34B: Nontoothed dissecting forceps.

### Toothed

**Use**

To hold tough structures like rectus sheath, cut margins of vaginal vault or margins of vaginal flaps in pelvic floor repair or the skin margins during suturing.

### Plain or non-toothed

**Use**

To hold soft tissues like peritoneal margins during suturing.

## SCALPEL BLADE WITH THE HANDLE (FIG. 16.35)

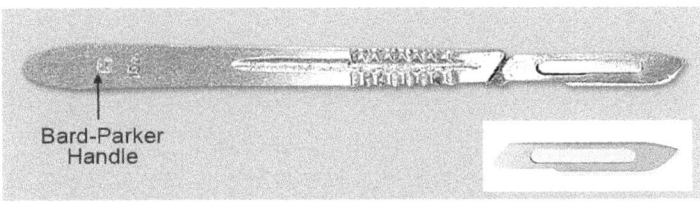

**Fig. 16.35:** Scalpel blade with the handle, Inset: Scalpel blade size 10.

The instrument is detachable—handle (Bard-Parker Handle) and blade. Scalpel blades are of various sizes and shapes. The available sizes are 10, 11, 12, 15, 20 and 22. Size 10 is commonly used as it is most versatile. Size 11 is used to perform stab incision for making laparoscopic point incision.

### Uses
- To cut the abdominal wall—skin, subcutaneous tissue, rectus sheath and opening the peritoneum.
- To cut the mucous coat in vaginoplasty operation and to cut tissues during surgery.
- To cut pedicles during hysterectomy.

## NEEDLES (FIGS. 16.36A TO C)

**Surgical needles have three areas:** The eye, the body and the point. The needles are made of stainless steel. The needles may be eyed or eyeless. Eyeless (atraumatic) needles are swaged. The body of the needles may be curved or straight. The disadvantages of eyed needles are—difficulties in threading and the tissue trauma. **Reverse cutting** needle has an additional sharp edge on the outside. Curved needles may be 1/2 circle (1/2 of a full circle) or 3/8 circle.

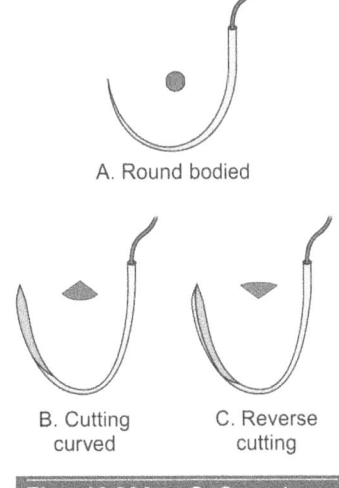

**Figs. 16.36A to C:** Curved needles.

### Round bodied (curved)

It is used while suturing soft structures like:
- Peritonization and suturing muscles.
- Suturing the pedicles in hysterectomy.
- Suturing the pubocervical fascia.
- Tubectomy or salpingectomy.

**Cutting (curved):** It is used while suturing tough structures like:
- Suturing the vaginal wall margins in PFR.
- Closure of the vaginal vault in abdominal hysterectomy.
- Repair of the rectus sheath.
- Suturing the skin.

## SCISSORS (FIGS. 16.37 TO 16.40)

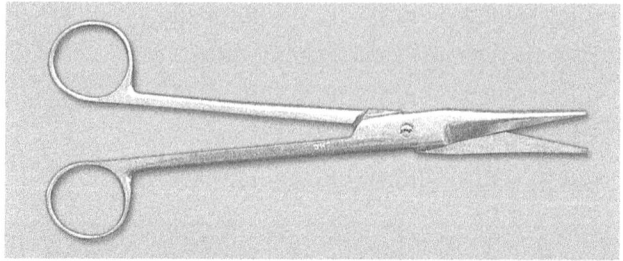

**Fig. 16.37: Scissors (Mayo's type):** This is used in almost every operation requiring tissue dissection and excision.

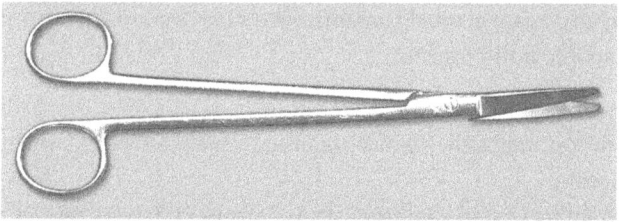

**Fig. 16.38:** Scissors (Bent on flat—Bonney type): This is used conveniently in anterior colporrhaphy to dissect the vesicovaginal space and also for tissue dissection.

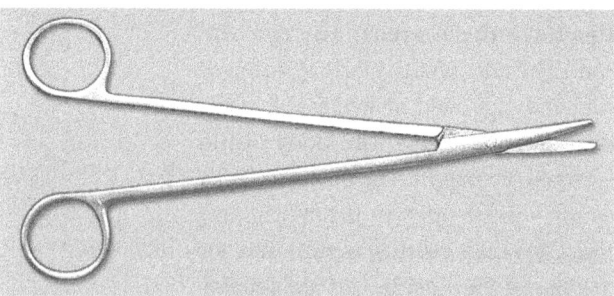

**Fig. 16.39:** Scissors (Metzenbaum): This is used for tissue dissection.

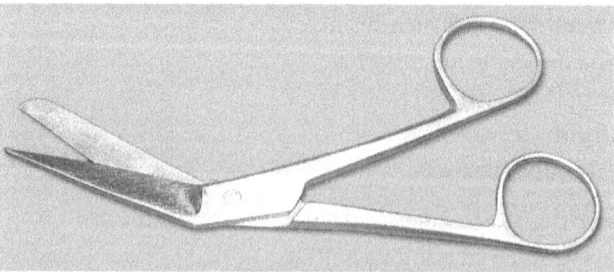

**Fig. 16.40:** Scissors (perineorrhaphy): It is comfortably used in perineorrhaphy operation; also used in episiotomy.

*Self-assessment:*

**Q. What are the indications of perineorrhaphy?**
**Ans.**
- Relaxed perineum
- Rectocele
- Enterocele.

**Q. What are indications of pelvic floor repair (PFR)?**
**Ans.** Cystocele, rectocele and relaxed perineum.

**Q. What are the complications of PFR?**
**Ans.** (a) **Operative:**
- Hemorrhage
- Injury to bladder, urethra, rectum, VVF or RVF.

(a) **Postoperative:**
- Urinary retention
- Infection—cystitis.

(c) **Late:**
- Dyspareunia
- VVF
- RVF
- Recurrence of prolapse
- Principal steps of perineorrhaphy, PFR and CPT repair.

# TOWEL CLIPS (FIG. 16.41)

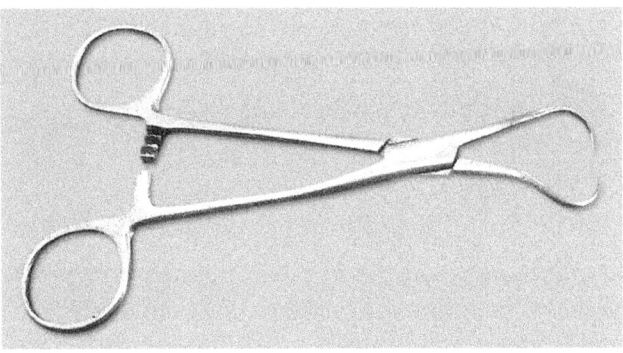

Fig. 16.41: Towel clip.

## Uses
These are used in draping the operative area—abdominal or vaginal. The towels or sheets are fixed to the skin and each other with these clips.

*Self-assessment:*

**Q. How antiseptic cleaning is done before any abdominal or vaginal operation?**

**Ans.** Antiseptic cleaning is done using povidone iodine 7.5% solution or Savlon (chlorhexidine) solution.

## LOOP HOOK (FIG. 16.42)

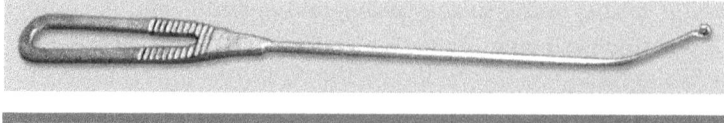

Fig. 16.42: Loop hook.

**Use**

To remove IUCD from the uterine cavity when the threads are missing.

**Method of use**

Cervical canal is dilated if needed. The hook is introduced within the uterine cavity. The IUCD is felt and is grasped within the hook. It is then pulled out.

**Precautions**

Location of the IUCD within the uterine cavity must be confirmed. Trauma (perforation) to the uterus is to be avoided. Hysteroscopic removal can also be done.

## ELECTROCAUTERY (FIG. 16.43)

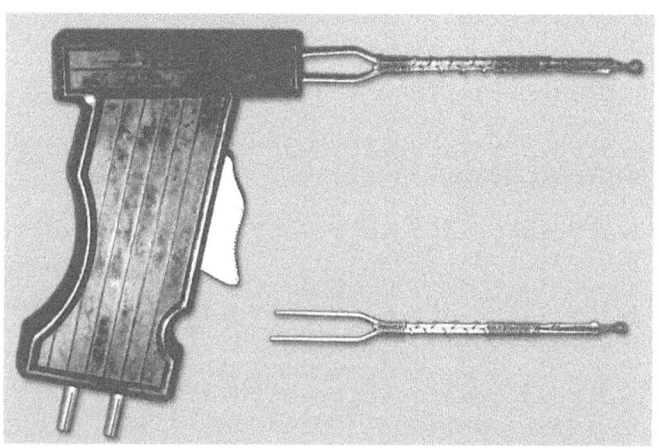

Fig. 16.43: Electrocautery (inset—the cautery probe).

**Use**

Thermal cauterization of the cervix for cervical ectopy (erosion).

*Self-assessment:*

Q. *Mention the steps of thermal cauterization.*

Ans. Radial strokes are made to burn the epithelium of the ectopy area. The strokes are made about 2 mm deep and at a distance of 1 cm.

Q. *How tissue healing occurs?*

Ans. The burn area sloughs out. Re-epithelialization occurs by growth of squamous epithelium.

**Q. How the patient is counseled for the postoperative care?**

**Ans.** Patient is counseled about the serosanguinous discharge for about 2-3 weeks. Thereafter it heals with the epithelialization by squamous epithelium.

**Q. What are the complications of the procedure?**

**Ans.** Excessive vaginal discharge, slight vaginal bleeding and pelvic pain.

## HODGE-SMITH PESSARY (FIG. 16.44)

It is made up of volcanite or ebonite. It is sterilized by keeping it in lysol for 24-48 hours.

**Indications of use**
- Puerperal retroversion of the uterus
- Retroversion in early pregnancy
- Pessary test to relieve symptoms of retroversion.

**Contraindications**
- Fixed retroversion of uterus
- Presence of infection.

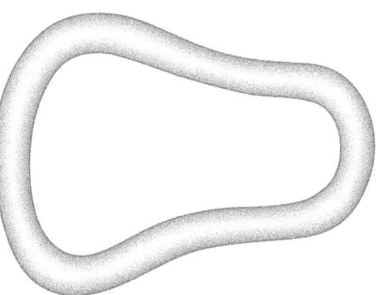

Fig. 16.44: Hodge-Smith pessary.

*Self-assessment:*

**Q. How to determine the size of a pessary?**

**Ans.** Patient lies in dorsal position after evacuation of the bladder. Bimanual pelvic examination is done by introducing two fingers of the right hand. The tip of the middle finger lies at the apex of the stretched posterior fornix. The fingers are mobilized to bring the radial border of the index finger underneath the symphyisis pubis. The point is marked by the index finger of the left hand. The fingers are withdrawn. The length of the tip of the middle finger and this mark is taken as the diameter of the pessary.

Usually 3 sizes of the pessaries are considered:
 (i) One with the same size
 (ii) One with one size lesser
 (iii) One with one size bigger.
With trial method, the one which is more comfortable and effective is selected.

**Q. Describe the method of insertion of a pessary.**

**Ans.** The patient lies in dorsal position with an empty bladder. The pessary is held collapsed or folded to make the insertion easy. A lubricant may be used. It is introduced inside the vagina and is pushed high. The broad end lies in the posterior fornix, the narrow end behind the symphysis pubis and the concavity is directed upwards.

**Q. What instructions should be given to the patient while inserting a pessary?**

Ans. 
- To have vaginal douche at least twice a week.
- To check after 1 month.
- To be removed or reintroduced after 3 months.

## RING PESSARY (FIG. 16.45)

It is made up of watch-spring with rubber. It is sterilized by boiling for half an hour.

**Uses**
- Prolapse in early pregnancy—it is kept for 18 weeks.
- Prolapse in puerperium.
- Prolapse in a woman who is unfit surgery.

**Contraindications**
- Presence of sepsis
- Gross relaxation of pelvic floor muscles.

**Measurements:** As in Hodge-Smith pessary.

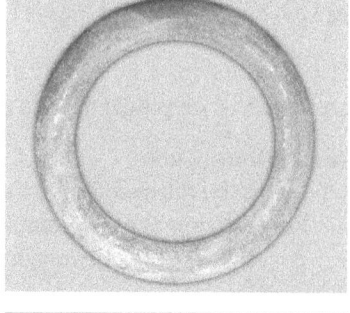

Fig. 16.45: Ring pessary.

**Instructions:** As in Hodge-Smith pessary.

*Self-assessment:*

**Q. What are the indications of insertion of ring pessary?**

Ans. *See* p. 396.

**Q. What is the mechanism of action?**

Ans. Pessary cannot cure prolapse. It relieves symptoms by stretching the hiatus urogenitalis. Thus, it prevents vaginal and uterine descent.

**Q. How do you this disinfect, clean and sterilize the instruments?**

Ans. (a) **Disinfection** is done by any one of the methods: Immersing instruments in:
- (i) Boiling water for 20 minutes
- (ii) 2% glutaraldehyde (cidex) solution for 20 minutes
- (iii) 0.5% chlorine solution for 20 minutes (0.5% of chlorine solution is made by adding 3 teaspoons (15 g) of bleaching powder in one liter of water).

(b) **Cleaning:** Instruments are disassembled and washed from all surfaces in running (preferably warm) water. The cannulas should be flushed repeatedly.

(c) **Sterilization:** Either by:
- (i) Autoclaving at 121°C (250°F), under pressure of 15 lbs/in$^2$ (106 kPa) for 30 minutes
- (ii) Immersing in 2% glutaraldehyde (cidex) solution for 10 hours.

## SUTURE MATERIALS

The suture materials used in a particular surgical step depend on the strength of the tissues to be sutured and the time required for the wound to regain its strength. Depending on diameter, sutures are categorized into no. 0, 1, 2, etc. Sutures when smaller than no. 0, are indicated as 1-0, 2-0 and so forth. Due considerations also to be given on tensile strength of the suture, the rate at which the suture material loses its strength in vivo and the interaction expected between suture and tissues.

**Classification:** The suture materials may be classified either as absorbable or nonabsorbable. Their biological origin or synthetic preparations are mentioned briefly.

|  | Absorbable | Nonabsorbable |
|---|---|---|
| Biological | Catgut | Silk |
|  | Collagen | Cotton |
| Synthetic | Dexon } Delayed absorbable<br>Vicryl<br>PDS | Terelene/Dacron<br>Polyamide<br>Polypropylene<br>Steel |

**Sutures:** Sutures may be **monofilament** (Dexon, PDS, nylon) or **polyfilament** (vicryl, silk). It is based on the number of fiber strands. Monofilament (single stranded fiber) sutures need 5 to 6 throws to make knots secured. Polyfilament sutures are braided and their knots are secured with usual ( 2 to 3 ) throws. Risks of infection are high with polyfilament sutures. However, the tensile strength of polyfilament sutures is high.

### (A) Absorbable
(i) **Biological**
- **Catgut** (derived from the word kitgut—strings of a musical instrument known as kit) is obtained from the submucosa of sheep or ox intestines. Treatment with chromic sulfate produces chromic catgut and the untreated material produces plain catgut. Chromic catgut is degraded and phagocytosed by proteolytic enzymes of white blood cells (inflammatory cells) slowly. Chromic catgut loses half of its tensile strength by 10 days and maintains some strength up to 21 days. Plain catgut loses 70% of its tensile strength by 7 days.
- **Collagen** is derived from ox Achilles tendon.
- Both are available in plain and chromic form.

(ii) **Synthetic**
- **Dexon**—Dexon (polyglycolic acid) is a copolymer of glycolic acid and is degraded by hydrolysis with minimal inflammation. It loses half of its tensile strength in 15 days and is absorbed in 4 months.
- **Vicryl (polyglactin):** It is a copolymer of lactide and glycolide. It loses its tensile strength in 30 days. It is absorbed by 70 days. It produces less tissue reaction than catgut.
- **Vicryl rapide (coated) (Fig. 16.46):** It is also a polyglactin suture. It is similar to plain catgut. Absorption is rapid with minimal tissue inflammation. 70% of its tensile strength is lost by 7 days. It is used for soft tissues, episiotomy repair and skin.

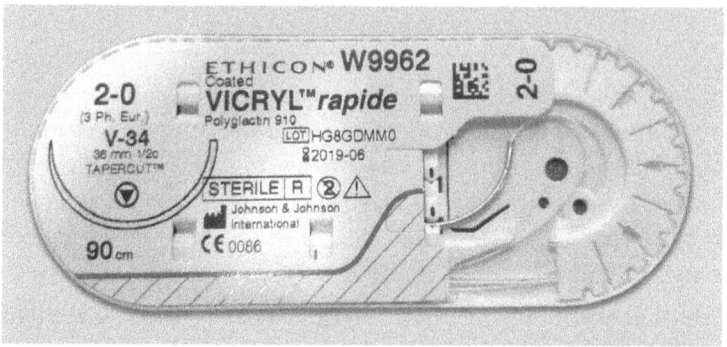

**Fig. 16.46:** Vicryl rapide 2-0 suture, length 90 cm with round bodied needle, 36 mm, half circle.

- The tensile strength of the above sutures is much greater than that of catgut. But these sutures need more throws to secure knots compared to catgut.
- **Polydioxanone suture (PDS)** is a pliable monofilament made of polydioxanone. It loses half of its tensile strength in 28 days. Tissue inflammation is minimal. Monofilament sutures have no interstices to lodge any bacteria. So infections are rare.
- **Polyglyconate sutures** have got similar properties. These are used for fascial closure.

All the synthetic absorbable materials are sterilized by ethylene oxide.

| | | Sutures | | | |
|---|---|---|---|---|---|
| Nature | Type | Wound support | Complete absorption | Tissue where used | |
| Absorbable | • Plain catgut | 7–10 days | 4–8 weeks | • Subcutaneous tissue and its blood vessels | |
| | • Chromic catgut | 3 weeks | 8–12 weeks | • Vascular pedicle, vaginal wall, rectus sheath | |
| Delayed absorbable | • Dexon | 3 weeks | 8–12 weeks | • Subcuticular<br>• Fascial structure<br>• Skin | |
| | • Vicryl | 3–4 weeks | 8–10 weeks | • Microsurgery<br>• Vaginal vault, | |
| | • PDS | 6–7 weeks | 4–6 months | • Rectus sheath<br>• Uterine muscles | |
| | • Vicryl rapide | 7–10 days | 5–6 weeks | • Episiotomy, subcuticular tissues | |
| Non-absorbable | • Nylon | | | • Skin herniorrhaphy | |
| | • Prolene | | | • Herniorrhaphy<br>• Rectus sheath | |
| | • Silk | | | • Skin of the abdomen<br>• Ligation of internal iliac artery | |
| | • Dacron | | | | |

***(B) Nonabsorbable:***
  (i) **Biological**
    - **Silk** suture can be handled and tied easily. It has excellent knot security. It is sterilized by gamma radiation. It is a foreign protein and initiates strong inflammatory response and loses half of its tensile strength by 1 year. It should not be used in contaminated or infected tissue.
    - **Cotton** is the weakest nonabsorbable suture. It loses 50% of the tensile strength by 6 months. Wet cotton is stronger (10%) than dry cotton. It is rarely used now.
  (ii) **Synthetic**
    - **Terelene or dacron**—these are extruded from a homopolymer.
    - **Polyamide (nylon)**—this is a man-made and may be monofilament or multifilament. It is very much nonreactive in tissues. Monofilament nylon has greater tensile strength, incites less tissue reaction and is less prone to infection than braided nylon.
    - **Polypropylene (prolene)** is a hydrocarbon polymer and is monofilament. It has least tissue reaction. Knot security is greater. It is sterilized by ethylene oxide.
    - **Steel** suture is nonreactive and has highest tensile strength. It is not commonly used now in obstetrics and gynecology. This is used in orthopedic and dental surgery.

Nonabsorbable sutures maintain their tensile strength for a long time. However, there may be suture related pain or rarely sinus formation.

# INSTRUMENTS USED FOR ENDOSCOPIC SURGERY

## LAPAROSCOPIC INSTRUMENTS (FIGS. 16.47A TO C):

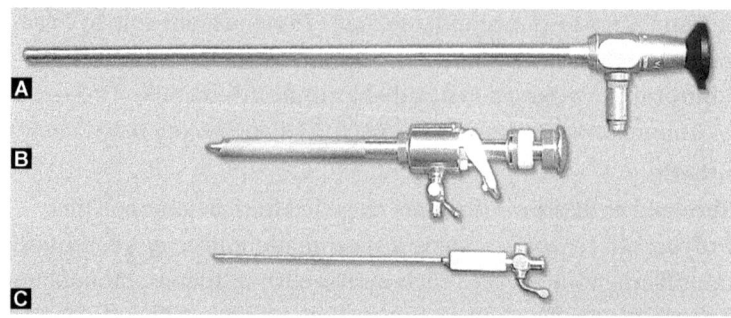

Figs. 16.47A to C: (A) Telescope; (B) Trocar and cannula; (C) Veress needle.

(a) **Telescope:** Rigid telescopes are used with rod lens system. Caliber varying from 4 to 12 mm. Angle of view may be either straightforward (0°) or oblique (30°) (Fig. 16.47A).

(b) **Trocar and cannula.**

(c) **Veress needle:** The Veress needle consists of a spring loaded blunt perforated trocar within a sharp cannula. Resistance allows the sharp cannula to protrude but when the resistance disappears, the blunt trocar protrudes out. This prevents injury to the viscera (Figs. 16.47B and C).

**Use**

It is used in laparoscopy operation to produce pneumoperitoneum. The common site of puncture is through a small incision made in the lower rim of the umbilicus.

## TROCAR AND CANNULA (FIG. 16.48)

The instrument is introduced through the same infraumbilical incision through which Veress needle is passed at an angulation of 45° towards the pelvis.

After its introduction, trocar is withdrawn and the telescope is introduced. It is then attached to the cold light source.

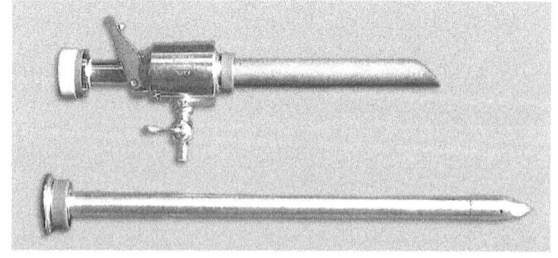

Fig. 16.48: Cannula and trocar—separated.

## Self-assessment:

**Q. What are the indications of laparoscopy?**

**Ans.** See p. 530.

**Q. What are the complications of laparoscopy?**

**Ans.** See p. 531.

**Q. What distension media is used in laparoscopy?**

**Ans.** Carbon dioxide gas is commonly used.

**Q. Mention the advantages and disadvantages of laparoscopic sterilization operation over conventional methods.**

**Ans.** See p. 542.

**Q. Discuss briefly the pneumoperitoneum?**

**Ans.** Pneumoperitoneum is created with a especially designed needle called Veress needle. It is introduced into the peritoneal cavity making a small incision (1.25 cm) below the umbilicus. Abdomen is inflated with about 1–4 L of carbon dioxide gas. Intraperitoneal pressure should not increase >20 mm Hg.

**Q. Why $CO_2$ is preferred for the creation of pneumoperitoneum?**

**Ans.** (a) $CO_2$ is a gas soluble in blood and is rapidly absorbed
(b) Risk of embolism is less
(c) It does not support combustion when electrodiathermy is used inside.

**Q. How the correct placement of Veress needle is ascertained?**

**Ans.** Different methods are there to ascertain the correct placement of the needle;
(a) Hanging drop method.
(b) Syringe barrel test: Aspiration is done to exclude inadvertent injury to any organ. (examples are: Blood from vessel puncture, urine from bladder puncture and fecal matter from bowel puncture).
(c) Low intra-abdominal pressure (<10 mm Hg) on correct placement of the needle.
(d) Obliteration of liver dullness on percussion when there is free flow of $CO_2$ inside the abdominal cavity.

**Q. What are the different methods of hemostasis used during laparoscopic surgery?**

**Ans.** (1) Electrocoagulation:
  (a) Monopolar electrosurgery
  (b) Bipolar electrosurgery
(2) Laser coagulation (using $CO_2$, KTP-532, Nd-YAG lasers)
(3) Ligasure—to cut and seal blood vessels
(4) Enseal vessels fusion where tissues are desiccated and cut
(5) Mechanical clips and staples (titanium clips and staples)
(6) Sutures as used in open surgery.

**Q. What are the complications of laparoscopic surgery?**

**Ans.** Complications may be specific to laparoscopic surgery. These are:

(a) Extraperitoneal insufflation leading to surgical emphysema.

(b) Cardiac arrhythmias due to $CO_2$ absorption.

(c) Injury to blood vessels (mesenteric and inferior epigastric vessels)

(d) Injury to viscera: Bowel and bladder

(e) Complications due to electrosurgical methods: Thermal injury to bowel, bladder and ureter.

(f) Other complications are due to anesthesia, infections, hemorrhage, etc.

**Q. What are the contraindications of laparoscopy?**

**Ans.** (a) Severe cardiopulmonary disease

(b) Patient hemodynamically unstable

(c) Extensive peritoneal adhesions

(d) Generalized peritonitis.

## HYSTEROSCOPIC INSTRUMENTS (FIGS. 16.49A TO C)

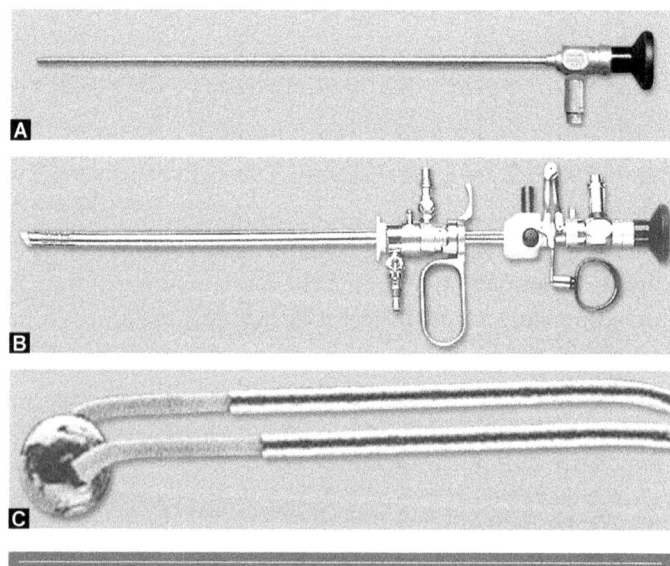

**Figs. 16.49A to C:** Hysteroscopic instruments.

(a) **Telescope:** Rigid telescopes are commonly used. The telescope may be either straight on (0°) or for oblique view 30°. Flexible telescopes are also used (Fig. 16.49A).

(b) **Telescope with working elements (Fig. 16.49B).**

(c) **Electrodes (coagulating roller ball electrode) (Fig. 16.49C).**

## Self-assessment:

**Q. What is hysteroscopy?**

**Ans.** Endoscopic visualization of the cervical canal as well as the uterine cavity, is known as hysteroscopy. Hysteroscopy may be done for diagnostic as well as therapeutic purposes.

**Q. What are the indications of hysteroscopy?**

**Ans.** *See* p. 537.

**Q. What distension media is used in hysteroscopy?**

**Ans.** Commonly used liquid media—glycine 1.5%. It does not conduct electricity. Other media used for hysteroscopy are:
- Liquid media: Normal saline, mannitol (5%)
- Gas media: Carbon dioxide ($CO_2$).

**Q. What are the complications of hysteroscopy?**

**Ans.** *See* p. 538.

**Q. What is the distension media used in hysteroscopy?**

**Ans.** (a) $CO_2$
(b) Normal saline
(c) Glycine 1.5%
(d) Mannitol (5%).

**Q. What are the contraindications of hysteroscopy?**

**Ans.** (a) Pelvic infection
(b) Pregnancy
(c) Cervical cancer
(d) Cardiopulmonary disorders.

## 16B. SPECIMENS

### Chapter Objectives
**Good knowledge and understanding of:**
- Description of the specimen based on the anatomical structures
- Macroscopic description of organ(s) with associated pathology
- Surgical procedures done in relation to such pathology
- Expected histopathology
- Management options
- Follow-up management

## SPECIMENS IN GYNECOLOGY

**Description:**

The description of a specimen includes:
- Identification of the organ(s)
- To describe the pathology as seen on naked eye examination.

**Identification of the organ(s)**

*Uterus*

*The uterus is identified by:*
- Pear-shaped structure
- Adnexal attachment
- Cervical opening: Circular in nulliparous—transverse slit in parous.

*Anterior surface is identified by:*
- Attachment of round ligament
- Loose attachment of uterovesical peritoneum.

*Posterior surface is identified by:*
- Attachment of ovarian ligament with or without ovary.
- Cut margin of the posterior peritoneum which is densely attached and placed at a lower level than the cut edge of the anterior peritoneum.

*Uterine tubes:* Tubular structures with abdominal ostium surrounded by fimbriae and mesosalpinx.

*Ovary:* Fallopian tube is usually attached to the ovarian specimen. If the uterine tube is not mounted, even then the specimen is likely to be ovarian as there is no other pelvic organs resembling it, exception being a parovarian cyst (*see* Fig. 16.67).

*Structures attached at the cornu of the uterus:*
(1) Round ligament—a cord-like structure attached anteriorly and running laterally.
(2) Fallopian tube—round and a tube-like structure and extending laterally towards the ovary as fimbrial end. It lies in the middle.
(3) Ligament of the ovary—a small and cord-like structure attached posterolaterally going to the ovary (*see* p. 513, Fig. 15.18).

## SPECIMEN — 1 (FIG. 16.50) AND SPECIMEN — 2 (FIGS. 16.51 AND 16.52)

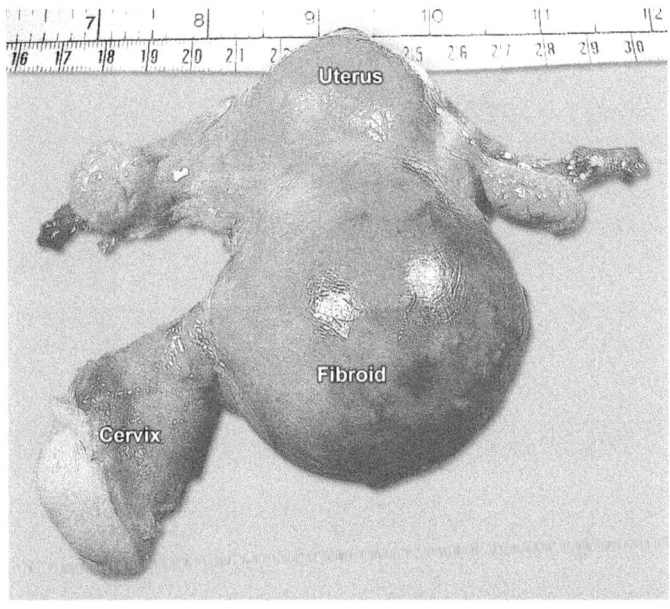

**Fig. 16.50:** Huge fibroid uterus.

**Description:** This is a specimen of uterus with tubes and ovaries of both the sides (Fig. 16.50).

There is alteration in the size (enlarged) and shape (irregular) of the uterus due to (multiple) fibroid(s). The fibroids are of different sizes. Some are cut open to show whorled appearance (Fig. 16.52). A capsule is seen surrounding it (interstitial fibroid) or part of the tumor is covered by endometrium (submucous fibroid Fig. 16.51) or a part is covered by serous coat (subserous fibroid Fig. 16.52). One subserous fibroid has got a pedicle (Fig. 16.52)—pedunculated.

The tubes and the ovaries are looking normal.
**Operation done:** Total hysterectomy with bilateral salpingo-oophorectomy.
**Diagnosis:** Multiple fibroids of the body of the uterus.

*Self-assessment*

**Q. What are the causes of menorrhagia?**

**Ans.**
- Increased surface area of the endometrium
  - Interference with normal uterine contractility due to interposition of fibroid
  - Pelvic congestion
  - Hyperplastic endometrium due to hyperestrogenism.

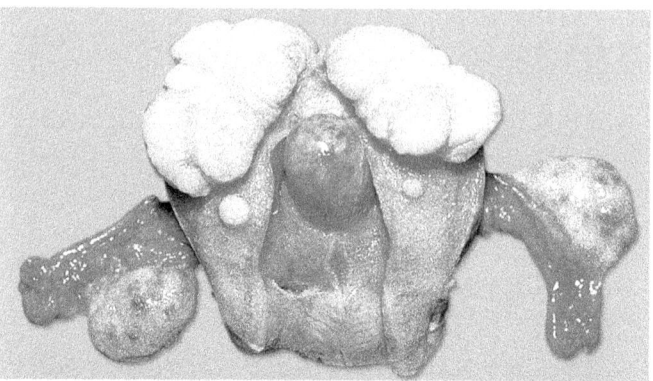

**Fig. 16.51:** Fibroid uterus — Subserous, interstitial and submucous variety. Specimen 2, fig. 16.52 has got a huge subserous (arrow) and also a pedunculated subserous variety of fibroid (arrow). Both the specimens are cut-opened to show the endometrial cavity. Both the cavities are increased and distorted.

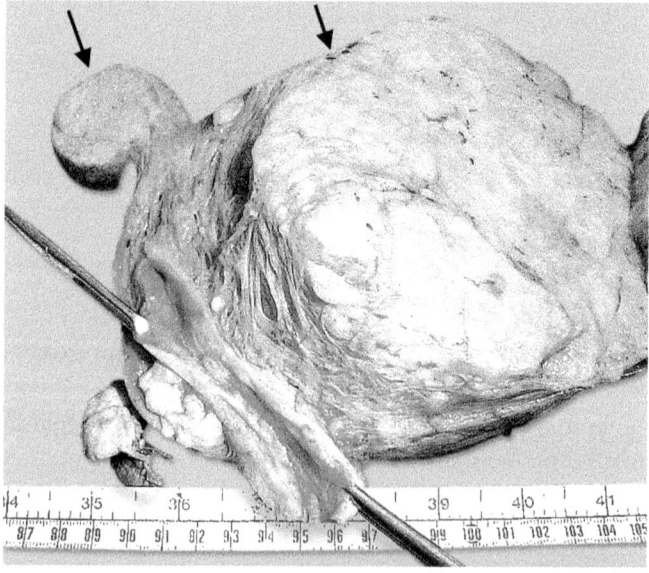

**Fig. 16.52:** Uterine cavity is shown with Allis tissue forceps.

**Q. What are the causes of infertility?**

**Ans.**
- Distortion of uterine cavity
- Endometrial congestion causing failure of nidation
- Ulceration of endometrium (endometritis) causing defective nidation
- Associated anovulation
- Associated tubal block.

**Q. What are the causes of pelvic pain?**

**Ans.**
- Degeneration of fibroid
- Extrusion of polyp
- Associated with endometriosis
- Pelvic infection (PID).

**Q. How to differentiate a fibroid from an ovarian tumor on clinical examination?**

**Ans.** Detailed history taking and clinical examination are helpful to differentiate the two.

**History** of menorrhagia, dysmenorrhagia, slow growth favors fibroid.

**Abdominal examination :** On palpation—fibroid feels firm in consistency and may be with irregular surface. Ovarian mass is cystic in feel and the surface is smooth.

| Uterine (fibroid) | Ovarian tumor |
|---|---|
| Abdominal examination difficult to differentiate at times ||
| Bimanual examination ||
| • Uterus is not felt separated from the mass <br> • On moving the cervix by vaginal fingers: The mass felt per abdomen also moves simultaneously <br> • On moving the mass per abdomen: The cervix moves as felt by the vaginal fingers | • Uterus is felt separated from the mass <br> • The mass felt by the abdominal hand does not move <br><br><br><br> • The cervix does not move |
| **Exception:** Pelvic adhesions that may fix the mass to the uterus ||

**Q. What is the place of medical management?**

**Ans.** Medical management is aimed to improve the symptoms of the woman. The common indications of medical management are:
(a) To improve menorrhagia
(b) To correct anemia
(c) To relieve pelvic pain.

**Q. What are the different types of medical management available?**

Ans.
- Prostaglandin synthetase inhibitors
- COCs
- LNG-IUS
- GnRH analogs:
  - Agonists
  - Antagonists
- Danazol
- Antiprogesterone (mifepristone)
- Progesterone receptor modulators.

**Q. What is the place of hysterectomy?**

Ans. Elderly women (>40 years) with symptomatic fibroid who have completed their family are considered for hysterectomy. There is no risk of recurrence of either fibroid or menorrhagia following hysterectomy.

**Q. What could be the presentation of the woman in the clinic?**

Ans. **NB:** As these specimens are obtained following total hysterectomy, such women are unlikely to suffer from infertility. As bilateral oophorectomy had been done, their probable age would be >45 years.

**Q. What are the different treatment options available for fibroids?**

Ans. (a) Surgery—
    (i) Myomectomy
    (ii) Hysterectomy
    (iii) Myolysis.

    Myomectomy may be done by:
    (i) Laparotomy
    (ii) Laparoscopy
    (iii) Hysteroscopy

(b) Medical therapy (*see* p. 378)

(c) Interventional radiology—uterine artery embolization.

(d) MRI-guided High intensity focussed ultrasound *see* p. 378)

(e) Myolysis (*see* p. 378).

**Q. How do you differentiate fibroid uterus from adenomyosis?**

Ans. *See* p. 486, 637.

**Q. What are the indications of myomectomy?**

Ans. *See* p. 516.

**Q. What are the prerequisites to myomectomy?**

Ans. *See* p. 568.

**Q. What are the contraindications to myomectomy?**

**Ans.** *See* p. 516.

## SPECIMEN — 3 (FIG. 16.53)

**Description:** This is a specimen of uterus with tubes and ovaries of both the sides.

Anterior surface of the uterus is cut open to show a mass arising from the fundus protruding into the uterine cavity. Another mass is seen to come out of the uterus through the cervical canal with a long pedicle.

**Operation done:** Total hysterectomy with bilateral salpingo-oophorectomy.

**Diagnosis:** Submucous fibroid-polyps—sessile and pedunculated.

*Self-assessment:*

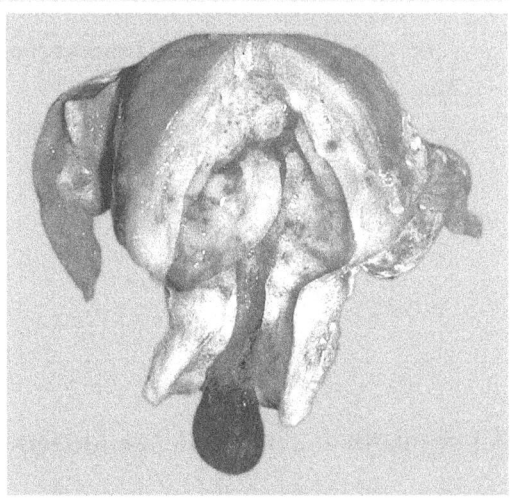

Fig. 16.53: Submucous fibroid polyps (sessile and pedunculated). Patient suffered menorrhagia, metrorrhagia and dysmenorrhea.

**Q. What would be the clinical presentation in such a case (Fig. 16.53)?**

**Ans.** Common clinical presentation in such a woman is:

(A) Menstrual abnormality:
- Menorrhagia
- Dysmenorrhea
- Metrorrhagia.

(B) Pain abdomen.

**Q. How do you confirm the diagnosis?**

**Ans.** (A) Clinically, the pedunculated polyp can be seen on speculum examination
(B) Ultrasonography can be helpful in the diagnosis
(C) Sonohysterography
(D) Hysteroscopy with direct visualization of the polyps.

**Q. When do myomas require to be removed (indications of myomectomy)?**

**Ans.** (i) Any myoma growing during the follow-up period.
(ii) Menorrhagia not responding to medical therapy.
(iii) Excessive pain or pressure symptoms.
(iv) Woman with infertility or recurrent miscarriage when no cause other than fibroid is present.

**Q. What are the secondary changes in a fibroid?**

**Ans.** (A) Degenerations (common = hyaline 65%)

(B) Atrophy (postmenopausal age)

(C) Necrosis

(D) Sarcomatous charge (rare).

**Q. What are the different treatment options available for fibroids?**

**Ans.** (A) Medical and (B) Surgical

(A) Medical: Drugs used are—prostaglandin synthetase inhibitors, GnRH analogues, antiprogesterone (mifepristone) and LNG-IUS.

(B) Surgical methods include:
- Myomectomy
- Embolotherapy
- Myolysis
- Hysterectomy.

## SPECIMEN — 4 (FIGS. 16.54A AND B)

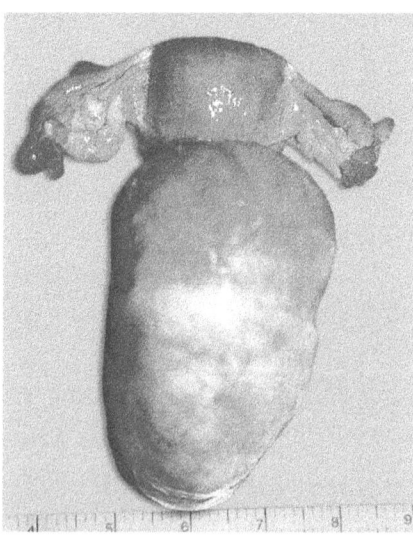

**Fig. 16.54A:** A huge posterior cervical fibroid.

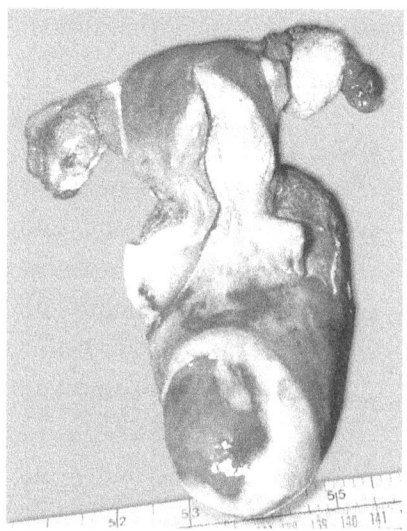

**Fig. 16.54B:** Same specimen as in Fig. 16.54A, is seen from the anterior surface.

**Description:** This is a specimen of uterus (Fig. 16.54A) with tubes and ovaries of both the sides. There is a huge mass arising from the posterior cervical wall. The small uterus sits on the top of the huge mass. (Lantern on dome of St. Paul's).

The anterior surface of the uterus (Fig. 16.54B) is cut open to show the anterior cervical wall and the uterine cavity.

**Operation done:** Total hysterectomy with bilateral salpingo-oophorectomy with removal of the mass.

**Diagnosis:** Cervical fibroid (posterior).

*Self-assessment:*

**Q. What are the types of cervical fibroid?**

**Ans.** (1) Anterior cervical: May produce urinary symptoms (retention).
(2) Posterior cervical: May cause rectal symptoms (constipation).
(3) Lateral cervical: Compression effect to blood vessels and displacement of the ureter.
(4) Central cervical: (Lantern on the dome of St Paul's).

**Q. Modes of presentation in a case with cervical fibroid?**

**Ans.** Woman often present with pressure symptoms depending upon the location of the fibroid.

**Q. Approach for surgical removal of cervical myoma?**

**Ans.** It depends upon the location of the myoma—anterior approach for anterior cervical myoma, posterior approach for posterior cervical myoma. For central cervical myoma, central approach through uterovesical pouch is done otherwise hemisection of the uterus is done to reach the myoma. The myoma is enucleated (intracapsular).

**Q. What type of uterine fibroid has the risks of ureteric injury?**

**Ans.** Cervical fibroids may compress the ureters. There is lateral displacement of the ureter in a lateral cervical fibroid. Ureter lies outside the capsule of the fibroid. Myomectomy should be done intracapsular.

**Q. What are the common gynecological pathologies where ureteric injury is more likely?**

**Ans.** Common pelvic pathology to cause ureteric injury are:
- Cervical fibroid
- Broad ligament tumor
- Pelvic endometriosis
- Gynecological malignancy
- Radical hysterectomy
- Colposuspension.

## SPECIMEN — 5 (FIGS. 16.55A AND B)

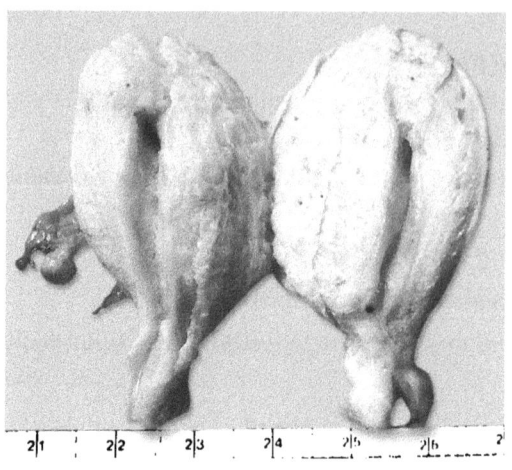

Fig. 16.55A: Specimen of adenomyosis.

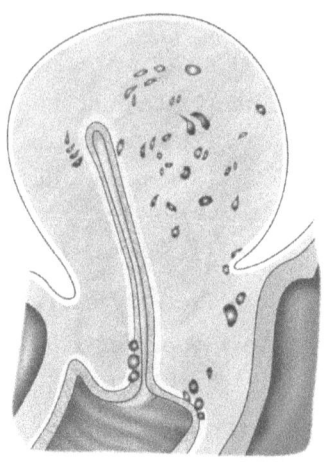

Fig. 16.55B: Adenomyosis (diagrammatic).

**Description:** This is a specimen of the uterus, the tubes and ovaries of both the sides. The uterus is enlarged and is cut open to show a diffuse growth located at one wall. The growth presents a striated appearance with scattered dark hemorrhagic spots. It has got no capsule (whereas in a case with fibroid uterus, it has whorled appearance and a capsule).

**Operation done:** Total hysterectomy with bilateral salpingo-oophorectomy.

**Diagnosis:** Adenomyosis.

*Self-assessment:*

    **Q. Mention the clinical features of pelvic endometriosis.**

**Ans.** See p. 445-446.

    **Q. Causes of infertility in endometriosis.**

**Ans.** Common causes are: Anovulation, luteal phase defect, dyspareunia, adhesion formation, poor oocyte quality, implantation failure, immunological.

    **Q. Mention the clinical features of adenomyosis.**

**Ans.** See p. 448.

    **Q. Describe the histological picture of adenomyosis.**

**Ans.** See p. 637.

    **Q. Outline the treatment for pelvic endometriosis.**

**Ans.** See p. 446-447.

    **Q. Outline the treatment for adenomyosis.**

**Ans.** See p. 448.

## SPECIMEN — 6 (FIG. 16.56)

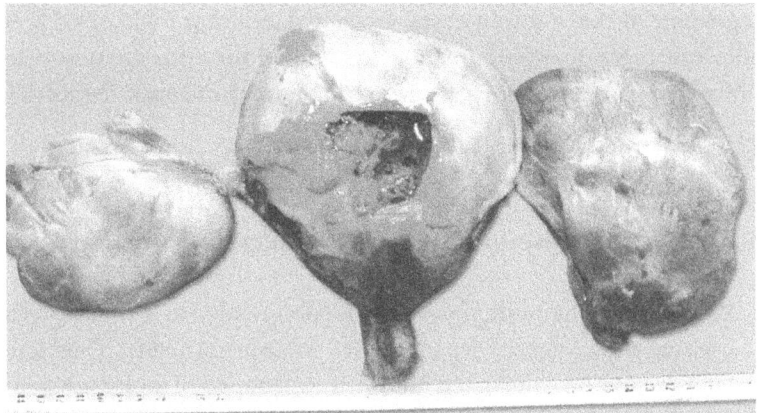

**Fig. 16.56:** Hydatidiform mole with bilateral large theca lutein cysts.

**Description:** This is a specimen of the uterus with tubes and ovaries of both the sides. The ovaries are hugely enlarged, lobulated with a yellowish tinge. The uterus is also enlarged. Vesicular mass is seen protruding out through the window of the incised uterus.

**Operation done:** Total hysterectomy with bilateral salpingo-oophorectomy.

**Diagnosis:** Hydatidiform mole with large theca lutein cysts of both the ovaries.

*Self-assessment:*

*Q. What are the high-risk factors for gestational trophoblastic neoplasia (GTN)?*

Ans.
- Duration of disease >4 months
- Initial serum β–hCG >40,000 mIU/mL
- Metastasis to brain or liver
- Failure of prior chemotherapy
- GTN developing following a term pregnancy
- WHO score is ≥7.

*Q. Mention the clinical features of GTN.*

Ans.
- Persistent ill health
- Irregular vaginal bleeding, at times heavy
- Symptoms due to metastasis
- Lung: Cough, hemoptysis
- Cerebral: Convulsions, headache, coma
- Liver: Jaundice
- Vagina: Bleeding.

*Q. What is the management protocol of GTN?*

Ans. Management protocol includes:
  (A) Chemotherapy (single agent or multiple agent)
  (B) Surgery: Hysterectomy

(C) Radiation therapy for brain metastasis

(D) Combination therapy.

- **Management of theca lutein cysts:** Once hydatidiform mole or GTN is treated, spontaneous regression (within a few months) of the cysts are observed. Rarely, they are removed when complications like torsion or intracystic hemorrhage occur.

*Q. What are the common sites of metastasis?*

Ans. See p. 484.

*Q. What is the place of prophylactic chemotherapy and what are its limitations?*

Ans. Prophylactic chemotherapy is not recommended as a routine as the drugs used are toxic. Majority of patients (80–90%) do not need it. Therefore, women "at risk" may be considered following evacuation of molar pregnancy.

*Q. WHO scoring system for risk assessment.*

Ans. (a) Age is >35 years

(b) Initial serum levels of hCG is ≥100,000 IU/mL

(c) Failure of hCG to become normal by 7–9 weeks, time or there is re-elevation

(d) Evidence of metastatic disease

(e) Recurrent molar pregnancy

(f) Patient unreliable for follow-up.

*Q. Reproductive behavior of women following treatment of GTN.*

Ans. Usually, there is no adverse effect on subsequent pregnancy. However, risk of premature ovarian failure and secondary malignancy have been observed.

## ▋ SPECIMEN — 7 (FIG. 16.57)

**Description:** This is the specimen of a uterus with the tubes and ovaries. The uterus is enlarged. The anterior surface of the uterus is cut open to show a purplish growth invading the myometrium. The tube and the ovary are looking healthy.

*This 43-year-old parous lady was admitted with irregular bleeding PV following a miscarriage. She underwent D and C thrice. Her serum β-hCG level following the present admission was 2,09,755 mIU/mL. Even following courses of multiagent chemotherapy, the serum hCG level remained persistently elevated.*

**Operation done:** Total hysterectomy. Histology confirmed choriocarcinoma.

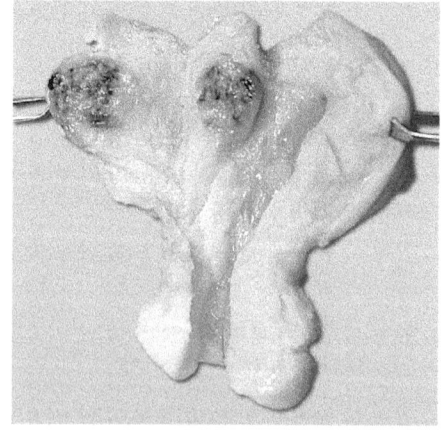

**Fig. 16.57:** Hemorrhagic growth is seen within the myometrium. Patient was resistant to chemotherapy.

**Diagnosis:** Choriocarcinoma of the uterus.

*Self-assessment:*

**Q. How the selection of chemotherapy regimen is done?**

**Ans.** In general, patients with nonmetastatic (low-risk) and good prognosis disease are treated with single agent therapy. Methotrexate or actinomycin D is commonly used. However, patients with poor prognosis, high-risk and or metastatic disease are treated with combination drug (EMACO) regimen.

**Q. What is the place of hysterectomy in GTN?**

**Ans.**
- Elderly females, family completed
- Placental site trophoblastic tumor
- Lesion resistant to chemotherapy.

**Q. How is the follow-up done in such case?**

**Ans.** Follow-up is done for all patients at least for 2 years. Serum β-hCG is measured weekly till negative → monthly for 6 months → 6 monthly thereafter.

## SPECIMEN — 8 (FIG. 16.58)

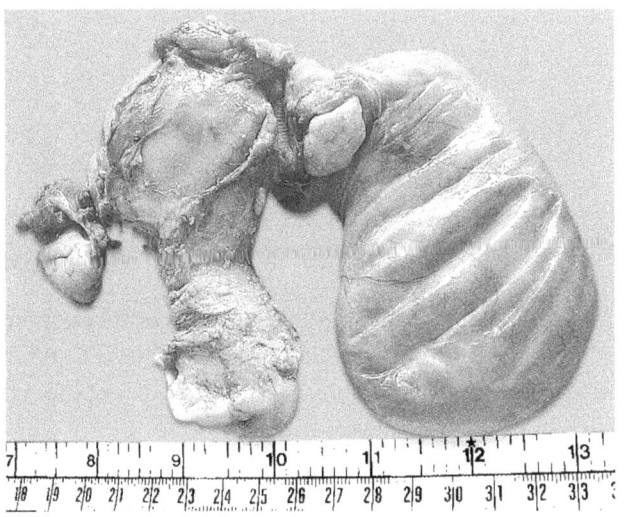

**Fig. 16.58:** Specimen of total hysterectomy with bilateral salpingo-oophorectomy showing a large hydrosalpinx (retort-shaped) of the left tube.

**Description:** This is a specimen of uterus, tubes and ovaries of both the sides. The left tube is markedly enlarged especially towards the outer half. The shape looks like a 'retort'. The inside fluid appears to be clear.

**Diagnosis:** Hydrosalpinx of the left tube.

*Self-assessment:*

**Q. Mention the pathogenesis of hydrosalpinx.**
**Ans.** See p. 493.

**Q. Mention the common organisms involved in pathology.**
**Ans.** See p. 413.

**Q. How is the mode of affection in gonococcal infection?**
**Ans.** See p. 413.

**Q. Explain the cause of the 'retort' shape.**
**Ans.** See p. 493.

**Q. Mention the steps of salpingectomy.**
**Ans.** (Dutta Gyne 7/e, p. 496).

## SPECIMEN — 9 (FIG. 16.59)

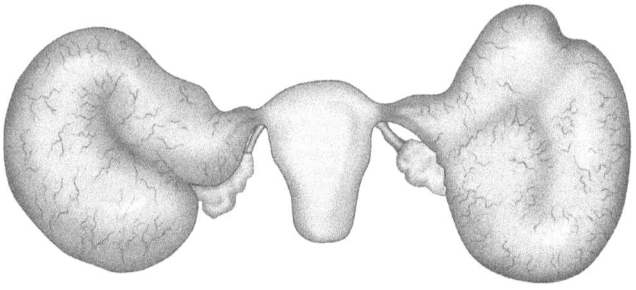

**Fig. 16.59:** Specimen of bilateral pyosalpinx.

**Description:** This is a specimen of the uterus, tubes and ovaries of both the sides. The tubes of both sides are hugely dilated, coiled, wall is thickened and matted with the ovaries. There are evidences of adhesions over the surfaces of the tubes and uterus. Pus is coming out of through the fimbrial end of the tube.

**Diagnosis:** Bilateral pyosalpinx.

*Self-assessment:*

**Q. What is the pathogenesis of bilateral hydrosalpinx?**
**Ans.** It is usually the end result of repeated attacks of endosalpingitis by pyogenic organisms. The common organisms *E. coli*, chlamydia treatments or Gonococcus.

**Q. Mention the clinical presentation of such a case.**
**Ans.** (a) Abdominal tenderness
(b) Adnexal tenderness
(c) Formation of tubo-ovarian mass.

**Q. What is the mode of spread for pyogenic, tuberculosis of other infections?**

**Ans.** (a) Pyogenic: Through lymphatic of pelvic viscera
(b) Tubercular: Through bloodstream
(c) Gonococcal: Through continuity.

**Q. Mention the complications of acute PID and the late sequelae.**

**Ans.** (a) Dyspareunia
(b) Infertility
(c) Adhesion formation
(d) Chronic pelvic pain.

## SPECIMEN — 10 (FIG. 16.60)

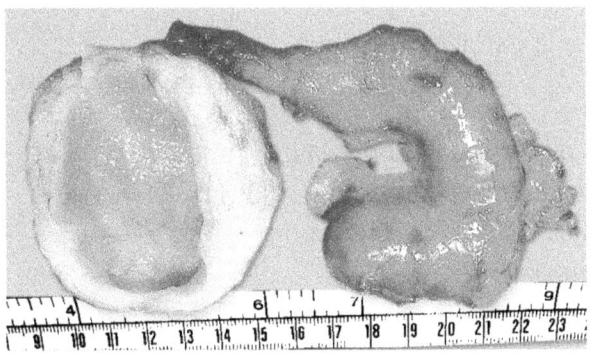

**Fig. 16.60:** Hematosalpinx of the right tube.

**Description:** This is a specimen of a noncommunicating horn of a bicornuate uterus (cut-opened) with the tube. The tube is elongated, sausage-shaped and purplish in color. The cut-open uterus shows the cavity which was filled with blood. The tube is filled with blood.

**Operation done:** Excision of the noncommunicating horn and the tube (salpingectomy).

**Diagnosis:** Rudimentary horn of the uterus with hematosalpinx.

*Self-assessment:*

**Q. Mention the causes of hematosalpinx.**

**Ans.** Tubal ectopic pregnancy, endometriosis, cryptomenorrhea and rarely primary tubal carcinoma (0.3% of all genital malignancies).

**Q. What are the causes of cryptomenorrhea?**

**Ans.** (1) Imperforate hymen
(2) Cervical stenosis
(3) Vaginal stenosis or atresia.

**Q. What is the clinical presentation of a tubal carcinoma?**

**Ans.** **Triad of** lower abdominal pain (colicky), profuse watery discharge (hydrops tubae profluens) and vaginal bleeding. Preoperative diagnosis is rare and often mistaken as an ovarian tumor.

## SPECIMEN — 11 (FIGS. 16.61A AND B)

**Description:** These are the specimens of the uterus with tube and ovary of the right side. The ovarian cysts (right) are cut open to show inspissated sebaceous material, hair and other mature (mesenchymal) tissues. Teeth is present in about a third (*see* Figs. 16.61A and B, and 16.85 and 16.86).

**Operation done:** Total hysterectomy with bilateral salpingo-oophorectomy.

**Diagnosis:** Dermoid cyst of the right ovary.

*Self-assessment*

Q. *Name the tissues arising from the three germ cell layers.*

**Ans.** Ectoderm: Hair, Mesoderm: Cartilage, Endoderm: Glands.

Q. *What is the frequency of bilaterality in dermoid cyst?*

**Ans.** Frequency of bilaterality is about 15–20%.

Q. *Common complication of dermoid.*

**Ans.** Torsion.

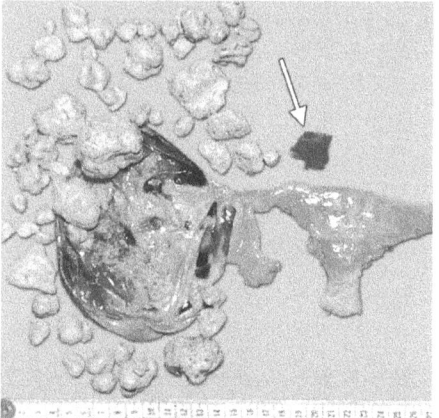

**Fig. 16. 61A:** Gross appearance of a dermoid cyst of the ovary showing hair, teeth (arrow) and butter balls (sebum aggregated to form spherules).

Q. *Management of dermoid in a young patient.*

**Ans.** Cystectomy.

Q. *Risk of malignant change in dermoid.*

**Ans.** Risk of malignant change is about 1–2%.

Q. *What are strumal carcinoids?*

**Ans.** These are teratomas and secrete serotonin (5-HT), and bradykinin. Patients usually present with the symptoms of abdominal pain, facial flushing, diarrhea or bronchospasm.

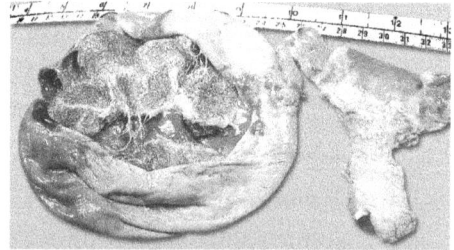

**Fig. 16.61B:** Gross appearance of dermoid cyst of the ovary with hair and sebaceous material (cut section).

**Q. How carcinoid tumors of the ovary are treated?**

**Ans.** Excision of the tumor (ovariotomy) causes rapid fall in the serum level of serotonin and disappearance of 5-hydroxyindoleacetic acid in the urine. There is rapid remission of symptoms.

## SPECIMEN — 12 (FIG. 16.62)

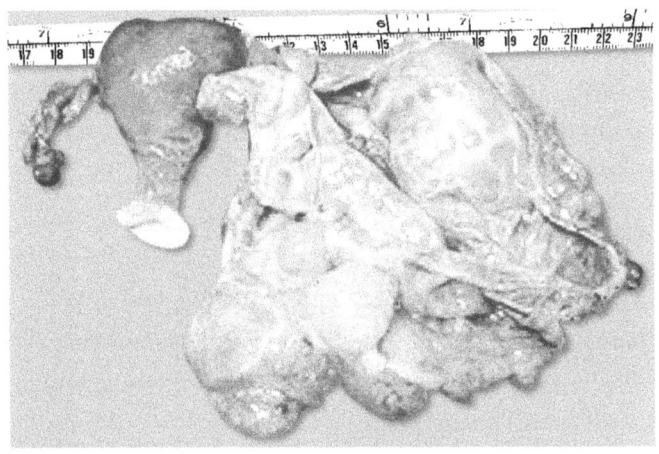

**Fig. 16.62:** Left-sided mucinous cystadenoma (gross appearance on cut specimen).

**Description:** This is a specimen of the uterus with tubes and ovaries of both the sides. The left-sided ovarian cyst is cut-open to show many septa. There are few smaller cysts projecting inside.

**Operation done:** Total hysterectomy with bilateral salpingo-oophorectomy.

**Diagnosis:** Mucinous cystadenoma.

*Self-assessment:*

**Q. What are the common epithelial tumors of the ovary?**

**Ans.** See p. 384, 487.

**Q. Discuss the differential diagnosis of a pelvic abdominal lump.**

**Ans.** See p. 490.

**Q. Mention the clinical presentation of a benign ovarian tumor.**

**Ans.** See p. 387.

**Q. What are the features of a functional cyst?**

**Ans.** See p. 384.

**Q. How a benign ovarian tumor could be differentiated from a malignant one clinically?**

**Ans.** See p. 385.

**Q. How laparotomy findings could be helpful to differentiate a benign tumor from a malignant one?**
Ans. See p. 385.

**Q. What are psammoma bodies?**
Ans. See p. 490.

**Q. What are the complications of a benign ovarian tumor?**
Ans. See p. 383.

**Q. Outline the management of a benign ovarian tumor.**
Ans. See p. 386.

**Q. What are the structures forming the ovarian pedicle?**
Ans. Structures forming the ovarian pedicle are:
Laterally: (a) Infundibulopelvic ligament
Medially:
(a) Ovarian ligament
(b) Medial end of the fallopian tube
(c) Mesosalpinx containing utero-ovarian anastomosis.
Middle: Part of broad ligament.

## SPECIMEN — 13 (FIG. 16.63)

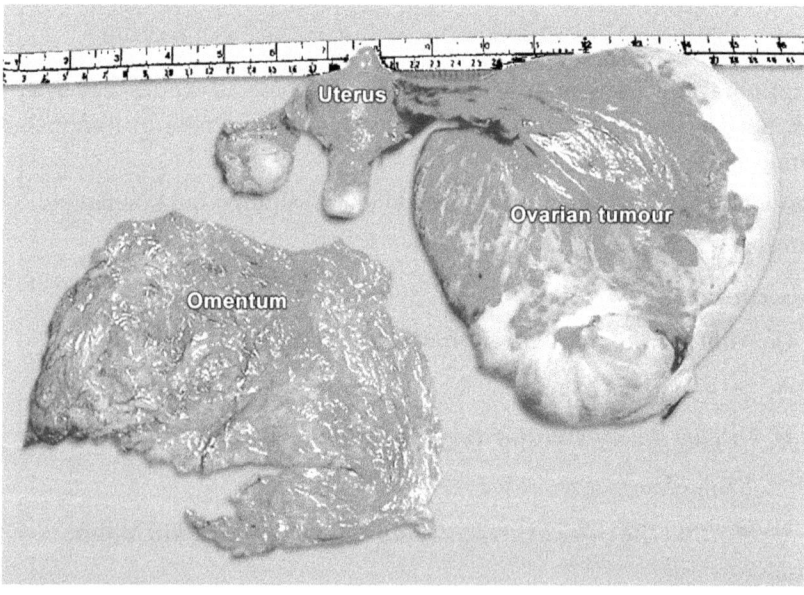

**Fig. 16.63:** Bilateral mucinous cystadenocarcinoma (confirmed on histology). Total hysterectomy, bilateral salpingo-oophorectomy with total omentectomy done.

**Description:** This is a pathological specimen of the uterus and both the ovaries. The ovaries are: Enlarged are lobulated with the walls being irregular and shaggy. Cut section shows solid areas with hemorrhage and necrosis at places.

**Diagnosis:** Most likely malignant ovarian tumors.

## Self-assessment:

**Q. Mention the clinical features of a malignant ovarian tumor.**

**Ans.** See p. 387.

**Q. Describe the FIGO staging of ovarian, tubal and peritoneal cancer.**

**Ans.** Current FIGO staging considers all the three organs under the same staging category and the management approach (see Table 16.1 for FIGO staging 2018).

**Table 16.1.** Figo staging of carcinoma of the ovary, tube and peritoneum (2018).

| |
|---|
| **Stage I: Tumor confined to ovaries or fallopian tube(s)** |
| T1-N0-M0 |
| IA: Tumor limited to 1 ovary (capsule intact) or fallopian tube; no tumor on ovarian or fallopian tube surface; no malignant cells in the ascites or peritoneal washings |
| T1a-N0-M0 |
| IB: Tumor limited to both ovaries (capsules intact) or fallopian tubes; no tumor on ovarian or fallopian tube surface; no malignant cells in the ascites or peritoneal washings |
| T1b-N0-M0 |
| IC: Tumor limited to 1 or both ovaries or fallopian tubes, with any of the following: |
| IC1: Surgical spill |
| T1c1-N0-M0 |
| IC2: Capsule ruptured before surgery or tumor on ovarian or fallopian tube surface |
| T1c2-N0-M0 |
| IC3: Malignant cells in the ascites or peritoneal washings |
| T1c3-N0-M0 |
| **Stage II: Tumor involves 1 or both ovaries or fallopian tubes with pelvic extension (below pelvic brim) or peritoneal cancer** |
| T2-N0-M0 |
| IIA: Extension and/or implants on uterus and/or fallopian tubes and/or ovaries |
| T2a-N0-M0 |
| IIB: Extension to other pelvic intraperitoneal tissues |
| T2b-N0-M0 |
| **Stage III: Tumor involves 1 or both ovaries or fallopian tubes, or peritoneal cancer, with cytologically or histologically confirmed spread to the peritoneum outside the pelvis and/or metastasis to the retroperitoneal lymph nodes** |
| T1/T2-N1-M0 |
| IIIA1: Positive retroperitoneal lymph nodes only (cytologically or histologically proven): |
| IIIA1(i) Metastasis up to 10 mm in greatest dimension |
| IIIA1(ii) Metastasis more than 10 mm in greatest dimension |
| IIIA2: Microscopic extrapelvic (above the pelvic brim) peritoneal involvement with or without positive retroperitoneal lymph nodes |
| T3a2-N0/N1-M0 |

*Contd...*

*Contd...*

| |
|---|
| IIIB: Macroscopic peritoneal metastasis beyond the pelvis up to 2 cm in greatest dimension, with or without metastasis to the retroperitoneal lymph nodes |
| T3b-N0/N1-M0 |
| IIIC: Macroscopic peritoneal metastasis beyond the pelvis more than 2 cm in greatest dimension, with or without metastasis to the retroperitoneal lymph nodes (includes extension of tumor to capsule of liver and spleen without parenchymal involvement of either organ) |
| T3c-N0/N1-M0 |
| **Stage IV: Distant metastasis excluding peritoneal metastases** |
| Stage IVA: Pleural effusion with positive cytology |
| Stage IVB: Parenchymal metastases and metastases to extra-abdominal organs (including inguinal lymph nodes and lymph nodes outside of the abdominal cavity) |
| Any T, any N, M1 |

| 1.2.2.1 \| **Regional lymph nodes (N)** | 1.2.2.2 \| **Distant metastasis (M)** |
|---|---|
| 1. NX: Regional lymph nodes (N) cannot be assessed<br>2. N0: No regional lymph node metastasis.<br>3. N1: Regional lymph node metastasis | 1. MX: Distant metastasis cannot be assessed<br>2. M0: No distant metastasis<br>3. M1: Distant metastasis (excluding peritoneal metastasis) |

**Q.** *What are the common malignant ovarian tumors?*

**Ans.** *See* p. 484.

**Q.** *How omentectomy is helpful in the management of ovarian malignancies?*

**Ans.** Omentum is the common site of metastasis either microscopic or in the form of nodules. In advanced cases, omental cake is formed. Removal of omentum removes the bulk of the tumor as much as possible. This improves the result of subsequent chemotherapy or radiotherapy.

**Q.** *Is epithelial ovarian cancer hereditary?*

**Ans.** About 5-10% of all epithelial ovarian cancers are familial. There are three different syndromes of hereditary ovarian cancer:

(i) Breast/ovarian familial cancer (75-90%) (Gene mutation: *BRCA1* and *BRCA2*)

(ii) Site specific ovarian cancer (5%)

(iii) Lynch II syndrome (2%)—(Gene mutation: *MLH1*, *MSH2*, and *MSH6*). Family history of nonpolyposis colorectal cancer, endometrial cancer, ovarian cancer

**Q.** *Mention the preventive measures against ovarian malignancy.*

**Ans.** *See* p. 388.

**Q.** *Mention the high-risk factors as well as the protective factors for ovarian malignancy.*

**Ans.** *See* p. 387.

**Q. How the staging of fallopian tube cancer differ from that of ovarian cancer?**

**Ans.** Current FIGO staging considers all the three organs under the same staging category and the management approach (see Table 16.1 for FIGO staging 2018).

**Q. What are the principles of surgical approach (guidelines) in a malignant ovarian tumor?**

**Ans.** See p. 389.

**Q. What is the primary surgery done in a case of advanced malignant ovarian tumor?**

**Ans. Staging laparotomy** → Maximum cytoreductive surgery (debulking procedure) is done. This includes: Total abdominal hysterectomy, bilateral salpingo-oophorectomy, infracolicomentectomy and resection of any metastatic tumor. Cytoreductive surgery is aimed at reducing the tumor load. Lesser the residual tumor volume (<1 cm), better is the response with chemotherapy and better is the survival.

**Q. Why maximum cytoreduction is targeted?**

**Ans.** (a) Abnormal proliferation of neoplastic cells produces cell clones that are chemoresistant.
(b) Excision of huge necrotic tissues improves drug delivery to the cancer cells.
(c) Removing bulk of cancer cells, improves the immunological defense.
(d) Maximum cytoreduction removes this large volume of chemoresistant cell mass.

**Q. How serum CA-125 measurement is helpful?**

**Ans.** It is helpful with a known case of ovarian cancer to assess the prognosis of the disease:
(i) Serum CA-125 is a glycoprotein and has got more prognostic value than diagnostic.
(ii) To know the response of treatment.
(iii) To know tumor resistance to chemotherapy.
(iv) Early detection of tumor recurrence.

**Q. What other tumor markers are helpful in the management of ovarian cancer?**

**Ans.** Other tumor markers used are : HE4, CA153, TP53.

**Q. What is the place of prophylactic oophorectomy during hysterectomy?**

**Ans.** See p. 379.

## SPECIMEN — 14 (FIG. 16.64)

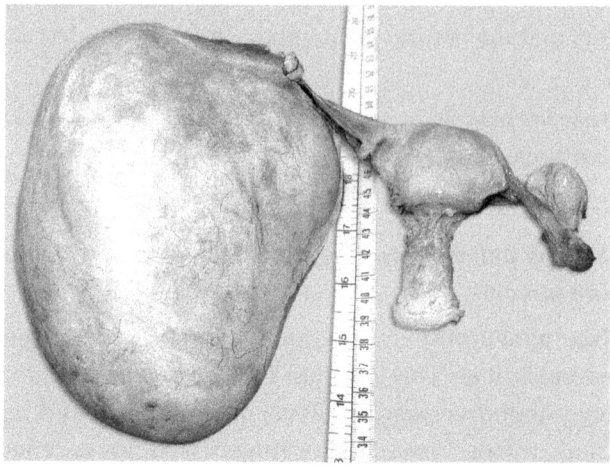

**Fig. 16.64:** Gross appearance of a solid ovarian tumor (right).

**Description:** This is a specimen of uterus with tubes and ovaries of both the sides. The right ovary is hugely enlarged and cut-opened to show its solid texture and a yellowish hue. The surface of the tumor is bosselated and glistening.

**Operation done:** Total hysterectomy with bilateral salpingo-oophorectomy.

**Diagnosis:** Solid ovarian tumor.

*Self-assessment:*

**Q. Common solid tumors of the ovary.**

**Ans. *Benign*:** Fibroma, the coma, Brenner tumor.

*Malignant:* Primary ovarian carcinoma, dysgerminoma, immature teratoma, mesonephroma.

**Q. What is Meigs' syndrome?**

**Ans.** It is a triad of findings including ascites, pleural effusion and benign ovarian fibroma. The cause is unknown. The ascites and pleural effusion resolve spontaneously when the ovarian tumor is removed.

**Q. What are the hormone producing tumors of the ovary?**

**Ans.**
- **Feminising tumors:** Granulosa cell and theca cell.
- **Masculinizing tumors:** Sertoli-Leydig cell and Hilus cell.
- **Others:** Struma ovarii (thyroid hormones) carcinoids (rare specialized germ cell ovarian tumors that secrete 5-HT).

**Q. What are germ cell tumors of the ovary?**

**Ans.** *See* p. 384.

## SPECIMEN — 15 (FIG. 16.65)

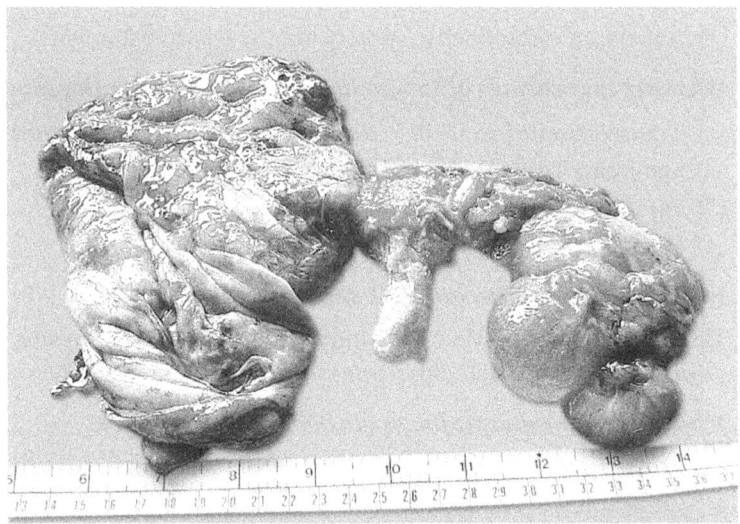

**Fig. 16.65:** Bilateral mucinous adenocarcinoma of the ovaries (gross appearance on cut specimen).

**Description:** This is a specimen of the uterus with tubes and ovaries of both the sides. The ovaries are enlarged with capsules ruptured. There is exophytic papillary growth on the surface and the growth infringes the surrounding organs. The cut surfaces show solid texture, extensive areas of hemorrhage and necrosis.

**Operation done:** Total hysterectomy with bilateral salpingo-oophorectomy.

**Diagnosis:** Bilateral ovarian carcinoma (papillary serous cystadenocarcinoma).

*Self-assessment:*

Q. *What are the reasons for difficulties in the management of ovarian cancers?*

Ans. *See* p. 491.

Q. *What are the chemotherapeutic agents commonly used?*

Ans. Commonly used drugs are:
   (1) Platinum group drugs (Cisplatin, carboplatin)
   (2) Taxane group (paclitaxel and docetaxel).
   Other newer chemotherapeutic drugs are:
   (a) Bevacizumab (antiangiogenic drug)
   (b) Pazopanib (multikinase inhibitor)
   (c) Gemcitabine.

Q. *What is the place of neoadjuvant chemotherapy for ovarian malignancy?*

Ans. Neoadjuvant chemotherapy is done in few advanced cases of epithelial ovarian cancers. This is followed by interval primary cytoreductive surgery. This is done in a case with advanced ovarian malignancy associated some comorbidity.

Benefits are:
(i) Rapid clinical improvement
(ii) Maximum cytoreductive surgery may be possible thereafter.

**Q. What are the methods of spread in a case of ovarian malignancy?**

**Ans.** (1) Transcoelomic (exfoliated cells in the peritoneal cavity) spread
(2) Lymphatic (para-aortic and superior gastric)
(3) Direct (adjacent tube and peritoneum)
(4) Hematogenous (late feature).

**Q. What is the place of second look surgery?**

**Ans.** This is less commonly done. Secondary surgery may be done in a case after primary suboptimal debulking procedure and chemotherapy.

**Q. What are the prognostic factors in ovarian malignancy?**

**Ans.** Important prognostic factors for ovarian malignancy are:
(i) Surgical stage (FIGO) of the disease (worse > stage II).
(ii) Histological type (endometrioid is better when compared to papillary serous) and grade (higher the grade, poorer the prognosis) of the tumor.
(iii) Presence of ascites: Poor outcome.
(iv) Presence of metastatic disease.

## SPECIMEN — 16

### Krukenberg tumor (Fig. 16.66)

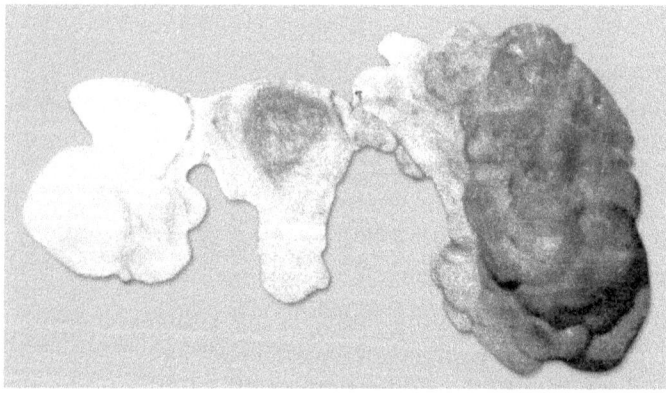

Fig. 16.66: Krukenberg tumor.

**Description:** This is a specimen of the uterus with tubes and ovaries of both the sides. The ovaries are found enlarged with lobulated appearance and are free of adhesions. The shape of the ovary is maintained. The color is pinkish with smooth surfaces. Uterus and tubes are found normal.

**Operation done:** Total hysterectomy with bilateral salpingo-oophorectomy.

**Diagnosis:** Probably Krukenberg's tumor.

## Self-assessment:

**Q. What is a Krukenberg's tumor?**

**Ans.** This is a metastatic adenocarcinoma of the ovary. Almost all metastasize from the stomach. Few arise in the breast, colon or biliary tract.

**Q. What is the suggestive appearance of the tumor for diagnosis?**

**Ans.** The tumor is usually bilateral, lobulated, solid in appearance with smooth surfaces. Usually adhesions are absent. Cut section is homogenous and may have degenerative cystic spaces.

**Q. What are the primary sites?**

**Ans.** Common primary sites are: GI tract (stomach, pylorus and colon), gallbladder, breast and endometrial carcinoma.

**Q. What is the mode of spread to the ovaries?**

**Ans.** (a) Retrograde lymphatic
(b) Transcoelomic spread

**Q. What is the histological picture of the tumor?**

**Ans.** The epithelial cells of the tumor look like 'signet ring'. These cells are characteristic of Krukenberg's tumor.

**Q. What is the prognosis of the tumor?**

**Ans.** Poor.

**Q. What is the survival rate?**

**Ans.** Median survival is less than a year in majority of the cases.

## SPECIMEN — 17 (FIG. 16.67)

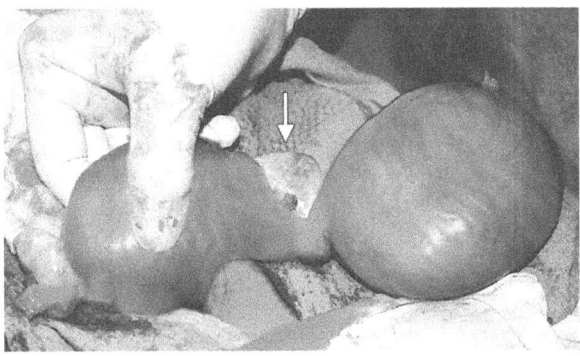

**Fig. 16.67:** At a glance, it seems to be a twisted ovarian cyst but careful inspection reveals the ovary (see arrow) is separated from the cyst.

**Description:** This is a specimen of the uterus with the tubes and ovaries. A hugely enlarged cyst is attached to the fimbrial end of the left tube which is stretched out. Left ovary is seen clearly (see arrow) behind the tube.

**Operation done:** Total hysterectomy with bilateral salpingo-oophorectomy with removal of the cyst is done.

**Diagnosis:** Paraovarian cyst (left).

*Self-assessment:*

**Q. How do you diagnose a paraovarian cyst?**

**Ans.** The ovary is seen separated from the cyst. The uterine tube is stretched over the cyst.

**Q. What is the embryological origin of the cyst?**

**Ans.** From the remnant of the Wolffian body, situated in the mesosalpinx.

**Q. Describe the appearance of the cyst.**

**Ans.** Usually, the cyst is unilocular, has a thin wall and is filled with clear fluid.

**Q. Discuss the clinical features and management of the cyst.**

**Ans.** Same as ovarian cyst.

**Q. Management.**

**Ans.** Excision of the cyst.

**Q. What is the risk of malignancy?**

**Ans.** Rare.

## SPECIMEN — 18 (FIG. 16.68)

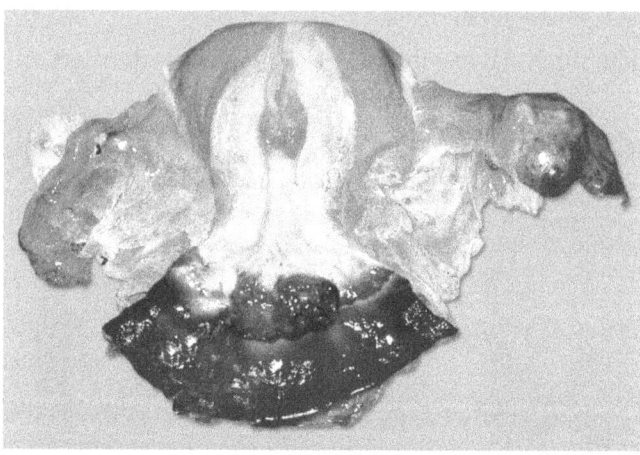

**Fig. 16.68:** A nodular growth (squamous cell carcinoma) occupies the posterior lip of the cervix in this specimen — Wertheim's radical hysterectomy done.

**History:** *Wertheim, Ernst (1864-1920)—Wertheim is best known for his radical abdominal hysterectomy, although he had many other contributions in vaginal surgery, especially for prolapse. He started his work as an assistant to Friedrich Schauta at German University. Later on he became the Professor of Gynecology in Vienna University.*

**Description:** This is a pathological specimen of the uterus, tubes and ovaries (both the sides) with upper vagina and parametrium of both the sides. The uterus is cut open to show a nodular growth on the ectocervix (lymph nodes are not shown in the photograph).
**Operation done:** Radical hysterectomy (Wertheim's operation) for carcinoma cervix.
**Diagnosis:** Carcinoma cervix.

*Self-assessment*:

Q. *What are the common histological types?*

Ans. Common histological types are:
(a) Squamous cell carcinoma (85–90%)
(b) Adenocarcinoma (10–15%)
(c) Clear cell adenocarcinoma
(d) Adenosquamous carcinoma
(e) Small cell carcinoma
(f) Undifferentiated carcinoma.

Q. *How the diagnosis of early carcinoma is made?*

Ans. See p. 468, 480.

Q. *What are the current changes in the staging of carcinoma cervix?*

Ans. See Table 16.2 for FIGO staging of carcinoma cervix (2018).

| Stage | Description |
|---|---|
| I | The carcinoma is strictly confined to the cervix (extension to the uterine corpus should be disregarded) |
| IA | Invasive carcinoma that can be diagnosed only by microscopy with maximum depth of invasion <5 mm[a] |
| IA1 | Measured stromal invasion <3 mm in depth |
| IA2 | Measured stromal invasion ≥3 mm and <5 mm in depth |
| IB | Invasive carcinoma with measured deepest invasion ≥5 mm (greater than Stage IA), lesion limited to the cervix uteri[b] |
| IB1 | Invasive carcinoma ≥5 mm depth of stromal invasion, and <2 cm in greatest dimension |
| IB2 | Invasive carcinoma ≥2 cm and <4 cm in greatest dimension |
| IB3 | Invasive carcinoma ≥4 cm in greatest dimension |
| II | The carcinoma invades beyond the uterus, but has not extended onto the lower third of the vagina or to the pelvic wall |
| IIA | Involvement limited to the upper two-thirds of the vagina without parametrial involvement |
| IIA1 | Invasive carcinoma <4 cm in greatest dimension |
| IIA2 | Invasive carcinoma ≥4 cm in greatest dimension |
| IIB | With parametrial involvement but not up to the pelvic wall |

*Contd...*

**Table 16.2:** FIGO staging of carcinoma of the cervix uteri (2018).

*Contd...*

| | |
|---|---|
| III | The carcinoma involves the lower third of the vagina and/or extends to the pelvic wall and/or causes hydronephrosis or nonfunctioning kidney and/or involves pelvic and/or para-aortic lymph nodes[c] |
| IIIA | The carcinoma involves the lower third of the vagina, with no extension to the pelvic wall |
| IIIB | Extension to the pelvic wall and/or hydronephrosis or nonfunctioning kidney (unless known to be due to another cause) |
| IIIC | Involvement of pelvic and/or para-aortic lymph nodes, irrespective of tumor size and extent (with r and p notations)[c] |
| IIIC1 | Pelvic lymph node metastasis only |
| IIIC2 | Para-aortic lymph node metastasis |
| IV | The carcinoma has extended beyond the true pelvis or has involved (biopsy proven) the mucosa of the bladder or rectum. (A bullous edema, as such, does not permit a case to be allotted to Stage IV) |
| IVA | Spread to adjacent pelvic organs |
| IVB | Spread to distant organs |

When in doubt, the lower staging should be assigned.

[a] Imaging and pathology can be used, where available, to supplement clinical findings with respect to tumor size and extent, in all stages.

[b] The involvement of vascular/lymphatic spaces does not change the staging. The lateral extent of the lesion is no longer considered.

[c] Adding notation of r (imaging) and p (pathology) to indicate the findings that are used to allocate the case to Stage IIIC. Example: If imaging indicates pelvic lymph node metastasis, the stage allocation would be stage IIIC1r, and if confirmed by pathologic findings, it would be Stage IIIC1p. The type of imaging modality or pathology technique used should always be documented.

### Q. Outline the lymphatic drainage of the cervix.

**Ans.** The lymphatic vessels from the cervix drain into the following groups of primary lymph nodes:

a. (i) Parametrial group
 (ii) Internal iliac group
 (iii) Obturator group
 (iv) External iliac group
 (v) Sacral group.

b. Secondary groups include:
 (i) External iliac
 (ii) Common iliac
 (iii) Para-aortic nodes

**Q. What is the management of CIS, microinvasive and early stage carcinoma?**

**Ans.** *See* p. 451.

**Q. Mention the advantages and disadvantages of radiotherapy.**

**Ans.**

| Radiotherapy | |
|---|---|
| Advantages | Disadvantages |
| (a) Can be used for all stages for cancer cervix stages | (a) Intestinal and urinary tract strictures, radiation hazards |
| (b) Say overall survival rate is 85% and it is comparable with that of surgery | (b) Vaginal fibrosis |
| (c) Less primary mortality and morbidity | (c) Radiation menopause in a young patient unless ovaries are transposed |

**Q. What are the tissues removed in radical hysterectomy?**

**Ans.** (a) Uterus and cervix
 (b) Wide tissues of parametrium
 (c) Periureteral tissues
 (d) Superior vesical artery
 (e) Cardinal and uterosacral ligaments
 (f) Upper three fourth of vagina
 (g) Thorough pelvic lymphadenectomy.

**Q. What are the procedures that may be used as per FIGO for staging?**

**Ans.** The following procedures may be used and should be mentioned when used.
- Ultrasonography
- Lymphangiography
- CT
- MRI
- PET
- Radionuclide imaging
- Laparoscopy or laparotomy
- Histopathology

**Q. What are the complications of radical hysterectomy?**

**Ans.** (a) Complications are similar to that of total abdominal hysterectomy (*see* p. 512)
 (b) Specific complications of radical procedures are:
   (i) Ureteric fistula
   (ii) Vesicovaginal fistula
   (iii) Bladder dysfunction
   (iv) Lymphocyst formation.

**Q. What are the preventive measures of carcinoma cervix?**

**Ans.** (1) **Primary prevention:**
- Identifying high-risk women
  (a) Early sexual intercourse
  (b) Early age of first pregnancy
  (c) High-risk HPV infection
- Prophylactic HPV vaccine
- Use of condom.

(2) **Secondary prevention:**
  (a) Screening of cervical pathology for early detection in CIN and microinvasive stage and appropriate treatment
  (b) Down staging (WHO 1996).
  (c) Screening for high-risk HPV infection.

**Q. What is the place of vaccine in prevention of cancer cervix?**

**Ans.** See p. 394.

**Q. What are the causes of death in carcinoma cervix?**

**Ans.** Causes of death are:
(a) Uremia
(b) Hemorrhage
(c) Sepsis
(d) Cachexia
(e) Complication due to metastasis.

**Q. What is the differential diagnosis of carcinoma cervix?**

**Ans.** Cervical cancer needs to be differentiated from:
(a) Tubercular ulcer of the cervix
(b) Syphilitic ulcer
(c) Cervical ectopy
(d) Products of conception in incomplete abortion
(e) Fibroid polyp (ulcerated).

**Q. What is the place of laparoscopic-assisted vaginal trachelectomy?**

**Ans.** Indications are:
(a) To preserve the reproductive function of the woman
(b) In early stage disease (stage IAI, A2, IBI).

## SPECIMEN — 19 (FIG. 16.69)

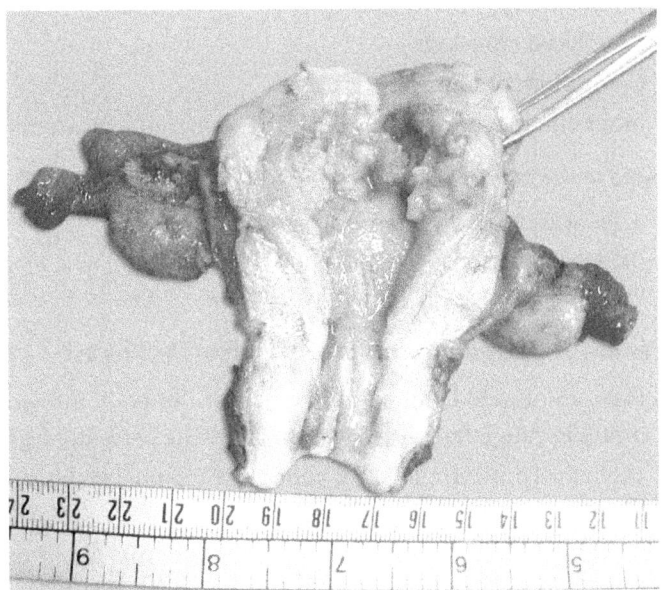

**Fig. 16.69:** The uterus is cut-open to show a diffuse and partly necrotic growth of adenocarcinoma filling the uterine cavity.

**Description:** This is a specimen of the uterus with tubes and ovaries of both the sides. The uterus is uniformly enlarged. The anterior surface is cut-open to show a fungating growth confined to the body. The tubes and ovaries are healthy.

**Operation done:** Total hysterectomy with bilateral salpingo-oophorectomy.

**Diagnosis:** Endometrial carcinoma.

*Self-assessment:*

> **Q. Discuss the specimen as seen in Figure 16.69.**
>
> **Ans.** It is a specimen of the uterus cut-opened to show a diffuse endometrial growth covering the region of the fundus. The growth is ulcerated. The rest of the cavity and endocervix appears free of the tumor.
>
> **Q. Mention the methods of diagnosis.**
>
> **Ans.** (a) **History**—any case of the postmenopausal bleeding is considered to be endometrial cancer unless proved otherwise
>
> (b) **Transvaginal ultrasonography (TVS)**—endometrial thickness ≥4 mm is suggestive endometrial cancer

(c) **Endometrial biopsy** using a pipellele cannula or with a Sharman's curette
(d) **Hysteroscopy** and targeted biopsy
(e) **Fractional curettage**
(f) **Computed tomography (CT)**
(g) **Magnetic resonance imaging (MRI)** are used for myometrial invasion.

**Q. What are the histological types of endometrial carcinoma?**

Ans. (a) Adenocarcinoma (endometrioid 80%)
(b) Adenocarcinoma with squamous elements
(c) Papillary serous carcinoma.

**Q. What are the lymphatic drainage of body of the uterus?**

Ans. (a) From the fundus and adjoining part of the body through lymphatics draining along the ovarian lymphatics to the para-arotic group of nodes
(b) From the cornu-drains in the superficial inguinal nodes along the round ligament
(c) Rest of the body of the uterus drains into external iliac group of nodes
(d) Adjacent to the cervix → along the cervical lymphatics (see below).

**Q. Who are the high-risk women?**

Ans. (a) Persistent stimulation of endometrium with unopposed estrogen
(b) Age: Median age of 60
(c) Party: Nulliparous woman
(d) Late menopause
(e) Corpus cancer syndrome (obesity, hypertension and diabetes)
(f) Obesity
(g) Family history of ovary, breast or colon cancer.

**Q. What are the surgical procedures in the management?**

Ans. (a) Extrafascial hysterectomy with bilateral salpingo-oophorectomy is commonly done for endometrial cancer confined to the body.
(b) Combined therapy is considered for cases depending upon the FIGO stage of the disease (myometrial invasion). Adjuvant radiotherapy is usually given in cases with myometrial invasion.

**Q. Describe the FIGO staging of carcinoma endometrium.**

Ans. See Table 16.3 for FIGO staging of carcinoma endometrium (2018).

**Table 16.3:** Cancer of the corpus uteri.

**FIGO STAGING FOR CARCINOMA ENDOMETRIUM (2018)**

| Stage I[a] | Tumor confined to the corpus uteri |
|---|---|
| IA[a] | No or less than half myometrial invasion |
| IB[a] | Invasion equal to or more than half of the myometrium |
| Stage II[a] | Tumor invades cervical stroma, but does not extend beyond the uterus[b] |
| Stage III[a] | Local and/or regional spread of the tumor[c] |
| IIIA[a] | Tumor invades the serosa of the corpus uteri and/or adnexae[c] |
| IIIB[a] | Vaginal involvement and/or parametrial involvement[c] |
| IIIC[a] | Metastases to pelvic and/or para-aortic lymph nodes[c] |
| IIIC1[a] | Positive pelvic nodes |
| IIIC2[a] | Positive para-aortic nodes with or without positive pelvic lymph nodes |
| Stage IV[a] | Tumor invades bladder and/or bowel mucosa, and/or distant metastases |
| IVA[a] | Tumor invasion of bladder and/or bowel mucosa |
| IVB[a] | Distant metastasis, including intra-abdominal metastases and/or inguinal nodes) |

[a]Either G1, G2, or G3.
[b]Endocervical glandular involvement only should be considered as stage I and no longer as stage II.
[c]Positive cytology has to be reported separately without changing the stage.

**Q. What is the place of chemotherapy and radiotherapy?**

**Ans.** (a) Combined therapy with radiation followed by extended hysterectomy at an interval of 6 weeks is done in a case with stage II carcinoma

(b) Chemotherapy is used in advanced cases. Commonly used drugs are: Progestogens, adriamycin, carboplatin and paclitaxel.

## SPECIMEN — 20 (FIG. 16.70)

**Description:** This is a specimen of the vulva. The vulva shows a large exophytic growth and biopsy revealed squamous cell carcinoma.

**Operation done: Radical vulvectomy.** Vulvectomy specimen is obtained by the skin sparing "long horn" incisions. Tips of the horns rest on the anterior superior iliac spines. The upper margin of incision is interspinous, the lower margin is along the inguinal skin creases and the labiocrural folds. Three incision technique is currently used in most of the centers.

**Diagnosis:** Carcinoma of the vulva.

*Self-assessment:*

**Q. What are the common sites of vulval malignancy?**

Ans. (a) Labium majus
(b) Clitoris
(c) Labium minus.

**Q. What are the different histological types?**

Ans. (a) Squamous cell carcinoma
(b) Melanoma
(c) Adenocarcinoma
(d) Basal cell carcinoma
(e) Sarcoma.

**Q. What is the clinical presentation of a case?**

Ans. (a) May be asymptomatic
(b) Pruritus vulvae
(c) Swelling of vulva with discharge
(d) Vulval ulceration
(e) Bleeding
(f) Inguinal mass (enlarged lymph nodes).

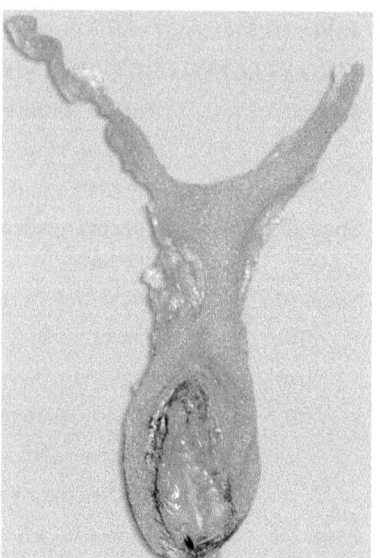

**Fig. 16.70:** Carcinoma of the vulva — radical vulvectomy done using "long horn" incisions.

**Q. What are the types of vulvectomy?**

Ans. (a) **Simple vulvectomy:** Tissues removed are mons pubis, clitoris, labia-majora and minora
(b) **Radical vulvectomy:** Removal of entire tissues of vulva along with bilateral inguinofemoral lymphadenectomy.

**Q. What are the complications of radical vulvectomy?**

Ans. (A) Early: Hemorrhage, groin, wound infection, wound dehiscence and delayed healing
(B) Late: Leg edema, dyspareunia, femoral or inguinal hernia and recurrence of malignancy.

**Q. Mention the lymphatic drainage of the vulva?**

Ans. Vulval lymphatics communicate freely on either side.
(A) (i) Labia majora (anterior half) → superficial inguinal nodes
(ii) Labia majora (posterior half) → superficial inguinal → deep inguinal → external iliac group of nodes.

(B) Labia minora, prepuce of clitoris → superficial inguinal nodes
(C) Glans clitoris → deep inguinal and external iliac nodes
(D) Bartholin's gland → superficial inguinal nodes
(E) Node of Cloquet: Located at the femoral canal, medial to the femoral vein. It receives lymphatic drainage from superficial inguinal nodes. May be absent in some.

**Q. Significance of a sentinel node.**

**Ans.** Sentinel node is the first node that drains a primary tumor. This node can be detected intraoperatively by lymphatic mapping.

**Q. What are the prognostic factors?**

**Ans.** (a) Clinical stage (FIGO) of the disease
(b) Depth of stomal invasion
(c) Involvement of lymph nodes.

**Q. Describe the FIGO staging of vulval carcinoma.**

**Ans.** See Table 16.4 for FIGO Staging of Vulval Cancer (2018).

| Table 16.4: FIGO staging for carcinoma of vulva (2018). | |
|---|---|
| Stage I | Tumor confined to the vulva |
| IA | Lesions ≤2 cm in size, confined to the vulva or perineum and with stromal invasion ≤1.0 mm[a], no nodal metastasis |
| IB | Lesions > 2 cm in size or with stromal invasion >1.0 mm[a], confined to the vulva or perineum with negative nodes |
| Stage II | Tumor of any size with extension to adjacent perineal structures (1/3 lower urethra, 1/3 lower vagina, anus) with negative nodes |
| Stage III | Tumor of any size with or without extension to adjacent perineal structures (1/3 lower urethra, 1/3 lower vagina, anus) with positive inguinofemoral lymph nodes |
| IIIA | (i) With 1 lymph node metastasis (≥5 mm), or<br>(ii) 1–2 lymph node metastasis (es) (<5 mm) |
| IIIB | (i) With 2 or more lymph node metastases (≥5 mm), or<br>(ii) 3 or more lymph node metastases (<5 mm) |
| IIIC | With positive nodes with extracapsular spread |
| Stage IV | Tumor invades other regional (2/3 upper urethra, 2/3 upper vagina), or distant structures |
| IVA | Tumor invades any of the following:<br>(i) 2/3 upper urethra, 2/3 upper vagina, bladder mucosa, rectal mucosa, or fixed to pelvic bones<br>OR<br>(ii) Fixed or ulcerated inguinofemoral lymph nodes |
| IVB | Any distant metastasis including pelvic lymph nodes |

[a]The depth of invasion is defined as the measurement of the tumor from the epithelial-stromal junction of the adjacent most superficial dermal papilla to the deepest point of invasion.

# 16C. IMAGING STUDIES IN GYNECOLOGY

**Chapter Objectives**
**Basic knowledge and understanding with:**
- Skiagram (X-ray images)
- Ultrasonogram
- Computed Tomograms (CT)
- Magnetic Resonance Images
- Rational use
- Diagnosis of pelvic pathology
- Interpretation of results
- Adverse effects (if any)

## HYSTEROSALPINGOGRAM

### FIG. 16.71

Hysterosalpingogram (HSG) showing radiopaque shadow demarcating the uterine cavity. The radiopaque dye is visible in the lumen of both the tubes. There is peritoneal spillage on both sides. The HSG cannula is in situ.

**Diagnosis:** Normal hysterosalpingogram (normal cavity) with bilateral patent tubes (free peritoneal spill).

*Self-assessment:*

Q. *What are the indications of* HSG?
Ans. *See* p. 476.

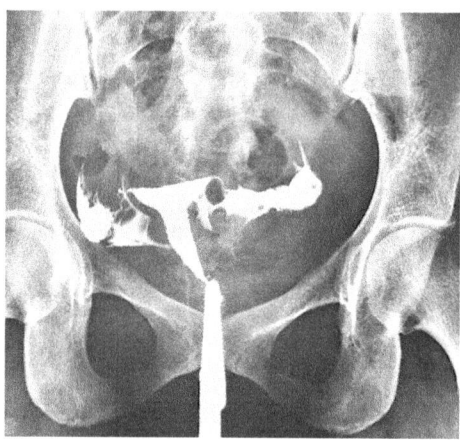

Fig. 16.71: Hysterosalpingogram with bilateral peritoneal spillage.

Q. *What are the* contraindications of HSG?
Ans. *See* p. 478, 570.

Q. *What is the* timing of HSG?
Ans. *See* p. 570.

**Q. What are the steps of operation of HSG?**

**Ans.** *See* p. 502.

**Q. What are the complications?**

**Ans.** *See* p. 502 and 570.

**Q. What is the next step of investigation in this case?**

**Ans.** As the tubes are patent, the couple should be investigated to **assess** the **ovarian** (whether she is ovulating or not) and **male factors** (semen analysis) for **infertility.**

**Q. What are the methods to detect ovulation?**

**Ans.**
- Regular menstruation
- Basal body temperature—biphasic pattern
- Cervical mucus study (loss of fern pattern in scraping)
- Vaginal cytology—progestational effect
- Levels of serum progesterone (rising level) at LH surge
- Endometrial biopsy: Secretory changes (D21–D23)
- Serial sonography: Detection of dominant follicle as other follicles collapse following ovulation.

## FIG. 16.72

Hysterosalpingogram showing radiopaque shadow demarcating the uterine cavity. No radiopaque shadow is visible in either tube.

**Diagnosis:** Hysterosalpingogram showing bilateral cornual block.

*Self-assessment:*

**Q. What are the causes of cornual block?**

**Ans.** Commonly, it is due to infections. Genital tuberculosis often causes cornual block.

**Q. What are the alternative investigations?**

**Ans.** Alternative investigations for assessment of tubal patency are:
(a) Laparoscopic chromopertubation
(b) Sonohysterosalpingography.

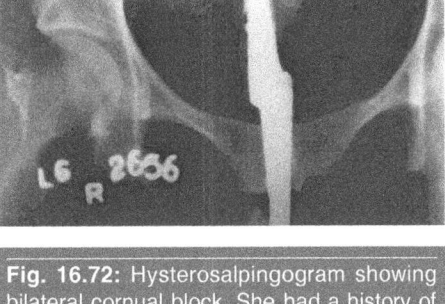

Fig. 16.72: Hysterosalpingogram showing bilateral cornual block. She had a history of MTP.

**Q. What is the management if tubes are damaged?**

**Ans.** If the tubes are damaged, assisted reproductive technology (ART) is the option. This may be in vitro fertilization and embryo transfer (IVF-ET).

**Q. What are the results of tuboplasty?**

**Ans.** Results of tuboplasty depend on the underlying pathology, method of tuboplasty (macro-or microsurgery). Overall success rate following tubal anastomosis is 75%.

**Q. What are the different methods of ART?**

**Ans.**
- IVF-ET: In vitro fertilization and embryo transfer
- ICSI: Intracytoplasmic sperm injection.

**Q. What is the management if tubes are normal?**

**Ans.** To assess the male factor (semen analysis) and ovarian factor (detection of ovulation) for infertility.

**Q. What other information can be obtained from HSG?**

**Ans.** See p. 502.

**Q. What are the causes of tubal block?**

**Ans.** Salpingitis, salpingitis isthmica nodosa, benign polyps within the tubal lumen, tubal endometriosis, tubal spasm and intratubal mucous debris.

## FIG. 16.73

Hysterosalpingogram showing radiopaque shadow filling the uterine cavity. The tubes of both sides are distended with the radiopaque dye. There is no evidence of peritoneal spillage.

**Diagnosis:** Bilateral hydrosalpinx (fimbrial block).

**Self-assessment:**

**Q. What are the causes of bilateral fimbrial block?**

**Ans.** Salpingitis (acute or chronic infection of the tube) is the common cause.

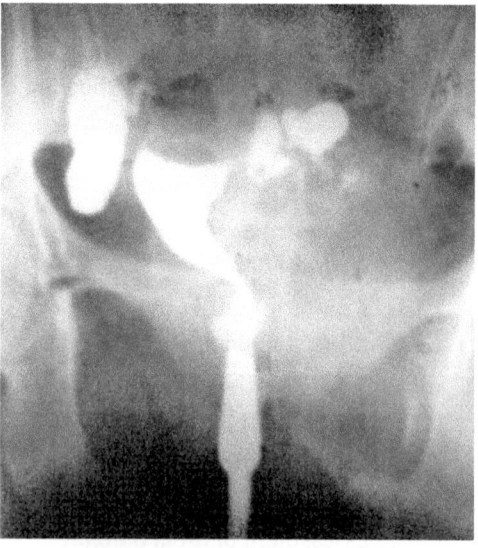

Fig. 16.73: Hysterosalpingogram showing bilateral hydrosalpinx (fimbrial block). Bilateral salpingostomy was done. Thereafter, she had an ectopic pregnancy.

**Q. What is the management for proximal, distal and midtubal block?**

**Ans.** **(A) Proximal tubal block** may be overcome by hysteroscopic cannulation. This is done using a hysteroscope.

(B) **Distal tubal block** may be treated by:
   (i) Fimbrioplasty
   (ii) Fimbryolysis.

(C) **Midtubal block**—tubotubal anastomosis may be done.

**Q. What is the appearance of the tube on HSG when infected with tuberculosis?**

**Ans.** The appearance on HSG are:
  (a) Vascular or lymphatic extravasation of dye
  (b) Rigid tubes with nodulations at places
  (c) Beaded appearance of the tubes
  (d) Coiling or clarification of tubes.

**Q. What is the reproductive outcome in a woman with pelvic tuberculosis?**

**Ans.** Chances of conception in such a case is remote. Even if she conceives, the risk of ectopic pregnancy is high.

**Q. Does the presence of hydrosalpinx impair the result of IVF?**

**Ans.** Hydrosalpinges reduce the pregnancy rates of IVF by about 50%. Endometrial receptivity is reduced resulting in implantation failure. Salpingectomy improves the outcome.

### FIG. 16.74

Hysterosalpingogram showing markedly dilated tube with retention of dye (right).

**Diagnosis:** Hydrosalpinx of the right tube.

*Self-assessment:*

**Q. What are the other methods of diagnosis?**

**Ans.** USG and laparoscopy.

**Q. What are the dangers of HSG in such a case?**

**Ans.** Risk of flaring up of pelvic infection is very high in such a case. Therefore, HSG is contraindicated in a case with hydrosalpinx.

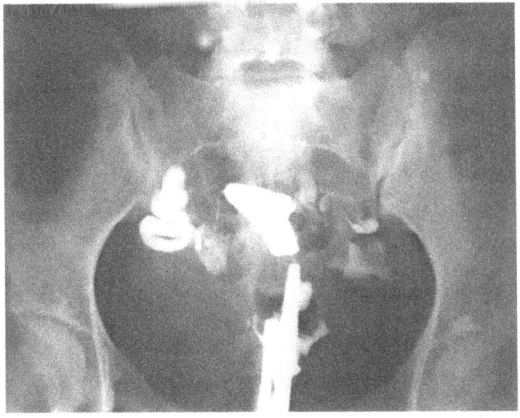

Fig. 16.74: Hysterosalpingogram showing markedly dilated tube with retention of dye (*right*).

**Q. What are the common types of tubal reconstructive surgery?**

**Ans.** Different types of tubal reconstructive surgery are:
(a) Salpingolysis
(b) Fimbrioplasty
(c) Salpingostomy
(d) Tubotubal anastomosis
(e) Tubocornual anastomosis.

**Q. What factors are related to the success of tuboplasty?**

**Ans.** Success of tubal reconstructive surgery depend upon the following factors:
(a) Underlying pathology of the tube; tubercular salpingitis has got poor outcome.
(b) Presence of adhesions.
(c) Presence of hydrosalpinx.
(d) Length of the reconstructed tube is <4 cm.

**Q. What are the guidelines for tubal surgery?**

**Ans.** (a) Tubal surgery may be considered in young women with mild disease or after previous tubal sterilization.
(b) IVF is considered as the treatment option for the any complicated tubal occlusive disease.

## FIG. 16.75

Hysterosalpingogram showing a radiopaque shadow filling both the horns of the uterus. The radiopaque dye is visible within the tubes. There is peritoneal spillage on both the sides (Fig. 16.75).

**Diagnosis:** It seems to be a case of bicornuate uterus with bilateral patent tubes.

*Self-assessment:*

**Q. How do you confirm a bicornuate uterus from septate uterus?**

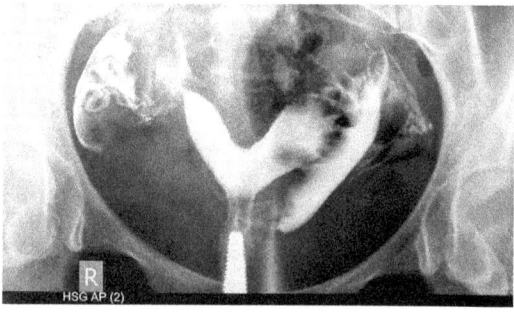

Fig. 16.75: Hysterosalpingogram showing bicornuate uterus. Metroplasty was done for recurrent midtrimester miscarriage. Subsequently, she had a live birth at term, delivered by lower segment cesarean section (LSCS).

**Ans.** For confirmation one needs to see both the internal and external architecture of the uterus. Combined hysteroscopy and laparoscopy are helpful in this regard.

**Q. How do you manage a case of septate uterus in recurrent miscarriage?**

**Ans.** Hysteroscopic resection of the uterine septum is most effective. Successful pregnancy following hysteroscopic septum resection is about 90%.

**Q. What are the gynecological symptoms in bicornuate uterus?**

**Ans.** Important symptoms are: Dysmenorrhea, dyspareunia, infertility and menstrual abnormality (menorrhagia).

**Q. What is the management of a bicornuate uterus?**

**Ans.** It is difficult. Metroplasty or unification (Strassman or Tompkins) operation has been recommended.

### FIG. 16.76

Hysterosalpingogram showing a radiopaque shadow filling a single horn of the uterus. There is peritoneal spillage from the tube.

**Diagnosis:** It seems to be a case of unicornuate uterus with patent tube.

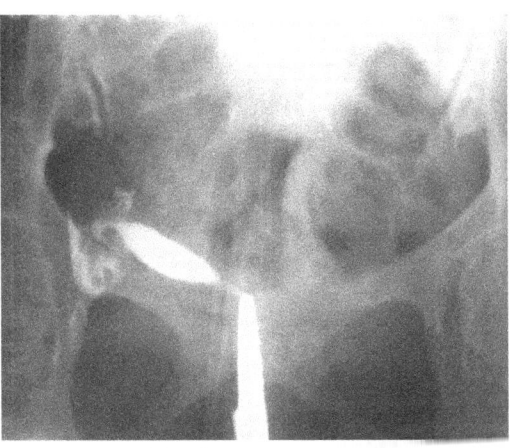

Fig. 16.76: Hysterosalpingogram showing a unicornuate uterus.

*Self-assessment:*

**Q. How do you confirm the diagnosis?**

**Ans.** Confirmation of diagnosis is by:
(1) Laparoscopic method of visualization.
(2) 3D ultrasonography or MRI is also helpful.

**Q. What type of Müllerian anomaly is this unicornuate uterus?**

**Ans.** It is due to failure of development of the other Müllerian duct.

**Q. What is the reproductive outcome with unicornuate uterus?**

**Ans.** Often it is poor. This is due to poor uterine capacity, less muscle mass and inability to expand.

## FIG. 16.77

Hysterosalpingogram showing irregular filling of radiopaque dye without any outline of uterine tubes.

**Diagnosis:** Uterine synechiae (Asherman's syndrome).

*Self-assessment:*

Q. **What are the common causes of uterine synechiae?**

Ans. (a) Excessive (overzealous) curettage following abortion or childbirth
(b) Excessive curettage in a case with DUB
(c) Tubercular endometritis.

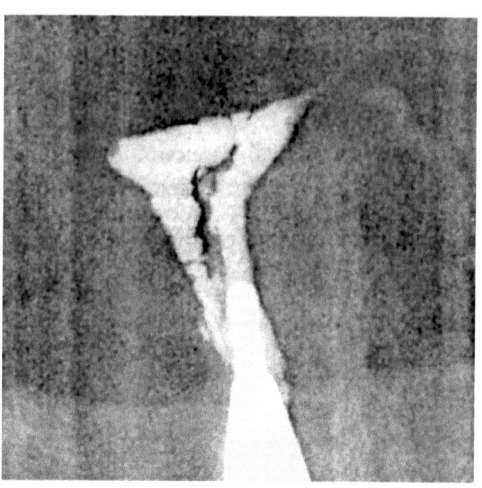

Fig. 16.77: Hysterosalpingogram showing intrauterine adhesion.

Q. **What are the other methods of diagnosis?**

Ans. Hysteroscopic visualization of the endometrial cavity is a useful method for the diagnosis. Adhesiolysis could be done at the same sitting hysteroscopically.

Q. **What is the management of uterine synechiae?**

Ans. Hysteroscopic adhesiolysis is to be done. This procedure may be followed by insertion of an intrauterine contraceptive device (IUCD) to prevent readhesion.

Q. **What are the uterine causes of amenorrhea?**

Ans. (a) Mayer-Rokitansky-Küster-Hauser (MRKH) syndrome
(b) Tubercular endometritis
(c) Uterine synechiae
(d) Surgical removal of uterus (hysterectomy)
(e) Postradiation.

Q. **In what conditions of amenorrhea karyotyping is needed?**

Ans. (i) Patients with uterus but no breasts and high FSH levels–Gonadal failure
(ii) Patients with no uterus but breasts present—androgen insensitivity syndrome
(iii) Premature ovarian failure if <30 years of age
(iv) Short stature (<60") with Turner stigmata—Turner's syndrome.

## Chapter 16 • Practical Gynecology 633

## ULTRASONOGRAPHY

### FIG. 16.78

Ultrasonographic view of a septate uterus.

*Self-assessment:*

Q. *What are the different types of uterine abnormalities?*

Ans. (a) Agenesis
(b) Hypoplasia
(c) Unicornuate uterus
(d) Bicornuate uterus
(e) Didelphys uterus
(f) Septate uterus
(g) Arcuate uterus.

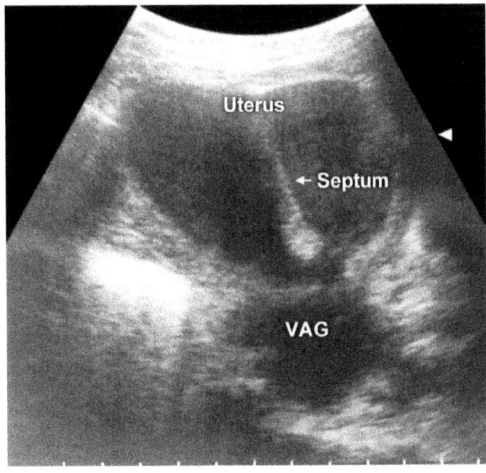

Fig. 16.78: Ultrasonographic view of a septate uterus.

Q. *What may be the clinical presentation of such a case?*

Ans. Clinical presentation varies with the type of abnormalities. Sometimes, it may remain asymptomatic.

**Gynecological:**
(a) Infertility
(b) Menstrual abnormalities (menorrhagia).

**Obstetrical:**
(a) Miscarriage (may be recurrent)
(b) Cervical incompetence
(c) Preterm labor.

Q. *What are the different obstetric complications?*

Ans. See p. 540, Fig. 15.56.

Q. *What are the different modes of diagnosis?*

Ans. Different combinations of methods are done:
(a) Hysterosalpingography
(b) Hysteroscopy
(c) Laparoscopy
(d) Ultrasonography (3D)
(e) Magnetic resonance imaging (MRI).

**Q. What are the treatment options available?**

**Ans.** Many cases do not need any surgical intervention: Few cases may need:

(a) Hysteroscopic metroplasty (septal resection)

(b) Excision of rudimentary horn

(c) Unification operation (bicornuate uterus).

### FIG. 16.79

*Self-assessment:*

**Q. What are the causes of symmetrical enlargement of the uterus?**

**Ans.** (a) Pregnancy

(b) Submucous or intramural (solitary) fibroid, adenomyosis

(c) Hematometra

(d) Pyometra.

**Q. How a couple should be counseled before proceeding to myomectomy?**

**Ans.** The operation should be done for preservation of reproductive function:

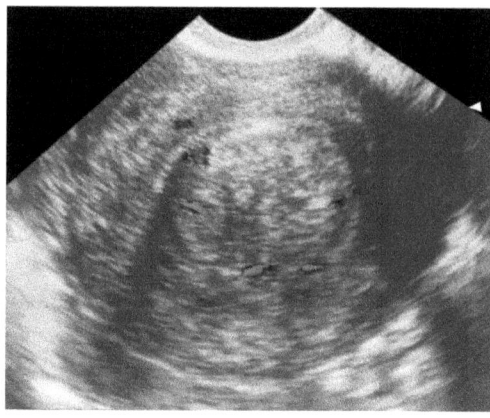

Fig. 16.79: Ultrasonographic (TV) view of a leiomyoma.

(a) Myomectomy should be done for presentation of reproductive function

(b) Pregnancy rate following myomectomy is about 40–60%.

(c) Myomectomy is a more risky operation especially when fibroid(s) are too big or too many.

(d) Risk during operation: Hemorrhage.

(e) Remote complications are: Persistence of menorrhagia, recurrence of fibroid and risks of relaparotomy.

**Q. What are the drugs used to control menorrhagia?**

**Ans.** (a) Antiprogesterones (mifepristone)

(b) Danazol

(c) GnRH analogs

(d) LNG-IUS

(e) Prostaglandin synthetase inhibitors (mefenamic acid).

**Q. What are the principal steps of myomectomy?**

**Ans.** (a) Uterine incision: A linear midline incision is made on the anterior wall.

(b) Incision is deepened through the myometrium, and the capsule to reach the myoma.

(c) The myoma is grasped with a single-toothed vulsellum. The dissection is continued. Myoma is enucleated from its capsule by sharp and blunt dissection. The fibroid is removed.

(d) Myoma bed is closed by interrupted mattress sutures.

**Q. What are the measures that can be adopted to minimize blood loss during myomectomy operation?**

**Ans.** During operation:
(a) Local injection of vasopressin over the myoma
(b) Use of tourniquet—to occlude the uterine vessels
(c) Use of Bonny's myomectomy clamp.

**Q. What are the different methods of surgery?**

**Ans.** (a) Laparotomy
(b) Laparoscopy
(c) Hysteroscopy
(d) Others—myolysis, radiology intervention (embolotherapy).

**Q. What are the different types of surgery done for leiomyoma?**

**Ans.** See p. 378.

**Q. What are the common complications of myomectomy?**

**Ans.** See p. 517.

**Q. What are the long-term results of myomectomy in respect of recurrence and others?**

**Ans.** Risk of recurrence: 30–50%
Persistence of hemorrhage: 1–5%
Risk of relaparotomy: 20–25%.

**FIG. 16.80**

*Self-assessment:*

**Q. What are the different modalities of treatment options for pelvic endometriosis?**

**Ans.** Also *see* p. 445. Endometriosis
(a) *Expectant (observation only)*
(b) *Medical therapy:*
  • Hormones
  • Others
(c) *Surgery:*
  • Conservative
  • Definitive

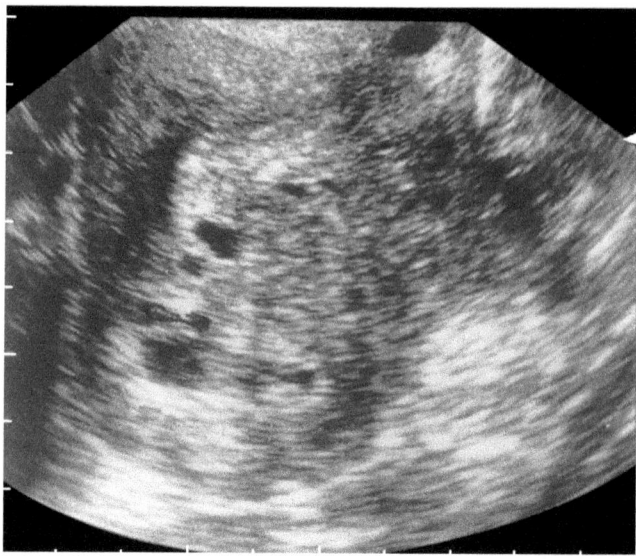

Fig. 16.80: Sonographic view of adenomyosis showing diffusely enlarged uterus with cystic spaces.

(d) *Combined therapy:* Medical followed by surgical and surgical followed by medical therapy.

**Q. What are the common sites of pelvic endometriosis?**

**Ans.** Common sites are:
(a) Ovaries
(b) Pelvic peritoneum
(c) Pouch of Douglas
(d) Rectosigmoid septum.

**Q. Mention the indications and the different types of surgery that can be done for endometriosis?**

**Ans.** Indications of surgery are:
(a) Endometriosis with severe symptoms not responding to hormone therapy.
(b) Advanced stage disease to restore pelvic anatomy.
(c) Endometriomas >1 cm.

**Q. How do you manage a case of chocolate cyst (ovarian endometrioma) of the ovary?**

**Ans.** (a) Small endometrioma <3 cm—laparoscopic cyst aspiration and cyst wall epithelium is destroyed by diathermy or laser.
(b) Large endometrioma ≥4 cm—ovarian cystectomy with adhesiolysis.

**Q. What are the different hormones used in the management of endometriosis?**

**Ans.** Combined oral pills, progestogens (oral, IM or IUCD), danazol, gestrinone or GnRH analogues.

**Q. What is the treatment of scar endometriosis?**

**Ans.** It is done by excision of the endometriotic nodule in the scar tissue.

**Q. How fibroid uterus could be differentiated from adenomyosis?**

**Ans.**

| Differentiating features of fibroid uterus and adenomyosis | | |
|---|---|---|
| | Fibroid uterus (see Fig. 16.79) | Adenomyosis (*see* Fig. 16.80) |
| **Age** | • Usually observed in the reproductive age | • Commonly seen in women older than 40 years |
| **Pathology** | • It is the benign neoplasia of the smooth muscle and fibrous tissue of the uterus | • It is due to the presence of functioning endometrium within the muscle layers of the uterus |
| **Uterus** | • Irregularly enlarged depending upon the site, size and number of myomas. It is firm and nontender (unless degeneration) | • Diffusely enlarged due to myohyperplasia. Uterus is soft and tender<br>• Size is usually <16 weeks size of pregnancy |
| **Symptoms** | • Menorrhagia and dysmenorrhea—often present | • Menorrhagia—present. Dysmenorrhea often begins a week before and it continues even after the period is over |
| **Diagnosis** | • **Sonography (TVS)**: Homogeneous echogenic area over the fibroid | • Cystic spaces within the myometrium<br>• MRI low signal intensity junctional zone (JZ) thickness ≥12 mm is suggestive of adenomyosis |
| | • **Cut section:** *Capsule* present, smooth and whitish surface with whorled appearance<br>• **Histology:** Proliferation of smooth muscle and fibrous tissue | • *Capsule* absent. Diffuse trabeculated appearance, cystic spaces with hemorrhagic spots<br>• Proliferation of endometrial glands and stroma. Phagocytic cells laden with hemosiderin pigment are present |

## FIG. 16.81

Ultrasonographic view of CuT inside the uterine cavity. Thread was missing in this case.

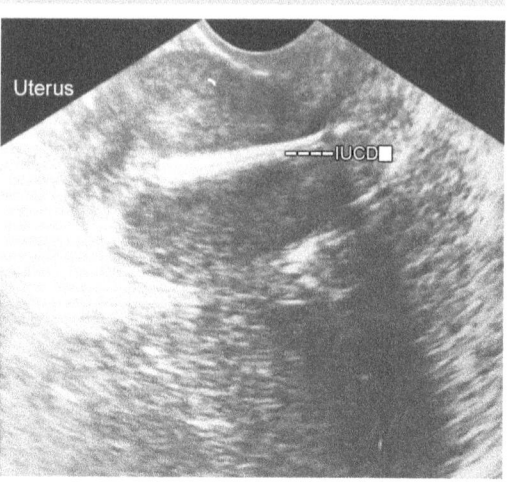

Fig. 16.81: Ultrasonographic view of a Cu T inside the uterine cavity, in a case of missing thread.

*Self-assessment:*

**Q. What are the possible causes of missing thread?**

**Ans.** (a) Thread coiled inside
(b) Threads torn and expelled out
(c) IUCD expelled out unnoticed
(d) Perforation of the uterus
(e) Pregnancy when the threads are drawn inside the uterus.

**Q. How do you investigate such a case with missing thread?**

**Ans.** (a) Ultrasonography can locate IUCD in the abdominal cavity or within the uterine cavity.
(b) Hysteroscopy can help in direct visualization and can remove it at the same time.

**Q. What are the indications of removal of IUCDs?**

**Ans.** (a) Missing thread
(b) Persistent pelvic pain
(c) Persistent menorrhagia
(d) Woman desirous of pregnancy.

**Q. What are the complications of IUCD use?**

**Ans.** (A) *Immediate:*
(i) Cramp-like pain
(ii) Perforation of the uterus
(iii) Syncopal attack.

(B) *Remote:*
(i) Pelvic pain
(ii) Abnormal bleeding
(iii) Pelvic infection
(iv) Perforation of the uterus.

**Q. What are the specific advantages of the third generation of IUCDs over the others?**

**Ans.** (a) Higher efficacy
(b) Longer duration of action
(c) Low expulsion rate
(d) Reduced risk of ectopic pregnancy
(e) Reduced risk of PID.

**Q. Mention some of the noncontraceptive benefits of LNG-IUCD?**

**Ans.** (a) Reduction of menorrhagia, dysmenorrhea
(b) Used in the management of endometrial hyperplasia
(c) Used as an alternative to hysterectomy for menorrhagia
(d) Used as hormone replacement therapy.

### FIG. 16.82

Ultrasonographic view of an ovarian hyperstimulation syndrome (OHSS). Multiple follicles are seen.

*Self-assessment:*

**Q. What are the different grades and the clinical features of OHSS?**

**Ans.** Ovarian hyperstimulation syndrome (OHSS) could be of three grades depending upon severity.
(a) Mild (10-20%)
(b) Moderate (5-10%)
(c) Severe (1-2%).

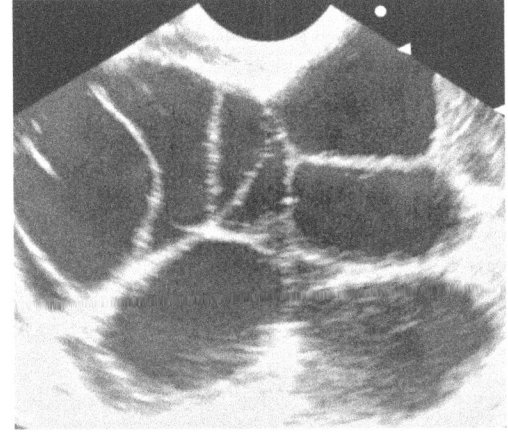

Fig. 16.82: Sonographic view of OHSS.

**Q. How the woman usually presents?**

**Ans.** The woman usually presents with: Abdominal pain, nausea, vomiting, ascites, ARDS, oliguria, renal failure and there is raised WBC count (>15,000/mL), liver dysfunction and thromboembolism.

**Q. How could this problem be prevented?**

**Ans.** (a) Low dose gonadotropins use
(b) Close monitoring of super ovulation cycles
(c) Not to be use ovulatory dose of hCG in susceptible cases.

**Q. What are the indications of gonadotropins use in infertility?**

Ans. Indications are:
  (a) Hypogonadotropic hypogonadism
  (b) Clomiphene failed or resistant cases
  (c) Unexplained infertility
  (d) Subfertile women who are elderly (>35 years).

**Q. What is ovarian reserve?**

Ans. It means the quantity as well as the quality of follicles present in the ovary.

**Q. Who are the high responders?**

Ans. High responders are those who have exaggerated response in follicular development when follicular stimulation is done.

**Q. What is coasting?**

Ans. It is done in high responders to prevent OHSS. Gonadotropin stimulation is stopped. GnRH agonist is continued. Once the level of estradiol is within normal range, hCG is given.

**Q. How do you manage a case of OHSS?**

Ans. (a) To monitor the patient within complete hemogram, LFTs, RFTs, coagulation profile and urine output.
  (b) Oral fluids to continue.
  (c) Abdominal paracentesis to relieve respiratory distress.
  (d) Human albumin may be given.
  (e) Intensive care management may be needed.
  (f) Surgery is rarely indicated.

## X-RAY

**FIG. 16.83**

*Self-assessment:*

**Q. What are the secondary changes in a fibroid?**

Ans. (a) Degenerations: Hyaline, cystic, calcific and red degeneration
  (b) Infection
  (c) Atrophy
  (d) Necrosis
  (e) Sarcomatous change.

**Q. What are the degenerations in fibroid?**

**Ans.** (a) Hyaline degeneration is the most common.
(b) Cystic degeneration is seen in menopause. Cystic spaces are seen within the fibroid.
(c) Fatty degeneration.
(d) Calcific degeneration (10%). The whole of fibroid changes into a calcific mass, called as 'womb stone'.
(e) Red degeneration is usually seen in pregnancy and puerperium. It is vascular in origin. It is often associated pain abdomen.
(f) Atrophy—usually occurs in menopause.
(g) Necrosis—may occur due to inadequate vascular supply.
(h) Infection is commonly seen in submucous fibroid.
(i) Sarcomatous change occur in <0.1% of cases.

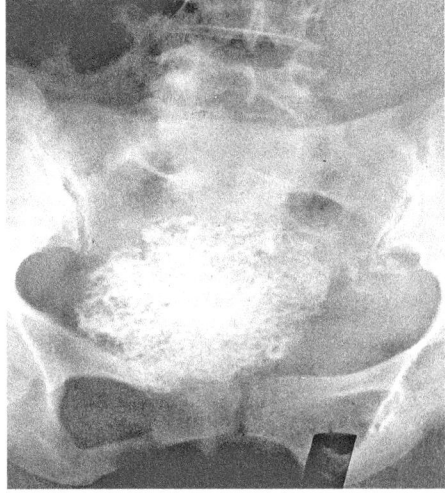

**Fig. 16.83:** Plain X-ray of the pelvis and lower abdomen showing the calcific degeneration of a fibroid (popcorn appearance).
(*Courtesy:* Dr P Panigrahi Senior Consultant Gynecologist, JLN Hospital, Bhillai)

### FIG. 16.84

**Description:** It is a skiagram of the pelvis showing radiopaque shadow (tooth). Most likely, it is a dermoid cyst of the ovary.

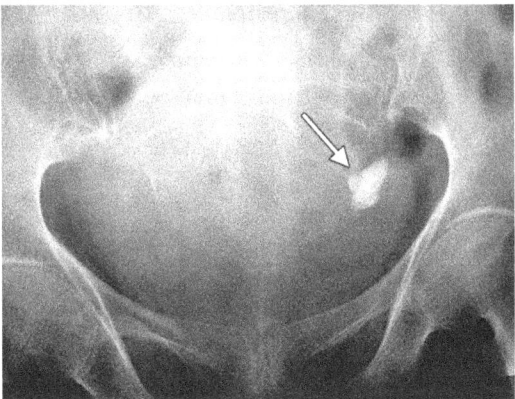

**Fig. 16.84:** Straight X-ray of the pelvis showing a tooth within an ovarian dermoid.

*Self-assessment:*

**Q. Describe the cut section of an ovarian dermoid cyst.**

**Ans.** On cut section—mainly sebaceous material is found. There is a solid area which often contains hair, bones, cartilage or teeth.

**Q. What is the risk of malignancy in a dermoid cyst of the ovary?**

**Ans.** About 1-2%.

**Q. What is struma ovarii?**

**Ans.** Struma ovarii is composed of thyroid tissue. It is a rare variety of ovarian tumor.

## CT SCAN

### FIG. 16.85

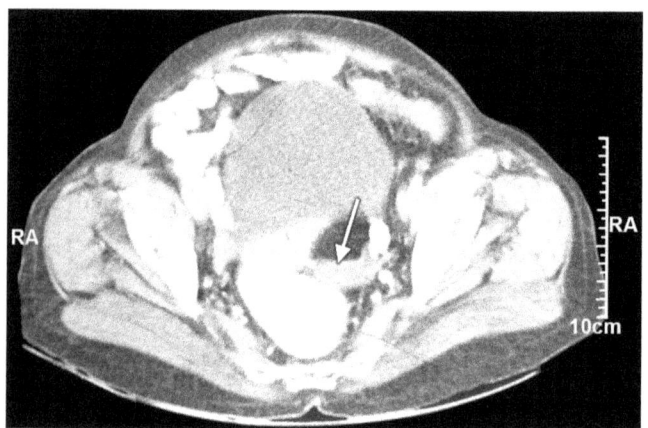

**Fig. 16.85:** Showing fat, fat-fluid level and dental element (arrow).

**Q. Describe typical findings of an ovarian dermoid cyst in CT.**

**Ans.** Characteristics of a dermoid cyst in CT include the mixture of low density areas due to fat, high density areas from dental elements or calcification (arrow) and a fat-fluid level.

### FIG. 16.86

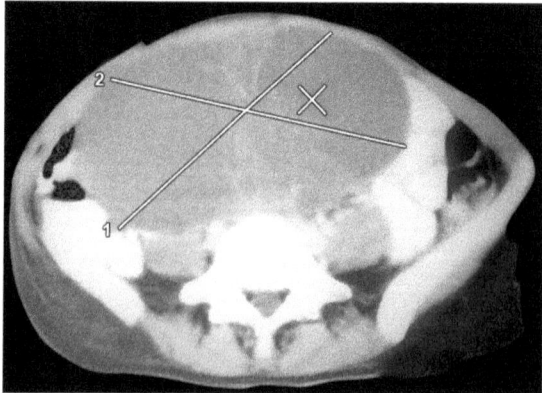

**Fig. 16.86:** Computed tomographic (CT) view of an ovarian tumor.

Chapter 16 • Practical Gynecology    643

**Q. What special advantages CT has got in gynecology?**

**Ans.** CT can be useful in staging of ovarian carcinoma as it can detect peritoneal, omental and serosal deposits. It is superior to ultrasound.

**Q. What is the place of sonography and positron emission tomography (PET) in the management of ovarian malignancy?**

**Ans.** USG especially color Doppler sonography can detect the blood flow velocity within the tissues. Presence of mural nodules, papillary excrescence, solid components suggest malignancy.

PET: It is more sensitive and specific for detection of metastatic disease and recurrence of ovarian or cervical malignancy. It is superior to CT or MRI.

**Q. What is the limitation of USG?**

**Ans.** Compared to CT or MRI, USG is not sufficient for accurate staging of any pelvic malignancy.

**Q. What is the value of CT in the evaluation of pelvic or periaortic lymph node metastasis?**

**Ans.** For most pelvic malignancies lymph nodes more than 8 mm in maximum short axis dimension (MSAD) are regarded as abnormal. CT is helpful to detect retroperitoneal metastatic nodes. However, results may be false-negative due to micrometastasis or false-positive due to lymphadenitis or reactive hyperplasia.

## MRI

**FIG. 16.87**

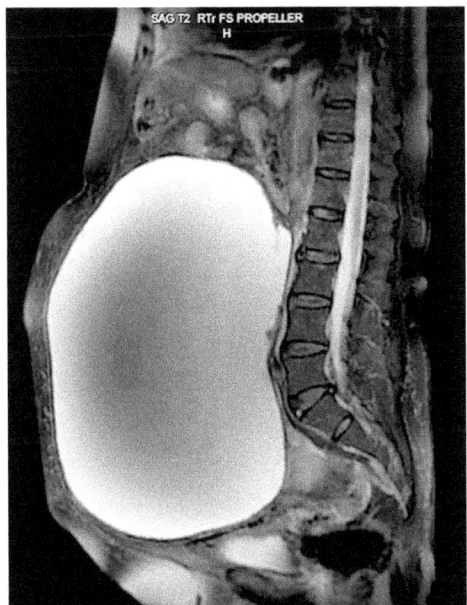

Fig. 16.87: Sagital view of MRI showing a huge ovarian tumor occupying the whole abdomen.

**Description:** MRI of an ovarian tumor.

*Self-assessment:*

**Q. How magnetic resonance imaging (MRI) is useful as a diagnostic tool in gynecology?**

**Ans.** See below

**Q. What are the advantages of MRI in the management of ovarian neoplasms?**

**Ans.** MRI has the advantages of determining the nature of the neoplasm (benign or malignant). It can detect the retroperitoneal lymph nodes and the metastasis also. It can detect the recurrence of the tumor early.

### FIG. 16.88

*Self-assessment:*

**Q. How normal endometrium and myometrium could be studied with MRI?**

**Ans.** With MRI endometrium is shown as the inner zone of high-signal intensity stripe. The deeper myometrium is recognized as a very low-signal intensity zone. The junctional zone demarcates the two (Fig. 16.88). The myometrium appears as the intermediate signal intensity zone. In postmenopausal women, the contrast between the junctional zone and the myometrium decreases.

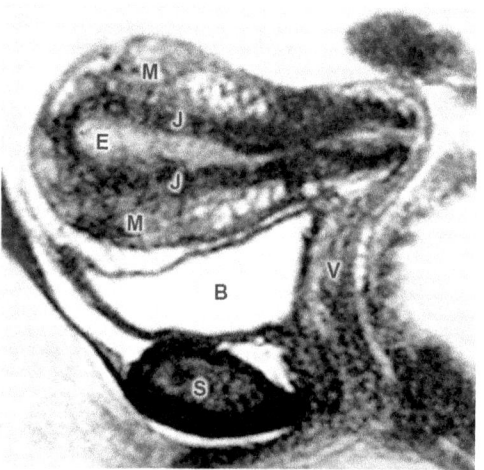

Fig. 16.88: MRI plate of a normal uterus on a sagittal T2-weighted spin-echo image showing endometrium (E), the junctional zone (J), the myometrium (M), urinary bladder (B) and the vagina (V).

**Q. What special advantages MRI has got in gynecology?**

**Ans.** (1) MRI offers multiplaner images.
(2) Gadolinium enhanced $T_2$-weighted images can determine:
  (i) Depth of myometrial invasion and that of pelvic and periaortic (retroperitoneal) nodal metastasis in endometrial carcinoma.
  (ii) Invasion of malignant process in the cervix accurately.
  (iii) It can detect recurrence of pelvic tumor.
  (iv) It is superior to CT in detecting metastatic nodes.
(3) MRI is safe in pregnancy.

# 16D. DRUGS IN GYNECOLOGY

> **Chapter Objectives**
> **To demonstrate the knowledge and understanding of:**
> - Commonly used drugs, indications, contraindications and the side effects
> - Hormonal preparations including combined oral pills
> - Anticancer drugs

## CLOMIPHENE CITRATE

**Clomiphene citrate (CC)** is the drug used for induction of ovulation.

**Indication:** Women suffering from anovulatory infertility.

**Dose:** It is prescribed 50 mg once or twice daily between D3 and D7 of the cycle (5 days).

**Mechanism of action:** CC is an antiestrogenic as well as weakly estrogenic. It causes increased gonadotropin secretion. Ovulation is expected to occur 5–7 days after the last day of therapy.

**Result:** Successful ovulation rate is as high as 90%, but pregnancy rate is about 50%.

**Side effects:** Hot flushes, nausea, visual symptoms and ovarian hyperstimulation (rare).

## LETROZOLE

**Letrozole** is used for ovulation induction. It inhibits the enzyme aromatase. It suppresses estrogen synthesis. It is given 2.5 mg once or twice daily D3–D7 of the cycle. Pregnancy rate is similar or better than that of clomiphene. Multiple pregnancy rates are low (*see* more on p. 443).

## DANAZOL

**Danazol** is an isoxazole derivative of 17-α ethinyl testosterone. It is strictly an antigonadotropin but also has androgenic action.

**Mechanism of action:** It suppresses the frequency of GnRH pulses → suppression of pituitary follicular stimulating hormone (FSH) and luteinizing hormone (LH) surge. Serum estrogen (estradiol) level is reduced.

**Indications of use:**
- Endometriosis
- DUB
- Symptomatic fibroid
- Precocious puberty (*See* Dutta Gyne 7/e, p. 40) and
- Premenstrual tension syndrome.

**Side effects are:** Acne, weight gain, hirsutism and hot flushes.

## PROGESTERONE

**Progesterone (PGN)** is a natural hormone (C-21 steroid) produced mainly by the corpus luteum of the ovary. Placenta is another major source during pregnancy.

**Synthetic progesterones (progestins)** are available.

**Commonly used progesterones are:**

(A) Natural: Progesterone.

(B) Synthetic: Progestins = Medroxyprogesterone, norethisterone, levonorgestrel, gestodene.

**Uses in gynecology:**

(1) **Progesterone challenge test**—done in cases with pathological amenorrhea. Medroxy progesterone 10 mg daily for 5 days is given orally.

(2) **Contraception:**
   (a) Minipill
   (b) Combined oral pill
   (c) DMPA
   (d) LNG—IUS (IUCD)
   (e) Implant.

(3) **Endometriosis**—progestins cause atrophy of the ectopic endometrial tissues.

(4) **Endometrial hyperplasia** and endometrial carcinoma.

(5) **Luteal support**—micronized progesterone is used as vaginal suppository or given orally 200 mg twice daily.

## COMBINED (ESTROGEN AND PROGESTERONE) ORAL CONTRACEPTIVE PREPARATIONS (COC)

**Uses:** (1) Contraception
(2) Dysfunctional uterine bleeding
(3) Endometriosis
(4) Dysmenorrhea
(5) Hirsutism.

**Q. When to start a pill for the purpose of contraception?**

**Ans.** New users should normally start a pill packet on D-1 of the cycle. Next pack should be started on the 8th day (same day of the week the pill finished, irrespective of the bleeding).

**Q. When to use additional contraception?**

**Ans.** To ensure efficacy, additional method (condom) may be used when other drugs are used. These drugs are:
 (a) Broad spectrum antibiotics (ampicillin)
 (b) Enzyme inducers (rifampicin, nevirapine).

**Q. What are failure rates of the commonly used contraceptives?**

**Ans.**

| Methods | Pregnancy rate per 100 women year |
|---|---|
| CuT 380A | 0.8 |
| LNG 20 | 0.1 |
| Combined oral Contraceptives (COCs) | 0.1 |
| Norplant | 0.05 |
| Implanon | 0.01 |
| Vasectomy | 0.15 |
| Tubectomy | 0.15 |

**Q. What are the contraindications of combined oral contraceptives (COCs)?**

**Ans.**

| Absolute | | Relative | |
|---|---|---|---|
| a. | Arterial and venous thrombosis | a. | Age >40 |
| b. | Severe hypertension | b. | History of jaundice |
| c. | Valvular heart disease | c. | Hyperlipidemia |
| d. | Diabetes with vascular complications | d. | Breastfeeding |
| e. | Pregnancy | e. | Diabetes |
| f. | Undiagnosed genital tract bleeding | | |
| g. | Smoker >35 years | | |

**Q. How do you counsel a woman when she misses her pill(s)?**

**Ans.** When she missed one pill in the row, she is advised to take the missed pill as soon as she remembers it (within 24 hours). She should take the rest as per schedule.

**Q. When she missed two pills?**

**Ans.** (A) **In the first week.**
- She should take 2 pills at each of the next two days and continue the rest as scheduled.
- At the same time, she should also take extra precaution for the next 7 days (either to use condom or avoid sex).

(B) **When** two pills are missed in the third week or more than two active pills are missed at any time:
- To use another method of contraception for next 7 days (to use condom or avoid sex)
- Next pack to start without a break.

## TRANEXAMIC ACID

**Tranexamic acid** is an antifibrinolytic agent. It is an analog of aminocaproic acid (ACA). It blocks the conversion of plasminogen to plasmin. It is used in cases with abnormal uterine bleeding (menorrhagia), bleeding following IUCD use (and after prostatic surgery). It reduces menstrual blood loss by 50%. It counteracts the endometrial fibrinolytic system (Fig. 16.88).

**Dose schedule:** Loading dose 15 mg/kg orally, followed by 30 mg/kg orally every 6 hours.

**Contraindications:** It should not be used in cases with disseminated intravascular coagulopathy.

**Side effects:**
- **Gastrointestinal**
  - Nausea
  - Diarrhea
  - Abdominal discomfort
- **Others**
  - Postural hypotension
  - Intravascular thrombosis.

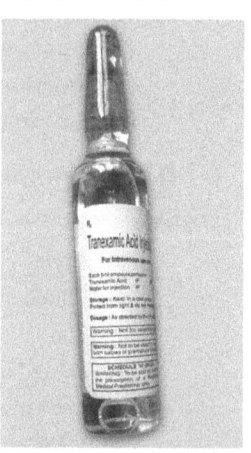

Fig. 16.88: Tranexamic acid.

## MIFEPRISTONE

**Mifepristone:** It is an antiprogestogenic steroid. It sensitises the myometrium to prostaglandins and initiates uterine contractions. It softens and dilates the cervix.

**Indications:**
(a) Medical termination of pregnancy up to 63 days of gestation.
(b) Along with prostaglandins ($PGE_1$), it is for MTP of 13-20 weeks.
(c) Induction of labor in cases with intrauterine fetal death.
(d) Endometriosis to arrest the growth and to relieve pain.
(e) Fibroid uterus to arrest the growth.

**Dose:**
(i) For MTP: 600 mg single dose, by mouth
(ii) Labor induction: 600 mg daily for 2 days by mouth.
(iii) Treatment of leiomyomas: 2.5 to 10 mg given orally daily for 3 to 6 months.

**Side effects:**
- Nausea
- Vomiting
- Abdominal cramps
- Vaginal bleeding and uterine contractions.

**Contraindications:**
- Uncontrolled severe asthma
- Suspected ectopic pregnancy and
- Chronic adrenal failure.

## METFORMIN

**Metformin** is a biguanide group of drug. It reduces hepatic glucose production. It improves peripheral glucose utilization by increasing insulin sensitivity.

**It is used as an insulin sensitizer in cases with polycystic ovarian disease who are often insulin resistant.** These women suffer from anovulation and infertility. Metformin is found to reduce hyperinsulinemia and hyperandrogenemia. Ovulation induction is more successful when CC or letrozole is combined with metformin. Metformin is given in a dose of 500 mg twice or thrice daily. It does not induce hypoglycemia in a normal individual (*see* more on p. 443).

**Side effects:** Anorexia, epigastric discomfort, diarrhea and lactic acidosis (rare).

## METHOTREXATE

**Methotrexate** is a folic acid antagonist. It prevents reduction of folic acid to folinic acid by inhibiting the enzyme dihydrofolate reductase.

**Indications:**
(1) Management of persistent GTN
(2) Choriocarcinoma
(3) Medical management of tubal ectopic pregnancy
(4) Management of ovarian germ cell cancers
(5) Management of cases with morbid adherent placenta following delivery, to inhibit growth of trophoblastic tumor cells.

**Side effects:**
- Nausea
- Vomiting
- Oral ulceration
- Mucositis
- Stomatitis
- Alopecia
- Anemia and
- Hepatitis.

## CISPLATIN/CARBOPLATIN

**Cisplatin/carboplatin** are the platinum group of compounds. Platinum group of drugs are most effective against epithelial ovarian cancer.

**Mechanism of action:**
- Like alkylating agents, they cause cross linkage of DNA strands and prevent cell division.
- They may be used in combination with paclitaxel.
- Carboplatin is less toxic compared to cisplatin.

**Side effects:**
- Nausea
- Vomiting
- Anemia
- Granulocytopenia
- Azotemia
- Renal failure
- Compared to cisplatin and carboplatin has less toxicity.

# Single Best Answer and Multiple Choice Questions

CHAPTER 17

**Chapter Objectives**

Total 207 SBAs in gynecology, are there for comprehensive revision of subject with added explanations.
- It is a good practice area to test individual's level of knowledge.
- To detect area of weakness and to make it up.

❖ Single Best Answer (SBA)      651
❖ Multiple Choice Questions (MCQs)      651

## Chapter 17 • Single Best Answer and Multiple Choice Questions

# 1. SURGICAL ANATOMY

## QUESTIONS

Q.01 *The following are in relation with pudendal artery except:*
(a) It is a branch of anterior division of internal iliac artery
(b) One of its branches is middle rectal artery
(c) Its main supply is to the perineal and vulval structures
(d) It anastomoses with superficial and deep pudendal arteries, branches of femoral artery

Q.02 *The following statements are related to Bartholin's gland except:*
(a) Bartholin cyst is usually located in the duct or ductules
(b) Marsupialization is an effective surgery
(c) Incision is made on the outside skin
(d) Complete excision of the gland is needed in 10–15% due to recurrence

Q.03 *Germ cells arise from:*
(a) Germinal epithelium
(b) Yolk sac endoderm
(c) Wolffian duct
(d) Müllerian duct

Q.04 *The followings are developed from mesonephric duct:*
(a) Uterus
(b) Fallopian tubes
(c) Upper vagina
(d) None of the above

Q.05 *Complete failure of fusion of Müllerian ducts results in:*
(a) Uterine didelphys
(b) Subseptate uterus
(c) Bicornuate uterus
(d) Absence of uterus

## ANSWERS

Ans 01. (b) Middle rectal artery is one of the visceral branches of anterior division of internal iliac artery. One of the branches of the pudendal artery is inferior rectal.

Ans 02. (c) Incision is made on the vaginal mucosa below the hymenal ring.

Ans 03. (b) *See* Dutta Gyne 7/e, p. 30.

Ans 04. (d) All are developed from paramesonephric duct (Müllerian duct). *See* Dutta Gyne 7/e, p 27, Table 3.1.

Ans 05. (a) *See* Dutta Gyne 7/e, p. 35.

## QUESTIONS

**Q.06** *The followings are related correctly to embryology except:*
(a) Germ cells within the genital ridge are developed from the germinal epithelium
(b) Ovarian ligaments and round ligaments are developed from genital ligament (gubernaculum)
(c) Clitoris is developed from genital tubercle
(d) Labia majora are developed from labioscrotal swelling

**Q.07** *Rectocele is confirmed by:*
(a) Bimanual examination
(b) Speculum examination
(c) Digital vaginal examination
(d) Rectal examination

**Q.08** *The ovary is attached with all except:*
(a) Ovarian ligament
(b) Posterior leaf of the broad ligament
(c) Infundibulopelvic ligament
(d) Round ligament

**Q.09** *Vestigeal structures in the broad ligament are all except:*
(a) Duct of Gartner
(b) Epoophoron
(c) Paroophoron
(d) Round ligament

**Q.10** *The definitive kidney is developed from:*
(a) Pronephros
(b) Mesonephros
(c) Metanephros
(d) None of the above

**Q.11** *Histologically, the labia minora contains:*
(a) Hair follicles
(b) Sweat glands
(c) Sebaceous glands
(d) All of the above

## ANSWERS

**Ans 06.** (a) Germ cells are derived from the endoderm of yolk sac and they migrate to the genital ridge along the dorsal mesentery between 20 and 30 days (*see* Dutta Gyne 7/e, p. 30).

**Ans 07.** (d)

**Ans 08.** (d) *See* Dutta Gyne 7/e, p. 9.

**Ans 09.** (d) Round ligament and ovarian ligament are gubernaculum of the ovary (*see* Dutta Gyne 7/e, p. 27).

**Ans 10.** (c)

**Ans 11.** (c) The labia minora is devoid of hair follicles or sweat glands (*see* Dutta Gyne 7/e, p. 26).

## QUESTIONS

**Q.12** *The followings are the different parts of the broad ligament except:*
(a) Mesovarium
(b) Mesosalpinx
(c) Infundibulopelvic ligament
(d) Round ligament

**Q.13** *Length of the round ligament is:*
(a) 5 cm
(b) 10 cm
(c) 15 cm
(d) 20 cm

**Q.14** *Distinction between bicornuate and septate uterus can be made most accurately by:*
(a) Hysterosalpingography (HSG)
(b) Bimanual examination to find the presence or absence of median raphe
(c) Laparoscopy
(d) Combination of laparoscopy and hysteroscopy

**Q.15** *The followings are related to labia except:*
(a) Labia majora are homologous with the scrotum in male
(b) Labia minora contain numerous hair follicles
(c) Round ligaments terminate in the upper-third of labia majora
(d) Branches of femoral artery supply the vulva

**Q.16** *The followings are related to the anatomy of vagina except:*
(a) Long axis of vagina almost lies parallel to the plane of the pelvic inlet
(b) Posterior vaginal wall is longer than the anterior wall
(c) The posterior fornix is deeper than the others
(d) The entire posterior wall is directly related to the rectum and anal canal

**Q.17** *Arterial supply of the vagina is derived from all except:*
(a) Uterine artery
(b) Vaginal artery
(c) Superior rectal artery
(d) Internal pudendal artery

## ANSWERS

**Ans 12.** (d)
**Ans 13.** (b) *See* Dutta Gyne 7/e, p. 18.
**Ans 14.** (d) The combination of the knowledge of the internal and external uterine contour defines the precise nomenclature and the degree of the particular anomaly.
**Ans 15.** (b) Hair follicle is absent in labia minora.
**Ans 16.** (d) The middle-third of the vagina is related to rectum whereas the lower-third is separated from the anal canal by perineal body. (*see* Dutta Gyne 7/e, p. 3).
**Ans 17.** (c) It should be middle or inferior. Superior rectal is a branch of inferior mesenteric artery (*see* Dutta Gyne 7/e, p. 5).

## QUESTIONS

**Q.18** *The followings are related to the crossing of uterine artery and ureter except:*
 (a) The crossing occurs about 1.5 cm away at the level of internal os
 (b) The ureter crosses the uterine artery posteriorly
 (c) The uterine artery crosses the ureter from above and in front
 (d) The crossing occurs just after the ureter enters the ureteric tunnel

**Q.19** *The followings are related to the fallopian tube except:*
 (a) Length measures about 10 cm
 (b) Isthmus measures about 2.5 cm
 (c) Uterine ostium measures 1 mm in diameter
 (d) There is shedding of tubal epithelium during menstruation

**Q.20** *The followings are in relation to ovarian attachment except:*
 (a) The ovary lies intraperitoneally
 (b) It is attached to the broad ligament by the mesovarium
 (c) Attached to the lateral wall by infundibulopelvic ligament
 (d) Attached to the uterus by the round ligament

**Q.21** *The followings are related to urethral (female) anatomy except:*
 (a) The length is about 4 cm
 (b) The lining epithelium is transitional and at the meatus stratified squamous
 (c) The arterial supply is from inferior vesical and internal pudendal
 (d) Nerve supply is entirely from pudendal

**Q.22** *Lymphatics of the cervix drain primarily into the following glands except:*
 (a) Internal iliac (b) Inguinal
 (c) Obturator (d) External iliac

## ANSWERS

**Ans 18.** (d) The ureter is crossed by the uterine artery prior to its entrance into the ureteric tunnel (*see* Dutta Gyne 7/e, p. 11).

**Ans 19.** (d) There is no shedding (*see* Dutta Gyne 7/e, p. 8).

**Ans 20.** (d) The ovary is attached to the uterus by the ovarian ligament (*see* Dutta Gyne 7/e, p. 9).

**Ans 21.** (d) The pudendal nerve supplies the lower part but the upper part is supplied by the autonomic fibers from the hypogastric and pelvic plexuses.

**Ans 22.** (b) Lymphatics from the cervix do not directly drain into the inguinal group of glands (*see* Dutta Gyne 7/e, p. 23, Fig. 2.3).

## QUESTIONS

**Q.23** *The ureter*
(a) Lies superior in the lateral vaginal fornix
(b) Has a squamous epithelial lining
(c) Passes behind the external iliac vessels
(d) Is crossed by the genitofemoral nerve

**Q.24** *The Müllerian duct:*
(a) Develops medial to the Wolffian duct
(b) Is also known as the mesonephric duct
(c) Starts to form at 6 weeks of embryonic life
(d) Opens into the urogenital sinus separately

**Q.25** *Regarding the arterial supply of the pelvis all are correct except:*
(a) The posterior trunk of internal iliac supplies the gluteal muscles
(b) Medial sacral artery arises from aorta
(c) The inferior vesical artery arises from the posterior trunk of internal iliac
(d) The inferior rectal artery arises from the internal pudendal artery

**Q.26** *Vagina develops from:*
(a) Müllerian duct only
(b) Sinovaginal bulb only
(c) Both Müllerian duct and sinovaginal bulb
(d) Gartner's duct

**Q.27** *The following arteries in the pelvis are the branches of internal iliac artery except:*
(a) Middle rectal artery
(b) Superior rectal
(c) Internal pudendal artery
(d) Uterine artery

## ANSWERS

**Ans 23.** (a)
**Ans 24.** (c) *See* Dutta Gyne 7/e, p. 27.
**Ans 25.** (c) *See* Dutta Gyne 7/e, p. 21.
**Ans 26.** (c)
**Ans 27.** (b)

## QUESTIONS

**Q.28** Length of the fallopian tube is:
(a) 10 cm
(b) 7 cm
(c) 5 cm
(d) 3 cm

**Q.29** Left ovarian vein drains into:
(a) Inferior vena cava
(b) Left common iliac vein
(c) Left renal vein
(d) Left hypogastric vein

**Q.30** Regarding female urethra, all are correct, except:
(a) It measures 4 cm in length
(b) It is related to the anterior vaginal wall
(c) Mucous membrane is lined by columnar epithelium
(d) It opens below the clitoris

**Q.31** Prostate in male is homologous to which organ in female?
(a) Cervical glands
(b) Bartholin's gland
(c) Skene's glands
(d) Bulbourethral glands

**Q.32** Bartholin's gland is situated in the:
(a) Superficial perineal pouch
(b) Deep perineal pouch
(c) Urogenital diaphragm
(d) None

**Q.33** The gonad which is palpable outside abdominal cavity is almost always:
(a) Ovary
(b) Testis
(c) Ovotestis
(d) Supernumerary

**Q.34** The organ which has complete origin from Müllerian ducts is:
(a) Uterus
(b) Vagina
(c) Round ligament
(d) Ligament of ovary

## ANSWERS

**Ans 28.** (a)
**Ans 29.** (c)
**Ans 30.** (c) *See* Dutta Gyne 7/e, p. 10.
**Ans 31.** (c) Skene's glands or paraurethral glands are situated adjacent to the distal urethra (*see* Dutta Gyne 7/e, p. 10).
**Ans 32.** (a)
**Ans 33.** (b)
**Ans 34.** (a)

## 2. REPRODUCTIVE ENDOCRINOLOGY

### QUESTIONS

**Q.35** *The following are associated with carcinoma cervix except:*
(a) Early sexual intercourse
(b) Use of condom
(c) Combined oral pills
(d) HPV 31, 45 infection

**Q.36** *The functions of LH are all except:*
(a) Activation of theca cells to produce progesterone
(b) Helps the physical act of ovulation
(c) Initiates luteinization of the granulosa cells
(d) Completion of first meiotic division and extrusion of first polar body

**Q.37** *The commonest use of combined estrogen and progestogen preparations:*
(a) Dysmenorrhea
(b) Endometriosis
(c) Diagnosis of pregnancy
(d) Oral contraception

**Q.38** *Source of estrogen production is:*
(a) Adrenal
(b) Placenta
(c) Peripheral tissue
(d) All of the above

**Q.39** *The followings are the changes in the endometrium in a regular 28 day cycle except:*
(a) Subnuclear vacuolation is the evidence of high LH activity
(b) On the 21st day, the glands become tortuous with visible secretion in the lumen
(c) On the 22nd day, stromal edema is maximum
(d) Leukocytic infiltration is maximum at about 2 days before menstruation

### ANSWERS

**Ans 35.** (b) It is a protective factor (*see* Dutta Gyne 7/e, p. 264, Table 23.2).

**Ans 36.** (a) LH stimulates theca cells for androgen precursor production which are converted into estrogens in the granulosa cells (*see* Dutta Gyne 7/e, p. 57).

**Ans 37.** (d)

**Ans 38.** (d) Ovarian and adrenal androstenedione can be converted to estrone in the peripheral tissue. This is an important site of estrogen production after menopause.

**Ans 39.** (a) Subnuclear vacuolation is due to progesterone and appears on D 18, 36–48 hours after ovulation (*see* Dutta Gyne 7/e, p. 72).

## QUESTIONS

**Q.40** Raised serum levels of FSH are found in:
(a) Oral contraceptive pill use
(b) Postmenopausal women
(c) With the use of GnRH analogs
(d) Turner syndrome

**Q.41** Withdrawal bleeding following administration of progestogen in a case of secondary amenorrhea indicates all except:
(a) Absence of pregnancy
(b) Production of endogenous estrogen
(c) Endometrium is responsive to estrogen
(d) Defect in pituitary-gonadal axis

**Q.42** The following condition is aggravated by the use of combined oral contraceptives:
(a) Hirsutism
(b) Endometriosis
(c) Premenstrual tension
(d) Cervical ectopy

**Q.43** Serum FSH level in postmenopausal women is:
(a) 0.5–2 IU/L
(b) 5–10 IU/L
(c) 15–20 IU/L
(d) Above 40 IU/L

**Q.44** Androgen production in testis occurs in:
(a) Leydig's cells
(b) Sertoli cells
(c) Tunica albuginea
(d) Rete testis

**Q.45** Female infertility is mostly due to:
(a) Anovulation
(b) Tubal block
(c) Luteal phase defect
(d) Tuberculous endometritis

**Q.46** Mean blood loss during usual menstrual flow is:
(a) 15 mL
(b) 35 mL
(c) 90 mL
(d) 150 mL

## ANSWERS

**Ans 40.** (b and d)
**Ans 41.** (d) *See* Dutta Gyne 7/e, p. 386.
**Ans 42.** (d)
**Ans 43.** (d)
**Ans 44.** (a)
**Ans 45.** (a)
**Ans 46.** (b) *See* Dutta Gyne 7/e, p. 66.

## QUESTIONS

**Q.47** *The following findings will be present in Turner's syndrome, except:*
(a) Short stature
(b) Absence of sex chromatin body
(c) Cubitus valgus
(d) Normal ovaries

**Q.48** *As per WHO standard, oligospermia means:*
(a) Sperm count less than 10 million per cc
(b) Sperm count less than 20 million per cc
(c) Sperm count less than 40 million per cc
(d) Sperm count less than 60 million per cc

**Q.49** *Gonadectomy is indicated in:*
(a) Klinefelter's syndrome
(b) Androgen insensitivity syndrome
(c) Turner's syndrome
(d) Isosexual sexual precocity

**Q.50** *Uterus is absent in primary amenorrhea of patients with:*
(a) Turner's syndrome
(b) Testicular feminization syndrome
(c) Imperforate hymen
(d) Premature ovarian failure

**Q.51** *Commonest cause of oligomenorrhea in an adolescent female is:*
(a) Hypothyroidism
(b) PCOS
(c) Hyperprolactinemia
(d) Tuberculous endometritis

**Q.52** *Ovulation can be detected by all, except:*
(a) Basal body temperature change
(b) Cervical mucus study
(c) Cervical cytology
(d) Serum progesterone

**Q.53** *All are the causes of menorrhagia except:*
(a) Fibroid uterus
(b) IUCD
(c) Cervical polyp
(d) Adenomyosis

## ANSWERS

**Ans 47.** (d) *See* Dutta Gyne 7/e, p. 363.
**Ans 48.** (b) *See* Dutta Gyne 7/e, p. 190.
**Ans 49.** (b)
**Ans 50.** (b)
**Ans 51.** (b)
**Ans 52.** (c) *See* Dutta Gyne 7/e, p. 192.
**Ans 53.** (c) *See* Dutta Gyne 7/e, p. 152.

## QUESTIONS

**Q.54** *Secondary amenorrhea is due to all, except:*
(a) Polycystic ovarian disease
(b) Imperforate hymen
(c) Thyroid dysfunction
(d) Tuberculosis

**Q.55** *All are the high-risk factors for endometrial carcinoma, except:*
(a) Obesity
(b) Multiparity
(c) Use of estrogen
(d) Women with PCOS

**Q.56** *Rokitansky-Kuster-Hauser syndrome is associated with:*
(a) Ovarian agenesis
(b) Tubal agenesis
(c) Bicornuate uterus
(d) Vaginal agenesis

**Q.57** *Sequence of pubertal development in girls is:*
(a) Thelarche, menarche, pubarche
(b) Menarche, thelarche, pubarche
(c) Thelarche, pubarche, menarche
(d) Menarche, pubarche, thelarche

**Q.58** *Masculinizing tumor of the ovary is:*
(a) Granulosa cell tumor
(b) Dysgerminoma
(c) Arrhenoblastoma
(d) Clear cell carcinoma

**Q.59** *Commonest cause of secondary amenorrhea is:*
(a) PCOD
(b) Pregnancy
(c) Genital tuberculosis
(d) Lactation

**Q.60** *Usually, the first endocrinal evidence of approaching menopause is:*
(a) Raised FSH
(b) Raised LH
(c) Raised testosterone
(d) Decreased estrogen

## ANSWERS

**Ans 54.** (b) *See* Dutta Gyne 7/e, p. 457, Table 28.3.
**Ans 55.** (b) *See* Dutta Gyne 7/e, p. 292.
**Ans 56.** (d) *See* Dutta Gyne 7/e, p. 373, Table 29.1.
**Ans 57.** (c) *See* Dutta Gyne 7/e, p. 39.
**Ans 58.** (c) *See* Dutta Gyne 7/e, p. 318.
**Ans 59.** (b) *See* Dutta Gyne 7/e, p. 376.
**Ans 60.** (a) *See* Dutta Gyne 7/e, p. 46.

## 3. BENIGN LESIONS IN GYNECOLOGY

### QUESTIONS

Q.61 **The commonest site of pelvic endometriosis is:**
 (a) Uterosacral ligament
 (b) Ovary
 (c) Rectovaginal septum
 (d) Pelvic peritoneum

Q.62 **Treatment of mild endometriosis in a patient aged 30 years with infertility is:**
 (a) Symptomatic treatment to relieve pain
 (b) Producing pseudopregnancy state by using danazol (17α ethyl testosterone)
 (c) Producing pseudomenopause by using combined 'pill'
 (d) GnRH analog monthly

Q.63 **Scar endometriosis is most common except followings:**
 (a) Abdominal hysterotomy for MTP
 (b) Cesarean section
 (c) Vaginal delivery with episiotomy
 (d) Appendicectomy

Q.64 **The followings are related to scar endometriosis:**
 (a) It is always associated with pelvic endometriosis
 (b) Implantation occurs through vascular and lymphatic dissemination
 (c) It is cured by hormone therapy
 (d) Excision is usually the treatment

### ANSWERS

**Ans 61.** (b)

**Ans 62.** (a) Danazol acts by producing pseudomenopause and combined pill acts by producing pseudopregnancy. There is no place of ovulation suppression by medical management for such a patient. There is no such well-controlled study to show the superiority of surgery or medical therapy over expectant management in mild or minimal endometriosis.

**Ans 63.** (a) *See* Dutta Gyne 7/e, p. 256

**Ans 64.** (d) *See* Dutta Gyne 7/e, p. 256.

## QUESTIONS

**Q.65** *Irrespective of age, the best noninvasive method of control of bleeding in dysfunctional uterine bleeding:*
(a) Estrogen
(b) Androgen
(c) Progestogen
(d) D + C

**Q.66** *Regarding retroversion of the uterus:*
(a) Occurs in 20% of normal women
(b) It is a common cause of infertility
(c) May be corrected by Fothergill's operation
(d) It is caused by heavy lifting

**Q.67** *Primary dysmenorrhea can be treated by all except:*
(a) Antiprostaglandins
(b) Cyclic combined estrogen and progestogen preparations
(c) Presacral neurectomy
(d) Uterine curettage

**Q.68** *For cytohormonal study which of the index is most informative?*
(a) Eosinophilic
(b) Karyopyknotic
(c) Cornification
(d) Maturation

**Q.69** *Causes of pyometra at the age of 35 are all except:*
(a) Infected lochiometra
(b) Infected polyp blocking the cervical canal
(c) Endocervical carcinoma
(d) Senile endometritis

## ANSWERS

**Ans 65.** (c) *See* Dutta Gyne 7/e, p. 157.
**Ans 66.** (a)
**Ans 67.** (d) Curettage is not the treatment but dilatation of the cervix may be of help.
**Ans 68.** (d) See Dutta Gyne 7/e, p. 192, Table 9.4.
**Ans 69.** (d) Senile endometritis is a problem of the postmenopausal lady.

## Chapter 17 • Single Best Answer and Multiple Choice Questions

### QUESTIONS

**Q.70** *Uterine synechiae is commonly due to all except:*
- (a) Puerperal curettage
- (b) Following cesarean section
- (c) Tubercular endometritis
- (d) Following IUCD insertion

**Q.71** *Postmenopausal vaginal bleeding may be due to all except:*
- (a) Urethral caruncle
- (b) CIN 3
- (c) Carcinoma of the fallopian tube
- (d) Atrophic vaginitis

**Q.72** *The diagnosis of pelvic endometriosis is confirmed by:*
- (a) Congestive dysmenorrhea
- (b) Painful defecation
- (c) Nodular feel of the uterosacral ligaments
- (d) Laparoscopy

**Q.73** *Commonest cause of male infertility among the following is:*
- (a) Defective spermatogenesis
- (b) Genital tract infection
- (c) Genital tract obstruction
- (d) Sperm autoimmunity

### ANSWERS

**Ans 70.** (d) Rarely, it occurs following myomectomy or even after insertion of IUCD when infection sets in. However, IUCD is used for treatment of synechiae (*see* Dutta Gyne 7/e, p. 378).

**Ans 71.** (b) CIN is an asymptomatic lesion.

**Ans 72.** (d) *See* Dutta Gyne 7/e, p. 251.

**Ans 73.** (a)

# 4. GENERAL GYNECOLOGY

## QUESTIONS

**Q.74** *Cytohormonal maturation index of a woman during a menstrual cycle (28 day ovulatory cycle) and life time, is as mentioned except:*

(a) Day 5—0/50/50
(b) Day 14—0/40/60
(c) Day 28—0/70/30
(d) Childhood—80/20/0

**Q.75** *Regression of the corpus luteum starts from:*

(a) Just prior to menstruation
(b) 4-6th day prior to menstruation
(c) With the onset of menstruation
(d) After the menstruation

**Q.76** *Preferred method for collection of material for cytohormonal study is:*

(a) Scraping from the upper one-third of lateral vaginal wall
(b) Vaginal pool specimen by pipette
(c) Cervical scraping
(d) Scraping from lower third of vagina

**Q.77** *Functional cyst of the ovary is characterized by:*

(a) It does not usually exceed 6 cm
(b) It may persist even after the cure of the functional disorder to which it is associated
(c) It is more associated with patient taking oral 'pill'
(d) It is usually multilocular

## ANSWERS

**Ans 74.** (a) Estrogenic effect is much less on day 5, as such maturation index should be ideally 0/60/40.

**Ans 75.** (b) *See* Dutta Gyne 6/e, p. 70.

**Ans 76.** (a) Contaminated cells from other sites are avoided (*see* Dutta Gyne 7/e, p. 92).

**Ans 77.** (a) *See* Dutta Gyne 7/e, p. 235.

## Chapter 17 • Single Best Answer and Multiple Choice Questions

### QUESTIONS

**Q.78** The cavity of the uterine body becomes smaller in all except:
(a) Endometrial carcinoma
(b) Menopause
(c) Inversion
(d) Hypoplastic uterus

**Q.79** For cytohormonal study which of the index is most informative?
(a) Eosinophilic
(b) Karyopyknotic
(c) Cornification
(d) Maturation

**Q.80** The optimal pH for maintenance of active motile spermatozoa is:
(a) 4.5–5.5
(b) 6–7
(c) 7.2–7.8
(d) 8–9

**Q.81** Rectocele is confirmed by:
(a) Bimanual examination
(b) Speculum examination
(c) Digital vaginal examination
(d) Rectal examination

**Q.82** The causes of retention of urine in female are all except:
(a) Hematocolpos
(b) Fundal fibroid uterus
(c) Mucocolpos
(d) Retroverted gravid uterus

**Q.83** Mature Graafian follicle measures:
(a) 5–10 mm
(b) 15–20 mm
(c) 25–30 mm
(d) More than 30 mm

**Q.84** In relation to Bartholin's gland all are correct except:
(a) It is a compound racemose gland
(b) It is partly covered by bulbospongiosus
(c) Its duct measures about 20 mm
(d) It lies deep to urogenital diaphragm

### ANSWERS

**Ans 78.** (a)
**Ans 79.** (d) *See* Dutta Gyne 7/e, p. 92, Table 9.4.
**Ans 80.** (c) *See* Dutta Gyne 7/e, p. 190. Table 17.3
**Ans 81.** (d)
**Ans 82.** (b) Cervical fibroid can cause retention of urine (*see* Dutta Gyne 7/e, p. 338, Table 25.7).
**Ans 83.** (b) *See* Dutta Gyne 7/e, p. 69.
**Ans 84.** (d) The Bartholin glands lie superficial to urogenital diaphragm in the superficial perineal pouch.

## QUESTIONS

**Q.85** *These terms are related to semen analysis except:*
(a) Oligospermia means reduction in sperm count
(b) Asthenospermia means reduction in spermatozoa vitality
(c) Teratospermia means malformed sperm
(d) Necrozoospermia means deformed sperm

**Q.86** *Cervical ectopy can be effectively treated by:*
(a) Electrocauterization (b) Cryosurgery
(c) Amputation of the cervix (d) All of the above

**Q.87** *Asymptomatic puerperal ectopy should be treated by:*
(a) Expectant management for about 3 months postpartum
(b) Electrocauterization
(c) Chemical cauterization
(d) Cryocauterization

**Q.88** *The following statements are related to dysmenorrhea except:*
(a) Spasmodic dysmenorrhea is estrogen related
(b) Fibroid is related to congestive dysmenorrhea
(c) Pre- and co-menstrual dysmenorrhea is characteristic of pelvic endometriosis
(d) Congestive dysmenorrhea is usually secondary

**Q.89** *Hidradenomas are tumors which originate in the sweat glands situated on all except:*
(a) Mons (b) Labia majora
(c) Labia minora (d) Perineum

## ANSWERS

**Ans 85.** (d) Necrozoospermia means spermatozoa are dead or motionless.
**Ans 86.** (d)
**Ans 87.** (a) In majority, there is spontaneous regression.
**Ans 88.** (a) Spasmodic dysmenorrhea is related to progesterone which causes synthesis and release of PGF2α.
**Ans 89.** (c) As because there is no sweat gland in labia minora, hidradenoma cannot develop.

## Chapter 17 • Single Best Answer and Multiple Choice Questions

### QUESTIONS

**Q.90** Indications of rectal examination in gynecology are:
(a) Genital prolapse
(b) Carcinoma cervix
(c) Cases with atresia vagina
(d) All of the above

**Q.91** All are true about acquired immunodeficiency syndrome (AIDS) except:
(a) The infection is due to a DNA virus
(b) The virus binds to the CD4 molecule on T cells
(c) Transmission can be by artificial insemination
(d) Mother-to-child transmission is about 30%

**Q.92** In a normal human female, the number of oocytes is greatest at:
(a) Intrauterine life
(b) Birth
(c) Puberty
(d) Peak reproductive period

**Q.93** The zygote enters the uterine cavity in:
(a) 4 cell stage
(b) 6–16 cell stage
(c) 32–64 cell stage
(d) None of the above

**Q.94** Commonest cause of oligomenorrhea in adolescent female is:
(a) Hypothyroidism
(b) Polycystic ovarian disease
(c) Hyperprolactinemia
(d) Tuberculous endometritis

**Q.95** Vaginal pH is maintained by which organisms?
(a) Anaerobic streptococci
(b) Doderlein's bacillus
(c) E. coli
(d) Diphtheroids

**Q.96** Metrorrhagia is caused by all except:
(a) Submucous myoma
(b) Subserous fibroid uterus
(c) Intrauterine contraceptive device
(d) Submucus polyp

### ANSWERS

**Ans 90.** (d) In genital prolapse, it is done to differentiate rectocele from enterocele.
**Ans 91.** (a)
**Ans 92.** (a)
**Ans 93.** (b)
**Ans 94.** (b)
**Ans 95.** (b)
**Ans 96.** (b)

## QUESTIONS

**Q.97** In which day of cycle endometrial biopsy is best taken for detection of ovulation:
(a) 5th–7th day
(b) 10th–14th day
(c) 9th–11th day
(d) 21st–24th day

**Q.98** Menstruation is defined as precocious, if it starts before the age of:
(a) 8 years
(b) 10 years
(c) 14 years
(d) 12 years

**Q.99** Spinnbarkeit is mostly demonstrated in which phase of menstrual cycle?
(a) Proliferative
(b) Secretory
(c) Just before menstruation
(d) Menstrual

**Q.100** Bartholin's ducts open into:
(a) Labia majora
(b) Labia minora
(c) Lower vagina
(d) Groove between minora and hymen

**Q.101** "Peg cells" are seen in:
(a) Vagina
(b) Vulva
(c) Ovary
(d) Fallopian tubes

**Q.102** Cystic swelling in anterolateral wall of the vagina, impulse on coughing negative, most likely diagnosis is:
(a) Bartholin's cyst
(b) Gartner duct cyst
(c) Cystocele
(d) Adenocarcinoma vagina

**Q.103** Which is the deepest fornix of the vagina:
(a) Anterior
(b) Left lateral
(c) Right lateral
(d) Posterior

## ANSWERS

Ans 97. (d)
Ans 98. (a)
Ans 99. (a) *See* Dutta Gyne 7/e, p. 93.
Ans 100. (d)
Ans 101. (d)
Ans 102. (b) *See* Dutta Gyne 7/e, p. 172.
Ans 103. (d)

## 5. GENITAL TRACT INFECTION

### QUESTIONS

**Q.104** *The following are related to Trichomonas vaginitis except:*
(a) It is a sexually transmitted disease
(b) The organism is a flagellated parasite
(c) The discharge is curdy white with flakes
(d) Strawberry appearance of the posterior fornix and the cervix is characteristics

**Q.105** *The following are related to Monilial vaginitis except:*
(a) The causative organism is *Candida albicans*
(b) Recurrence rate following initial cure is very low
(c) The relative concentrations of lactobacilli and *Candida albicans* in the vagina are inversely related
(d) Associated with hormonal factors, depressed immunity and antibiotic use

**Q.106** *The following statements are related to salpingitis except:*
(a) Gonococcal infection is usually limited to endosalpinx
(b) Pyogenic infection involves whole thickness of the tube
(c) Tubercular infection involves all the layers of the tube
(d) Tubal infection is usually unilateral

**Q.107** *Common modes of tubal infection are all except:*
(a) Gonococcal infection—by continuity and contiguity
(b) Pyogenic—through parametrial lymphatics
(c) Tubercular—by pelvic lymphatics causing perisalpingitis
(d) Chlamydia—colonize the cervix initially

### ANSWERS

**Ans 104.** (c) The discharge is frothy, yellowish and offensive (*see* Dutta Gyne 7/e, p. 134).
**Ans 105.** (b) Recurrence rate varies from 20–80%.
**Ans 106.** (d) Tubal infection is usually bilateral.
**Ans 107.** (c) Hematogenous infection leading to interstitial salpingitis.

## QUESTIONS

**Q.108** The most reliable method of diagnosis of genital tuberculosis is:
(a) Endometrial curettage in late secretory phase followed by histological and bacteriological examination
(b) Hysterosalpingography
(c) Hysteroscopy and laparoscopy
(d) PCR for nucleic acid amplification from specimen

**Q.109** Normal inhabitants of vaginal flora are all except:
(a) *Streptococcus*
(b) Chlamydia
(c) Doderlein's bacillus
(d) *Candida* species

**Q.110** Surgical treatment options for chronic cervicitis may be:
(a) Cauterization
(b) Cold knife conization
(c) Hysterectomy
(d) All of the above

**Q.111** The followings are the sexually transmitted diseases except:
(a) Trichomonas vaginitis
(b) Herpes simplex type 2 vaginitis
(c) Parvovirus B19
(d) Chlamydia trachomatis

**Q.112** Tubercular ulcer of the cervix should primarily be treated by:
(a) Amputation
(b) Hysterectomy
(c) Antitubercular therapy
(d) Electrocauterization

**Q.113** The followings are related to Chlamydia trachomatis (C. trachomatis):
(a) It is an obligate, intracellular bacteria
(b) The organism mainly affects the squamous epithelium
(c) Fitz-Hugh-Curtis syndrome is more due to Chlamydia than *Gonococcus*
(d) Symptoms include dysuria and postcoital bleeding

## ANSWERS

**Ans 108.** (d) Genital TB is paucibacillary and smears and cultures are usually negative. PCR can detect even less than 10 organisms in a specimen. Histology is suggestive but not diagnostic. (See Dutta Gyne 7/e, p. 116).

**Ans 109.** (b)

**Ans 110.** (d)

**Ans 111.** (c)

**Ans 112.** (c)

**Ans 113.** (a, c, d) Chlamydia affects the columnar and transitional epithelium.

## QUESTIONS

**Q.114** *The followings are the late sequelae of acute PID except:*
 (a) Increased infertility rate
 (b) Chronic pelvic pain and ill health
 (c) Recurrent fetal loss
 (d) Increased rate of ectopic pregnancy

**Q.115** *Strawberry vagina is seen in infection with:*
 (a) Trichomonas vaginalis
 (b) Bacterial vaginosis
 (c) *Candida albicans*
 (d) Herpes simplex

**Q.116** *Ectopic pregnancy is associated with all except:*
 (a) Salpingitis
 (b) IUCD
 (c) Reconstructive plastic operations on the tube
 (d) Clomiphene citrate therapy

**Q.117** *Monilial vaginitis is commonly associated with all except:*
 (a) Prolonged antibiotic therapy
 (b) Diabetes mellitus
 (c) Treatment of malaria with chloroquine
 (d) Pregnancy

**Q.118** *Treatment of Asherman's syndrome is:*
 (a) Dilatation and curettage
 (b) Hysterotomy
 (c) Adheslolysis and IUCD
 (d) Hysterectomy

**Q.119** *Most common site for genital tuberculosis is:*
 (a) Ovary
 (b) Uterus
 (c) Cervix
 (d) Fallopian tube

## ANSWERS

**Ans 114.** (c) *See* Dutta Gyne 7/e, p. 111.
**Ans 115.** (a)
**Ans 116.** (d)
**Ans 117.** (c)
**Ans 118.** (c)
**Ans 119.** (d)

## QUESTIONS

**Q.120** Greenish yellow discharge per vaginam with strawberry vagina is suggestive of infection with:
(a) Trichomonas vaginalis
(b) Gonococcal infection
(c) Atrophic vaginitis
(d) Monilial

**Q.121** Asymptomatic carrier of gonococcal infection in female lodges the organism in:
(a) Endocervix
(b) Vagina
(c) Urethra
(d) Fornix

**Q.122** What is not a criteria for diagnosis of bacterial vaginosis?
(a) Presence of 'clue-cells'
(b) Fishy odor of vaginal secretion on alkalinization
(c) Plenty of lactobacilli
(d) Vaginal pH greater than 4.5

**Q.123** The following are related to trichomonas vaginitis except:
(a) It is a sexually transmitted disease
(b) The organism is a flagellated parasite
(c) The discharge is curdy white with flakes
(d) Hanging drop preparation is helpful to the diagnosis

## ANSWERS

**Ans 120.** (a)
**Ans 121.** (a)
**Ans 122.** (c) *See* Dutta Gyne 7/e, p. 125.
**Ans 123.** (c) *See* Dutta Gyne 7/e, p. 134.

## 6. BENIGN TUMORS

### QUESTIONS

**Q.124** *The following are related to submucous fibroid except:*
(a) It constitutes about 5% of all uterine fibroids
(b) Sarcomatous degeneration is less than in other variety of fibroid
(c) Even a small fibroid produces maximum symptoms
(d) Menorrhagia is the classic symptom

**Q.125** *The following statements are related to degeneration of fibroid except:*
(a) Calcification occurs in the center of myoma of old women
(b) Infection commonly occurs in submucous fibroid
(c) Red degeneration is solely confined to pregnancy
(d) Fatty degeneration is quite rare

**Q.126** *Diagnosis of a small submucous fibroid can be best done by:*
(a) Saline infusion sonography (SIS)
(b) Hysterography
(c) Hysteroscopy
(d) Sonography

**Q.127** *The following statements are related to dermoid cyst of the ovary except:*
(a) It is the commonest of all ovarian teratomas
(b) It is bilateral in about 15%
(c) It may turn to malignancy
(d) It contains only ectodermal element

### ANSWERS

**Ans 124.** (b) *See* Dutta Gyne 7/e, p. 222.
**Ans 125.** (c) Red degeneration can occur in puerperium. It is seen most often in the second trimester of pregnancy.
**Ans 126.** (a) *See* Dutta Gyne 7/e, p. 226.
**Ans 127.** (d) Ectodermal, endodermal and mesodermal tissues are present.

## QUESTIONS

**Q.128** Commonest benign tumor of ovary is:
 (a) Dermoid cyst  (b) Serous cystadenoma
 (c) Mucinous cystadenoma  (d) Endometrioma

**Q.129** Commonest secondary change found in uterine fibromyoma is:
 (a) Fatty degeneration  (b) Red degeneration
 (c) Hyaline degeneration  (d) Sarcomatous change

**Q.130** Which variety of ovarian cyst is more likely to undergo torsion?
 (a) Dermoid cyst  (b) Serous cystadenoma
 (c) Mucinous cystadenoma  (d) Serous cystadenocarcinoma

**Q.131** Psammoma body is characteristically found in:
 (a) Serous cystadenoma of ovary  (b) Mucinous cystadenoma of ovary
 (c) Follicular cyst of ovary  (d) Luteal cyst of ovary

**Q.132** The components of Meigs' syndrome are:
 (a) Fibroma of ovary  (b) Ascites
 (c) Hydrothorax  (d) All of the above

**Q.133** Attacks of flushing and cyanosis occur in which type of ovarian tumor?
 (a) Struma ovary  (b) Krukenberg tumor
 (c) Carcinoid tumor of ovary  (d) Granulosa cell tumor

**Q.134** In mucinous ovarian tumor, all are true except:
 (a) Arises from surface epithelium of ovary
 (b) Contain thick viscid mucin
 (c) Tumor may grow to a large size
 (d) Presence of psammoma bodies

## ANSWERS

Ans 128. (b)
Ans 129. (c)
Ans 130. (a)
Ans 131. (a)
Ans 132. (d)
Ans 133. (c)
Ans 134. (d)

## QUESTIONS

**Q.135** *Virilizing tumors of the ovary are all except:*
- (a) Sertoli Leydig cell tumor
- (b) Arrhenoblastoma
- (c) Adrenal like tumors of ovary
- (d) Granulosa cell tumor

**Q.136** *Call-Exner bodies are formed in:*
- (a) Arrhenoblastoma
- (b) Granulosa-theca cell tumor
- (c) Brenner's tumor
- (d) Endodermal sinus tumor

**Q.137** *Psammoma body is characteristically found in:*
- (a) Serous cystadenoma of ovary
- (b) Mucinous cystadenoma of ovary
- (c) Dysgerminoma of ovary
- (d) Luteal cyst of ovary

**Q.138** *Commonest degeneration during pregnancy in fibroid uterus is:*
- (a) Hyaline degeneration
- (b) Calcareous degeneration
- (c) Red degeneration
- (d) Fatty degeneration

**Q.139** *Commonest complication of ovarian cyst is:*
- (a) Torsion
- (b) Rupture
- (c) Malignancy
- (d) Meigs' syndrome

## ANSWERS

**Ans 135.** (d)
**Ans 136.** (b)
**Ans 137.** (a) *See* Dutta Gyne 7/e, p. 238.
**Ans 138.** (c) *See* Dutta Gyne 7/e, p. 224.
**Ans 139.** (a) *See* Dutta Gyne 7/e, p. 243.

## 7. GENITAL MALIGNANCY

### QUESTIONS

**Q.140** *The following are associated with carcinoma cervix except:*
(a) Early sexual intercourse
(b) Use of condom
(c) Combined oral pills
(d) HPV 31, 45 infection

**Q.141** *The early symptoms of carcinoma cervix are all except:*
(a) Intermenstrual bleeding
(b) Contact bleeding following coitus or vaginal examination
(c) Leukorrhea with often pinkish discharge
(d) Variable degrees of pain

**Q.142** *The commonest cause of death in cancer cervix is:*
(a) Renal failure following ureteric obstruction
(b) Hemorrhage
(c) Sepsis
(d) Hepatic failure

**Q.143** *The best procedure to diagnose carcinoma cervix following positive cytology is:*
(a) Four quadrant cervical biopsy
(b) Cone biopsy
(c) Ring biopsy
(d) Colposcopic directed biopsy

**Q.144** *Postmenopausal endometrial hyperplasia is due to hyperestrogenic state, the sources being:*
(a) Adrenal glands
(b) Hilus cells of the ovary
(c) Peripheral conversion of androgens
(d) All of the above

### ANSWERS

**Ans 140.** (b) It is a protective factor (*see* Dutta Gyne 7/e, p. 264, Table 23.2).

**Ans 141.** (d) Pain is a late symptom of carcinoma, indicating involvement of the parametrium (*see* Dutta Gyne 7/e, p. 284).

**Ans 142.** (a) *See* Dutta Gyne 7/e, p. 285.

**Ans 143.** (d)

**Ans 144.** (d) Androstenedione from the adrenal glands and testosterone from the hilus cells of the ovary are peripherally converted into estrogen.

## QUESTIONS

**Q.145** The preferred treatment of CIN-3/CIS in a parous woman aged 45 years is:
(a) Hysterectomy
(b) Cold knife conization
(c) Cryosurgery
(d) Cauterization

**Q.146** Pseudomyxoma peritonei is associated with all except:
(a) Mucinous cystadenoma of the ovary
(b) Mucocele appendix
(c) Carcinoma gallbladder
(d) Carcinoma of the large bowel

**Q.147** Germ cell ovarian tumors are all except:
(a) Choriocarcinoma
(b) Dysgerminoma
(c) Granulosa cell tumor
(d) Endodermal sinus tumor

**Q.148** The following are the chemotherapeutic drugs and the side effects—match them appropriately:
(a) Cyclophosphamide      1. Renal failure
(b) Cisplatin             2. Myocarditis
(c) Doxorubicin           3. Oral ulceration (mucositis)
(d) Methotrexate          4. Hemorrhagic cystitis

**Q.149** Regarding hydatidiform mole:
(a) Best diagnosed by ultrasonography
(b) May present with small for date uterus
(c) Chromosomes are derived entirely from the mother
(d) Initial β-hCG levels >100,000 IU/L is a risk factor for malignancy

## ANSWERS

**Ans 145.** (a) *See* Dutta Gyne 7/e, p. 270.
**Ans 146.** (c) It is associated with mucocele of gallbladder (*see* Dutta Gyne 7/e, p. 244).
**Ans 147.** (c) It is a sex cord stromal tumor (*see* Dutta Gyne 7/e, p. 237, Table 21.1).
**Ans 148.** (a) = 4; (b) = 1; (c) = 2; (d) = 3.
**Ans 149.** a, b, d. Q.(c) : Complete moles have 46 XX, both of which are derived entirely from the father (*see* Dutta Gyne 7/e, p. 298).

## QUESTIONS

**Q.150** *Followings are the tumor characteristics—match them appropriately.*

(a) Dysgerminoma           1. Often secrete estrogen
(b) Endodermal sinus cell tumor    2. Highly radiosensitive
(c) Granulosa cell tumor    3. Maximum cytoreduction
(d) Epithelial ovarian cancer    4. β-hCG and α fetoprotein

**Q.151** *Level of serum CA-125 is raised in:*

(a) Epithelial ovarian cancer    (b) Adenomyosis
(c) Pancreatitis    (d) All of the above

**Q.152** *The following conditions are associated with these names—match them appropriately.*

(a) Meigs    1. Intermenstrual pain
(b) Mittelschmerz    2. Pararectal deep perineal incision
(c) Schuchardt    3. Cysts attached to the abdominal ostium of the fallopian tube
(d) Kobelt    4. Ascites, hydrothorax and ovarian fibroma

**Q.153** *Side effects of chemotherapy include all except:*

(a) Nausea    (b) Alopecia
(c) Lymphoedema    (d) Myelosuppression

**Q.154** *Match the side effects according to the drug:*

(a) Bleomycin    1. Bone demineralization
(b) Cyclophosphamide    2. Hematuria
(c) Paclitaxel    3. Pulmonary fibrosis
(d) Heparin    4. Arrhythmias

## ANSWERS

**Ans 150.** (a) = 2; (b) = 4; (c) = 1; (d) = 3.
**Ans 151.** (d).
**Ans 152.** (a) = 4; (b) = 1; (c) = 2; (d) = 3.
**Ans 153.** (c)  It is observed following pelvic lymphadenectomy.
**Ans 154.** (a) = 3; (b) = 2; (c) = 4; (d) = 1. *See* Dutta Gyne 7/e, p. 427-428.

## Chapter 17 • Single Best Answer and Multiple Choice Questions

## QUESTIONS

**Q.155** *Factors considered in the epidemiology of cervical cancer include exposure to:*
(a) Herpes simplex virus
(b) Human papillomavirus
(c) Both of above
(d) None of above

**Q.156** *Nodal metastasis in cervical cancer may be better detected early by the following:*
(a) Ultrasound examination
(b) CT scan
(c) MRI
(d) PET CT

**Q.157** *The following statements in connections with carcinoma in situ of cervix are true except:*
(a) Human papillomavirus (HPV) may be causative agent
(b) Basement membrane is always invaded in all cases
(c) Common histopathological report is squamous cell carcinoma
(d) Usually spreads by lymphatics

**Q.158** *Which one is solid and malignant ovarian tumor?*
(a) Brenner's tumors
(b) Thecoma
(c) Mesonephroma
(d) Fibroma

**Q.159** *Causes of postmenopausal bleeding are all except:*
(a) Endometrial carcinoma
(b) Decubitus ulcer
(c) Carcinoma of bladder
(d) Atrophic endometritis

**Q.160** *Tumor marker of choriocarcinoma is:*
(a) Estrogen
(b) Progesterone
(c) Alpha fetoprotein
(d) hCG

## ANSWERS

**Ans 155.** (b)
**Ans 156.** (d)
**Ans 157.** (b)
**Ans 158.** (c)
**Ans 159.** (c)
**Ans 160.** (d)

## QUESTIONS

**Q.161** *Regarding cervical carcinoma, all are correct, except:*
(a) It is a preventable cancer
(b) Commonly, it is a squamous cell carcinoma
(c) Radical hysterectomy is the only treatment
(d) Cytology screening can prevent it

**Q.162** *Regarding female urethra, all are correct, except:*
(a) It measures 4 cm in length
(b) It is related to the anterior vaginal wall
(c) Mucous membrane is lined by columnar epithelium
(d) It opens below the clitoris

**Q.163** *Which investigation is not done in FIGO staging of carcinoma cervix?*
(a) IVP
(b) CECT
(c) MRI
(d) None of the above

**Q.164** *CIN grade II means:*
(a) Carcinoma cervix stage II
(b) Carcinoma in situ
(c) Involvement up to basal 2/3 of the epithelium
(d) Any CIN persisting for more than 2 years

**Q.165** *CA-125 is used as a tumor marker for:*
(a) Carcinoma cervix
(b) Carcinoma endometrium
(c) Carcinoma ovary
(d) Carcinoma vulva

## ANSWERS

**Ans 161.** (c)
**Ans 162.** (c) *See* Dutta Gyne 7/e, p. 10.
**Ans 163.** (d) *See* Dutta Gyne 7/e, p. 281, Table 24.7.
**Ans 164.** (c) *See* Dutta Gyne 7/e, p. 262, Table 23.1.
**Ans 165.** (c) *See* Dutta Gyne 7/e, p. 431, Table 31.9.

## Chapter 17 • Single Best Answer and Multiple Choice Questions

### QUESTIONS

**Q.166** Bilateral ovarian carcinoma, ascites with positive malignant cells. The FIGO stage is:
(a) Ib  
(b) IC3  
(c) IIb  
(d) IIc  

**Q.167** All may be etiologically related with endometrial cancer except:
(a) Long menstrual life  
(b) Late menarche  
(c) Late menopause  
(d) Nulliparity  

**Q.168** What is the correct descending order of incidence of malignancy of female genital organs in India?
(a) Endometrium, cervix, ovary  
(b) Cervix, ovary, endometrium  
(c) Ovary, cervix, endometrium  
(d) Cervix, endometrium, ovary  

**Q.169** According to the surgical staging of endometrial carcinoma, stage-IB means:
(a) Myometrial invasion less than 1/2  
(b) Uterine cavity length 8 cm or less  
(c) Tumor invades cervical stroma  
(d) Myometrial invasion equal to or more than 1/2  

**Q.170** The commonest ovarian malignancy is:
(a) Serous cyst adenocarcinoma  
(b) Mucinous cyst adenocarcinoma  
(c) Malignant teratoma  
(d) Endometrioid carcinoma  

**Q.171** Signet ring cell is diagnostic of:
(a) Brenner tumor  
(b) Serous cyst adenocarcinoma  
(c) Granulosa cell tumor  
(d) Krukenberg's tumor  

### ANSWERS

**Ans 166.** (b) *See* Dutta Gyne 7/e, p. 307, Table 24.24.  
**Ans 167.** (b) *See* Dutta Gyne 7/e, p. 292.  
**Ans 168.** (b) *See* Dutta Gyne 7/e, p. 333, Table 24.3.  
**Ans 169.** (d) *See* Dutta Gyne 7/e, p. 295, Table 24.14.  
**Ans 170.** (a) *See* Dutta Gyne 7/e, p. 305.  
**Ans 171.** (d) *See* Dutta Gyne 7/e, p. 319.

# 8. CONTRACEPTION

## QUESTIONS

**Q.172** *The following condition(s) is aggravated by the combined oral contraceptives is:*
(a) Hirsutism
(b) Endometriosis
(c) Premenstrual tension
(d) Cervical ectopy

**Q.173** *Regarding postpill amenorrhea is:*
(a) It is a side effect of combined oral contraceptive pill (COC)
(b) It may be due to hyperprolactinemia
(c) It should be investigated without delay
(d) It is due to prolonged use of pills

**Q.174** *Safe, effective and acceptable contraception in women over 40 years is:*
(a) Barrier contraception
(b) Combined estrogen-progestogen pill
(c) Progestin only pill
(d) Intrauterine device

**Q.175** *Prolonged use of combined estrogen-progestin contraceptive pill is likely to reduce the incidence of:*
(a) Ovarian cancer
(b) Cervical cancer
(c) Vaginal cancer
(d) Vulval cancer

**Q.176** *Complications of vasectomy for male sterilization:*
(a) Prostatic cancer
(b) Infection
(c) Antisperm antibody formation
(d) Decreased libido

## ANSWERS

**Ans 172.** (d)

**Ans 173.** (b) Amenorrhea following stoppage of COC is not a causal association. Overall incidence is less than 1% for duration of more than 6 months, Spontaneous resumption of menstruation occurs in majority by 6 months' time. Amenorrhea persisting >6 months should be investigated as any other case of secondary amenorrhea. Pituitary adenoma need to be excluded.

**Ans 174.** (c) *See* Dutta Gyne 7/e, p. 403.

**Ans 175.** (a) *See* Dutta Gyne 7/e, p. 401.

**Ans 176.** (b) *See* Dutta Gyne 7/e, p. 407.

## QUESTIONS

**Q.177** Contraindications to use of combined oral contraceptive includes the followings except:
(a) Active liver disease
(b) Thromboembolic disorders
(c) Gallbladder disease
(d) Nulliparity

**Q.178** Among the followings, Pearl index is highest with:
(a) Combined oral contraceptive
(b) Intrauterine contraceptive device
(c) Barrier contraception
(d) Calendar rhythm method

**Q.179** "Emergency contraception" includes the use of following except:
(a) Estrogen and progestogen pills
(b) Progestogen only
(c) IUCD only
(d) Coitus interruptus

**Q.180** Which IUCD needs to be replaced after 10 year:
(a) CuT-380
(b) LNG containing IUCD
(c) CuT-200
(d) Multiload-375

**Q.181** The method of sterilization least suited for recanalization is:
(a) Pomeroy's method
(b) Fallope rings
(c) Filshie clips
(d) Bipolar cauterization

**Q.182** Followings are contraindications of IUCD except:
(a) Irregular vaginal bleeding
(b) Pelvic inflammatory disease
(c) Following MTP
(d) Uterine didelphys

**Q.183** All are reasonably good time for insertion of IUCD except:
(a) Postmenstruation
(b) Postabortion
(c) Immediately after delivery
(d) One week after delivery

## ANSWERS

**Ans 177.** (d) *See* Dutta Gyne 7/e, p. 400.
**Ans 178.** (d)
**Ans 179.** (d)
**Ans 180.** (a) *See* Dutta Gyne 7/e, p. 397.
**Ans 181.** (a)
**Ans 182.** (c)
**Ans 183.** (d) *See* Dutta Gyne 7/e, p. 393.

## 9. OPERATIVE GYNECOLOGY

### QUESTIONS

**Q.184** *Hysteroscopy is used for all except:*
(a) Removal of IUD
(b) Diagnosis of uterine polyp
(c) To take endometrial biopsy from the appropriate sites
(d) To confirm patency of the fallopian tube

**Q.185** *Complete perineal tear occurs in all except:*
(a) Forceps delivery in undiagnosed occipitoposterior
(b) Extension of mediolateral episiotomy
(c) Shoulder dystocia
(d) Precipitate labor

**Q.186** *Rectovaginal fistula most commonly occurs in:*
(a) Congenital
(b) Following obstructed labor
(c) Carcinoma vagina
(d) A sequelae of repair of CPT

**Q.187** *The followings are related to vesicovaginal fistula except:*
(a) Sloughing fistula is common where obstetric care is suboptimal
(b) Fistula following irradiation or malignancy is difficult to repair
(c) Even for a sloughing fistula, spontaneous closure is a possibility
(d) Chance of successful repair is best when repair is done immediately

**Q.188** *Sequelae of vaginal hysterectomy with PFR are all except:*
(a) Vault prolapse
(b) Dyspareunia
(c) Tender perineal scar
(d) Early menopausal symptoms

### ANSWERS

**Ans 184.** (d) See Dutta Gyne 7/e, p. 512.
**Ans 185.** (b) It may occur as extension of central episiotomy (*See* Dutta Gyne 7/e, p. 354).
**Ans 186.** (d) See Dutta Gyne 7/e, p. 351.
**Ans 187.** (d)
**Ans 188.** (d) As the ovaries are generally preserved, symptoms are not early.

## QUESTIONS

**Q.189** *Complications of MTP in the first trimester are all except:*
 (a) Pelvic endometriosis
 (b) Asherman's syndrome
 (c) Cornual block
 (d) Preterm labor in subsequent pregnancy

**Q.190** *Material used to distend the uterine cavity during hysteroscopy is:*
 (a) Glycine dextran solution
 (b) Saline solution
 (c) Carbon dioxide gas
 (d) All of the above

**Q.191** *During anterior colporrhaphy, the lower limit of base of urinary bladder is best identified by:*
 (a) Most prominent bulge at vaginal introitus
 (b) Transverse vaginal sulcus
 (c) Lower limit of bulge in front of cervix
 (d) Passing a metal catheter in urinary bladder

**Q.192** *Appropriate surgical treatment of procidentia in a woman aged 40 years is:*
 (a) Fothergill's operation
 (b) Ward-Mayo's operation
 (c) LeFort's operation
 (d) Cervicopexy

## ANSWERS

**Ans 189.** (a) Endometriosis is observed with hysterotomy not with menstrual regulation or dilatation and evacuation.
**Ans 190.** (d)
**Ans 191.** (d)
**Ans 192.** (b)

## QUESTIONS

**Q.193** *Commonest of the following complications of laparoscopy is:*
 (a) Periumbilical hematoma formation
 (b) Surgical emphysema
 (c) Bowel injury
 (d) Injury to great vessels

**Q.194** *Part of the fallopian tube which is ideally excised in tubal sterilization is:*
 (a) Part of isthmus  (b) Part of ampullary part
 (c) Isthmo-ampullary junctional zone  (d) Infundibulum

**Q.195** *During routine laparotomy for gynecological surgery, the following structures are most liable to injury except:*
 (a) Intestines  (b) Omentum
 (c) Urinary bladder  (d) Inferior epigastric artery

**Q.196** *Tubal patency is judged by all of the followings except:*
 (a) Insufflation of tubes  (b) Hysterosalpingography
 (c) Laparoscopic dye test  (d) Hysteroscopy

**Q.197** *Which one is not the component of Fothergill's operation?*
 (a) Amputation of cervix
 (b) Anterior colporrhaphy
 (c) Tightening the Mackenrodt's ligament in front of the cervix
 (d) Shortening the uterosacral ligaments

**Q.198** *In a patient with 3rd degree perineal tear, presenting after one week of delivery, repair should be done:*
 (a) Immediately  (b) After two weeks
 (c) After 12 weeks  (d) After 6 months

## ANSWERS

**Ans 193.** (b)
**Ans 194.** (a) *See* Dutta Gyne 7/e, p. 408.
**Ans 195.** (d)
**Ans 196.** (d)
**Ans 197.** (d) *See* Dutta Gyne 7/e, p. 179, Table 16.5.
**Ans 198.** (c)

## QUESTIONS

**Q.199** In which day of cycle endometrial biopsy is best taken for detection of ovulation:
(a) 5th–7th day
(b) 10th–14th day
(c) 9th–11th day
(d) 21st–24th day

**Q.200** VVF in India is commonly due to:
(a) Carcinoma cervix
(b) Prolonged labor
(c) Gynecological surgery
(d) Carcinoma vagina

**Q.201** Which gas is most commonly used in laparoscopy?
(a) $O_2$
(b) $CO_2$
(c) $N_2O$
(d) $N_2$

**Q.202** Laparotomy should be done in a case of ovarian cyst with pregnancy is:
(a) Immediately on diagnosis
(b) Preferably in 2nd trimester
(c) Preferably in 3rd trimester
(d) Preferably after delivery

## ANSWERS

**Ans 199.** (d)
**Ans 200.** (b)
**Ans 201.** (b) *See* Dutta Gyne 7/e, p. 504.
**Ans 202.** (b) *See* Dutta Obs 8/e, p. 245.

# 10. DRUGS

## QUESTIONS

**Q.203** *Regarding the drugs all are true except:*
(a) Mifepristone is antiestrogenic
(b) Estrogen is antiandrogenic
(c) Ulipristal modulates progesterone
(d) Danazol is antigonadotropin

**Q.204** *Danazol is:*
(a) Estrogen derivative
(b) Progestogen derivative
(c) Combined estrogen and progesterone
(d) Androgen derivative

**Q.205** *All are true for Clomiphene citrate except:*
(a) It is an ovulation-inducing drug
(b) It is antiestrogenic
(c) It can cause multiple pregnancy
(d) It is weakly progestrogenic

**Q.206** *All of the following drugs are used in endometriosis except:*
(a) Danazol
(b) Medroxyprogesterone acetate
(c) Norethisterone
(d) Venlafaxine

**Q.207** *Medical management of fibroid includes all, except:*
(a) Danazol
(b) Progestogens
(c) Progesterone receptor modulators
(d) GnRH

## ANSWERS

**Ans 203.** (a) It is antiprogesterone.
**Ans 204.** (d)
**Ans 205.** (d)
**Ans 206.** (d)
**Ans 207.** (d) *See* Dutta Gyne 7/e, p. 228, Table 20.7.

# CHAPTER 18

# History in Obstetrics and Gynecology

**Chapter Objectives**
- Eminent personalities with their contributions in the specialty are a few.
- It is good for a candidate to have some knowledge about them.
- A candidate with this knowledge, certainly has an edge over to one who has not.

❖ Eponyms in Medicine 690

List of eminent personalities with their contributions in obstetrics and gynecology has been presented in this section. Sometimes, questions are asked by the examiner in relation to such personalities with their contributions. Failure to answer such question is not going to fail the candidate, but certainly this improves the impression upon the candidate if he/she could answer it.

## EPONYMS IN MEDICINE

| | |
|---|---|
| **Allis Oscar Huntington** | *See* p. 564 |
| **Andrews, Henry (1871–1942)** | Consultant Obstetrician and Gynecologist working at London Hospital. His name is associated with Brandt-Andrews maneuvers; which describes the procedure of delivery of the placenta by controlled cord traction and suprapubic pressure. **Brandt, Thure** (1819–1895) Obstetricians and Gynecologist from Stockholm. |
| **Apgar, Virginia (1909–1974)** | Anesthetist working in America. She introduced **"Apgar Score"** for assessment of cardiopulmonary and neurological status of the newborn at birth. This was described in 1953. Virginia Apgar's newborn score is used almost universally. Apgar was a popular musician and played cello and violin. Virginia Apgar died in her sleep on 7 August 1974. |
| **Bonney, William Frances Victor (1872–1953)** | *See* p. 568 |
| **Braxton-Hicks, John (1825–1997)** | Obstetrician and Gynecologist at Guy's Hospital, London. He described intermittent painless uterine contractions during pregnancy. "Braxton-Hicks Contractions" in 1871. He also described bipolar (combined external and internal) version in 1860. |
| **Christian Doppler, Johann (1803–1853)** | Austrian Physicist and Mathematician. Doppler effect of ultrasound was described by him in 1842. |
| **Das Sir KN** | Consultant Obstetrician and Gynecologist and Principal of Carmichael (now RG Kar) Medical College, Kolkata. He designed a special variety of long curved obstetric forceps suited for the Indian women, whose pelvis and baby sizes are comparatively small to the Western countries. This is popularly known as the Das's variety of obstetric forceps. |

| | |
|---|---|
| **Deaver John Blair** | *See* p. 574 |
| **Federich Shauta** | *See* p. 616 |
| **Foley Frederick Eugene Basil** | *See* p. 556 |
| **Green-Armytage, Vivian Bartly (1882–1961)** | MB, Captain Indian Medical Service. He was the resident surgeon at Eden Hospital, Kolkata (1912). Later, he became the Professor of Obstetrics in the same department. He also worked in West London Hospital. He devised the forceps, "Green Armytage forceps" for holding the uterine incision margins and the angles during cesarean section. |
| **Hegar, Alfred (1830-1914)** | Professor of Obstetrics and Gynecology in Freiburg. He designed the metallic-graded cervical dilators, Hegar's dilator. |
| **James Ire** | *See* p. 548 |
| **Herbert Trout** | *See* p. 548 |
| **Papanicolaou, George Nicholas (1883–1962)** | *See* p. 548 |
| **Krukenberg, Friedrich (1871–1946)** | Pathologist and Professor of Ophthalmology, Halle. He described Krukenberg tumor in 1896. |
| **Leventhal, Michael (1901–1973)** | American Obstetrician and Gynecologist. He along with Stein, Irving from Chicago, described Stein-Leventhal syndrome (Polycystic ovarian syndrome) in 1935. |
| **Menon, K Krishna (1908–1988)** | Gynecologist from Madras (presently Chennai), served the Indian Medical Service in the Second World War. He was the Professor of Obstetrics and Gynecology at Madras Medical College and Stanley Medical College. He became the Director Professor of the Institute of Obstetrics and Gynecology at Madras Medical College and Government Hospital for Women and Children. He was a Visiting Professor in Britain and United States. Menon became the President of Federation of Obstetrics and Gynecological Societies of India in 1961 and honorary Fellow of the Royal College of Obstetricians and Gynecologists. He was awarded "Padma Shri" in 1973 by the President of India. Menon presented his results using, Lytic Cocktail in the management of eclampsia at the University College Hospital, London in 1960. He spoke with his own experience from the hospital that he worked. Menon's monumental work on "lytic cocktail" using phenothiazine and pethidine in eclampsia was published in Jr Obstet Gynecol, Br Common W. 1961;68:417-26. |

| Mitra, Subodh (1896–1961) | Gynecological Cancer Surgeon and Vice-Chancellor, University of Calcutta, India. He is remembered for his new technique of operation, "Radical vaginal hysterectomy with bilateral extraperitoneal pelvic lymphadenectomy". This operation is popularly known as "Mitra's operation for cancer of the cervix". |
|---|---|
| Naegele, Franz Carl (1778–1851) | Franz Carl Naegele is remembered for three things: Pelvic deformity, Naegele's obliquity (anterior asyclitism). Franz Carl Naegele was born in Dusseldorf, Germany. He was the Director at the University of Heidelberg, succeeding his father-in-law in the position. |
| Palmer, Raoul (1905–1985) | Raoul Palmer used laparoscopy in Gynecology in 1943. Besides laparoscopy, he was also a noted surgeon for his skills in tubal and vaginal surgery, 'Palmer's Point' in laparoscopic surgery goes by this name. He assisted Vivian Green-Armytage, while in Paris, in vaginal hysterectomy operation. |
| Pantaleoni, D Commander C (1869) | Pantaleoni made the first report on the use of endoscope (hysteroscope) to diagnose and treat an intrauterine lesion in 1869. Initial works on hysteroscope was done by Philipp Bozzini in 1805.<br><br>Initial hysteroscopy use was made by paraffin lamp illumination as devised by Francis Cruse of Dublin in 1865. It took more than a century for diagnostic and operative hysteroscopy to become popular. |
| Papanicolaou, George Nicholas | See p. 548 |
| Purandare, BN (1911–1990) | Gynecologist from Mumbai, India, is recognized by his abdominal cervicopexy operation for cases with nulliparous prolapse (Prolapse without a cystocele). |
| Shirodkar, VN (1899–1971) | Gynecologist from Grant Medical College, Mumbai, India. He introduced "Shirodkar's Stitch" cervical cerclage operation in 1955, for cases with cervical incompetence and recurrent mid-trimester abortion. He was the President of the Federation of Obstetric and Gynecological Societies of India. |
| Sims, James Marion (1813–1883) | See p. 550 |
| Spencer Wells Thomas | See p. 574 |
| Turner Henry (1892–1970) | Professor of Medicine, Oklahoma University, USA. He described Turner's syndrome (Ovarian dysgenesis 45XO). He became the doyen of clinical endocrinology in United States. He diagnosed his own lung cancer as inoperable. He worked until his death on 4th August, 1970. |

| | |
|---|---|
| **Vigneaud, Vincent Du (1901–1978)** | Revolution in the use of oxytocic drugs was made with the identification and synthesis of oxytocin in 1953. Working in the Department of Biochemistry of Cornell University Medical College, Vigneaud and his colleagues identified and synthesized the hormone oxytocin and also vasopressin. Du Vigneaud received Nobel Prize for chemistry in 1955 for his landmark research in identification and synthesis of posterior pituitary hormones. |
| **Wertheim Ernst** | *See* p. 616 |

# Index of Section I Obstetrics

Page numbers followed by *f* refer to figure and *t* refer to table.

## A

Abdomen 12
   closure of 276*f*
   hugely enlarged 96*f*
   inspection of 8*f*
   uniform enlargement of 8*f*
Abdominal examination 184
Abdominal pain 105
   causes of 119
   lower 32
Abdominal transducers 232*f*
ABO and Rh grouping 251
Abortion
   complete 118
   incomplete 118
   induction of 331
   inevitable 118
   missed 118
   spontaneous 117
   threatened 118
   types of 113
   unsafe 239
Abruptio placenta 103, 104, 106
   causes of 104
   complications of 104
Acardiac fetus 89*f*
Accidental hemorrhage 104
Accredited social health activist 356
Accurate documentation 112
Acephalus 89*f*
Acetic acid test 79
Acid elution test 83
Allis's tissue forceps 275f, 285, 286*f*
Amenorrhea 33
   cause of 37
American Diabetic Association 55
Amniocentesis 81, 97
Amniotic fluid 81, 98
   analysis of 81*f*
   index 99
   volume 68
Amniotic membrane 272*f*

Anembryoinic pregnancy 113, 114
Anemia 49, 250
   causes of 48, 49
   complications of 250
   congenital 83
   deficiency 48, 250
   grades of 49
   prevalence of 53
   prevention 239
Angular cheilitis 48
Antenatal care 133, 253, 351
Antenatal checkup 351*f*
Antenatal clinic
   management in 204
   pregnant woman in 19
Antenatal corticosteroid therapy 192
Antenatal investigations, routine 10
Antenatal preventive measures 111
Antepartum hemorrhage 100, 239
   causes of 321
Anticoagulants 333
Anticonvulsant 333
   regime 76
Anti-D
   dose of 83
   immunoglobulin 119
   prophylactic 84
   prophylaxis 84
Antiepileptic drugs 362
Antihypertensives 331
Aorta, compression of 109, 109*f*
Apgar scoring 308
APH, causes of 284
Appendicectomy 5
Arrest disorders 213*f*
Arrhythmias 334
Arterial embolization, selective 111
Asphyxia neonatorum, causes of 308
Asphyxiated neonate 308
Assisted vaginal breech delivery 63, 202
Asynclitism 177, 186
   anterior 186
   posterior 186

Atonic postpartum hemorrhage, causes of 283
Atonic uterus 107
Atrophic glossitis 48
Auxiliary nurse midwives 192, 349
    role of 194

## B

Back, exercise for 13*f*
Balloon temponade 109*f*
Besides
    atonic hemorrhage 108
    breech presentation 59
Beta hCG tests 18
Betamethasone 191, 193, 242
Betamimetics 336
Birth
    attendant 349
    defects, cause 361
    planning and preparing for 353
    preparedness 353
    trauma 308
Bishop's score 25, 66, 70
Blood 97
    glucose, tests for 23
    pressure
        measurement of 7*f*
        of pregnant woman, measurement of 73*f*
    transfusion
        advantages of 52
        indications of 52
        risks of 52
B-lynch
    suture, procedure of 110
    technique, application of 110*f*
Bony pelvic outlet 173, 173*f*
BP apparatus 7*f*
Bradycardia 43
Breast
    engorgement 35
    examination 12
    infection 37
Breastfeeding
    after delivery, start 39
    difficulty in 36
    maternal benefits of 244
Breech delivery 60
Breech presentation 20, 59, 61, 202, 208
    causes of 60, 205
    cesarean
        delivery for 205
        section for 64
    denominator in 203
    diagnosis of 202
    incidence of 62
    management of 241
    varieties of 59, 205
Brow presentation 209
    denominator of 209
Burns-Marshall method 64, 202

## C

Calcium channel
    antagonists 336
    blocker 332
Caput succedaneum 189
Carbohydrate metabolism, alterations of 54
Carboprost 324f, 328
Cardiotocograph 232*f*-234*f*
    drawbacks of 229
    interpretation of 231
    trace 233
Cardiotocography 229, 232*f*
Cardiovascular system 11
Care after delivery 354
Cavum septum pellucidum 367*f*
Cephalhematoma 189
Cephalic presentation 10, 20
Cephalopelvic disproportion 27, 27f, 28, 186
Cerebral artery, middle 82
Cervical
    dilatation 214, 222, 290
        rate of 224
    dilators 258*f*, 291*f*
    scoring system, preinduction 289
    tear 293
Cervicograph 218
    plotting of 218
Cervix
    dilatation of 182
    favorable 66
    ripe 24
    unfavorable 66
Cesarean delivery 4, 41, 42, 211, 243, 246, 248
    delivery of floating head during 277
    indications of 58
    previous 41
Cesarean section 269
    complications of 270
    delivery of head in 273*f*
    elective repeat 47
    indications of 61, 90, 269
    instruments for 270*f*
    lower segment 269, 270
Chignon 306, 306*f*
Cho square sutures technique 111*f*

Choriocarcinoma 18
Chorionicity 91
Chromosomal anomaly, type of 119
Clinical pelvimetry 28
Clinical thermometer 280, 280*f*
Compound presentation 211
Compressus 89
Conception, control of 163
Conjoint twins 88*f*
Contraception
    choice of 33
    pill, emergency 356
    start 33
Contraceptive advice 58
Coombs' test 85
Cord attachment, abnormalities of 309
Cord clamp (disposable) 309, 309*f*
Cord clamping
    delay in 188
    early 188
    procedure of 188
Cord presentation 210
Cord prolapse 210, 211
    causes of 211
    complications of 211
    exclude 185
    management of case with 211
Cord round neck, management of 308
Cord traction, controlled 190
Cordocentesis, risks of 82
Corticosteroid 5
    contraindications for using 193
    indications for 193
    injection 191
    therapy 192
Couvelaire uterus 106
Craniotomy
    contraindications of 278, 310
    indications of 277, 310
Critical titer 81
Crown rump length 318, 318*f*, 365*f*
    measurement 318
CTG
    abnormal 322
    advantages of 229
Curve of carus 170
Cusco's bivalve 284, 284*f*
Cusco's speculum 283
Cystitis 37

# D

Das dilators 290
Das/Hegar's dilator 258*f*, 290, 291*f*
Deaths among children, causes of 341

Deep transverse arrest 201
Deep vein thrombosis 40
Deflexion 186
    causes of 200
    mild 199
    severe 199
Deliver fetal head 187
Delivery
    method of 70
    mode of 209
    pull during 302
Depot medroxyprogesterone acetate 356
Destructive operation 277, 278
    complications of 278, 310
Deviation bulge 81*f*
Dexamethasone 191-193, 242
    injection 193
Diabetes
    during labor, effects of 55
    effects of 55
    hypertension and 240
    mellitus 98
Diabetic mother, uncontrolled 93*f*
Diagonal conjugate, measurement of 172*f*
Diamniotic twin gestation 91*f*
Diazepam therapy 236
Dichorionic twin gestation 91*f*
Digital innovations 347
Dinoprostone gel 329
Dipstick test 22*f*
Disposable delivery kits 353
Dizygotic twins, membrane status of 90
Doppler 7*f*
    (ultrasound) fetal monitor 322, 322*f*
    flow study 69
    velocimetry 68, 69*f*
Double decidual sign 317, 317*f*
Doyen's retractor 292, 292*f*
Dystocia 213
    causes of 213

# E

Eclampsia 72, 75, 248
    management of 236
    maternal complications of 75
    prognostic factors of 76
    severe 249
    stages of convulsion in 75
    types of 75
Eclamptic convulsions 76*f*
Ectopic pregnancy
    diagnose 115
    tubal 116
Edema, causes of 20

EFM, advantages of 322
Embryo appears 318
Embryonic cardiac activity 319
    detection of 319
Embryonic development, critical periods in 365
Embryonic heart, rate of 319
Endocrine, causes 117
Epidural analgesia 248
Episiotomy 33, 261, 285
    common indications of 34
    complications of 262, 305
    cut during 305
    indications of 261, 305
    repair of 262
    scissors 262f, 305, 305f
    structures cut in 262
    types of 262, 305
    use of 33
    wound 31
Erb's palsy 60
External cephalic version 241
    advantage of 61
    benefits of 204
    chance of 62
    complications of 62, 204, 205
    contraindications of 61, 241
Extraplacental bleeding 100
Face presentation 20, 206, 207f, 208
    causes of 207
    diagnosis of 208
    positions of 207

## F

Female pelvis, types of 171
Female sterilization 356
Female urethra, length of 281
Femur length 368f
Fetal
    abdominal circumference 368f
    anomaly detection 247
    axis pressure 182
    biometry 247
    biophysical profile 23
    bradycardia, causes of 230t, 322
    cardiac activity 319
    death 105f
    factors 200
    femur, sonographic view of 368f
    malformation 98, 362
    parameters 68
    reduction, selective 91
    risk categories 360
    tachycardia, causes of 229
Fetal complications 83, 99
    common 88
Fetal congenital
    anomalies 97
    malformation 98
Fetal distress 28, 201, 254
    appearance of 43
Fetal growth
    parameters and charts 363
    restriction 68
        causes of 69
        types of 71
Fetal head
    engagement of 209
    engaging diameter of 206f
    internal rotation of 169
    level of 224
    station of 184
Fetal heart
    rate 224
        normal 319
    sound 22
        auscultation, procedure of 7f
Fetal movement
    count, daily 23
    woman's perception of 4
Fetal skull 125, 174, 175, 178, 179
    landmarks of 174f
Fetal well-being
    antenatal assessment of 135
    antenatal clinic to assess 6
Feticide, selective 92
Fetomaternal hemorrhage, risk of 85
Fetus 125
    and newborn, hemolytic disease of 83
    cardiac activity of 366f
    effects on 215
    excess mobility of 205
    papyraceus 88f, 89
FGR
    baby 69
    fetuses 71
Flexion point 268, 306
Floating head, causes of 26
Flow velocity waveform 69f
Flushing curette 291, 291f
Foley's catheter 40, 282f
Foley's self-retaining catheter 282
Folic acid supplementation 240
Food and drug administration 360
Foramen magnum 178f

Forceps
    application of 264, 302
        types of 301
    axis traction devices 304, 304f
    before applications of 302
    delivery 64, 202, 263
        complications of 264
        difficulties in 302
        indications of 263, 302
        low 265, 302
        procedure of low 265
        types of 263
    failed 264, 303
    green armytage 275f
        hemostatic 307, 307f
    Kocher's 188
        hemostatic 287, 288f
    left blade of 265f
    Little wood's 286, 286f
    long
        curved obstetric 300, 300f
        straight hemostatic 287, 287f
    long-curved 304
    over ventouse, advantages of 269
    ovum 294, 294f
    parts of 301
    sponge holding 293, 293f
    tent introducing 296, 296f
    trial of 264, 303
    uterine dressing 295, 295f
    Wrigley's 277, 277f, 301f, 303
Forewater, formation of bag of 182
Frank breech 59f
Fundal grip 9, 9f

## G

Genetic causes 117
Gestation age 71
Gestation embryonic heart 319
Gestation sac
    diagnosis of 317
    normal 316
    shape of 317
Gestational age 23
    assessment of 23
    assignment 369
    calculate 18
    small for 71
Gestational diabetes mellitus 54
    baby of 57
    diagnosis of 55
    prevalence of 55
    woman with 58

Gestational hypertension 78
Gestational sac 316, 316f
    location of 316
Giant vulsellum 311, 311f
Grand mother's theory 85

## H

Hawkin-Ambler dilator 258f, 290, 291f
Head circumference, measurement of 367f
Head, delivery of 272f
Health care systems 357
Heart disease 248
Hegar's dilators 290
HELLP syndrome 77
    complications of 77
    management of 78
    medical management 78
    observations in 77
Hematoma, large 40
Hemoglobin
    estimation 250
        during antenatal 250
    level 49
Hemoglobinopathy, case of 250
Hemorrhage 239
    control 330
    in early pregnancy, causes of 113
Heparin 333
Hepatitis B 39
Hepcidin 49
HIV positive mother, breastfeeding in 39
Homan's sign 40
Hydatidiform mole 18
    case of 322
    evacuation of 295
Hydralazine 74, 332
Hydrops fetalis 83
Hypertension 239
    chronic 78, 79
Hypochromic microcytic anemia 48f
Hypomagnesemia 334
Hypothermia 191
Hysterectomy 111
    indication of 106

## I

Iatrogenic rupture 313
Ibuprofen 11, 40
Icterus gravis neonatorum 83
Iliac artery ligation, internal 111
Iliopectineal line 167f
Iliopubic eminence 167f

Inevitable abortion, case of 114
Infection 239
Injection dexamethasone, administration of 193
Institutional delivery 355
Instruments, processing of 311
Insulin therapy 57
Intrapartum electronic fetal monitoring 229
Intrapartum fetal monitoring 229
    methods of 229
Intrapartum preventive measures 111
Intrauterine
    contraceptive device 356
    fetal death 93
        causes of 93
        clinical features of 94
        diagnosis of 319
    growth restriction 68*f*
        diagnose 68
        woman with 70
Iron
    absorption of 50, 245
        reduces 245
    balance, negative 48
    deficiency anemia 49, 245
        causes of 49
        diagnosis of 49
        signs of 48
    deficiency, mother suffers from 245
    loss 245
    salts of 51
Ischial spines, level of 184
Isoimmunization status 80

## J

Janani Shishu Suraksha Karyakram 350

## K

Karman's type 259*f*, 299
Kelly's long forceps 34*f*
Kick chart, maintain 66
Kielland's forceps 301*f*, 304
Kleihauer count 83
Klumpkey's palsy 60
Knee chest exercise 13*f*
Koilonichia 48

## L

Labetalol 74, 331
Labor 50, 139
    abnormal 198

acceleration of 331
active management of 216, 218
active phase of 212*f*, 213*f*, 224
advantages
    of partographic management of 218
    of trial of 30
after cesarean section, trial of 45
analysis of 219
and delivery 165
and puerperium 239
arrest 213
    disorder in 212, 213
assess progress of 184
augmentation of 224, 326, 331
causes of obstructed 214
clinical stages of 180
complicated 139
contraindications of induction of 221
course of 209, 224
    normal 229
dangers of induction of 288
effects of obstructed 214
end, trial of 30
fetal head during 184
first stage of 181
in brow presentation 209
incidence of prolonged 243
indications of induction of 221, 288
induction of 221, 222
latent phase of 214
manage third stage of 189
management of third stage of 237, 254, 255
mechanism of 176, 177
methods of induction of 221
monitoring-partography 217
nonprogress of 28
normal 139, 180, 218
obstructed 214, 215, 226, 239, 243, 252
onset of 185
pain, false 183
partograph
    for abnormal 224
    for normal 222
posterior position in 201
preterm 88, 191, 195
primary dysfunctional 213
problems 308
progress of 185
prolonged 212
second stage of 183, 187, 214
spontaneously 66
stage of 180, 184
surgical induction of 288

third stage of 98, 188
    complication in 90
    management 255
    trial of 29
    types of dysfunctional 213
    with cord prolapse
        with true knot 210*f*
        woman in 210*f*
Laminaria tent 296, 296*f*
Laser photocoagulation 92
Lean's regimen 236
Left occiput
    anterior 179*f*
    posterior 198*f*
    transverse 179, 179*f*
Leg cycling exercise 14*f*
Leg over ankle, pitting edema of 20*f*
Leopold's first maneuver 9*f*
Leopold's fourth maneuver 10*f*
Leopold's maneuvers 9
Leopold's second maneuver 9*f*
Leopold's third maneuver 10*f*
Linea nigra 8*f*
Live fetus, umbilical cord of 88*f*
Live virus vaccines 20
Liver enzymes, elevated 77
Lovset's maneuver 64, 206
Low birth weight 71
Lower segment
    cesarean section, operative procedure of 270
    transverse scar 42, 42*f*

# M

Magnesium
    sulfate 196, 236, 333
        side effect of 79
        toxicity of 335
    toxicity 335
        management of 335
Magnetic resonance imaging 323
Malar flexion 64, 202
Malaria 48
    and jaundice 5
Maneuvers and operative obstetrics 160
Manual vacuum aspiration 260, 299*f*
    advantages of 297
    cannula 261*f*
    complications of 297
    procedure of 260
    syringe 260*f*, 296, 297*f*
        parts of 298, 298*f*

Massive vulval edema 72*f*
Mastitis 37
    acute 36
Maternal bony pelvis, method of holding 177
Maternal conditions 308
Maternal death 253, 342
    causes of 238f, 255, 340
    in eclampsia, causes of 76
    reducing 346
    surveillance 347
Maternal health 338, 341
    beyond 2030 357
    antenatal clinic to assess 6
Maternal medications 308
Maternal morbidity, severe acute 343
Maternal mortality 238
    ending preventable 346
    rate 339, 342
    ratio 339, 342
        levels of 339
        statewise 340
    reduced 236
Maternal near miss 343
Maternal pelvis 125, 166, 178*f*
Maternal pubic symphysis 184
Maternal red cell alloimmunization,
    pregnancy with 80
Maternal sensorium 236
Mauriceau Smellie-Veit technique 64
McAfee regimen 102
Mechanical stretching, progressive 182
Membranes, prelabor rupture of 197
Menon's regimen 236
Metal catheter 282
Metallic cervical dilator, single-ended 290
Methergin 324*f*, 325
Methyldopa 74, 332
Methylergometrine 325, 330
    side effects of 326
Micro-birth plan 353
Mini pill 33
Miscarriage 117, 119
    causes of recurrent 117
    complete 115
    diagnosed, threatened 113
    inevitable 114
    missed 115
    recurrent 115, 117
    silent 113
    threatened 113
    types of 118, 118*t*
Misoprostol 324*f*, 329
    dose schedule of 330

Molar pregnancy 321f
  case of 321
  complications of 322
Molecular weight heparin, low 333
Monochorionic twins, complications of 90
Monozygotic twins, membrane status in 90
Mother breastfeed 85
Mucus sucker 308, 308f
Multiple pregnancy 86, 249
Multiple toothed vulsellum 285, 285f
Myomectomy 5
Myometrial fibers 184

## N

Naegele's formula 5, 23
National Health Mission 348, 349
  guidelines 349
National Health Policy 357
National Population Policy 217
Neonatal intensive care unit 242
Neonates, preterm 191
Nerve injury 60
Neural tube defects, incidence of 240
Newborn
  care 267f, 355
    essential 354, 357
  exchange transfusion in 85
  infant 155
Nicardipine 336
Nifedipine 74, 332, 336
Nonstress test 23, 229, 233
  abnormal 233f
Normal delivery, fetal head during 176f
Normal placenta, weight of 313

## O

Obstetric auscultation 10
Obstetric care, emergency 252, 357
Obstetric case discussions 16
Obstetric charts 359
  and graphs 363
Obstetric complications 107
  common 97
Obstetric examination 8, 8f, 18
  position of woman during 186f
Obstetric forceps
  functions of 263, 302
  parts of long curved 263
  short-curved 277f, 301f, 303
  types of 300
  varieties of 263
Obstetric grips 9, 200

Obstetric hemorrhage 107, 252
Obstetric instruments 280
Obstetric intervention 247
Obstetric palpation 10, 12
Obstetric pelvic axis 170, 170f
Obstetric practice, modern 247
Occipitosacral arrest 199
Occiput posterior position 198
  causes of 200
Occiput-sacral position 199
Oligohydramnios 98, 99
  case of 99
  causes of 99
Oral iron 50
  preparations 51
  therapy 51
Organic cardiac disease 249
Outlet forceps 303
  delivery 302
Ovulation 33
Ovum, blighted 114f
Oxytocics 324, 324f
Oxytocin 94, 249, 254, 324, 324f
  administration, routes of 222
  dangers of 325
  infusion 222, 326
    dose calculation 221
  side effects of 325
  stress test 254

## P

Palpation 8, 12
Parent pelvis, types of 171
Parenteral iron therapy 51
  advantages of 51
  indications of 51
  side effects of 51
Parenteral oxytocin 237
Parietal presentation
  anterior 186
  posterior 186
Partograph 184, 218-220, 220f, 223f, 225f, 227f
  components of 219
  plotting of 217
Partographic observation 226
Parturition, phases of 181
Patwardhan's technique 276
Pawlik's grip 9, 10f, 20
Peak systolic velocity 82
Pectineal line 167f
Pelvic axis 169
  anatomical 170, 170f

Pelvic contraction 29
   degree of 29
Pelvic diameters, demonstrate 177
Pelvic dimension
   greatest 168
   least 169
Pelvic examination 194
Pelvic factors 200
Pelvic floor 169
Pelvic grip 9, 20, 185
Pelvic inclination, angle of 172, 172f
Pelvic outlet 173f
   anatomical 173
Pelvic pathology 28
Pelvis
   anatomical position of 177f
   anteroposterior diameters of 169f
   axes of 170
   brim of 166, 167f, 168
   constitute 170
   contracted 27
   different joints in 170
   false 167
   female 166f
   planes of 168, 168f
   transverse diameter of 199f
   types of 29
Perforator (Oldham's) 278f, 310, 310f
Perineal tear 286
   causes of 286
   degrees of 200
Perineum, pain in 39
Peripheral blood film 48f
Phenytoin therapy 236
Piles, bleeding 52
Pill 33
Pinard's stethoscope 309, 309f
Placenta
   abnormalities of 313
   accrete, incidence of 103
   amniotic fluid 123
   and membranes, delivery of 274f
   delivery of 47, 310
   expression of 190f
   low lying 100, 103
   normal 312, 312f
      attachment of 313
   previa 26, 52, 100, 102, 103, 105, 205, 321f
      anterior 102f
      case of 101, 103, 321
      cause of bleeding in 101
      complications of 101, 321
      management of 103
      risk of recurrence for 103
      types of 101, 321
      woman with 101
   separation of 189, 190
   succenturiata 312, 312f
      clinical significance of 313
Placental abruption 104, 105, 105f
   bleeding in 105
   case of 105
   recurrence for 106
Placental bleeding 100
Placental insufficiency 308
Plasma
   glucose, levels of 56, 58
   reagin test 352
   volume expansion 78
Plastic suction cannula 259f, 299
Pneumonia 37
Polyhydramnios 96-98
   common causes of 97
   diagnosis of 96
   pathology of 98
Pondral index 71
Postmaturity, diagnose 65
Postpartum
   contraception 356
   exercises 13
   period, detection of complication during 355
Postpartum hemorrhage 107, 255
   causes of 107, 283
   diagnose traumatic 284
   high-risk factors of 108
   management 107
   prevention 107
   primary 107, 108
   sites of traumatic 284
Povidone iodine 271f
Practical obstetrics 279
Preconceptional counseling 24
Pre-eclampsia 72, 78, 105
   case of 74
   complications of 74
   development of 73
   nonsevere 78
   pregnancy with 72f
   recurrence of 78
   severe 73, 78, 248, 249
   syndrome 74
Pregestational diabetes 58
Pregnancy 50
   and teratogenicity, drug therapy in 360
   anemia in 48, 49

case of normal 19
classify diabetes in 54
complicated 146
contraindicated in 20
danger signs during 354
demand of iron in 245
diabetes in 54, 57
early 119, 136
    diagnosis of 19
ectopic 115
effects of diabetes 55
hemorrhage in early 113
high-risk 242
history of present 11
hypertensive disorders complicating 78
in human, duration of 195
late 23, 119
maternal complications during 87
medical
    disorders in 239, 252
    illness during 153
normal 18
physiological
    anemia of 48
    changes in 129
post-term 65, 67
prolonged 65, 195
Rh grouping in 251
skin changes during 8*f*
surgical illness during 153
term 195
woman with diabetes in 58
Pregnant woman
    measurement of height of 6*f*
    registration of 353
Prelabor rupture of membranes, cause 197
Prenatal counseling 240
Preterm baby 191
Preterm birth
    concern for 195
    prevalence of 197
Preterm delivery 191
    previous 195
Preterm labor, threatened 194
Pretrem birth and prematurity, significance of 191
Primipara, common in 32
Progestin, injectable 33
Prophylactic
    ergometrine 326
    forceps 248, 264, 303
        delivery 248
    oxytocin 249

Prophylaxis 333
Prostaglandin 94, 327
    E1 329
    E2 328
    preparations of 328
    use of 328
Prostin 324*f*
    E2 gel 329
Pubic crest 167*f*
Pubic tubercle 167*f*
Pudendal nerve block analgesia 170
Puerperal emergencies 32
Puerperal pyrexia 37
    causes of 32, 37
Puerperal sepsis 32, 38, 355
    causes of 38
    predisposing factors for 38
Puerperium 31, 32, 50, 254
    abnormal 37, 143
    breast problems during 39
    cause of anovulation in 37
    normal 11, 12, 31, 37, 143
    urinary problems in 32
    with baby, normal 12*f*
Pulmonary infection 37
Pyopagus 88*f*

# R

Randomized control trial 361
Reproduction, fundamentals of 121
Respiratory
    distress syndrome 191
    system 11
Resuscitation 40
Retroplacental clots 105*f*
Rh
    hemolytic disease 81*f*
    incompatibility 84
    negative woman 80, 249
Rhesus alloimmunization 82
    pathology of 80
Right occiput posterior 198, 198*f*
Ringer's solution 108
Ritgen's maneuver 187, 266*f*
Rubber catheter 281
    simple 281*f*
    sterile simple 308
Rupture uterus 313, 313*f*
    case of 287, 313
    causes of 287, 313
    diagnosis of 313
    types of 313

## S

Sacrococcygeal joints 170
Sacroiliac articulation 167*f*
Sacroiliac joints 170
Safe mothorhood 164
Salpingostomy 315*f*
Scalpel vasectomy, no 356
Scar
  dehiscence 44*f*
  rupture 46, 313, 313
    during labor 43
    type of 42
  tenderness 42
    assessment of 42f, 43*f*
Scissors
  in obstetrics, prevention and control of 334
  long straight 289, 289*f*
  prevents 236
Sepsis 252
Septic abortion 115, 118
Septostomy 92
Shoulder
  delivery of 266*f*
  traction 64, 202
Sims' double-bladed posterior vaginal speculum 283, 283*f*
Single umbilical artery, significance of 288
Skin condition 8
Sonography 65
Specimens 312
Spine and limbs stretching 14*f*
Square sutures 110
Staphylococcus pyogenes 38
Stethoscope 6f, 22*f*
Straight leg raising 13*f*
Striae gravidarum 8*f*
Suction and evacuation
  complications of 260
  operation trolley for 300, 300*f*
Symphysis pubis 167*f*, 170, 266*f*
Symphysis-fundal height 20
  measurement 9*f*
Systemic examination 18

## T

Teratogen 361
Teratogenicity, determine 361
Term pregnancy, classification of 65
Termination of pregnancy, methods of 297
Thalassemia 48
Thrombophlebitis 37

Tocograph 233
Tocolytic drugs 336
TOLAC 45
  benefits of 45
Total dose infusion 52
  advantages of 52
  iron for 52
Total maternal deaths, percentage of 340
Transabdominal sonogram 102*f*
Transverse lie 22, 209
True labor pain 183
True pelvis 167
  parts of 167
Trunk rotation exercise 14*f*
Trunk, delivery of 267*f*
Tubal ectopic pregnancy
  acute 314, 315
  unruptured 314, 314f, 315, 315*f*
Tuberculosis 37
Tuberous sclerosis 76*f*
Twin
  interlocking of 90*f*
  monochorionic 242
  peak sign 91*f*
  presentations, combinations of 87
  type of 90
Twin pregnancy 89, 89f, 90, 320, 366*f*
  complications of 242
  diagnose chorionicity of 91
  diagnosis of 87, 320
  fetal heads in 320
  management of 320
  second stage complications of 89
  two fetal heads in 320*f*
  ultrasonography of 86*f*
Twin-to-twin transfusion
  complications of 92
  pathology of 92
  pregnancy with 92
  syndrome 90

## U

Ultrasonogram 316, 320, 321
  hydatidiform mole 321
  placenta previa 321
Umbilical cord 95, 205, 287
  structures of 288
  true knot in 95*f*
Umbilical grip 9
Umbilical vein, level of 368*f*
Urinalysis, dipsticks for 280, 280*f*
Urinary tract infection 32, 37

Urine
  during pregnancy, causes of retention of 282
  formation of 98
  incontinence of 32
  retention of 32
  test 18
Uro-dip reagent strips 280, 280f
USG machine 7f
Uterine
  compression sutures 109
  contractions 181, 182, 185, 224, 237, 327
  curette 294, 295f
  devascularization procedures 111
  enlargement, excessive 96
  factors 200
  hyperstimulation 254
  incisions, types of 292
  muscle incision 272f
  musculature 249
  retractions 182
  rupture 44, 254
    complications of 44
    risk of 44
  scar 47
    dehiscence 43, 313
    types of 42
  segment, lower 182
  sound 290
  tamponade 109
  vessels 236
  wound
    methods of suturing 307
    suturing of 275f
Uterus 205
  causes of subinvolution of 32, 35
  contour of 8
  involution of 32, 35, 37
  lower segment of 272f
  massaging 237
  with ulnar border of left hand, height of 9f

# V

Vaginal birth after cesarean 44, 46
  advantages of 246
  benefits of successful 246
  contraindications of 45
  counseled for 47
Vaginal bleeding 46
  causes of 100

Vaginal breech delivery 62, 63, 63f, 202, 204, 205
  complications of 60, 63
  methods of 61
Vaginal delivery 103, 199, 201, 206f
  and management 180
  operative 305
  prospect of 208
  safe 201
Vaginal examination 186
Vaginal pessary (propess) 329
Vaginal speculum 284
  self-retaining 284f
Valve cup 298f
Valve liner 298f
VBAC-TOL, women for 246
Venereal disease research laboratory 352
Ventouse
  application of 268
  over forceps, advantages of 268
Ventouse cup 268f, 306f
  with traction device 306
Ventouse delivery 201, 268
  complications of 269
  contraindications of 268
  hazards of 306
  indications of 268
Vertex presentation 20
Vigorous curettage, drawbacks of 295
Vital statistics 346
Vulval hematoma
  case of 40
  diagnose 39

# W

Weight and height measurement tools 6f
WHO partograph 220f
Wound infection 37

# Y

Yolk sac 317, 318f
  detection of 317
  functions of 317

# Z

Zuspan regimen 79

# Index of Section II Gynecology

Page numbers followed by *f* refer to figure and *t* refer to table.

## A

Abdomen, burst 512
Abdominal hysterectomy 379, 509, 511*f*
    common indications of 509, 559
    indications of 571
    operation 510, 513
    steps of 511
    types 509
Abdominal operation 581
Abdominal ostium 535*f*
Abdominal wound, common complications of 512
Abnormal uterine bleeding
    classification of 420
    common causes of 420
    management of 421, 422
    medical management of 421
Abortion, recurrent midtrimester 477*f*
Acetic acid 468
Acquired prolapse 401
Adenocarcinoma filling uterine cavity 621*f*
Adenomyosis 377, 418*f*, 445, 448, 486, 596, 600, 600*f*, 637
    clinical features of 600
    sonographic view of 636*f*
    specimen of 600*f*
    treatment for 600
Adjuvant therapy 442
    place of 432
Alli's tissue forceps 498*f*, 499*f*, 516*f*, 524*f*, 564, 564*f*, 594*f*
    pair of 522*f*
    uses 565
Amenorrhea 453, 466
    common causes of 453, 454
        primary 453
        secondary 454
    diagnosis of 454
    karyotyping 632
    primary 453
    secondary 454
    uterine causes of 632
Androgen producing tumors 388
Anesthetic complications 531
Anovular bleeding 419
Anovulation
    causes of 431
    common causes of 442
Anovulatory infertility 432
Anti-Müllerian hormone 470
Antituberculous chemotherapy 417
Armed surgical robotic system, four 546*f*
ART, different methods of 628
Artery forceps, long straight 513*f*
Ascites 490
Asherman's syndrome 538, 539*f*
    common causes of 538
Auvard's self-retaining posterior vaginal speculum 553, 553*f*
Ayre's spatula 478, 479*f*, 548

## B

Babcock's forceps 575, 575*f*
Bacterial vaginosis 414
Balfour self-retaining retractor 573, 573*f*
Barkelay Bonney vaginal clamp 576
Barrier methods 467
Bartholin's cyst 505*f*
    marsupialization of 504
Basal body temperature 562
Basal layer 434
Basal zone 438
Benign ovarian tumor 386, 607
    clinical presentation of 607
    complications of 383, 388, 490, 608
    management of 491, 608
Benign tumor 490, 673
    differentiate 608
Bethesda classification system 553
Bicornuate uterus 477*f*, 478, 630, 630*f*, 631
    laparoscopic view of 534*f*
    management of 478, 631
Bilateral fimbrial block 477*f*
    causes of 628

Biopsy 421
  endometrial 422, 431, 483, 537, 562, 622
Bivalent vaccine 472
Bladder during surgery 555
Blood loss, amount of 434
Blunt curette 483, 561
Body of uterus, lymphatic drainage of 622
Bonney's myoma screw 568*f*
Bonney's myomectomy clamp 569, 569*f*
  uses 569

## C

Cancer cervix 468, 526, 527
  prevention of 452, 620
Cancer death
  causes of 472
  common causes of 468
Cannula 531, 531*f*, 588, 588*f*
Carboplatin 649
Carcinoma
  diagnosis of early 617
  early stage 619
  endometrial 622
  endometrium, FIGO staging of 622, 623
  of cervix uteri, FIGO staging of 617*t*
  of vulva, FIGO staging for 625*t*
Carcinoma cervix
  causes of 527, 620
  different histological types of 577
  differential diagnosis of 527, 620
  measures for 526
  preventive measures of 620
  staging of 617
Carcinoma of ovary
  FIGO staging of 609*t*
  management of 491
Catheterization, procedure of 554
Cells, collection of 548
Cervarix 472
Cervical
  canal 500*f*
  cancer screening, guidelines 450
  cytology screening 450, 479, 549
  ectopy 482, 553
  lip 558
  mucus study 431, 562
  myoma, surgical removal of 599
  pathology 468
  polyp, large 482*f*
  screening programs 468
  smear 478, 550
  softening and dilatation, causes of 469
Cervical artery 522*f*
  ascending 515*f*

Cervical biopsy 503
  complications of 504, 578
  different types of 577
  indications 503
  procedure for 503
  types 503
Cervical dilators 557
  uses 557
  varieties 557
Cervical fibroid 599
  huge posterior 598*f*
  types of 599
Cervical intraepithelial neoplasia 449, 468, 478
  cases with 452
  diagnose case with 449
  significance of detection of 449
  site of origin for 449
Cervical occlusion clamp 567, 567*f*
  uses 567
Cervicovaginal junction 515*f*, 521*f*
Cervix 428*f*, 501*f*
  amputation of 507, 558, 559
  anterior lip of 521*f*
  congenital elongation of 401
  conization of 451
  dilatation of 501
  lesions in 552
  lymphatic drainage of 618
  posterior lip of 558, 616*f*
  premalignant state of 468
  supravaginal part of 395
  thermal cauterization of 504
Cesarean section, lower segment 630*f*
Chemotherapy 461, 602*f*
  place of 623
  regimen, selection of 603
Chlamydial infection 492
Chocolate cyst 377, 382, 533*f*
Choriocarcinoma 424, 461, 484
Chromopertubation 432
Chromosomal pattern, abnormal 453
Cisplatin 649
Clamps
  fifth pair of 511
  first pair of 511
  fourth pair of 511
  pair of 511
  second pair of 511
  third pair of 511
Clomiphene citrate 442, 645
  dose 645
  indication 645
  mechanism of action 645
  side effects 645

Clomiphene therapy, result of 442
Clue cells 493
Coagulating roller ball electrode 590
Collagen 585
Colpoperineorrhaphy 523, 524
    indications 523
    preliminaries 524
    principal steps 524
Colporrhaphy
    anterior 523, 580$f$
        indications 523
        preliminaries 523
Colposcopy 451, 468
Combined oral contraceptive 467
    contraindications of 647
    preparations 646
Combined oral pill 646
Combipack 469
Complete perineal tear 411
    operation 411
    patient on discharge 412
    preventive measures 412
    principal steps of 411
    repair of 412
    special postoperative care 411
Conservative surgical management 447
Contact bleeding, causes of 419
Contraception 646, 682
    method of 467
    pill for purpose of 646
    use additional 647
Contraceptives 647
Cornual block
    bilateral 477$f$, 627$f$
    causes of 627
Corpus luteum 437
Corpus uteri, cancer of 623$t$
Cotton suture 587
Cryptomenorrhea 455
    causes of 605
    common causes of 455
Cu T, ultrasonographic view of 638$f$
Cusco's bivalve adjustable self-retaining vaginal speculum 552, 552$f$
Cusco's speculum 482$f$
    advantages of 481
    benefit of 482
Cyst
    appearance of 616
    embryological origin of 616
    features of functional 384, 607
    management of 616
Cystic glandular hyperplasia 419
Cystocele 392$f$, 401, 404, 555

Cytobrush 479$f$, 548, 548$f$
    methods 548
Cytology
    Bethesda classification system of 553
    screening 548
    testing, procedure of 450
Cytoreduction, maximum 611

## D

Danazol 645
    indications of use 645
    mechanism of action 645
    side effects 645
Deaver's retractor 574, 574$f$
Decubitus ulcer 395
Dental element 642$f$
Dermoid
    common complications of 606
    cyst 606
    management of 606
Dexon 585
Dilatation and curettage 421, 498, 551
    complications 499
    indication of 498, 551
    instrument trolley for operation 498
    steps of operation 498, 499
Dilatation and insufflation 501
    complications 502
    contraindications 502
    indications of 501
    steps 502
Dilatation operation, complications of 557
Dissecting forceps 578
    tooth of 578$f$
Distal tubal block 566, 629
Distant metastasis 610
Distended tube 493
Distension media 538, 591
    used in hysteroscopy 529, 591
Doyen's retractor 573, 573$f$
    uses 573
Drugs 688
Dye test 404
Dyskaryotic smear 479, 549
    different types of 479, 549
Dysmenorrhea 597$f$

## E

Ectopic pregnancy 477$f$, 628$f$
Ectopy heal 504
Electrocautery 582, 582$f$
Electrodes 590

Electrodiathermy 541
　set 510
Electrosurgical complications 531
Endocervix 482f
Endometrial
　ablation 537
　cancer 537
　cycle 438
　pathology 455
　polyp 429
　sampling 421
Endometriosis 445, 447f, 646
　common sites of 445
　examination 445
　management of 637
Endometriotic lesions 532
Endometriotic nodule 447f
　excision of 446f
Endometrium 419, 500f, 644f
　ahedding of 455
　different phases of 439
　normal 644
Endosalpingitis 416
Endoscopic surgery 378, 471, 528, 588
Enterocele 396
Episiotomy 580f
Epithelial cell
　carcinomas 491
　tumors 383
Epithelial ovarian
　cancer
　　hereditary 610
　　management of 389
　　treatment of 391
　　tumors 487, 488
Epithelial tumor 384
Estrogen 646
　deficiency, symptoms of 464
　producing tumors 388
　progesterone challenge test, result of 455
　replacement therapy 379
Ethylene oxide 586
Evisceration 512
Excisional methods 451
　different 452
Exfoliative cytology screening 468
Extrafascial hysterectomy 622

# F

Fallopian tube 416, 513f, 522f, 535f, 543f, 609
　cancer, staging of 611
　loop of 544f

Falope ring 542, 543f, 544, 544f
　applicator 543f
　lower end of 544
　upper end of 543f
Female infertility 460, 463
　causes of 430
Female metal catheter 498f, 555, 555f
　uses 555
Female rubber catheter 554, 554f
　uses 554
Female sterilization 505, 506
　abdominal route 505
　steps of operation 505
Female urethra, length of 555
Feminising tumors 612
Fetal loss, recurrent 534f
Fibroid 380, 595, 596, 598
　calcific degeneration of 641f
　capsule of 518f
　classification of 375f
　complications of 376
　degenerations in 641
　differentiate 595
　multiple 485f
　pedunculated subserous variety of 594f
　polyp 402
　　huge 428f
　secondary changes in 598, 640
　uterus 374, 374f, 376, 382, 385, 486f, 517f, 518f, 594f, 637
　　bimanual examination 377
　　case of 377
　　causes of infertility 377
　　clinical presentation for 485
　　diagnosis 374
　　differential diagnosis 377
　　differentiate 486, 596
　　huge 593f
　　management of 377
　　medical management of 377
　　operation 485, 486
　　signs of 375
　　specimen 485, 486
　　symptoms of 375, 486
　　treatment of choice for 379
　　treatment options for 380
　　types of 375
Fitz-Hugh Curtis syndrome 414
Flushing curette 561f, 562
Foley's catheter 480f, 556, 556f
Follicle 437
　recruitment of 435
Follicular growth and maturation 436

Formol saline 501*f*
Fothergill's operation 398, 402, 508
    complications of 398, 508, 560, 571
    indication of 398, 560
    principal steps of 571
    steps of 508, 560
Fothergill's stitch 398, 508
Fractional curettage 622

## G

Gartner's duct cyst 401, 555
Gauze pieces 498*f*
Genital hiatus 394
Genital malignancy 676
Genital prolapse, common symptoms
    associated with 565
Genital ridge 434
Genital symptoms 459
Genital tract infection 669
Genital tuberculosis 416, 492, 495
    diagnose 494
    symptoms of 416
Genitourinary fistula 403
    diagnosis 403
Genitourinary prolapse 392*f*, 395-397
    classification of 393
    factors aggravate 399
Germ cell 434
    carcinomas 491
    layers 606
    neoplasm, treatment of 391
    tumors 383, 487, 488
Gestational trophoblastic neoplasia 601
    clinical features of 601
    management protocol of 601
    place of hysterectomy 603
    treatment of 602
Glandular cell abnormalities 553
Gonadotropin-releasing hormone
    advantages of 378
    disadvantages of 378
Gonadotropins 436
    indications of 640
Gonococcal infection 604
Gonococcus infection, spread of 413
Graafian follicle, mature 435
Grasp fallopian tube 544
Gynecological pathologies, common 599
Gynecological surgery 406
Gynecology
    drugs in 645
    instruments 548
    operative 496, 684

## H

HAIR-AN syndrome 440
Hawkin-Ambler dilator 500*f*, 557*f*
Hegar's dilator 557*f*
Hematosalpinx, causes of 605
Hemorrhage 487*f*, 517
Hemorrhagic growth 602*f*
Hemostasis, different methods of 589
Hemostatic forceps 510
    long straight 511*f*, 574, 574*f*
Hodge-Smith pessary 583, 583*f*
    contraindications 583
    indications of use 583
Hormonal responsiveness 434
Hormone replacement therapy 459
HPV infection, pathogenesis of 527
Huffman-Graves speculum 481, 481*f*
Human immunodeficiency virus 458
    infection, screening for 458
    treatment of 493
Human papilloma virus 468
    infection 550
    role of 526
    types of 449
    vaccine 472
Hydatidiform mole 423, 423*f*, 427, 601*f*
    complications of 424
    diagnosis of 423, 424
    karyotype pattern of complete 426
Hydrops tubal profluens 493
Hydrosalpinx 413*f*, 493
    bilateral 628*f*
    impair, presence of 629
    large 382*f*, 603*f*
    pathogenesis of 604
        bilateral 604
Hydrotubation 569
Hymen 394*f*
    plane of 394*f*
Hyperandrogenemia 440
Hyperplasia, endometrial 646
Hypogonadism
    hypergonadotropic 453
    hypogonadotropic 453
Hypothalamic factors 454
Hysterectomy 388, 422, 489, 611
    place of 596
    primary 461
Hysterosalpingogram 476*f*, 477*f*, 626, 626*f*-632*f*
    common contraindications of 478
    complications 627
    contraindications of 626
    dangers of 629

indications of 626
obtained from 477
step of
  investigation 627
  operation of 627
timing of 626
Hysterosalpingograph 476
Hysterosalpingography 431, 502, 460
  advantages of 570
  alternatives to 570
  cannula 503f, 569, 569f
    uses 569
  complications of 502, 570
  contraindications of 502, 570
  indication of 502, 570
  over laparoscopy 570
  steps 502
Hysteroscope 536f
Hysteroscopic instruments 590, 590f
Hysteroscopic metroplasty, benefits of 541
Hysteroscopic procedure, operative 541f
Hysteroscopy 421, 529, 536, 591, 622
  complications of 538, 591
    operative 541
  contraindications of 529, 591
  indications of 537, 591
  management option for 539
  operative 537
  symptoms of 539
  type of abnormality 540

# I

Iatrogenic drugs 454
Incision, abdominal 518f
Infection, risk of 463
Infertility 416, 430, 492, 540, 562
  causes of 595
  diagnosis 430
  in endometriosis 600
  ovarian
    causes of 483, 562
    factors for 430
    primary 430
    proportion of 430
    secondary 430
    work up 466, 537
Infundibulopelvic ligament 513f
Insufflation cannula 572, 572f
  use 572
Insufflation test 431
Intermittent hydrosalpinx 493
Interstitial salpingitis 416

Intrauterine
  adhesion 537, 539f, 632f
  contraceptive device 632
    complications of 638
  foreign body, removal of 537
Invasive procedure 460, 466
Ischemic fistula, pathology of 403

# K

Kidney dish 510
Kocher's artery forceps 571, 571f
  tooth of 571f
  use 571
Koilocyte 480
Koilocytosis 549
Krukenberg's tumor 384, 387, 487, 614, 615

# L

Labor, preterm 540
Landon's bladder retractor 521f, 571, 571f
  uses 572
Lanes tissue forceps 566, 566f
  uses 566
Langenback's and Czerney's retractors 510
Laparoscopic chromopertubation 432f, 535f
  over hysterosalpingography, advantages
    of 535
Laparoscopic instruments 531f, 588
Laparoscopic ovarian drilling 509
Laparoscopic procedures 542
Laparoscopic sterilization 543, 543f
  advantages of 589
  disadvantages of 589
Laparoscopic surgery 528, 589
  complications of 529, 590
Laparoscopic surgical procedures 530
Laparoscopic tubal sterilization 541, 542
Laparoscopic tubectomy 471
  advantages of 542
Laparoscopic-assisted vaginal trachelectomy
  620
Laparoscopy 421, 432, 460, 466, 530, 532,
  537, 562, 589
  benefits of 532
  complications of 531, 589
  contraindications of 529, 590
  indications of 530, 589
  operative 530
  over laparotomy, advantages of 530
Laparotomy 378, 381f, 385, 491
  staging of 611
Leech Wilkinson variety 503f, 569, 569f

Leiomyoma 635
  ultrasonographic view of 634*f*
Letrozole 443, 645
  place of 443
Levator ani muscles 524*f*
Levator plate 400
Leydig cells 470
Little Wood's forceps 565, 565*f*
  use 565
Lletz procedure, loops for 525*f*
Loop excision, procedure of 525*f*
Loop hook 582, 582*f*
Lugol's iodine 468
Luteal phase 438
  defect 438
Luteal placental shift 438
Luteal support 646
Lymph nodes
  regional 610
  retroperitoneal 609
Lymphoma 553

# M

Mackenrodt's ligament 522*f*
Male infertility, common causes of 430
Malignancy, risk of 616, 642
Malignant ovarian tumor 389, 390, 488, 611
  clinical features of 390 488, 609
  common 491, 610
  treatment of 489
Marsupialization, advantages of 505
Mayer-Rokitansky-Küster-Hauser syndrome 453
Medical management, different types of 596
Meigs' syndrome 385, 612
Menarche 434
  mean age of 434
Menorrhagia 597*f*
  causes of 376, 594
  common causes of 418
  drugs used to control 634
Menstrual abnormality 416, 492
Menstrual bleeding, heavy 422
Menstrual cycle 435, 439, 483
  endometrial biopsy 431, 562
  normal 434
Menstruation
  normal 434
  physiology of 434
  regular normal 431
Mesenteric cyst 382, 382*f*
Mesosalpinx 493, 506*f,* 513*f*

Metal catheter 404
Metastasis, common sites of 484, 602
Metastatic tumor, secondary 384, 487
Metformin 443, 649
  functions of 443
  lowers blood glucose 443
  place of 442
  side effects 649
  works 443
Methotrexate 649
  indications 649
  side effects 649
Methylene blue dye 535*f*
Metropathia hemorrhagica 419
Metroplasty 477*f,* 537, 630*f*
Metrorrhagia 597*f*
Midtubal block 629
Mifepristone 473, 648
  contraindications 648
  dose 648
  indications 648
  lower dose 469
  side effects 648
  use of 473
Minimally invasive surgery 528
Minipill 646
Miscarriage 484*f*
  recurrent 537, 540, 631
    midtrimester 630*f*
Misoprostol 469, 473
  benefits of 469
  complications of 469
  higher dose 469
Missing thread, causes of 638
Molar pregnancy 423
  clinical features of 423
Molar tissue 423
Moles, complete 426
Mother-to-child transmission 458
Mucinous cystadenocarcinoma, bilateral 608*f*
Mucinous cystadenoma, left-sided 607*f*
Müllerian abnormalities 466
Müllerian anomaly 537
  types of 631
Müllerian duct 470
Multiple follicles, development of 443
Multiple toothed vulsellum 521*f,* 558, 558*f*
  uses 558
Myoma 518*f*
  screw 510, 568
    uses 568
Myomectomy 378, 380, 516, 517, 537, 568, 634, 635

common complications of 635
complications of 517, 568
contraindications of 486, 516, 597
indications of 516, 596, 597
operation, blood loss during 635
principal steps of 516, 634
principles of 568
results of 517
Myometrial contractions 469
Myometrial receptors, stimulates 469
Myometrium 602f, 644, 644f

# N

Necrosis 487f
Needle 579
    curved 579f
    holder 576
        uses 576
Neoadjuvant chemotherapy 391, 613
Nodular growth 616f
Nodular masses, solid 487f
Nonconception cycle 438
Nontoothed dissecting forceps 578f
Nuclear abnormalities 479
Nulliparous prolapse 398

# O

Obstetric fistula 403
Oligomenorrhea, causes of 419
Olive pointed malleable graduated metallic uterine sound 560
    uses 560
Omentectomy, total 608f
Oocyte 437
Oophorectomy 379, 509
    benefits of 379
Oral contraceptive preparations, uses 646
Organ, identification of 592
Ovarian biopsy 509
Ovarian cancer 462, 611
    correct staging of 465
    diagnosis of 465
    early diagnosis of 462
    management of 488, 491, 611, 613
    poor outcome of 391
    staging of 465
Ovarian carcinoma 389
Ovarian cycle 435, 436
Ovarian cyst 615f
    features of functional 490
    torsion of left 384f
    types of 388

Ovarian cystectomy 509
Ovarian dermoid cyst 641f, 642
    cut section of 642
Ovarian endometrioma 636
Ovarian factors 454
Ovarian hyperstimulation syndrome 443, 639
    clinical features of 639
    manage case of 640
Ovarian ligament 513f
Ovarian malignancy 387, 465, 488, 610, 613, 614
    management of 610, 643
    methods for 489
    protective factors for 388, 488, 610
    risk of 390
Ovarian neoplasms, management of 644
Ovarian pedicle, structures forming 608
Ovarian reserve 640
Ovarian steroidogenesis, concept of 436
Ovarian syndrome 379
Ovarian tumor 377, 381, 381f, 385, 386, 386f, 387, 595
    advanced malignant 611
    bilateral malignant 385f
    borderline 389
    common symptoms of 387
    computed tomographic view of 642f
    diagnosis 382
    different types of surgery 387
    differential diagnoses 382
    gross appearance of solid 612f
    huge 643f
    investigations 383
    management of 386, 388
    on clinical examination 595
    surgical treatment 383
    twisted 382f
    ultrasonographic view of 383f
Ovariotomy 509
Ovary 592
    bilateral
        malignant epithelial tumors of 487f
        mucinous adenocarcinoma of 613f
    carcinoid tumors of 607
    chocolate cyst of 636
    common
        epithelial tumors of 607
        malignant tumor of 387, 488
        solid tumors of 612
        tumors of 487
    dermoid cyst of 606f, 642
    epithelial carcinoma of 389
    germ cell tumors of 384, 612

hormone producing tumors of 612
Krukenberg's tumor of 387
ligament of 522*f*
non-neoplastic cysts of 384
removed during hysterectomy 379
tumors of 388, 487
wedge resection of 509
Ovulation 437
  detect 431, 562, 627
  diagnosis of 483
  evidence of 483, 562
  induction 441-443
    management option 442
    risk of 443
  precede 437
Ovum forceps 564*f*
  dangers 564
  methods 564
  uses 564

# P

Pain, acute 383
Pap test screening 468
Papanicolaou's smear, grading of 479, 549
Paracervical tissue 515*f*
Paraovarian cyst, diagnose 616
Partial mole 426, 427*f*
  triploid chromosomal pattern of 427*f*
Pelvic abdominal
  lump, differential diagnosis of 490, 607
  mass 381*f*
    huge 517*f*
Pelvic abscess 494
  causes of 560
  different causes of 494
Pelvic brim, below 609
Pelvic endometriosis 445, 446, 466, 533*f*, 635
  clinical features of 600
  common sites of 636
  diagnose 532
  treatment for 600
Pelvic examination 446
Pelvic extension 609
Pelvic floor repair 555
  complications of 581
  indications of 581
  operation 399
Pelvic infections 413
  antibiotic therapy for 415
  bacterial vaginosis 414
  clinical features of acute 414
  important causes of infertility 415

indications of surgery 415
protective factors for 414
risk factors for 413
Pelvic inflammatory disease, complications of 414
Pelvic lesion, acute 466
Pelvic organ
  laparoscopic view of 531
  prolapse 392, 394
    different types of surgery 397
    quantitative scoring 393
    prolapse-quantification 394
Pelvic pain
  causes of 595
  chronic 466
Pelvic surgery 466
Pelvic tuberculosis 495, 629
Pelvis
  normal 532*f*
  plain X-ray of 641*f*
  straight X-ray of 641*f*
Periaortic lymph node metastasis 643
Perineal body 394
Perineal tear
  diagnosis 410
  different degrees of 410
  old complete 410, 410*f*
Perineorrhaphy 580*f*
  indications of 581
  operation 580*f*
Perineum, deficient 396
Peritoneal cancer 609
Peritoneal metastases 610
Peritoneal spillage, bilateral 476*f*, 626*f*
Persistent gestational trophoblastic neoplasia 425
Pessary
  method of insertion of 583
  size of 583
Pills, missed 647
Pituitary factors 454
Pneumoperitoneum 528, 531, 589
  creation of 528, 589
Polyamide 587
Polycystic ovarian syndrome 440
  abnormalities associated with 440
  diagnosis 440
  features of 440
  long-term sequelae of 441
  woman with 440
Polydioxanone suture 586
Polyglactin 585
Polyglyconate sutures 586

Polyp, different types of 553
Polypectomy 537
Polypropylene 587
Pomeroy's method 505
Popcorn appearance 641*f*
Pop-Q system 394, 394*t*
Pouch of Douglas 521*f*, 532*f*
Povidine iodine 498*f*
Preantral follicle 435
Pregnancy
   corpus luteum of 438
   methods of termination of 469, 473
   termination, second trimester 469
Primordial follicle 435
Procidentia 393*f*
Progesterone 646
   challenge test 455, 646
      bleeding on 456
   level of 438
   uses in gynecology 646
Prolactin, aerum levels of 456
Prolapse
   classification of 400
   different types of 402
   nonsurgical treatments of 572
   treatment for 400
   types of 400
Prolene 587
Proliferation, phase of 439
Proliferative phase, main features of 436
Prophylactic chemotherapy
   indications of 424
   place of 602
Prophylactic oophorectomy 388
   place of 489, 611
   risk of 379
Proximal tubal block 566, 629
Psammoma bodies 490, 608
Pseudobroad ligament fibroid 485*f*
Pseudocapsule 375*f*
Pseudomyxoma peritonei 385
Pubertal ovary 434
Punch biopsy forceps 503*f*, 577, 577*f*
   uses 577
Purse-string suture 523*f*
Pyometra, causes of 558
Pyosalpinx, specimen of bilateral 492*f*, 604*f*

## Q

Quadrivalent vaccine 472

## R

Radical hysterectomy 526
   complications of 526, 619
   tissues removed in 526, 619
Radical vulvectomy 623, 624*f*
   complications of 624
Radiotherapy 619
   advantages of 619
   disadvantages of 619
   place of 623
Rectocele 396
Rectovaginal fistula 408, 408*f*
   common causes of 408
   diagnosis 408
   repair of 409
Regeneration, phase of 439
Reproductive endocrinology 657
Resectoscope 537*f*
Retort shape, causes of 604
Retractors, abdominal 573
Reverse cutting needle 579
Revised National Tuberculosis Control Program 417
Ring loader 544
Ring pessary 584, 584*f*
   insertion of 584
Ring pusher 544
Robotic surgery 545
Robotics in gynecology 545
   disadvantages 546
Rubin's test 501

## S

Saline infusion sonography 421
Salpingectomy
   indications of 575
   steps of 604
Salpingitis isthmica nodosa 416
Salpingolysis 460
Salpingo-oophorectomy 575
   bilateral 382*f*, 485*f*, 603*f*, 608*f*
Salpingostomy, bilateral 477*f*, 628*f*
Sarcoma 553
Scar endometriosis, treatment of 637
Schiller's test 577
Scissors 580, 580*f*
Secretary phase, features of 436
Secretory endometrium, phase of 439
Semen analysis, normal values of 431
Sentinel node, significance of 625

Septate uterus  478, 540, 540*f*, 630, 631
    ultrasonographic view of  633*f*
Septum, resection of  540*f*
Serous cystadenoma  491*f*
Sertoli cells  470
Serum
    estradiol  431
    progesterone  431, 562
        estimation  431
Sex cord stromal tumor  384, 388, 487, 488
Sharman's curette  483, 483*f*, 561*f*, 562
Sharp curette  561
Silk suture  587
Sims' double-bladed posterior vaginal
        speculum  550, 550*f*
Sims' position  551
Sims' posterior vaginal speculum  482, 498*f*, 499*f*, 521*f*
Sims' speculum introduced  551
Sims' triad  405, 551
Single-toothed vulsellum  559, 559*f*
    uses  559
Skiagram  476
Skin
    incision, site of  505
    retractors  510
Snow storm  424
Sonography  643
Sonohysterosalpingography  477, 570
Sound test  428
Spatula  548, 548*f*
Spencer Well's clamps  574, 574*f*
Sponge holding forceps  498*f*, 563, 563*f*
    uses  563
Spongiosum  434
Squamous cell
    abnormalities  553
    atypical  553
    carcinoma  553, 616*f*, 624
Squamous intraepithelial lesion
    high-grade  553
    low-grade  553
Steel suture  587
Sterilize instruments  584
Stratum compactum  434
Struma ovarii  642
Strumal carcinoids  606
Sturmdorf suture  508
Submucous fibroid polyp  539*f*, 597*f*
Subserous fibroid uterus, multiple  375*f*
Subtotal hysterectomy, indications of  559
Surgery
    different methods of  635
    different types of  494, 635
    endometriosis, different types of  636
Suture materials  585
    absorbable  585
    nonabsorbable  585, 587
Swab test  404
Synechiolysis  537
Synthetic progesterones  646

## T

Telescope  531*f*, 588, 588*f*, 590
Testosterone, aecretion of  470
Theca lutein cysts
    bilateral large  601*f*
    management of  602
Thermal cauterization, steps of  582
Thermal cautery  504*f*
Thyroid  454
    function, evaluation of  456
Tissue healing  582
Toothed dissecting forceps  578*f*
Total abdominal hysterectomy  571, 575
    complications of  512, 575
Total hysterectomy  485*f*, 608*f*
    specimen of  382*f*, 603*f*
Towel clips  510, 581, 581*f*
    uses  581
Tranexamic acid  648
    contraindications  648
    dose schedule  648
    side effects  648
Transformation zone  451, 452
    large loop excision of  525
Transvaginal ultrasonography  621
Transverse vaginal sulcus  392*f*
Traumatic forceps delivery  408*f*
Trocar  531, 531*f*, 588, 588*f*
Tubal block
    causes of  628
    hysteroscopic method of  542
Tubal cancer  609
Tubal cannulation  537
Tubal carcinoma, clinical presentation
    of  606
Tubal factors  431
Tubal occlusion, laparoscopic methods for  541
Tubal patency, assessment of  477
Tubal reconstructive surgery
    common types of  630
    different types of  567
Tubal sterilization  537, 542, 544*f*
    different methods of  541
    laparoscopic view of  544*f*
Tubal surgery, guidelines for  630

Tube
  anatomical patency of 431
  delivery of 505
Tubectomy 505, 506
Tuberculosis 494, 605, 629
Tubo-ovarian mass 377
Tuboplasty
  operations, types of 567
  results of 628
  success of 630
Tumor 615
  appearance of 615
  growth 490
  markers 390, 462, 611
  masculinizing 612
  presence of 465
  prognosis of 615
Turner's syndrome 453

# U

Ultrasonography 374*f*, 633
Umbilicus, endometriosis in 445*f*
Unicornuate uterus 631, 631*f*
Unruptured tubal ectopic pregnancy 533*f*, 534
  diagnosis of 533
  management of 533
Ureteric injury 406, 599
  different types of 406
  management approach 407
  repair of 407
  risk of 599
Urethrocele, junction of 392*f*
Urinary bladder 644*f*
Urinary fistula, different types of 403
Urinary incontinence
  different causes of 554
  different types of 403
Urinary symptoms 395, 459
Urinary tract infections, symptoms of 407
Urine
  acute retention of 480
  chronic retention of 480, 554
  retention of 480, 481, 554
Uterine 595
  abnormalities, different types of 633
  artery 522*f*
    ascending branch of 514*f*
  bleeding
    abnormal 418, 420, 537
    different types of 419
    dysfunctional 419
    type of abnormal 418

  cavity 594*f*, 638*f*
    hysteroscopic view of 538
    normal 538*f*
  curette 561, 561*f*
    types 561
    uses 561
  dressing forceps 563, 563*f*
    uses 563
  factors 454
  fibroid, types of 599
  mass, huge 518*f*
  ostium 540*f*
  perforation, detection of 466
  polyp 428
    alternative treatment 429
    diagnosis 428
    method of treatment 428
  prolapse 396, 400, 401
    congenital 401
    degrees of 392
  septum, resection of 537
  sound 498*f*
  synechiae
    causes of 632
    management of 632
  tubes 592
  vessels 513*f*
Uterocervical canal, length of 561
Uterosacral ligament 515*f*, 522*f*, 532*f*
Uterovesical fold, loose peritoneum of 514*f*
Uterovesical peritoneum 521*f*
Uterus 419, 485*f*, 592, 621*f*
  body of 374*f*
  chronic inversion of 401
  cornu of 513*f*, 531, 593
  holding forceps 566, 566*f*
    use 566
  inversion of 428
  laparoscopic view of 533*f*
  MRI plate of normal 644*f*
  symmetrical enlargement of 634

# V

Vaccines 468, 472, 620
Vagina 644*f*
  lateral angles of 512
  remaining vault of 515*f*
  vault of 511, 515*f*
Vaginal bleeding, episodes of irregular 484*f*
Vaginal cytology 562
Vaginal flaps, triangular 521*f*
Vaginal hysterectomy 519, 521, 572, 575

actual steps 520
advantages of abdominal over 512
complications of 399, 520
indications of 559
preliminaries 519
Vaginal length, total 394
Vaginal operation 581
common 563
Vaginal over abdominal hysterectomy, advantages of 512
Vaginal part 395
Vaginal prolapse 400
Vaginal route 397
misoprostol 469
Vaginal specula, types of 481
Vaginal speculum 481
Vaginal wall 521f
anterior 392f, 393f, 514f
lesions in 552
posterior 521f, 524f
prolapse 395
retractor, anterior 560, 560f
Vault prolapse 397, 400
correction of 397

Veress needle 531, 531f, 588, 588f
correct placement of 528, 589
Vesicovaginal fistula 403, 404, 404f
diagnosis of 404
Vicryl rapide 585
2-0 suture 586f
Violin string 414
Vulsellum 498f
Vulva
carcinoma of 624f
lymphatic drainage of 624
Vulval carcinoma, FIGO staging of 625
Vulval malignancy, common sites of 624
Vulvectomy, types of 624

## W

Wertheim's radical hysterectomy 616f
Whiff test 492
Wolffian duct 470
Wound dehiscence 512

## Y

Y chromosome 470

EU GSPR Authorised Reprsentative
Logos Europe, 9 rue Nicolas Poussin
1700, La Rochelle, France
Phone: +33 (0) 6 67 93 73 78
E-mail: contact@logoseurope.eu

www.ingramcontent.com/pod-product-compliance
Ingram Content Group UK Ltd.
Pitfield, Milton Keynes, MK11 3LW, UK
UKHW050455150426
5217IPUK00025B/1699